SECOND EDITION

The World of the Counselor

An Introduction to the Counseling Profession

Ed Neukrug
Old Dominion University

THOMSON
BROOKS/COLE™

Australia • Canada • Mexico • Singapore • Spain
United Kingdom • United States

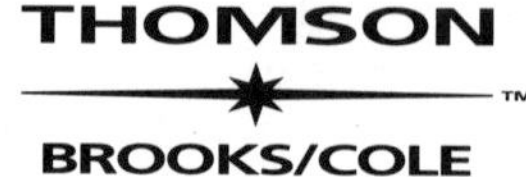

Sponsoring Editor: Julie Martinez
Assistant Editor: Shelley Gesicki
Editorial Assistant: Mike Taylor
Marketing Manager: Caroline Concilla
Marketing Assistant: Mary Ho
Project Manager, Editorial Production: Janet Hill
Print/Media Buyer: Vena Dyer
Permissions Editor: Sue Ewing
Production Service/Compositor: Scratchgravel Publishing Services
Text Designer: John Edeen
Illustrator: Scratchgravel Publishing Services
Cover Designer: Denise Davidson
Cover Photo: Stock Market
Cover/Interior Printer: Phoenix Color Corp.—BTB

Printed in the United States of America

1 2 3 4 5 6 7 06 05 04 03 02

For more information about our products, contact us at:

Thomson Learning Academic Resource Center
1-800-423-0563

For permission to use material from this text, contact us by:

Phone: 1-800-730-2214
Fax: 1-800-730-2215
Web: http://www.thomsonrights.com

Library of Congress Control Number: 2002104266

ISBN 0-534-54950-0

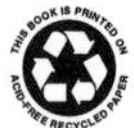

Brooks/Cole–Thomson Learning
511 Forest Lodge Road
Pacific Grove, CA 93950
USA

Asia
Thomson Learning
5 Shenton Way #01-01
UIC Building
Singapore 068808

Australia
Nelson Thomson Learning
102 Dodds Street
South Melbourne, Victoria 3205
Australia

Canada
Nelson Thomson Learning
1120 Birchmount Road
Toronto, Ontario M1K 5G4
Canada

Europe/Middle East/Africa
Thomson Learning
High Holborn House
50/51 Bedford Row
London WC1R 4LR
United Kingdom

Latin America
Thomson Learning
Seneca, 53
Colonia Polanco
11560 Mexico D.F.
Mexico

Spain
Paraninfo Thomson Learning
Calle/Magallanes, 25
28015 Madrid, Spain

To my mom,

my first counselor

About the Author

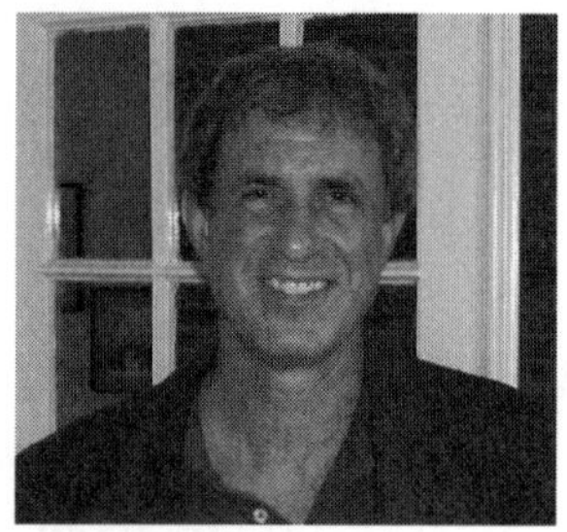

Born and raised in New York City, Dr. Ed Neukrug obtained his B.A. in psychology in 1973 from SUNY Binghamton, his M.S. in counseling from Miami University of Ohio in 1974, and his doctorate in counselor education from the University of Cincinnati in 1980.

After teaching and directing a graduate program in counseling at Notre Dame College in New Hampshire, he accepted a position at Old Dominion University in Norfolk, Virginia, where he currently is a Professor of Counseling and Chair of the Department of Educational Leadership and Counseling. In addition to teaching, Dr. Neukrug has worked as a counselor at a crisis center, an outpatient therapist at a mental health center, an associate school psychologist, a school counselor, and as a private practice psychologist and licensed professional counselor.

Dr. Neukrug has held a variety of positions in local, regional, and national professional associations in counseling and human services. Books he has written include *The World of the Counselor* (2nd ed.); *Experiencing the World of the Counselor: A Workbook for Counselor Educators and Students; Theory, Practice, and Trends in Human Services: An Introduction to An Emerging Profession* (2nd ed.); and *Skills and Techniques for Human Service Professionals: Counseling Environment, Helping Skills, Treatment.* In addition, he has published numerous articles and has received a number of grants and contracts with school systems and professional associations.

Dr. Neukrug ran the New York marathon in 1987 and someday would like to run another. He is married to Kristina Williams-Neukrug, who is an elementary school counselor. They have two children, Hannah and Emma.

Brief Contents

Contents

SECTION IV
The Development of the Person 223

Preface

They brought the fireman (now firefighter) to my school. I wanted to be just like him. They brought the policeman (now police officer)—that's a pretty fun job, I thought. My father, a building contractor, came and talked about building bridges. I was very proud. Maybe I would be a building contractor. The doctor, of course, was very impressive also. But they didn't bring the counselor. In fact, few of us knew about counselors—what they did, who they were. Despite this, I became one. And now, I want the world to know who they are and what they do. That is what this book is about.

Since publication of the first edition of *The World of the Counselor*, many reviewers, faculty, and students have remarked that the text is one of the most comprehensive yet readable of its kind. Often, faculty and students have suggested that it is a book that could be used when studying for comprehensive exams or when taking a certification or licensing exam. In revising the text I have attempted to maintain its comprehensiveness. However, I have also shortened it by eliminating what I found to be some redundant and extraneous materials. I think you will now find the text to be much "tighter." In addition, I have updated references, added relevant information related to changes in the field of counseling, added URLs for numerous Web sites, and added questions for relevant electronic searches (e.g., InfoTrac, PsychINFO, ERIC).

The text presents an overview of the counseling profession by offering relevant content, vignettes, and think pieces for students to ponder. The book loosely follows the common-core curriculum guidelines of the Council for Accreditation of Counseling and Related Programs (CACREP): (1) human growth and development, (2) helping relationships, (3) social and cultural foundations, (4) group work, (5) career and lifestyle development, (6) appraisal, (7) research and program evaluation, and (8) professional orientation (see http://www.counseling.org/cacrep). The text also offers specific content in the specialty areas of community agency counseling, school counseling, and higher education. Having the text adhere to the CACREP-accredited common-core areas assures compliance with a standard in the profession and offers the student a broad knowledge base.

Organization of the Text

The book is separated into seven sections. In writing the text I have attempted to weave all of the eight common-core areas listed above into the first six sections, with the seventh section focusing on the student's future in the counseling profession:

SECTION I, PROFESSIONAL ORIENTATION The name of this section reflects the CACREP common-core curriculum guideline of the same name, "Professional Orientation." Three chapters in this section include:

Chapter 1 The Counselor's Idenity: What, Who, and How?

Chapter 2 A History of the Counseling Profession

Chapter 3 Standards in the Profession: Ethics, Accreditation, and Credentialing

SECTION II, THE HELPING RELATIONSHIP I: THEORIES AND SKILLS Section II loosely follows the CACREP common-core curriculum guideline entitled, "Helping Relationships," although consultation, which is listed under this guideline, is covered in Section III. The two chapters in this section are:

Chapter 4 Individual Approaches to Counseling

Chapter 5 Counseling Skills

SECTION III, THE HELPING RELATIONSHIP II: THE COUNSELOR WORKING IN SYSTEMS This section draws from a number of CACREP curriculum guidelines that in some fashion address counseling within systems, including: marriage and family counseling (from CACREP specialty guidelines called "Marriage and Family Counseling"), group work (from CACREP common-core curriculum guideline "Group Work"), and consultation and supervision (drawn from CACREP common-core curriculum guideline, "Helping Relationships"). The three chapters in this section are:

Chapter 6 Family Counseling

Chapter 7 Group Work

Chapter 8 Consultation and Supervision

SECTION IV, DEVELOPMENT OF THE PERSON The broad spectrum of human development issues in counseling are examined in Section IV. Loosely following two of the CACREP common-core curriculum guidelines of "Human Growth and Development" and "Career and Lifestyle Development," this section includes the following three chapters:

Chapter 9 Development across the Lifespan

Chapter 10 Abnormal Development, Diagnosis, and Psychopathology

Chapter 11 Career Development: The Counselor and the World of Work

SECTION V, RESEARCH, PROGRAM EVALUATION, AND APPRAISAL This section is based on the two CACREP common-core curriculum guidelines: "Research and Program Evaluation" and "Appraisal." The two chapters in this section include:

Chapter 12 Testing and Assessment

Chapter 13 Research and Evaluation

SECTION VI, SOCIAL AND CULTURAL FOUNDATIONS IN COUNSELING Section VI loosely follows the CACREP common-core curriculum guideline of the same name. The two chapters included in this section are:

Chapter 14: Theory and Concepts of Multicultural Counseling

Chapter 15: Knowledge and Skills of Multicultural Counseling

SECTION VII, YOUR FUTURE IN THE COUNSELING PROFESSION: CHOOSING A SPECIALTY AREA, FINDING A JOB, AND TRENDS IN THE FUTURE This final section examines the three most popular specialty areas in counseling: School Counseling, Community Agency/Mental Health Counseling, and Student Affairs Practice (Counseling in a Higher Education Setting). Specific to each of these specialty areas, each chapter provides history, defines roles and functions, presents theory and practice issues, and provides the counselor with specific examples of what it's like to work in each of these specialty areas. Places of employment and potential salary are also given. The final chapter in this section examines trends in the future as well as ways that you can optimize your future choices when looking for a job or continuing on to graduate education. The section includes:

Chapter 16 School Counseling
Chapter 17 Agency and Mental Health Counseling
Chapter 18 Student Affairs Practice in Higher Education
Chapter 19 A Look toward the Future

A Focus on Multicultural, Ethical, Professional, and Legal Issues

In recent years there has been rising interest in multicultural issues and in ethical, professional, and legal issues in counseling. This interest has been highlighted by continual focus and debate in the literature and at conferences on these issues. Because of my belief in the importance of these issues to our profession, particular emphasis has been placed on them throughout the text. Thus, a separate chapter is offered on ethical and professional issues (Chapter 3), and two chapters—an entire section of the text—are devoted to multicultural counseling (Chapters 14 and 15). In addition, at the end of each chapter I have included a focus on multicultural counseling and on ethical, professional, and legal issues. Finally, I conclude each chapter with a segment entitled "The Counselor in Process," which stresses how the self-reflective counselor who is willing to risk change might deal with issues related to the chapter content.

I hope you enjoy this revised edition of *The World of the Counselor.*

Acknowledgments

My thanks to the following reviewers for their comments and suggestions: Jennifer Baggerly, University of South Florida, Tampa; Frank Biasco, University of West Florida; Ernie Biller, University of Idaho; Nils Carlson, California State University, Bakersfield; Arden Gale, University of Arkansas; Joshua M. Gold, University of South Carolina; Patricia Henderson, Henderson Consulting; Tracy Leinbaugh, Ohio University; Jackson Rainer, Gardner-Webb University; Lori Russell-Chapin, Bradley University; Maria Saxionis, Bridgewater State College; Thomas L. Walton, Warner Southern College; and Miguel Ybarra, Barry University.

A special thanks to my colleague and friend Chris Lovell, who has been using *The World of the Counselor* since it was first published and has made important suggestions for changes to this edition. He is truly a brilliant man and wonderful counselor educator! In addition, I would like to thank a number of individuals who have worked extremely long hours on the revision of *The World of the Counselor.* A very special heartfelt thanks to Margaret Pinette and Anne Draus, who have carefully copy edited the second edition with an exceptionally keen eye. Their hard work deserves particular praise. Also, I would like to thank my graduate assistant Debra Boyce, who did an initial edit of the new edition, sent away for permissions, worked hard on the index, and helped with numerous other tasks, many of which were crucial to improving the text. Thank you, Debra! Thanks also to Alaina Trott and Charles Fawcett, who assisted in finishing the indexes.

A number of individuals at Brooks/Cole deserve special attention. First, thanks to Julie Martinez, sponsoring editor, and Shelley Gesicki, assistant editor, who have supported my efforts toward completing this second edition. I am also grateful to Janet Hill, editorial project manager, who helped bring the team together to finish the text. Some of the staff who have particularly helped me along the way include Caroline Concilla in marketing; Margaret Parks in advertising; Sue Ewing in permissions; Vernon Boes, creative director, and designer Denise Davidson, who were key in creating the beautiful new cover. I appreciate the efforts of all of them.

Ed Neukrug

SECTION I

Professional Orientation

Overview

This first section of the text offers an overview of important professional issues in the field of counseling. A common theme running through each of the chapters is how the counseling profession has developed its unique professional identity. This is explored by looking at how we are the same as well as how we are different from other mental health professionals, by examining our unique history, and by stressing the standards of our profession.

In Chapter 1, I define *counseling* and distinguish it from related words such as *guidance* and *psychotherapy*. I also compare and contrast different kinds of mental health professionals who do counseling, and I examine some of the characteristics that are related to being an effective counselor. Chapter 2 reviews the history of the counseling profession, from the distant past, to the beginnings of the mental health field, to the current status of the profession. In Chapter 3, I present an overview, the development, and the implementation of three important standards in the counseling profession: ethics, accreditation, and credentialing.

At the conclusion of each of these three chapters, and every other chapter in the book as well, I will relate chapter content to important multicultural issues; ethical, professional and legal issues; and, in a section called "The Counselor in Process," to issues related to how the counselor lives as a person and professional in the world.

CHAPTER 1

The Counselor's Identity: What, Who, and How?

Surprisingly, counseling is not an easy concept to define. For one thing, it is a much overused term. We have financial counselors and employment counselors, camp counselors, retirement counselors, legal counselors, and nutrition counselors. With such a variety as this, what could these various practices have in common? [In fact] . . . they have little in common with . . . the practice of interpersonal/intrapersonal counseling. (Hackney & Cormier, 2001, p. 2)

When I had a temper tantrum as a kid, my mother would say, "I just don't understand why you get so angry; maybe I should take you to see a counselor." This threat intimated that there was something terribly wrong with me, but it also showed her love for me and deep desire to understand and help me.

I used to wonder what would it be like to see a counselor. It couldn't be a good thing if my mom was using it as a threat, I thought! On the other hand, maybe counseling would be a place where I could talk to someone who understood me, someone who could understand my moods, moods that felt normal to me yet were being defined as being wrong, kind of abnormal. Maybe seeing a counselor would be okay. In fact, maybe a counselor would say I was normal! But what exactly would a counselor do, I wondered?

Thankfully, over the years I've had the opportunity to be in counseling. And, irony of all ironies, I became a counselor. Well, maybe my mom intuited early that I was going to be intimately involved in counseling in one way or another!

This chapter is about understanding who is the counselor and what is counseling. I will attempt to define the word *counseling* and distinguish it from related words like *guidance* and *psychotherapy*. I will also compare and contrast counselors with other mental health professionals who do counseling. Next, I will examine some of the characteristics that are related to being an effective helper.

As we near the end of the chapter, we will examine the different professional associations in the field, with particular emphasis on the American Counseling Association

(ACA), the organization that serves counselors. I will conclude the chapter by highlighting the importance of multicultural issues in the field of counseling and by focusing on ethical, professional, and legal issues related to our identity as counselors.

Guidance, Counseling, and Psychotherapy: Variations on the Same Theme?

In spite of . . . [the] social consensus that counseling is a good thing and must be provided in ever-increasing quantity, there is some lack of agreement about what the word "counseling" means. (Tyler, 1969, pp. 9–10)

Deep, dark, secretive, sexual, unconscious, pain, hidden, long-term, reconstructive: These are some of the words I free-associate to when I think of the word *psychotherapy*. *Short-term, facilitative, here and now, change, problem-solving, being heard,* and *awareness* come to mind when I associate to the word *counseling*. And lastly, *advice, direction, on-the-surface, advocacy,* and *supportive* are words I think of when I associate to the word *guidance*. Are guidance, counseling, and psychotherapy different from one another, and which does the counselor do: guidance, counseling, or psychotherapy?

Over the years there have been a plethora of definitions of *counseling* that suggest it could be anything from a problem-solving, directive, and rational approach to helping normal people, an approach that is distinguishable from psychotherapy (Williamson, 1950; 1958); to a process that is similar to but less intensive than psychotherapy (Brown & Srebalus, 1996; Ivey & Simek-Downing, 1987; Nugent, 2000); to the assertion that there is no essential distinction between counseling and psychotherapy (Brammer, Abrego, & Shostrom; 1993; Corey, 2000a; Patterson, 1986).

An explanation for the confusion among the words rests in their historical roots. The word *guidance* first appeared around the 1600s and was defined as "the process of guiding an individual." Early guidance work involved individuals being directive and moralistic. This general definition continued into the 20th century when vocational guidance counselors used the word to describe the act of "guiding" an individual into a profession and when offering suggestions for life skills. Meanwhile, with the development of psychoanalysis near the end of the 19th century came the word *psychotherapy*. Meaning "caring for the soul," the word was derived from the Greek words *psyche*, meaning spirit or soul, and *therapeutikos*, meaning caring for another (Kleinke, 1994).

During the 20th century, vocational guidance counselors became increasingly dissatisfied with the word *guidance* and its heavy emphasis on direction and moral preaching. Consequently, the word *counseling* was adopted to describe the fact that, like their distant colleagues, the psychoanalysts who practiced psychotherapy, vocational counselors also dealt with social and emotional issues. As mental health workers became more prevalent during the mid-1900s, they too adopted the word *counseling*, rather than use the word *guidance* with its moralistic implications, or *psychotherapy*, which was increasingly associated with psychoanalysis. Tyler (1969) stated that "those who participated in the mental health movement and had no connection with vocational guidance used the word *counseling* to refer to what others were calling [psycho]therapy . . ." (p. 12).

In the training of counselors today, the word *guidance* has tended to take a back seat to the word *counseling*, while the words *counseling* and *psychotherapy* are generally used

FIGURE 1.1
Guidance, Counseling, and Psychotherapy Continuum

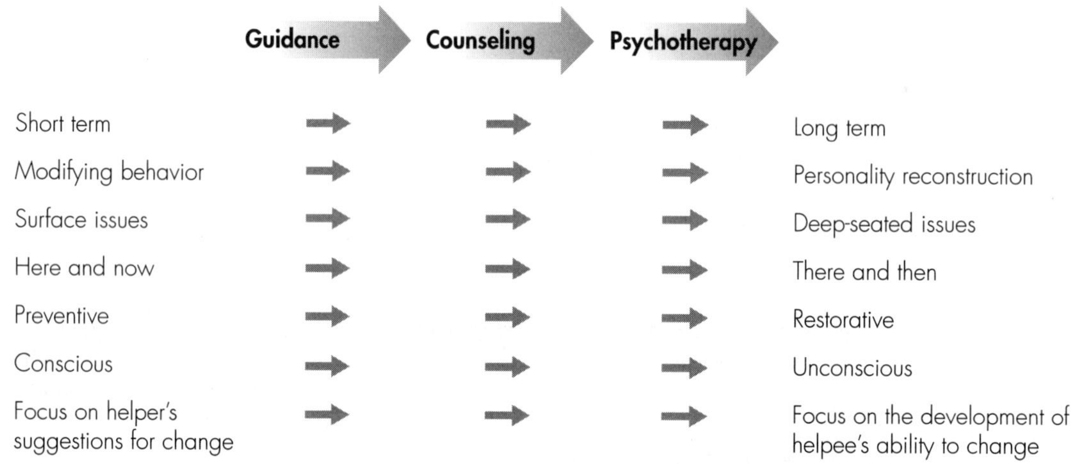

	Guidance	Counseling	Psychotherapy	
Short term	→	→	→	Long term
Modifying behavior	→	→	→	Personality reconstruction
Surface issues	→	→	→	Deep-seated issues
Here and now	→	→	→	There and then
Preventive	→	→	→	Restorative
Conscious	→	→	→	Unconscious
Focus on helper's suggestions for change	→	→	→	Focus on the development of helpee's ability to change

interchangeably in textbooks. Examine most texts that describe theories of counseling or psychotherapy, and you will find them to be texts on theories of counseling and psychotherapy; that is, the counseling theories and the theories of psychotherapy are the same, indistinguishable. For example, C. H. Patterson, who wrote a popular text, *Theories of Counseling and Psychotherapy*, stated that " . . . counseling and psychotherapy are both used in the title of this book because it appears to be impossible to make any clear distinction between them" (Patterson, 1986, p. xvii). Similarly, Baruth and Huber (1985) stated that they use the words *counseling* and *psychotherapy* equivalently throughout their book, and Corey (2000a), the author of the best-known text on theories of counseling and psychotherapy, simply does not address the issue, choosing to use the words interchangeably.

Despite the lack of distinction made in most texts, such a differentiation is likely to be made by the average person, perhaps by many counseling students, and even by professors of counseling. Therefore, some have suggested that the profession move toward a model that is in sync with public perception, one that views counseling and psychotherapy on opposite ends of the continuum (Hansen, Rossberg, & Cramer, 1994). An even broader, more complex model would place guidance and psychotherapy on opposite extremes, with counseling falling somewhere midway on the continuum (see Figure 1.1).

Comparison of Mental Health Professionals

Whether we call it guidance, counseling, or psychotherapy, in today's world we find a number of professionals practicing it. In fact, although differences in the training of the various mental health professionals exist, over the years the professional duties of the various mental health professionals have begun to overlap (Todd & Bohart, 1999). For instance, today some school counselors do therapy, counseling and clinical psychologists act as consultants to the schools, psychiatrists are social advocates, social workers and others can be psychoanalysts, mental health counselors do family therapy, and psychologists vie for the right to prescribe psychotropic medications (Foxhall, 2000). Let's examine some of the similarities and differences among counselors, psychologists, psychiatrists, social workers, psychiatric nurses, psychoanalysts, and psychotherapists.

Counselors

Over the years, the word *counselor* has simply meant any "professional who practices counseling" (Chaplin, 1975, p. 120). However, in recent years, most individuals who call themselves counselors will have master's degrees in counseling. Counselors can be found in a variety of settings serving in a variety of roles. We find them as school counselors, college counselors, agency counselors, private practitioners, rehabilitation counselors, and counselors in business and industry. The counselor's training is broad, and we find counselors doing individual and group counseling, administering and interpreting educational and psychological assessments, offering career counseling, consulting on a broad range of educational and psychological matters, and presenting developmentally appropriate guidance activities for individuals of all ages. Even though counselors are not generally experts in psychopathology, they usually have some knowledge of maladjustment and know to refer individuals who need more in-depth treatment.

Although there are many different kinds of counselors, all tend to have had common course work in professional orientation (e.g., history and ethics), the helping relationship, group work, human growth and development, social and cultural foundations, career and lifestyle development, appraisal, and research and program evaluation. In addition to these common core courses, counselors generally have had course work in a counseling specialty area, which might include classes in the history, roles and functions, and knowledge and skills of that specialty area. Finally, all counselors have had the opportunity to practice their acquired skills and knowledge at field placements (e.g., practicum and internship).

Today, most counseling programs at the master's level will offer specialty areas as recognized by the Council for the Accreditation of Counseling and Related Educational Programs (CACREP). These include community counseling, school counseling, college counseling, mental health counseling, career counseling, gerontological counseling, student affairs, and marriage, couple, and family counseling/therapy. Rehabilitation counseling is accredited by a separate accreditation body, the Council on Rehabilitation Education (CORE), and follows similar curriculum guidelines to those above with an added emphasis on courses related to working with individuals with disabilities. Not all programs use the exact names that CACREP suggests, and some programs will offer specialty areas outside of those delineated by CACREP. Generally, however, most programs will offer a core curriculum, field placement, and specialty course work.

All counselors can take an exam to become a National Certified Counselor (NCC), which is offered by the National Board for Certified Counselors (NBCC). NBCC also offers subspecialty certifications in clinical mental health counseling, school counseling, addictions counseling, and as an approved clinical supervisor (ACS). In addition, 46 states and the District of Columbia have legislated licensing laws that allow a counselor who has a master's degree, additional training, and supervision to practice as a Licensed Professional Counselor (LPC) (some states use a different title). Whereas certification is generally seen as acknowledging mastery of a content area, licensure allows counselors to practice independently and obtain third-party reimbursement for their practice (an in-depth discussion of credentialing can be found in Chapter 3). The counselor's professional association is called the American Counseling Association (ACA), which currently has

17 divisions and one organization affiliate that focus on a variety of counseling concerns (a further discussion of ACA and its divisions can be found on pp. 10–11).

While keeping in mind that a person with a master's degree in counseling is first a counselor and secondarily a school counselor, community counselor, and so on, the following are brief descriptions of some of the more prevalent counseling specialty areas.

School Counselors

A school counselor has a master's degree in counseling and a specialty in school counseling. Some states credential school counselors on the elementary, middle, and secondary levels, while other states offer credentialing that covers kindergarten through 12th grade (K–12). In recent years there has been a push by professional training programs, professional associations, and many in the field to replace the term *guidance counselor* with *school counselor*, as the latter term is seen as de-emphasizing the guidance activities of the school counselor (Hoyt, 1993). If they so choose, school counselors can become NCCs, and, in most states, LPCs. The school counselor's professional association is the American School Counselor Association (ASCA), which is a division of ACA, although ASCA has recently made attempts to become somewhat independent from its parent organization.

Mental Health, Agency, and Community Counselors

These counselors have master's degrees in counseling and a specialty in mental health counseling, community counseling, or agency counseling. Although CACREP distinguishes community counseling from mental health counseling, with the latter requiring more extensive training, individuals with these degrees generally work in agencies or in private practice conducting counseling and psychotherapy. These counselors can become NCCs, or, if they live in a state that offers licensing, LPCs. This counselor's professional association is the American Mental Health Counselors Association (AMHCA), which is a division of ACA, although AMHCA, like ASCA, has recently made attempts to become somewhat independent from its parent organization.

College Counselors and Counselors in Student Affairs Practices

These counselors may work in a variety of settings in higher education, including college counseling centers, career centers, residence life, advising, college crisis centers, and so forth. Usually, these counselors will have taken specialty course work in college student development. If they so choose, counselors who work in college settings can become NCCs, and, in most states, LPCs. The main professional associations of these counselors include the American College Personnel Association (ACPA) and the American College Counseling Association (ACCA), which is a division of ACA. Whereas ACPA's main focus is on administration of student services, ACCA tends to concentrate more on counseling issues in college settings. Both associations offer important services for the counselor who works in a higher-education setting.

Rehabilitation Counselors

Rehabilitation counselors offer a wide range of services to people with physical, emotional, and/or developmental disabilities. "Rehab" counselors work in state vocational rehabilitation agencies, unemployment offices, or private rehabilitation agencies. Whereas the accreditation for school, community, and student affairs counseling programs is provided by CACREP, the Council on Rehabilitation Education (CORE) is the accrediting body for rehabilitation counseling programs. Although the curricula in rehabilitation counseling programs largely parallel those in CACREP-approved programs, rehab programs include course work on vocational evaluation, occupational analysis, medical and psychosocial aspects of disability, legal and ethical issues in rehabilitation, and the history of rehabilitation counseling. Although rehabilitation counselors can become NCCs or LPCs, many choose to become Certified Rehabilitation Counselors (CRCs), which is a separate certification process. Many rehabilitation counselors will join the National Rehabilitation Counseling Association (NRCA) and/or the American Rehabilitation Counselor Association (ARCA), a division of ACA.

Marriage, Couple, and Family Counselors

Marriage, couple, and family counselors are specifically trained to work with systems and can be found in vast array of agency settings and in private practice. These counselors tend to have specialty course work in systems dynamics, family therapy, family life stages, and human sexuality, along with the more traditional course work in the helping professions. Today, there are 42 states that regulate the practice of marriage and family counseling. While some states follow the curriculum guidelines set forth by the American Association for Marriage and Family Therapy (AAMFT), others follow the CACREP guidelines for marriage, couple, and family counseling/therapy, and still others have set their own credentialing guidelines (AAMFT, 2001a). Most states that offer marriage and family counselor credentialing allow helping professionals with related degrees (e.g., counseling, social work, psychology) also to practice marriage and family counseling. AAMFT is one professional association for marriage and family counselors as is the International Association of Marriage and Family Counselors (IAMFC), a division of ACA.

Psychologists

There are many different types of psychologists practicing in a wide range of settings, including agencies, private practice, health maintenance organizations, universities, business and industry, prisons, and schools. Psychologists are often found administrating agencies, consulting with business and industry, or in supervisory roles for all types of mental health professionals. Generally, psychologists have an advanced graduate degree in psychology, usually a doctorate, postgraduate school supervision, and have passed a state licensing exam. Some of the many different kinds of psychologists include counseling psychologists, clinical psychologists, school psychologists, educational psychologists, neuropsychologists, and psychologists in academia. Today, each state determines the types of psychology licenses it authorizes as well as the requirements for those licenses.

Relative to the practice of psychotherapy, most states offer licensure in counseling and clinical psychology, and many states now allow individuals with a "Psy D.," a relatively new clinical doctorate in psychology, to become licensed as clinical or counseling psychologists (Robiner, Arbisi, & Edwall, 1994; Shapiro, 1994). The professional association for psychologists is called the American Psychological Association (APA). A brief discussion of clinical, counseling, and school psychologists, psychologists with whom the counselor is likely to have the most contact, follows.

Clinical Psychologists

Clinical psychologists have a strong background in science, theory, and practice, which enables them to alleviate maladjustment and promote psychological well-being (APA, 2001a). To obtain a license as a clinical psychologist, one must graduate from an APA-accredited doctoral program in clinical psychology and also complete additional requirements identified by state licensing boards. The professional association for clinical psychologists is Division 12 of the APA.

Counseling Psychologists

Historically, counseling psychologists have worked more with relatively healthy populations as compared to clinical psychologists' work with seriously impaired populations. Today, however, the difference between counseling and clinical psychologists is nominal. Just like clinical psychologists, to become a counseling psychologist one must obtain a doctoral degree from an APA-approved program and complete additional requirements as identified by the state licensing board. The professional association for counseling psychologists is Division 17 of the APA.

School Psychologists

School psychologists have the minimum of a master's degree in school psychology and are licensed by state boards of education, with their main interest focused on children, families, and the schooling process. Today, many school psychologists can be found conducting assessments and consultation for special education students. Because the training in school psychology tends to be in testing, human development, or system change (Todd & Bohart, 1999), school psychologists are usually not licensed by the state to do counseling and psychotherapy. The professional associations for school psychologists are the National Association of School Psychologists (NASP) and Division 16 of the APA.

Psychiatrists

A psychiatrist is a licensed physician who generally has completed a residency in psychiatry, meaning that in addition to medical school, he or she has completed extensive field placement training in a mental health setting. Being a physician, the psychiatrist has expertise in organic disorders, the identification and treatment of psychopathology, and the use of medication for psychiatric conditions. Although psychologists are hopeful that they will be able to prescribe psychotropic medication, currently only psychiatrists, and in some cases psychiatric nurses, can do so.

Because psychiatrists often have minimal training in techniques of individual and group counseling, assessment techniques, human development, and career counseling, they are sometimes not seen as experts in the delivery of counseling and psychotherapeutic services. Psychiatrists are employed in mental health agencies, hospitals, private practice settings, and health maintenance organizations. The professional association for psychiatrists is called the American Psychiatric Association (APA).

Social Workers

Although the term *social worker* can apply to those who have an undergraduate or a graduate degree in social work or a related field (e.g., human services), recently the term has become more associated with the master's degree in social work (MSW). Although social workers traditionally have been found working with the underprivileged and with family and social systems, today social workers provide counseling and psychotherapy for all types of clients in a wide variety of settings, including child welfare services, government-supported social service agencies, family service agencies, private practices, and hospitals. Although social workers have extensive training in counseling techniques, they usually are less well prepared in career counseling, assessment techniques, and quantitative research methods.

Although major theoretical distinctions exist between the MSW and the master's degree in counseling, the two degrees probably have more similarities than differences. With additional training and supervision, social workers can become nationally certified by the Academy of Certified Social Workers (ACSW). In addition, most states have specific requirements for becoming a Licensed Clinical Social Worker (LCSW). The professional association for social workers is the National Association of Social Workers (NASW).

Psychiatric Nurses

Primarily trained as medical professionals, psychiatric nurses are also trained in the delivery of mental health services (Davidson, 1992). Most psychiatric nurses work in hospital settings with lesser numbers working in community agencies, private practice, or educational settings. Psychiatric nurses can be found in a number of roles including nurse practitioner, clinical nurse specialist, head nurse, educator, administrator, director of nursing, researcher, staff nurse, therapist, and consultant (APNA, 2001). Currently holding prescriptive privileges in 36 states, psychiatric nurses provide a unique service for many mental health settings.

Although some psychiatric nurses have an associate or bachelor's degree in nursing, most hold an advanced degree in nursing. Because of their training in both medicine and basic counseling skills, they hold a unique position in the mental health profession. Certification of psychiatric nurses can be held in a number of mental health areas. The professional association of psychiatric nurses is the American Psychiatric Nurses Association (APNA).

Psychoanalysts

Psychoanalysts are trained in Freudian psychoanalysis from a number of recognized psychoanalytical institutes. Although the American Psychoanalytical Association (APsaA), the professional association of psychoanalysts, formerly would only endorse psychiatrists for training at psychoanalytical institutes (Turkington, 1985), they now allow other mental health professionals to undergo training (American Psychoanalytical Association, 2001). Because states do not license psychoanalysts, clients who are seeing a psychoanalyst should make sure that the analyst was trained at an institute sanctioned by the American Psychoanalytical Association and that he or she has a license in a mental health field (e.g., psychiatrist, psychologist, licensed professional counselor, licensed clinical social worker).

Psychotherapists

Because the word *psychotherapist* is not associated with any particular field of mental health practice, most states do not offer legislation that would create a license for "psychotherapists." One result of this lack of legislation is that, in many states, individuals who have no mental health training can call themselves psychotherapists. However, legislatures generally legislate the scope of psychotherapeutic practice, meaning that the practice of psychotherapy is generally limited to those individuals who are licensed mental health professionals within each state (e.g., psychologists, LPCs, LCSWs). The bottom line is that in most states any individual can call him- or herself a psychotherapist, but only licensed practitioners can practice psychotherapy.

Professional Associations in the Social Services[1]

In order to protect the rights of their members and as a method of supporting the philosophical beliefs of the membership, professional associations have arisen over the years for each of the major types of social service professionals discussed. These associations tend to:

- Offer national and regional conferences to discuss clinical issues and training issues.
- Provide access to malpractice insurance.
- Hire lobbyists to protect the interests of the membership.
- Provide newsletters and journals to discuss topics of interest to the membership.
- Provide opportunities for mentoring and networking.
- Provide codes of ethics and standards for practice.
- Provide job banks.
- Offer a wide variety of other membership benefits.

Most individuals reading this text are likely to be interested in joining the American Counseling Association, which will be discussed in detail shortly. However, for your professional knowledge and for those who might be interested in becoming members of related associations, some of the other major associations within the social service field will also be highlighted. Keep in mind that there are numerous organizations in the social services, and this list just features a few of the better-known associations.

The American Counseling Association

The beginnings of the American Counseling Association (ACA) can be traced back to 1913 with the founding of the National Vocational Guidance Association (NVGA). After many name and structural changes over the years, today's ACA is the world's largest counseling association. This 55,000-member, not-for-profit association is an umbrella organization that serves the needs of all types of counselors in an effort to "enhance the quality of life in society by promoting the development of professional counselors, advancing the counseling profession, and using the profession and practice of counseling to promote respect for human dignity and diversity" (ACA, 2001a).

Divisions of ACA

ACA currently sponsors 17 divisions and one organization affiliate. All of the divisions and the affiliate maintain newsletters, and most publish journals. The following is a list of ACA's divisions and the affiliate, the year they were founded, and the name of the journal(s) they publish. (Note: ACA has links to all of its divisions on its Web site.)

[1] Note: Web sites of professional associations can be found in Appendix B.

- AAC: Association for Assessment in Counseling (1965)
  Journal: *Measurement and Evaluation in Counseling and Development*
- AADA: Association for Adult Development and Aging (1986)
  Journal: *Adultspan*
- ACCA: American College Counseling Association (1992)
  Journal: *Journal of College Counseling*
- ACEG: Association for Counselors and Educators in Government (1984)
  Journal: None published
- ACES: Association for Counselor Education and Supervision (1952)
  Journal: *Counselor Education and Supervision*
- AGLBIC: Association for Gay, Lesbian, and Bisexual Issues in Counseling (1997)
  Journal: None published
- AMCD: Association for Multicultural Counseling and Development (1972)
  Journal: *Journal of Multicultural Counseling and Development*
- AMHCA: American Mental Health Counselors Association (1978)
  Journal: *Journal of Mental Health Counseling*
- ARCA: American Rehabilitation Counseling Association (1958)
  Journal: *Rehabilitation Counseling Bulletin*
- ASCA: American School Counselor Association (1953)
  Journal: *Professional School Counseling*
- ASERVIC: Association for Spiritual, Ethical & Religious Values in Counseling (1972)
  Journal: *Counseling and Values*
- ASGW: Association for Specialists in Group Work (1973)
  Journal: *Journal for Specialists in Group Work*
- C-AHEAD: Counseling Association for Humanistic Education and Development (1952)
  Journal: *The Journal for Humanistic Counseling Education and Development*
- CSJ: Counselors for Social Justice (Organizational Affiliate)
  Journal: None published
- IAAOC: International Association of Addiction and Offender Counselors (1974)
  Journal: *Journal of Addictions and Offender Counseling*
- IAMFC: International Association of Marriage and Family Counselors (1990)
  Journal: *The Family Journal: Counseling & Therapy for Couples & Families*
- NCDA: National Career Development Association (1985, formerly NVGA: 1913)
  Journal: *The Career Development Quarterly*
- NECA: National Employment Counseling Association (1966)
  Journal: *Journal of Employment Counseling*

Associations Related to ACA

ACA sponsors a number of affiliates and organizations that contribute to the betterment of the counseling profession in unique ways. A brief description of them follows. (Links to these associations can be found on the ACA Web site.)

- *The ACA Insurance Trust* provides liability insurance as well as a wide range of other kinds of insurance for its members.

- *The American Counseling Association Foundation (ACAF)* offers financial support for innovative research and services and fosters collaborative efforts in response to social needs.
- *The Council for Accreditation of Counseling and Related Educational Programs (CACREP)* develops standards for the accreditation of counseling programs.
- *The Legal Action Fund (LAF)* provides legal funding for cases in which counselors have been discriminated against and for cases that may impact greatly on the profession.
- *The Human Concerns Fund (HCF)* provides financial assistance to programs that assist the needy.
- *The National Board for Certified Counselors (NBCC)* offers accreditation as Nationally Certified Counselors (NCCs). In addition, specialty certifications are offered in school counseling, clinical mental health counseling, addictions counseling, and as approved clinical supervisors (APSs).
- *Chi Sigma Iota* provides recognition for outstanding academic achievement and service within the counseling profession.

Branches and Regions of ACA

In addition to the 18 divisions and affiliate, ACA has 56 branches, which consist of state associations, associations in Latin America, and associations in Europe. In addition, regional associations that represent broad areas of the United States also exist.

Membership Benefits of ACA

By becoming a member of ACA you have the opportunity to become actively involved in one or more of the divisions, receive the division's publications, and be involved with the affiliate organizations that ACA sponsors. Other benefits that ACA provides include:

- Professional development programs, such as conferences and continuing education workshops.
- Counseling resources, such as books, video and audio tapes, electronic news, and journals.
- Computer-assisted job search services.
- Professional liability insurance.
- Assistance in lobbying efforts at the local, state, and national levels.
- Networking and mentoring opportunities.
- Subscription to the *Journal of Counseling and Development* and other professional journals, based on division membership.
- A variety of discount and specialty programs (e.g., VISA, Air Travel, and so forth).
- Links to ACA Listservs for graduate students, international counseling issues, public policy issues, and counselor educators.

The American Psychological Association (APA)

Founded in 1892 by G. Stanley Hall, APA started with 31 members and now maintains a membership of 83,000. Undergraduate and graduate students can join as affiliate members. The main purpose of this association is "to advance psychology as a science, a profession, and as a means of promoting human welfare" (Associations Unlimited, 2001a). The association has 46 divisions in various specialty areas and publishes numerous psychological journals. The Counseling Psychology Division (Division 17) of the APA shares many of the same goals and purposes of some divisions of the American Counseling Association.

The American Psychiatric Association (APA)

Founded in 1844 as the Association of Medical Superintendents of American Institutions for the Insane, today the American Psychiatric Association (which also has the acronym APA) has close to 40,000 members. The association's main purpose is to "further the study of the nature, treatment, and prevention of mental disorders" (Associations Unlimited, 2001b). The association accomplishes this by offering programs and workshops on psychiatric disorders, evaluating and publishing statistical data related to psychiatric disorders, and supporting educational and research activities in the field of psychiatry. The association is active in advocacy work for mental health issues and has a number of councils and committees to focus on mental health concerns. The APA publishes journals in the field of psychiatry and is responsible for the development and publication of the *Diagnostic and Statistical Manual-IV-Text Revision (DSM-IV-TR)*, a major publication for mental health diagnosis.

The National Association of Social Workers (NASW)

The NASW was founded in 1955 as the result of the merger of seven membership associations in the field of social work. Servicing both undergraduate- and graduate-level social workers, NASW has nearly 155,000 members with its purpose being "to create professional standards for social work practice; advocate sound public social policies through political and legislative action; provide a wide range of membership services, including continuing education opportunities and an extensive professional program" (Associations Unlimited, 2001c). The association publishes four journals and other professional publications. Only practitioners with an undergraduate or graduate degree in social work or social work students are allowed to join this association.

The American Psychiatric Nurses Association (APNA)

A relatively young association, the American Psychiatric Nurses Association was founded in 1987 with 600 members. Today, APNA comprises close to 4000 members. The main purpose of APNA is to provide "leadership to advance psychiatric mental health nursing practice, improve mental health care for culturally diverse families, individuals, groups and communities, and shape health policy for the delivery of mental health services" (Associations Unlimited, 2001d). APNA offers a number of continuing education and professional development activities and publishes the Journal of the American Psychiatric Nurses Association. The association provides advocacy for psychiatric nurses to improve the quality of mental health delivery.

The American Association of Marriage and Family Therapists (AAMFT)

If you have a counseling degree, you might be interested in joining the International Association of Marriage and Family Counselors (IAMFC), which is a division of ACA, as noted earlier. However, in recent years the American Association of Marriage and Family

Therapy (AAMFT) has become prominent in the field of marriage and family counseling. Founded in 1945 as the American Association of Marriage and Family Counselors, AAMFT was established by family therapy and communication theorists to develop standards for their field and to offer an association that could bring together people with varying backgrounds who had an interest in marriage and family therapy (Associations Unlimited, 2001e). Today, AAMFT has 23,000 members, publishes the *Journal of Marital and Family Therapy*, sponsors a yearly conference, and is nationally active in a number of professional activities related to family counseling and family development.

The National Organization for Human Service Education (NOHSE)

Founded in 1975, NOHSE is a relatively new association whose main purpose is "to foster excellence in teaching, research and curriculum planning in the human service area; to encourage and support the development of local, state, and national human services organizations; to aid faculty and professional members in their career development" (Associations Unlimited, 2001f). This association is geared mostly toward undergraduate students and faculty in human service programs, although those who are involved in a graduate degree program in human services might also find this association interesting.

NOHSE has an active student membership and six regional associations (mid-Atlantic, midwest, northeastern, northwest, southern, and western). Each of these regions has its own professional meetings, and they operate somewhat independently, offering workshops, conferences, and other professional activities. NOHSE is still in the building stages, and there is still an opportunity to get involved on the ground floor of this organization.

Characteristics of the Effective Helper

How well counselors perform, what they do, and what they will become is a complex interaction of credentialing requirements, expectations of the settings in which they are employed, personal characteristics, and the quality and content of their preparation as counselors. (Herr, 1985b, p. 33)

In 1952, Eysenck looked at 24 uncontrolled studies that examined the effectiveness of psychotherapy on treatment outcomes and found that "roughly two-thirds of a group of neurotic patients will recover or improve to a marked extent within about two years of the onset of their illness, *whether they are treated by means of psychotherapy or not*" (p. 322, emphasis not included in original). Although Eysenck was justifiably criticized for methodological problems, his research did lead to debate concerning the effectiveness of counseling and resulted in hundreds of studies that examined its usefulness. The results of over 40 years of research showed:

> *When counseling effectiveness is calculated by determining the number of clients who improved, the results are amazingly similar across various studies. On the basis of both client and counselor ratings, approximately 22% of clients made significant gains, 43% made moderate changes, while 27% made some improvement . . .* (Sexton, 1993, p. 82)

But what is it that makes counseling effective? To answer this question, a number of reviews of the existing literature have examined the qualities necessary for an effective counseling relationship (Gladstein, 1983; Highlen & Hill, 1984; Lambert, Shapiro, & Bergin, 1986; Patterson, 1984; Rowe, Murphy, & De Csipkes, 1975; Sexton & Whiston, 1991; Sexton & Whiston, 1994). After examining this research, I have generated eight characteristics that seem to be either empirically or theoretically related to counselor effectiveness. There is little doubt that as research in these areas becomes more refined, some of these characteristics will change. The characteristics I have picked include: (1) empathy (2) genuineness, (3) acceptance, (4) open-mindedness, (5) mindfulness, (6) psychological adjustment, (7) relationship building, and (8) competence.

Empathy

Understanding, or being empathic,

> *. . . means that the therapist senses accurately the feelings and personal meanings that the client is experiencing and communicates this acceptant understanding to the client. When functioning best, the therapist is so much inside the private world of the other that he or she can clarify not only the meanings of which the client is aware but even those just below the level of awareness. Listening, of this very special, active kind, is one of the most potent forces of change that I know.*
> (Rogers, 1989a, p. 136)

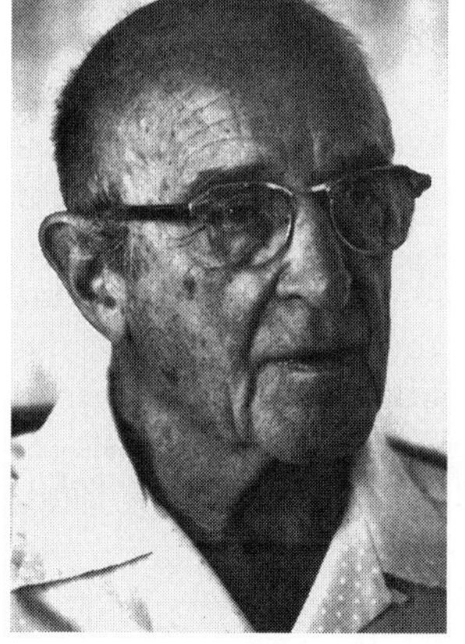

Carl Rogers

Whether or not one could truly understand the inner world of another has been discussed for centuries and was spoken of by such philosophers as Plato and Aristotle (Gompertz, 1960). Carl Rogers (1957) is given credit for bringing this concept to life in the 20th century in his discussions of empathic understanding. In respect to the counseling relationship, understanding through empathy is seen as a skill that can build rapport, elicit information, and help the client feel accepted (Egan, 1998). In addition, it has been shown to be related to positive client outcomes (Carkhuff, 2000; Luborsky, Crits-Christoph, Mintz, & Auerbach, 1988).

Whereas Rogers felt that empathy was a skill that should be used throughout the counseling relationship, some research suggests that it might be more effective at specific stages of the counseling relationship and only with certain clients (Gladstein, 1983). This would be somewhat supported by Robert Kegan's (1982, 1994) theoretical position that suggests that the ability to be empathic is a developmental skill accomplished more fully in adulthood and may increase as one grows older. Thus, one might conclude that, as a function of a counselor's cognitive development, some would be better at making empathic responses and others might be better at making other kinds of responses during varying points in the helping relationship. Also, some clients who are at lower developmental levels would not recognize an empathic person and would subsequently not gain from that person's understanding. A more detailed discussion of developmental levels can be found in this chapter and in Chapter 9, while empathy, as a counseling skill, will be discussed fully in Chapter 5.

Genuineness

Genuineness refers to the willingness on the part of the therapist to be authentic, open, and honest within the helping relationship. Humanists often speak of the importance of authenticity or genuineness in the establishment of healthy relationships, noting that individuals who embody such characteristics are transparent; that is, they readily show their feelings to others (Greenberg, 1994; Jourard, 1971; Rogers, 1957). On the other hand, they note that those who are nongenuine are closed off to their feelings and live fake, false lives. Rogers (1957) popularized the term *genuineness* (or *congruence*) and noted that it was a core condition in the counseling relationship, along with empathy and unconditional positive regard. While Rogers and other humanists have sung the praises of genuineness in the relationship, psychoanalysts and some behaviorists have traditionally downplayed the importance of a genuine relationship.

Gelso and Carter (1994) suggest that regardless of one's theoretical orientation, there exists an ongoing "real" relationship in which the client, to some degree, will see the therapist realistically, "even when the therapist tries to hide or make ambiguous his or her self" (p. 298). This real relationship has at its core the ability of the client to recognize the genuine (or nongenuine) self of the counselor. Although research on the relationship between genuineness and client outcomes has mixed results (Lambert et al., 1986), Gelso and Carter (1994) suggest all counselors should realize the importance of genuineness in the counseling relationship.

Acceptance

Being accepting is the ability to regard clients unconditionally despite differences in cultural heritage, values, or belief systems. Rogers (1957) called being able to accept clients "without strings attached" unconditional positive regard. Leo Buscaglia (1972) called this "responsible love":

> *Responsible love is accepting and understanding. . . . [L]ove helps us to accept the fact that the other individual is behaving only as he [or she] is able to behave at the moment.* (p. 119)

Unconditional acceptance of a client does not necessarily mean that one likes or condones everything a person does; however, such acceptance does show a deep understanding for another. For instance, one would assuredly not like the actions of a murderer or rapist; however, being accepting of this client would mean that the counselor has an understanding of the felon's world and how he or she came to be. This acceptance of another person is a likely by-product of the counselor's ability to be nondogmatic, empathic, and open-minded. The manifestation of these attitudes allows the client to feel safe enough to open a window into his or her soul, allowing the helper to see the client's hurts and pains. Research on acceptance and positive regard shows a relationship between these characteristics and positive client outcomes (Feitel, 1968; Patterson, 1984).

Open-Mindedness

Closely related to the ability to accept others is whether or not an individual is open-minded or nondogmatic (Rokeach, 1960). Belkin (1988) notes that "open-mindedness in the counseling setting may be defined as freedom from fixed preconceptions and an attitude of open receptivity to that which the client is expressing" (p. 66). The open-minded counselor is nondogmatic; he or she is not trying to convince the client of a certain point of view. Instead, the counselor is able to hear the client, be with the client, and be open to whatever the client might say. Dogmatic and closed-minded counselors are poor at showing empathy, are persistent in their way of viewing the world despite evidence to the contrary, and have difficulty forming positive counseling relationships (Allen, 1967; Anderson, Lepper, & Ross, 1980; Kemp, 1962; McAuliffe, Neukrug, & Lovell, 1998; Mezzano, 1969; Russo, Kelz, & Hudon, 1964; Tosi, 1970; Wright, 1975).

Probably one of strongest indications that a person is dogmatic is a belief in absolute truth. This individual sees no alternatives to his or her ways of viewing the world and believes there is just one right way of understanding reality. This absolutist, unequivocal thinking is highlighted by Carl Rogers, when he reviews a book by the theologian Reinhold Niebuhr:

> *As I lay the book down, I find that I am impressed most of all by the awesome certainty with which Dr. Niebuhr knows. He knows, with incredible assurance, what is wrong with the thinking of St. Thomas Aquinas, Augustine, Hegel, Freud, Marx, Dewey, and many, many others. He also knows what are the errors of communism, existentialism, psychology, and all the social sciences. His favorite term for the formulations of others is "absurd," but such other terms as "erroneous," "blind," "naive," "inane," and "inadequate" also are useful.*
> (Rogers, 1989b, p. 208)

Mindfulness (Internality)

Mindful people are focused, are capable of great sensitivity, are aware of how the context in which they live affects their lives and how they understand the world, and ultimately have great control over their lives (Langer, 2000). Such people have a high degree of internality; that is, they believe their fate is in their own hands, are free thinkers, have the ability to critically evaluate the opinions of others, and do not introject (swallow whole) other points of view. Although they may have strong opinions, they also respect the opinions of others and have a high regard for how their opinions might affect others (Lovell, 1999a; McAuliffe et al., 1998; Neukrug & McAuliffe, 1993).

Mindfulness tends to be a particularly important quality to model in the counseling relationship, as it highlights many attributes deemed important in Western culture. However, such an orientation may not be valued by clients from cultures that do not stress reliance on self (Pedersen, 2000; Sue, 1978; Yutrzenka, 1995).

Sue presents a continuum that reflects two aspects of internality, locus of control and locus of responsibility (see Figure 1.2). Based on this graphic presentation, one can

FIGURE 1.2
Locus of Control and Locus of Responsibility

SOURCE: Adapted from Sue, D. W. (1978). Counseling across cultures. *Personnel and Guidance Journal*. 56, 460. ACA. Reprinted with permission. No further reproduction authorized without written permission.

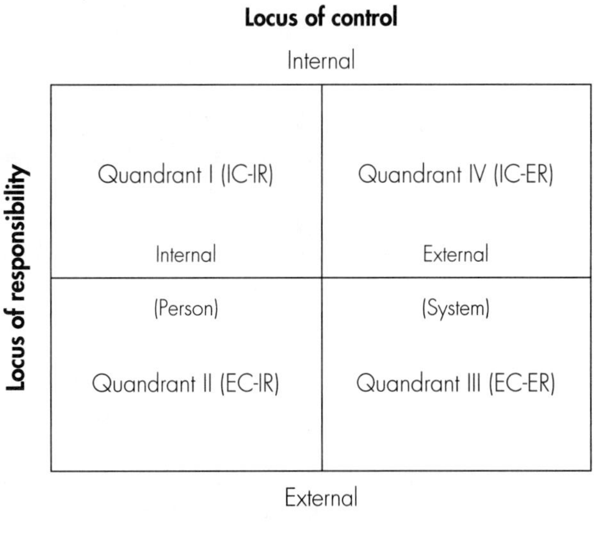

identify the quadrant within which can be found a specific culture's predominant style of relating. For instance, American culture's predominant style of relating would be in Quadrant I of Figure 1.2, which reflects an internal locus of control and internal locus of responsibility, whereas individuals from other cultures might locate themselves in one of the other quadrants. When working with clients, counselors should bear in mind that not all cultures may value the quality of internality.

Psychological Adjustment

> *My involvement in this [my own] therapeutic process brought about a turning point in my illness and a radical shift in my personal life. As a therapist myself, I now know how frightening it is for clients to take this step from the known into the unknown, to honestly experience and lovingly evaluate what they feel and who they are.* (Remen, May, Young, & Berland, 1985, p. 89)

With research showing that a well-adjusted counselor may have better client outcomes than counselors who are not well-adjusted (Lambert & Bergin, 1983), it is disturbing to find that therapists seem to have more than their share of psychological dysfunction (White & Franzoni, 1990). However, with 66% to 84% of varying types of therapists having participated in their own therapy (Deutsch, 1984; Neukrug, Milliken, & Shoemaker, 2001; Neukrug & Williams, 1993; Norcross, Strausser, & Faltus, 1988; Pope & Tabachnick, 1994; Prochaska & Norcross, 1983), it is heartening to see that therapists seem to want to work on their own issues. In fact, some research shows that positive client outcomes may be more likely if a therapist has been in his or her own personal therapy (Greenberg & Staller, 1981). It is also interesting that although only a small percentage of professional training programs in the mental health field require participation in therapy, an overwhelming percentage of therapists believe that therapy should be required by training programs, and a majority of therapists think it should be required by state licensing boards (Pope & Tabachnick, 1994).

Participation in one's own therapy has a number of benefits for the budding counselor. First, it obviously can assist the counselor in dealing with his or her own personal difficulties. "For counselor[s] to set themselves up as helper[s] to others, without having resolved major difficulties of their own, would appear to be farcical" (Wheeler, 1991, p. 199). Second, the counselor can gain a first-hand sense of whether what he or she does will work. Third, it enables the counselor to identify and empathize with the experience of sitting in the client's seat. Fourth, personal therapy yields great insight of self, which is likely to have a positive effect on the counseling relationship. Finally, it helps to prevent countertransference, "the process of [counselors] seeing themselves in their clients, of over identifying with their clients, or of meeting their needs through their clients" (Corey, 2000a, p. 19). In fact, Gelso and Carter (1994) suggest that whether or not the therapist is actively attending to countertransference, it will play an important role in the health and development of the relationship with the client.

Is therapy the only road to psychological adjustment? Probably not; however, it is a very special relationship not achievable through friendships or other significant relationships. Other activities, such as support groups, meditation, exercise, and journaling, have all been shown to have positive effects on our psychological adjustment. Therapy is not the only way, but it is one of a few activities that together can lead to good mental health and more effective counseling relationships.

Relationship Building

The relationship between the counselor and client may be the most significant factor in creating client change (Safran & Muran, 2000; Sexton & Whiston, 1991;Whiston & Coker, 2000). Gelso and Carter (1994) state that the "working alliance" is related to how the client presents and aligns his or her ego for the counseling relationship and how the client's ego is, or is not, joined with the counselor's " 'therapizing' self or ego" (p. 296). Such a relationship is closely related to the ability of the client and counselor to build an emotional bond and to work on setting attaining goals. The working alliance exists throughout the counseling relationship regardless of whether it is acknowledged by the counselor and the client.

The well-known family therapist Salvadore Minuchin (1974) stands apart from many other therapists in his acknowledgment and description of the importance of the building an alliance with clients. Using the term "joining" to describe the building of the client–helper relationship, he states:

> *The therapist's methods of creating a therapeutic system and positioning himself as its leader are known as joining operations. These are the underpinnings of therapy. Unless the therapist can join the family and establish a therapeutic system, restructuring cannot occur, and any attempt to achieve the therapeutic goals will fail.* (p. 123)

Generally, the ways in which the relationship is built are based on the theoretical orientation of the counselor in conjunction with his or her personality. For example, although psychoanalytical therapy stresses anonymity and distance on the part of the analyst early on in the relationship, many analysts are still able to quickly build a strong bond with their clients. Similarly, although humanists stress the importance of the relationship, there are many humanistically oriented therapists who have difficulty maintaining emotional bonds with clients because of their own personality style. The challenge for all counselors is to have the emotional fortitude to build strong relationships with their clients, to know how to build such bonds within the context of their theoretical framework, and to be able to understand how these bonds dramatically affect work with clients.

Competence

Counselor expertise has been shown to be a crucial element for client success in counseling (Whiston & Coker, 2000), and perceived competence has been consistently chosen by therapists as the most important factor in picking a therapist (Grunebaum, 1983; Neukrug & Williams, 1993; Neukrug, Milliken, & Shoemaker, 2001; Norcross et al., 1988). Thus it should not be surprising that being competent is the final characteristic I have chosen as crucial for counselors to embrace.

Competent counselors have a thirst for knowledge. They desire to examine the newest trends, the newest approaches, to be on the cutting edge of the field. Such counselors exhibit this thirst through their study habits, their desire to join professional associations, their reading of professional journals, their view that education is a lifelong process, and their ability to view their own approach to working with clients as something that is always broadening and deepening.

Counselors have both an ethical and legal responsibility to be competent (Corey, Corey, & Callanan, 1998; Welfel, 1998). For instance, the ACA ethical guidelines elaborate on seven areas of competence, including (1) practicing within one's boundary of competence, (2) practicing only in one's specialty areas, (3) accepting employment only for positions for which one is qualified, (4) monitoring one's effectiveness, (5) knowing when to consult with others, (6) keeping current by attending continuing education activities, and (7) refraining from offering services when physically or emotionally impaired (ACA, 1995a, Standard C). The legal system reinforces these ethical guidelines:

> *Psychotherapists commit professional malpractice if they are visibly less competent than the average of their peers . . . One function of lawsuits is to encourage competent therapy.* (Swenson, 1997, p. 166)

Thus being competent is our professional responsibility and necessitates that we continue the learning process throughout our lifetime.

The eight characteristics of (1) empathy, (2) genuineness, (3) acceptance, (4) open-mindedness, (5) mindfulness, (6) psychological adjustment, (7) relationship building, and (8) competence are qualities to which the effective counselor should strive. Few if any of us are already there. More than likely, each of these qualities can be nurtured and developed as we walk down our unique paths in life.

The Effective Counselor: A Constructive Development Perspective

What is it that enables one counselor to embody the qualities of the effective counselor while another counselor seems to struggle along? Two constructive developmental theories—William Perry's theory of intellectual and ethical development (King, 1978) and Robert Kegan's (1982, 1994) theory of the evolving self—offer a way of conceptualizing how counselors develop throughout their lives (see Chapter 10 for more on these theories).

Both theories conclude that, with certain opportunities in life, an adult's view of the world will change in a predictable fashion, from concrete, rigid thinking toward abstract, more flexible, "relativistic" thinking. Individuals at lower stages of development tend to want "answers" from authority figures, see others as holding the knowledge and answers to life's questions, and have not fully developed a separate sense of self. Individuals at the higher levels of development see knowledge as a mutual and reciprocal process whereby experts can share answers through an interactive learning process. Individuals at higher stages have a strong sense of self, listen to feedback about self from others, and are willing to learn, teach, share, and be open with others.

Recent research on adult cognitive development seems to support some of Perry and Kegan's hypotheses as it shows that individuals at higher stages tend to be more empathic and open-minded, have more of an internal locus of control, and have a thirst for knowledge. That is, they embrace many of the characteristics of the effective counselor noted earlier (Benack, 1988; Bowman & Allen, 1988; Bowman & Reeves, 1987; McAuliffe et al., 1998; Neukrug & McAuliffe, 1993; Reeves, Bowman & Cooley, 1989; Widick, 1977).

Because constructivist theory is developmental, it holds that all individuals are capable of moving to higher levels of development if placed in a nurturing and supportive environment that is challenging to the individual's view of the world. Counselor training programs hope to offer such an environment—one that supports students, yet challenges them to think about new ways of understanding self and others (McAuliffe & Erikson, 2000).

Multicultural Issues

The Helping Professions' Responsibility to Minority Clients

Research has consistently shown that clients from nonwhite backgrounds are frequently misdiagnosed, attend counseling at lower rates, terminate counseling more quickly, find counseling less helpful, and are more distrustful of white counselors and more trustful of counselors from their own ethnic/racial/cultural background (see Section 6). With relatively small numbers of minorities entering the helping professions (Axelson, 1999), it is imperative that the helping professions actively try to recruit counselors of color. Increased numbers of minority counselors along with better training in multicultural counseling are essential if culturally diverse clients are to feel comfortable seeking out and following through in counseling.

A Call to the Profession: Inclusion of Multiculturalism

Our identity as professionals has too long been based on a Western/European model that embraces the values and beliefs of white clients while negating the values and beliefs of minority clients. If counseling is to be an equal opportunity profession, counselors must graduate from training programs with more than a desire to help all people. As a profession, we will only have achieved competence in counseling diverse clients when each graduate of a training program has learned counseling strategies that can work for a wide range of clients, has worked with clients from diverse backgrounds, and leaves his or her program with an appreciation for diversity and an identity as a counselor that includes a multicultural perspective. Whitfield (1994) goes a step further, suggesting that each counseling graduate should be multilingual, have a multicultural view, be multiculturally literate, be ethnically informed, and be ecologically literate; that is, have knowledge of the environment from which the client comes (see Chapter 14). Most counseling programs would have much to change if they were to adopt all of these suggestions!

Ethical, Professional, and Legal Issues

Knowing Who We Are and Our Relationship to Other Professional Groups

Counselors have an identity, a body of knowledge that is unique to their profession. By knowing who we are, we also have a clear sense of who we are not. It is through our identity that we are able to define our limits, know when it is appropriate to consult with colleagues, and recognize when we should refer to other professionals. The ACA Code of Ethics (1995a) highlights these issues when it states:

> Boundaries of Competence: *Counselors practice only within the boundaries of their competence, based on their education, training, supervised experience, state and national professional credentials, and appropriate professional experience. . . .* (Standard C.2.a.)

> Ethical Issues in Consultation: *Counselors take reasonable steps to consult with other counselors or related professionals when they have questions regarding their ethical obligations or professional practice. . . .* (Standard C.2.e.)
>
> Inability to Assist Clients: *If counselors determine an inability to be of professional assistance to clients, they avoid entering or immediately terminate the counseling relationship. Counselors are knowledgeable about referral resources and suggest appropriate alternatives. . . .* (Standard A.11.b.)

Impaired Mental Health Professionals

All mental health professionals have a responsibility to be aware of the pressures and stresses that impinge on their lives and how these might affect their relationship with clients. A professional who is not attending to his or her own needs is likely to be ineffective in the counseling relationship. Incompetence is not only unethical but can lead to malpractice suits (Neukrug, Milliken, & Walden, 2001; Swenson, 1997).

> Impairment: *Counselors refrain from offering or accepting professional services when their physical, mental or emotional problems are likely to lead to harm to a client or others. They are alert to the signs of impairment, seek assistance for problems, and if necessary, limit, suspend, or terminate their professional responsibilities.* (ACA, 1995a, Standard C.2.g.)

The Counselor in Process: Personal Therapy and Related Growth Experiences

With research indicating that the mental health of the counselor is likely to be a crucial element to client improvement, it would seem imperative that counselors embrace the idea of entering their own counseling. Being in one's own counseling gives the counselor the "feel" for what it's like to be a client, the opportunity to learn from an *in vivo* model, and the ability to gain at close hand understanding of the format, structure, and boundaries of the counseling relationship. Being in one's own counseling allows the counselor to deal with unfinished business, prevent countertransference, and act as an effective model for clients.

Besides counseling, there are other growth experiences that may be beneficial to the counselor: meditation, relaxation exercises and stress reduction, discussion and support groups, exercise, journaling, and readings.

Your journey into the counseling profession may just be beginning, and I hope that it is a long and fruitful quest. During this journey consider engaging in personal growth activities that will foster your ability to understand yourself and have the added benefit of helping you work more effectively with your clients. And, most important, remember that the journey doesn't end until we die and maybe not then either.

Summary

In this chapter we attempted to define the somewhat elusive word *counseling* and distinguish it from the words *guidance* and *psychotherapy*. We then compared and contrasted some of the training, credentialing, and roles and functions of counselors, psychologists, psychiatrists, social workers, and psychiatric nurses. In addition, we also identified some of the benefits of professional associations, highlighted the American Counseling Association (ACA), and identified some related professional associations.

As the chapter continued we spent some time reviewing those aspects of the effective counselor, specifically identifying eight characteristics that may be related to positive client outcomes, including empathy, genuineness, acceptance, open-mindedness, mindfulness, psychological adjustment, relationship building, and competence. We examined how offering a supportive yet challenging environment is important for the development of these characteristics.

Near the end of this chapter we noted that clients from nonwhite backgrounds are generally not using and are more dissatisfied with counseling than white clients, and we discussed the ever-increasing and important role of multicultural issues within the counseling profession. We discussed the importance of learning how to approach clients from diverse backgrounds in ways that will make them more amenable to the counseling process. We also noted the importance for counseling programs to actively recruit more minority counseling students, because minority clients tend to be more trustful of counselors from their own cultural background.

In this chapter we discussed the importance of a number of ethical issues, including practicing in one's area of competence, the importance of consulting with other professionals, and the importance of terminating or referring clients when one is unable to work effectively with them. Finally, we discussed the importance of being in our own therapy and/or providing ourselves with growth experiences that could foster our own mental health as well as the mental health of our clients. We concluded by noting how our own personal growth is a lifelong process.

INFOTRAC and Other Information Resources (e.g., ERIC and PsycINFO)

Note: When relevant, key words are in quotation marks.

1. Search for information about the effect of "counselor characteristics" on the helping relationship. What characteristics, other than the ones in this chapter, are shown to be important in the helping relationship?
2. Examine the possible effects of treatment of an "impaired therapist" working with clients.
3. Review the kinds of "journals" in the varying professional associations.

CHAPTER 2

A History of the Counseling Profession

Can you imagine a woman hanged as a witch because she was mentally ill, or being placed in a straitjacket and thrown into a filthy, rat-infested cell for the remainder of her life? Or can you envision a man placed in a bathtub filled with iron filings to cure him of mental illness or bled to rid him of demons and spirits that caused him to think in demonic ways? What about having a piece of your brain scraped out in order to change the way you feel? Or being placed in a box that would receive "energy" and rid you of emotional and physical problems? These examples are a part of the history of our profession.

Unfortunately, I've taught long enough to know that when I teach history, it often is not as interesting as what you just read. In fact, my experience has been that half of the class mentally steps out. Why is this? Unfortunately, learning names, dates, and a few facts is just plain boring for some people. This used to be the case for me. It is no longer.

In 1962, Thomas Kuhn wrote a book called *The Structure of Scientific Revolutions* that changed the way I understood history and the accumulation of knowledge. What intrigued me in particular was his concept that knowledge builds upon prior knowledge and that, periodically, the time is ripe for a person to synthesize this prior knowledge and develop new, revolutionary ways of understanding what has come before. This he called the paradigm shift. This makes history more exciting for me, because I now see it as leading toward the next paradigm shift.

We are all part of history in the making. Some of us take an active role through research, scholarly pursuits, or leadership in professional organizations. Perhaps some of you will be instrumental in the next paradigm shift. Others go along for the ride, watching history unfold all around. Whether you are part of the next paradigm shift or an interested observer, you have been affected by the past; and, in your own unique way, you are affecting the future. Let's look at how history has made us what we are today, and then, later in the text, we can consider what we are moving toward in the future.

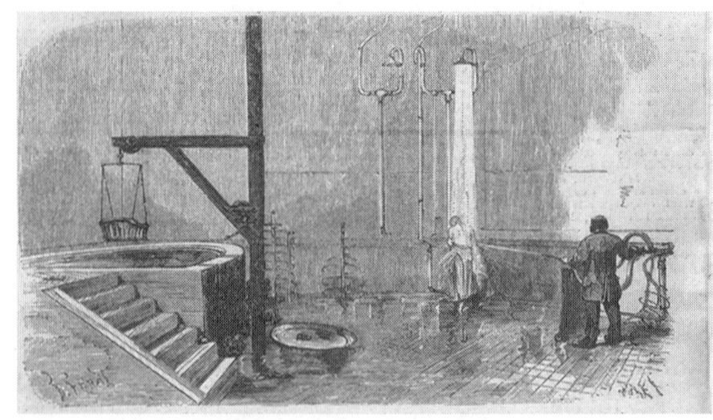

Early treatment of the mentally ill—hydrotherapy

We will start our look at history by going into the distant past, exploring some of the precursors to the mental health field. We will then take a brief look at the history of social work, psychology, and psychiatry, three fields that dramatically affected the counseling profession. We will examine the history of our profession in detail, from its early roots in vocational guidance to modern-day counseling. We will conclude the chapter by examining the relatively recent history of ethical standards and multicultural issues and examine how they have been important to our profession.

Understanding the Human Condition: From Early Antiquity to the Present

The first counselors were leaders of the community who attempted to provide inspiration for others through their teachings. They were religious leaders like Moses (1000 B.C.), Buddha (500 B.C.), and Mohammed (600). They were also philosophers like Lao-Tzu (600 B.C.), Confucius (500 B.C.), Socrates (450 B.C.), Plato (400 B.C.), and Aristotle (350 B.C.). (Kottler & Brown, 1999, p. 27)

Since the dawn of existence, people have attempted to understand the human condition. Myths, magic, beliefs in spirits, the use of ritualism, and sacred art have been some of the ways that people have made sense out of this complex world and have been implements for thought and introspection, "tools with which to think, talk, and know about self and world" (Ellwood, 1993, p. 20). Over the centuries shamans, or individuals who had special status due to their mystical powers, have been considered to be caretakers of the soul and thought to have knowledge of the future. Later in history, the concept of soul has often given way to the concept of psyche.

One of the first written treatises of a psychological nature can be traced back to an Egyptian papyrus of 3000 B.C.E. that shows a primitive attempt to understand some basic functions of the brain (Breasted, 1930). Almost 1000 years later, still in ancient Egypt, a wise man who was obviously psychologically minded wrote:

> *If thou searchest the character of a friend, ask no questions, (but) approach him and deal with him when he is alone. . . . Disclose his heart in conversation. If that which he has seen come forth from him, (or) he do ought that makes thee ashamed for him, . . . do not answer.* (Breasted, 1934, p. 132)

Such writings show that the "counseling way" clearly preceded modern times. However, it was Hippocrates (460–377 B.C.E.) who presented his reflections on the human condition that were to greatly change the Western world's view of the person. Whereas many contemporaries of Hippocrates believed that possession by evil spirits was responsible for emotional ills, his suggestions for the treatment of the human condition might even be considered modern by today's standards. For instance, for melancholia he recommended sobriety, a regular and tranquil life, exercise short of fatigue, and bleeding, if necessary. For hysteria, he recommended getting married, an idea with which many in today's world might argue.

With the advent of monotheistic religion, we see abundant examples of humankind's attempt to further understand self. The Old and New Testaments, the Quran, and other religious writings abound with such examples (Belgium, 1992). For instance, in Buddhism, the Sanskrit term *duhkha* speaks to the pain and suffering that people carry due to what is called "delusive perceptions" (Purton, 1993), and the Old and New Testaments offer us many reflections on the concept of guilt and sin—reflections that could very well come in handy today.

> *. . . Is no one any longer guilty of anything? Guilty perhaps of a sin that could be repented and repaired or atoned for? Is it only that someone may be stupid or sick or criminal or asleep. . . . Anxiety and depression we all acknowledge, and even vague guilt feelings; but has no one committed any sins?* (Menninger, 1973, p. 13)

The rise of Christianity and the development of Christian notions of the person were influenced by a number of philosophers and theologians who reflected on the nature of the person, the soul, and the human condition. For example, such philosophers as Plotinus (205–270), who believed the soul was separate from the body, had a lasting impact on the dualistic fashion in which the Western world views the mind and body.

The Renaissance in Europe might be considered the start of the modern era; with it came the printing press and the writings of modern philosophers. Individuals like Descartes (1596–1650), who believed that knowledge and truth come through deductive reasoning, and John Locke (1632–1704) and James Mill (1773–1836), who believed that the mind is a blank slate upon which experience generates ideas, set the stage for modern psychology labs to study human experience. These individuals, and others, led the way to the first professions that attempted to deal with the human condition. Thus, the 1800s saw the advent of modern psychology, the beginnings of modern-day social work and psychiatry, and the origins of the counseling field. Clearly, these fields were influenced by the contributions of great minds that preceded them.

A Brief History of Related Helping Professions: Social Work, Psychology, Psychiatry

Originating in the 19th century, the professions of social work, psychology, psychiatry, and counseling had somewhat different beginnings, with the counseling profession evolving out of early vocational guidance activities, the social work field developing out of the desire to assist the destitute, psychology starting as both a laboratory science and an attempt to understand the nature of the person, and psychiatry growing out of modern medicine's attempt to alleviate mental illness through medical interventions. Although originally evolving from quite different origins, they all have slowly moved toward many of the same theoretical conclusions and today can be seen on slightly different yet parallel paths (see Figure 2.1).

The Field of Social Work

Historical Background

The field of social work can be traced back to work with the poor and destitute in this country and in England. During the 1500s, the Elizabethan Poor Laws gave the Church

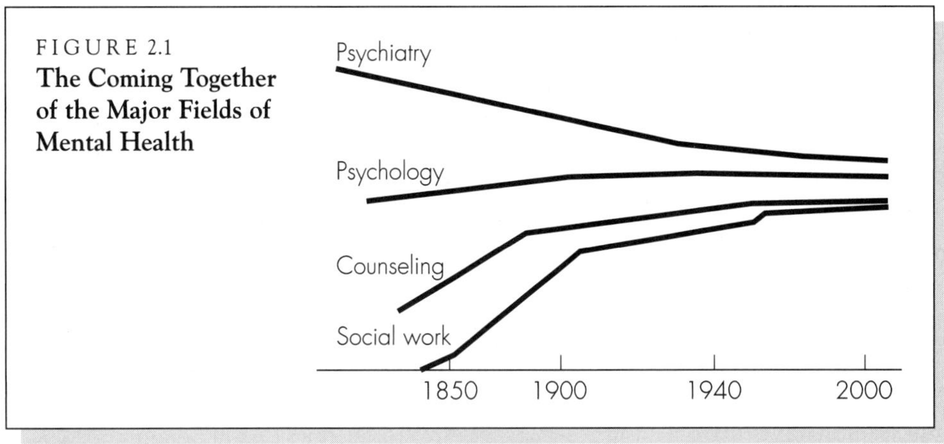

FIGURE 2.1
The Coming Together of the Major Fields of Mental Health

power to oversee the raising and administering of funds for the destitute. Until then, such relief was on a voluntary basis. As a carryover from this system, during the colonial period in America, local governments enacted laws to assist the poor. This same time also saw organized charities, usually affiliated with religious groups, begin to arise. In the 1800s, as populations in cities grew, an increasingly large underclass developed in this country whose needs could not be met by the traditional charitable organizations. Mounting political pressure thus led to the creation of specialized institutions such as reform schools, lunatic asylums, and other specialized institutions.

To assist the underprivileged who were not institutionalized, two major approaches evolved. Charity Organization Societies (COSs) had volunteers who would visit the poor, aid in educating children, give economic advice, and generally assist in alleviating the conditions of poverty. Generally the poor were given advice, support, small amounts of necessities, and a good dose of moral judgment and religious values. Sometimes these individuals, who became known as "friendly visitors," would spend years assisting one family. The COSs are seen as the beginnings of social casework, the process by which a client's needs are examined and a treatment plan is designed. In contrast to the COSs, the settlement movement had staff who actually lived in the poorer communities.

> *In essence it was simply a residence for university men in a city slum. . . . These critics looked forward to a society that encouraged people's social responsibility, not self-interest, to create a life that was kindly, dignified, and beautiful, as well as progressive and prosperous. Some of these thinkers rejected capitalism in favor of an idealized medieval community.* (Leiby, 1978, p. 129)

The idealistic young staff believed in community action and tried to persuade politicians to provide better services for the poor. One of the best-known settlement houses was Hull House, established by social activist Jane Addams (1860–1935) in 1889 in Chicago (Addams, 1910). Out of the involvement with the underprivileged arose articles and books concerned with methods of adequately meeting the needs of the underclass. At the turn of the 20th century, the first social work training programs arose. Over the next 30 years the social work field grew in many different directions with some of its main emphasis areas focusing on social casework, social group work, and community work.

During the 1940s and 1950s an increased emphasis on understanding the dynamics of social and family systems emerged. As social workers had already been working with social systems and families, this emphasis became a natural focus for many social work programs. Such programs stressed contextual or systems thinking, as opposed to seeing the individual as an island unto him- or herself, as did many of the early philosophers and psychologists. One social worker, Virginia Satir (1967), was particularly instrumental in reshaping the practices of the mental health profession to include a greater systems focus.

In 1955 a number of social work organizations combined to form the National Association for Social Work (NASW); and, in 1965, NASW established the Academy of Certified Social Workers (ACSW), which has set standards of practice for master's level social workers. Today, social workers can be found in a variety of social service settings from hospitals to mental health centers to homeless shelters, the roots of the social work profession. In addition, although many social workers today do individual psychotherapy and family therapy, others work in community settings doing advocacy work, and still others administer social service organizations.

Social Work's Influence on the Counseling Profession

The counseling profession has borrowed much from the field of social work. Social work, with its emphasis on understanding systems, has provided the counseling profession with an understanding of the individual from within the family and social system perspective. Because many of the major family therapists started out as social workers, counselors have learned to apply many of their concepts with clients. Also, social work's emphasis on field experience has rubbed off on counseling, as counselor education programs have increasingly offered more field experience in their training programs. Finally, social work's emphasis on advocacy is a constant reminder to counselors that their clients are greatly affected by the culture from which they come and the larger dynamics of society. It is a reminder to all of us that we must continually advocate for our clients on local, state, and national levels.

The Field of Psychology

Historical Background

The origin of the field of psychology can be traced back thousands of years. For instance, psychological thinking can be traced back to 7th century B.C.E. Greek philosophers who reflected on the nature of life and the universe. A few centuries later, the Greek philosopher Hippocrates offered notions on how to treat mental illness, and Plato (427–347 B.C.E.) suggested that introspection and reflection were roads to knowledge, that dreams and fantasies were substitute satisfactions, and that the human condition had physical, moral, and spiritual origins. Many consider Plato's student Aristotle (384–322 B.C.E.) to be the first psychologist because he used objectivity and reason to study knowledge and his writings were psychological in nature (Wertheimer, 1978).

Although Augustine (354–430) and Thomas Aquinas (1225–1274) highlighted consciousness, self-examination, and inquiry, there was little other "psychological thinking" during this 800-year period. This was partly due to the rise of Christianity, which downplayed reason and objectivity and highlighted the supernatural. However, the Renaissance of the 14th to 17th centuries saw a rediscovery of the Greek philosophies and a renewed interest in questions regarding the nature of the human condition. This was followed by philosophical discussions regarding the nature of the person as well as the beginning of the scientific method.

During the 19th century psychology was increasingly influenced by modern-day medicine, physics, and the new theory of evolution. Wilhelm Wundt (1832–1920) and Sir Francis Galton (1822–1911), two of the first experimental psychologists, developed laboratories to examine physical differences among people for such things as muscle strength, head size, and reaction time. This scientific orientation to the field of psychology quickly spread to the United States, where G. Stanley Hall (1846–1924) and James Cattell (1860–1940) opened laboratories at Harvard and the University of Pennsylvania in the late 1800s (Capshew, 1992). It was also during the 19th century that William James's (1842–1910) theory of philosophical pragmatism, or the concept that scientific theory could only be understood through the particular prism in which it was being examined, was published (Leary, 1992). Thus were mixed the two schools of psychology, the philosophical and the scientific.

One natural outgrowth of laboratory science was the development of psychological and educational tests at the end of the 19th century. For instance, Alfred Binet (1857–1911) developed, for the Ministry of Public Education in Paris, one of the first intelligence tests, which was used to assist in classroom placement of children who were mentally retarded (Drummond, 2000). The beginning of the 20th century saw the first use of school achievement tests, tests for vocational assessment, and some of the first "modern day" personality tests. Today, tests are found everywhere and are often an important component to a deeper understanding of our clients.

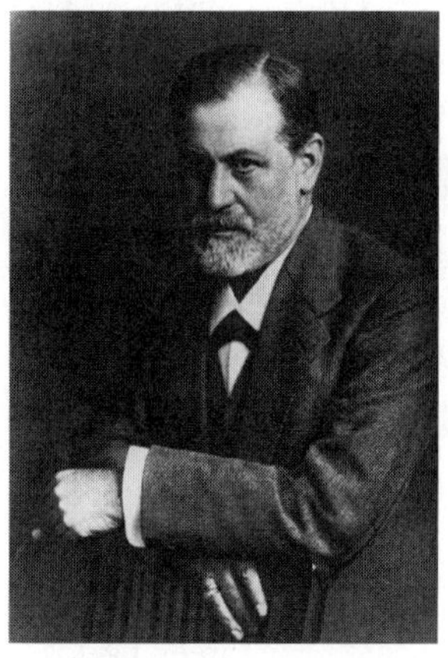
Sigmund Freud

The beginnings of the testing movement paralleled the rise of psychoanalysis, the first comprehensive psychotherapeutic system. Developed by Sigmund Freud (1856–1939), this movement was undoubtedly affected by the new emphasis on the scientific method. Freud had been greatly influenced by Anton Mesmer (mesmerize! 1734–1815) and Jean Martin Charcot (1825–1893), who were practicing a new phenomena called hypnosis. These early hypnotists showed that suggestion could play a powerful role in affecting an individual's mental state. In fact, Charcot showed that some physical disorders (e.g., some forms of paralysis), whose etiology was previously thought to only be of a physical nature, could be induced under hypnosis. Freud originally used hypnosis to uncover repressed and painful memories, but later stopped in favor of other techniques and subsequently developed his complex theory to understand the origins of human behavior. Freud's views on mental health and mental illness were revolutionary and continue to profoundly affect the ways in which we conceptualize client problems (Appignanesi, 1990). Although he was trained as a physician, Freud's concepts were very quickly adopted by the psychology profession.

Besides traditional psychoanalysis, the end of the 19th century saw the beginnings of other schools of psychology. Ivan Pavlov (1849–1936), in his experiments with classical conditioning of dogs, and others who followed, developed behaviorism, de-emphasized the importance of introspection, and stressed the importance of stimulus–response and environmental influences. During this same period, phenomenological psychology and existential psychology had their beginnings and stressed the nature of existence and the study of reality. Also around this time Gestalt psychology, which tried to answer questions about how individuals organize experience into reality, first emerged. The early days of behaviorism, existential psychology, phenomenological psychology, and Gestalt psychology are the roots of many of today's cognitive–behavioral and humanistically oriented therapies.

The American Psychological Association (APA) was founded in 1892 (Sokal, 1992) as an association mostly of experimental psychologists, but starting in the 1920s clinicians began to make a greater impact on the field and entered the association in large numbers.

During the mid-1940s APA went under a great revision and assimilated many new clinical associations such as Counseling Psychology (Division 17) (Finkel, 1994; Kelly, 1994; F.A. Young, 1992). This division, which shares much in common with the history and goals of the counseling profession, highlighted the fact that a vast majority of psychologists now viewed themselves as clinicians, not academics or scientists (Whiteley, 1984).

Today, we still find both experimental psychologists, who work in the laboratory trying to understand the psychophysiological causes of behavior, and clinical psychologists, who practice counseling and psychotherapy. In addition, we also find other highly trained psychologists doing testing in schools, working for business and industry with organizational concerns, and working in many other areas. Today, APA offers numerous benefits and scholarly activities, such as publishing journals that strive to understand human behavior, and, along with the American Psychiatric Association, it provides assistance in the development and continued refinement of the *Diagnostic and Statistical Manual IV-TR (DSM IV-TR)*, which is used in the diagnosis and treatment of psychiatric disorders (APA, 2000) (see Chapter 10).

Psychology's Influence on the Counseling Profession

The field of psychology has affected the counseling profession more than any other related mental health profession. Although psychology was the first profession to use a comprehensive approach to therapy, the counseling field was soon to follow and borrowed many of the theories used by early psychologists. Tests developed by psychologists at the turn of the 20th century were used by the early vocational guidance counselors and later adapted by counselors in many different settings. Research techniques developed by Wundt and others became the precursors to modern-day research tools used by counselors in their search for knowledge about the efficacy of counseling approaches and to evaluate programs they have developed. Finally, many modern-day counseling skills that were developed by psychologists during the early part of the 20th century were adapted by counselors in all differing settings. Psychology is truly our first cousin.

The Field of Psychiatry

Historical Background

Until the late 1700s mental illness was viewed as mystical, demonic, and generally not treatable. However, soon new ways of viewing the world and novel approaches to the understanding and treatment of mental diseases arose. In the late 1700s in France, Philippe Pinel (1745–1826), who is credited with being the founder of psychiatry, was one of the first of many to view insanity from a scientific perspective. Administering two mental hospitals, Pinel removed the chains that bound inmates and made one of the first attempts to treat inmates humanely.

During the 1800s great strides were made in the understanding, diagnosis, and treatment of mental illness. Emil Kraepelin (1855–1926) developed one of the first classifications of mental diseases, and Jean Martin Charcot (1825–1893) and Pierre Janet (1859–1947) both saw a relationship between certain psychological states and disorders that were formerly considered to be only of an organic nature.

In the United States, Benjamin Rush (1743–1813), a physician and dedicated social reformer, is considered to be the founder of American psychiatry. An impassioned believer in the abolition of slavery, a signer of the Declaration of Independence, and an ad-

BOX 2.1

The Beginnings of the Modern Mental Hospital

In 1773 the Publick Hospital for Persons of Insane and Disordered Minds admitted its first patient in Williamsburg, Virginia. The hospital, which had 24 cells, took a rather bleak approach to working with the mentally ill. Although many of the employees of these first hospitals had their hearts in the right place, their diagnostic and treatment procedures left a lot to be desired. For instance, some of the leading reasons that patients were admitted included masturbation, womb disease, religious excitement, intemperance, and domestic trouble—hardly reasons for admission to a mental institution. Normal treatment procedures were to administer heavy dosages of drugs, to bleed or blister individuals, to immerse individuals in freezing water for long periods of time, and to confine people to straitjackets or manacles. Bleeding and blistering was thought to remove harmful fluids from the individual's system (Zwelling, 1990). It was believed at that time that it was important to cause fear in a person, and even individuals like Dr. Benjamin Rush, known for his innovative and relatively benign treatment of the mentally ill, spoke of the importance of staring a person down (Woodside & McClam, 1990).

> *The first object of a physician, when he enters the cell or chamber of his deranged patient, should be to catch his EYE. . . . The dread of the eye was early imposed upon every beast of the field. . . . Now a man deprived of his reason partakes so much of the nature of those animals, that he is for the most part terrified, or composed, by the eye of a man who possesses his reason.*
> (Rush cited in Zwelling, 1990, p. 17).

vocate for the establishment of a peace institute as an alternative to the U.S. Military Academy, Rush appealed for humane treatment of the poor and mentally ill. Rush's text *Medical Inquiries and Observations upon the Diseases of the Mind,* published in 1812, became the seminal text in the field of psychiatry for the next 70 years (Baxter, 1994).

By the early 1800s, the Pennsylvania Hospital in Philadelphia and the Publick Hospital for Persons of Insane and Disordered Minds in Williamsburg, Virginia, had been established to treat the mentally insane. Early treatments for the mentally ill hardly resembled anything we might find in today's psychiatric hospitals; however, they were an acknowledgment that psychiatric disorders were real (see Box 2.1).

In the mid-1800s, Dorothea Dix (1802–1887) and others advocated the moral treatment of the mentally ill and suggested supportive care, encouragement and respect, removal from stressors, and vocational training as treatment of choice (Baxter, 1994). The spread of mental hospitals and the use of this new approach brought with it the founding of the Association of Medical Superintendents of American Institutions for the Insane in 1844. The forerunner of the American Psychiatric Association, this association had as its goals the improvement of diagnosis, care, and treatment of the mentally ill and developed standards for mental hospitals of the time.

In the first half of the 20th century, psychiatry developed in a number of different directions. Whereas many psychiatrists became entrenched in the psychoanalytic movement, others began to drift toward psychobiology as the treatment of choice for mental disorders, while still others became increasingly involved in social psychiatry (Sabshin, 1990). During the 1950s and 1960s a number of factors greatly affected the role and function of psychiatrists. First, during the 1950s there was a great expansion of the use of psychotropic medications. Then in the 1960s the deinstitutionalization of the mentally ill (e.g., Donaldson *v.* O' Connor, 1975; see p. 38) and the development of community-based mental health centers led to a greatly expanded role for psychiatrists in community agencies. Psychiatrists became increasingly less involved in doing psychoanalysis and more involved in the psychobiology of mental illness.

During the 1950s the American Psychiatric Association was instrumental in developing the first *Diagnostic and Statistical Manual of Mental Disorders (DSM-I)*, the forerunner of the *DSM-IV-TR*. The purpose of the *DSM-IV-TR* is to provide criteria for making clinical diagnoses that enhance agreement among clinicians (APA, 1994).

Today, with research indicating that some mental illness is predominantly or partially biologically based, psychiatrists have been playing an increasingly important role in the mental health field. In addition, with the advent of new and much improved psychopharmacological drugs, such as Prozac, psychiatrists have become very important consultants to counselors and other mental health professionals.

Psychiatry's Influence on the Counseling Profession

Psychiatry's focus on the classification of mental illness and on psychopathology has assisted counselors and other professionals in the diagnosis and development of treatment plans for clients, including the use of psychopharmacology. In addition, the awareness that some mental health problems may be organic has helped counselors understand that at times it is critical to make a referral to an expert in psychopharmacology and psychobiology.

An Early History of the Counseling Profession: The 1800s

Counseling represents the fusing of many influences. It brings together the movement toward a more compassionate treatment of mental health problems begun in the mid-nineteenth century France, the psychodynamic insights of Freud and psychoanalysis, the scientific scrutiny and methodology of the behavioral approach, the quantitative science of psychometrics, the humanistic perspective of client-centered therapy, the philosophical base of existentialism, and the practical insights and applications that evolved from the vocational guidance movement. (Belkin, 1988, p. 19)

In the 1800s, a number of forces came together that eventually led to the creation of the modern-day counseling profession. Such seemingly disparate forces as the social reform movements, the early days of vocational guidance, the beginning use of assessment instruments, and the first comprehensive approach to therapy came together to form the counseling profession. Let's take a brief look at each of these forces.

Social Reform Movements of the 1800s

During the 1800s a number of reform movements occurred simultaneously that eventually influenced the development of the counseling profession. Social workers, who were working with the poor and destitute; psychiatrists, who were trying to affect change in the treatment of the mentally ill; and educators, such as John Dewey (1859–1952), insisting on more humanistic teaching methods and access to public education—all had a common desire to help people in more humane and "modern" ways (Dewey, 1956; Dykhuizen, 1973; Neukrug, 2000). The counseling profession soon bore the fruits of these reform movements by embracing many of their ideals and some of their basic premises. Reform movements and their focus on caring for others no doubt had an affect on the *modus operandi* of the first professional counselors, the vocational guidance workers.

Vocational Guidance in the 1800s

Although modern-day vocational guidance activities and theory began in the latter part of the 1800s, as far back as the 10th century writings in an Iraqi text addressed occupational information, while the first job classification system was developed as early as 1468 by Sanchez de Arevalo, who wrote *Mirror of Men's Lives* (Carson & Altai, 1994). During the end of the 18th century, dramatic shifts took place in this country that were partially responsible for the beginnings of the vocational guidance movement and ultimately set the stage for the establishment of the counseling profession. This time in history saw the beginnings of the Industrial Revolution, social reform movements, and an increase in immigration, mostly to large northeastern cities. Perhaps for the first time, there was a large-scale need for vocational guidance. During the 1800s, prior to the development of vocational theory, a number of poorly written, moralistic books on occupational choice were written (Zytowski, 1972). However, now the stage was set for the development of the first comprehensive approaches to vocational guidance, guidance that would at least be partially based on the new science of testing (Herr & Cramer, 1995).

The Beginnings of the Testing Movement

Paralleling the rise of the vocational guidance movement were the beginnings of the testing movement. With the development of laboratory science in Europe and the United States came an increased interest in examining individual differences. Soon people were studying differences in intelligence, as it was then defined. For instance, Alfred Binet's intelligence test, developed in 1896, signified the beginning of the large-scale use of measurement instruments, soon to be used to assist individuals and institutions in decision making. Most significantly for the counseling profession, a number of these assessment instruments would soon be used in vocational counseling and would earmark the beginning of the counseling profession (Williamson, 1964).

Testing, vocational guidance theory, and the humane treatment approaches developed from the reform movements were three crucial elements to the formation of the counseling profession; however, the emergence of a comprehensive approach to psychotherapy may have been the most important component to the establishment of the counseling profession.

Psychoanalysis and the Development of Psychotherapy

Although for centuries philosophers and shamans reflected on the human condition and contributed treatises on psychological thought, it was not until the 1800s that a major shift took place in the understanding of mental illness. It was at this time that many challenged the notion that mental illness was caused by demons or was organic in nature. Instead, there evolved a consensus that at least some emotional problems were caused by unconscious psychological factors (Ehrenwald, 1976). Then, with the development of

Freud's theory of psychoanalysis in the late 1800s, we saw the first systematic and comprehensive approach to psychotherapy.

Freud's theory ushered in a new way of viewing the development of the person. Constructs never before discussed became commonplace and continue to be accepted in today's world. Freud and his disciples made terms like id, ego, superego, unconscious, and psychosexual development commonplace. Soon, these constructs permeated the western world, and this new "psychological" way of viewing the world affected the emerging field of counseling.

Modern-Day Counseling: Its Early Beginnings (1900–1950)

Early Vocational Guidance and the First Guidance Counselors

> *It is difficult even to imagine the difference of conditions now and in the early years of the century. . . . Think of what life would be without the railroad, only the stage-coach to carry our letters and ourselves across the country. Think of pulling oranges from Florida or California to Boston stores by team. Think of a city without a street-car or a bicycle, a cooking stove or a furnace, a gas jet or electric light, or even a kerosene lamp! Think of a land without photographs or photogravures, Christmas cards or color prints. . . .* (Parsons, cited in Watts, 1994, p. 267)

It was a different world at the beginning of the 20th century, but the rumblings of a new age were everywhere to be found. Social reformers were caring for the poor and demanding changes in education; psychiatry was changing its methods of treatment for the mentally ill; psychoanalysis and related therapies were the rage; the modern-day use of tests was beginning, and the Industrial Revolution was well underway. In some very subtle but important ways, each of these events would affect early vocational guidance and the emergence of the field of counseling.

The first part of the 20th century saw the beginnings of systematic vocational guidance in America. Although the concepts had been floating around in the latter part of the 1800s, the 1900s brought with it a comprehensive approach to vocational guidance. Then in 1907, troubled by the attitudes of youth, Jesse Davis (1871–1955) developed one of the first guidance curricula that focused on moral and vocational guidance and was presented during English composition classes in the Grand Rapids, Michigan, schools. At around the same time Eli Weaver (1862–1922), a New York City principal who had written a booklet called *Choosing a Career*, started vocational guidance in New York. Similarly, Anna Reed (1871–1946) soon established guidance services in the Seattle school system, and by 1910, 35 cities had plans for the establishment of vocational guidance in their schools (Aubrey, 1977). Although revolutionary in their thinking, many of these early vocational guidance reformers were motivated by moralistic thinking and theories of the time like social Darwinism, which suggested that individuals should fervently follow their supervisors and "fight their co-workers for advanced status" (survival of the fittest) (Rockwell & Rothney, 1961, p. 352).

The individual who undoubtedly had the greatest effect on vocational guidance in America was Frank Parsons (1854–1908) (McDaniels & Watts, 1994). Today seen as the founder of guidance in America, Parsons was greatly influenced by the reform movements of the time, such as the work of Jane Addams at Hull House. Eventually establishing the

Vocational Bureau, which assisted individuals in "choosing an occupation, preparing themselves for it, finding an opening in it, and building a career of efficiency and success" (Parsons cited in Jones, 1994, p. 288), Parsons hoped that vocational guidance would eventually be established in the public schools—a hope he would not see come to fruition due to his untimely death in 1908. In 1909 his book *Choosing a Vocation* was published posthumously. Soon after his death, perhaps as a tribute to the energy he gave to the vocational guidance movement, Boston became the site for the first vocational guidance conference. This conference resulted in the founding of the National Vocational Guidance Association (NVGA) in 1913, which is generally considered to be the distant predecessor of American Counseling Association (ACA).

Frank Parsons was a man with a vision. He envisioned systematic vocational guidance in the schools; he envisioned a national vocational guidance movement; he foresaw the importance of individual counseling; and he hoped for a society in which cooperation was more important than competition and where concern replaced avarice (Jones, 1994). It is clear that Parsons's principles of vocational guidance greatly affected the broader field of counseling.

Parsons's main thrust toward vocational guidance is usually presented as a three-part process:

> *(1) a clear understanding of yourself, your aptitudes, interests, ambitions, resources, limitations, and their causes; (2) a knowledge of the requirements and conditions of success, advantages and disadvantages, compensation, opportunities, and prospects in different lines of work; [and] (3) true reasoning on the relations of these two groups of facts.* (Parsons, 1989, p. 5)

However, a deeper examination of Parsons's work shows us that many of his principles eventually became some of the major tenets of the counseling profession (Jones, 1994). For instance, Parsons noted the importance of having an expert guide, while suggesting that a good guide cannot make a decision for a person who, ultimately, has to decide what's best for him- or herself. He also suggested that the counselor should be frank (genuine) and kind with the client and that it was crucial for the counselor to assist the client in the development of analytic skills. It is clear that Frank Parsons deserves the title Founder of Vocational Guidance, and in many ways he can be seen as founder of the counseling field.

With the beginnings of a theoretical orientation and the establishment of a national association, the vocational guidance movement was established. Although the spread of the movement did not occur as quickly as some might have liked (Aubrey, 1977), a number of acts were eventually passed to strengthen vocational education (Herr, 1985a). One such act, the Depression-era Wagner O'Day Act (1932), established the U.S. Employment Services and provided ongoing vocational guidance and placement to all unemployed Americans. Vocational counseling as part of the landscape of America was here to stay, and it would soon have an impact on all facets of counseling.

Although vocational guidance in the schools soon took hold, it was not long before individuals advocated for a broader approach that attended to a large variety of students' psychological and educational needs. For instance, John Brewer (1932) suggested that guidance should be seen in a total educational context and that guidance counselors should be involved in a variety of functions in the schools, including adjustment counseling, assistance with curriculum planning, classroom management, and of course, occupational guidance. One tool used by the counselor was the test (Aubrey, 1982).

The Expansion of the Testing Movement

> *It is doubtful that vocational guidance would have survived without a psychological support base in psychometrics.* (Aubrey, 1977, p. 290)

With the advent of the vocational guidance movement, testing was to become commonplace. Parsons, for instance, strongly advocated the use of tests in vocational guidance (Williamson, 1964). As a result of World War I, assessment of ability was applied on a large-scale basis, because tests such as the Army Alpha were used to determine placement of recruits (see Box 2.2). These ability tests would soon be adapted to use in vocational guidance.

The use of tests to assist in vocational counseling was promoted by the development of one of the first major interest inventories, the Strong Vocational Interest Blank, in 1927 (Campbell, 1968). This test, which in its revised form is still one of the most widely used instruments of its kind, was to revolutionize vocational counseling.

But tests were not just used with vocational assessment. For instance, Woodworth's Personal Data Sheet was an early personality instrument used by the military to screen out emotionally disturbed individuals. The successful large-scale military use of tests led to the development and adoption of similar instruments in the schools, business, and industry (Drummond, 2000). By the middle of the 20th century, tests to measure cognitive ability, interests, intelligence, and personality were commonplace. Although often used in vocational counseling, many of these tests soon found their way into all kinds of counseling practices.

The Spread of Psychotherapy and Its Impact on the Counseling Profession

> *Most sane people think that no insane person can reason logically. But this is not so. Upon reasonable premises I made most reasonable deductions, and that at the time when my mind was in its most disturbed condition.* (Beers, 1948, p. 57)

In 1908 Clifford Beers (1876–1943), a Yale graduate who had been hospitalized for years due to schizophrenia, wrote *A Mind That Found Itself*. In 1909 he helped to establish the National Committee for Mental Hygiene, which lobbied Congress to pass laws that would eliminate the deplorable conditions of mental institutions. Soon, this committee began to organize the first child guidance clinics, staffed by social workers, psychologists, and psychiatrists. At the same time psychoanalysis was beginning to come out of the elite office of the psychiatrist and work its way into the community. The end of World War I saw a number of psychologists offering their services to returning doughboys who had psychological problems associated with the war (today such problems are often diagnosed as posttraumatic stress syndrome). Since the long-term treatment approaches of the psychoanalysts were of little use to these clinicians, they soon began to develop new, shorter-term approaches.

As treatment approaches to the individual changed, and as mental health clinics spread, the need for psychological assistants, often with a bachelor's or master's degree, became evident. The master's level assistants often had degrees in social work, but increasingly there were individuals with a relatively new degree—a master's degree in counseling, which started as a degree in vocational guidance. It was a natural transition for individuals with this degree to move into the mental health field, because they were trained in both counseling techniques and in assessment.

BOX 2.2

The Army Alpha Test

The Army Alpha was used to determine placement in the armed forces during WWI. Below is an adaptation of the test, as printed in *Discover* magazine. Take the test and discuss your thoughts about it.

> *The average mental age of the recruits who took the Army Alpha test during WWI was approximately 13. Could you do better? You have three minutes to complete these sample questions, drawn verbatim from the original exam.* (McKean, 1985)

The following sentences have been disarranged but can be unscrambled to make sense. Rearrange them and then answer whether each is true or false.

1. Bible earth the says inherit the the shall meek. true false
2. a battle in racket very tennis useful is true false

Answer the following questions:

3. If a train goes 200 yards in a sixth of a minute, how many feet does it go in a fifth of a second?
4. A U-boat makes 8 miles an hour under water and 15 miles on the surface. How long will it take to cross a 100-mile channel if it has to go two-fifths of the way under water?
5. The spark plug in a gas engine is found in the:
   crank case manifold cylinder carburetor
6. The Brooklyn Nationals are called the:
   Giants Orioles Superbas Indians
7. The product advertised as 99.44 per cent pure is:
   Arm & Hammer Baking Soda Crisco Ivory Soap Toledo
8. The Pierce-Arrow is made in: Flint Buffalo Detroit Toledo
9. The number of Zulu legs is: two four six eight

Are the following words the same or opposite in meaning?

10. vesper–matin same opposite
11. aphorism–maxim same opposite

Find the next number in the series:

12. 74, 71, 65, 56, 44, Answer:
13. 3, 6, 8, 16, 18, Answer:
14. Select the image that belongs in the mirror:

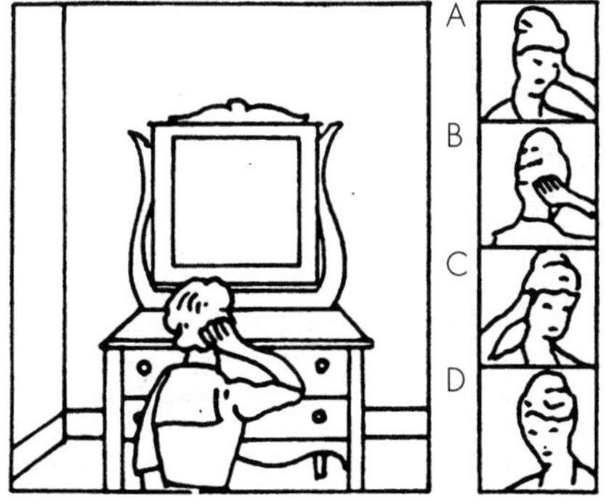

15. & 16. What's missing in these pictures?

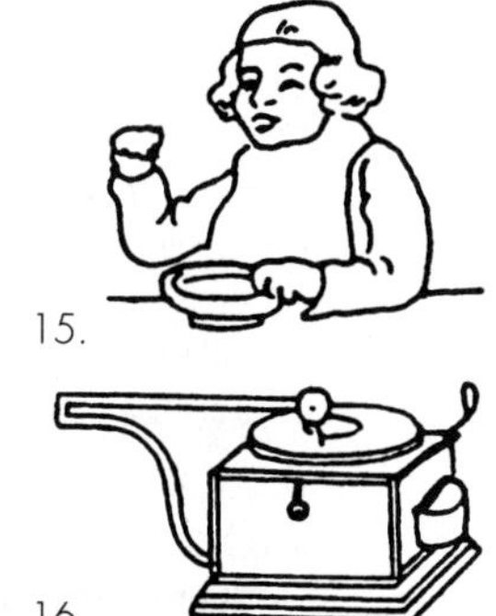

Answers: 1. true, 2. false, 3. twelve feet, 4. nine hours, 5. cylinder, 6. superbas, 7. Ivory Soap, 8. Buffalo, 9. two, 10. opposite, 11. same, 12. 29, 13. 36, 14. A, 15. spoon, 16. gramophone horn

Scoring: All item except 3, 4, 10, and 11 = 1.25 points. Items 3 and 4 = 1.875 points, Items 10 & 11 = .625 points. Add them all up, they equal your mental age. What is wrong with this test? Examine it for problems with content, history, cross-cultural contamination, and so forth.

The emergence of the counseling field as something other than pure vocational guidance had its biggest push when, during the 1930s, E. G. Williamson (1900–1979) developed what is considered to be the first comprehensive theory of counseling (as distinguished from Freud's theory of psychoanalysis). Known as the Minnesota Point of View (for the University of Minnesota), or trait and factor theory, Williamson's approach initially grew out of the ideas of Frank Parsons. Although originally vocationally oriented, the approach was modified and soon was seen as a generic approach to counseling and psychotherapy. The trait and factor approach involved a series of five steps, which included (1) analysis, examining the problem and obtaining available records and testing on the client; (2) synthesis, summarizing and organizing the information to understand the problem; (3) diagnosis, interpreting the problem; (4) counseling, aiding the individual in finding solutions; and (5) follow-up, assuring proper follow-up (Patterson, 1973).

As a result of Nazism, during the 1930s and 1940s many humanistic philosophers, psychiatrists, and psychologists fled Europe for the United States and dramatically influenced the field of psychotherapy and education here. Carl Rogers (1902–1987), who initially worked at the Rochester Guidance Center, was greatly affected by these humanists and would soon revolutionize the practice of counseling. His humanistic, client-centered, nondirective approach to working with individuals was viewed as shorter-term, more humane, more honest, and more viable for most clients. The early 1940s saw the publication of Carl Rogers's book *Counseling and Psychotherapy*, which was to have a major impact on the counseling profession (Rogers, 1942). Rogers and others in the newly established field of humanistic counseling and education were a major impetus for the counseling field moving from a vocational guidance orientation to one with a much broader base. Rogers's approach was ripe for the times, as it reflected the increased focus on personal freedom and autonomy of the post-WWII years (Aubrey, 1977). Although Rogers and other 1940s humanists had a great impact on the field of counseling, their influence was minor compared to what was about to occur during the second half of the century.

Modern-Day Counseling: Its Recent Past (1950–2000)

The 1950s: Emergence, Expansion, and Diversification

> *If one decade in history had to be singled out for the most profound impact on counselors, it would be the 1950s.* (Aubrey, 1977, p. 292)

During the 1950s the counseling profession had an increasingly greater shift toward a humanistic, nondirective orientation. This decade saw Carl Rogers become an even greater influence on the field as he published his second book, entitled *Client-Centered Therapy: Its Current Practice, Implications and Theory* (Rogers, 1951). In addition, affected by the push to depathologize individuals, this decade saw the promulgation of developmental theories in the areas of career counseling (e.g., Ginzberg, Ginsburg, Axelrad, & Herma, 1951; Super, 1953), child development (e.g., Piaget, 1954), and lifespan development (e.g., Erikson, 1950). These theories stressed the notion that individuals would face predictable tasks as they passed through the inevitable developmental stages of life and that knowledge of these developmental tasks could greatly aid counselors in their work with clients.

Perhaps the most important event that would affect counseling during this time was the 1957 launching of Sputnik. The launching of this Russian satellite sent a chill through many Americans and was the impetus for Congress passing the National Defense Education Act (NDEA) in 1958. The NDEA allocated funds for training institutes that would quickly graduate secondary school counselors. These counselors, it was hoped, would identify students gifted in math and science who could be future scientists. The obvious result of this legislation was the significant increase in secondary school counselors in the late 1950s and 1960s. The bill was extended to elementary school counselors in 1964.

Besides the dramatic increase in school counselors, the 1950s also saw the first full-time college counselors and the beginning of college counseling centers. A natural extension of secondary school counseling, college counseling centers often started as vocational administration counseling centers initiated after World War II (Nugent, 2000). As with other aspects of the counseling profession, college counseling centers quickly took on the humanistic and developmental approach to working with students and were generally staffed by counselors and psychologists. Other student services that employed counselors also saw a great expansion.

Community agencies also saw an influx of counselors and psychologists during the 1950s. The discovery of antipsychotic, antidepressant, and antianxiety medications and the controversial yet widespread use of electroconvulsive therapy enabled the release of large numbers of people from state hospitals who then found needed services at local community agencies (Kornetsky, 1976; Mehr, 2001). In addition, this decade saw counselors increasingly staffing vocational rehabilitation centers, working with both the physical and psychological needs of individuals, especially the many who had been seriously injured during World War II.

The changes in the field during the 1950s were reflected in changes in the professional associations. On the heels of the founding of the American Association of Marriage and Family Counseling in 1945 (AAMFC, later to be called AAMFT), the 1950s saw the formation of NASW, the changing of the name of Division 17 of the APA from the Counseling and Guidance Division to the Division of Counseling Psychology, and the formation of the American Personnel and Guidance Association (APGA) from a merger of four counseling related associations (see Chapter 1). Whereas Division 17 required a doctorate for full membership, APGA distinguished itself with its master's level requirement. APA was clearly moving full force into the clinical area, whereas APGA was keeping counseling at a second tier with an emphasis on guidance activities. This decade quickly saw the development of a number of APGA divisions that reflected the growing diversity of counselors in the field. Thus we saw the founding of divisions for school counselors (American School Counselor Association, ASCA), counselor educators (Association for Counselor Education and Supervision, ACES), career counselors (National Career Development Association, NCDA), rehabilitation counselors (American Rehabilitation Counseling Association, ARCA), and humanistic educators and counselors (Counseling Association for Humanistic Education and Development, C-AHEAD).

The 1960s: Increased Diversification

During the first half of the 20th century three main approaches to counseling and therapy existed: psychodynamic approaches (e.g., Freud), directive theories (e.g., Williamson), and client-centered theories (e.g., Rogers) (Gladding, 2000). However, during the late 1950s and continuing into the 1960s a number of new, at the time revolutionary, approaches to counseling began to take shape including the rational emotive (cognitive) approach of Albert Ellis (Ellis & Harper, 1961); the behavioral approaches of Bandura (1969), Wolpe (1958), and Krumboltz (1966a, b); the relational/behavioral approach of William Glasser's reality therapy (1961, 1965); the highly affective Gestalt approach of Fritz Perls (1969); the communication approach of transactional analysis (Berne, 1964); and the existential approaches of Arbuckle (1965), Frankl (1963), May (1950), and others. These counseling approaches were no doubt created at least partially because of the great demand for therapists during this time period

The need for counselors and other mental health professionals expanded as the direct result of the passage of many legislative actions related to President Johnson's "Great Society" initiatives (Kaplan & Cuciti, 1986). One such legislative action was the Community Mental Health Centers Act of 1963, which funded the establishment of nationwide mental health centers to provide short-term inpatient care, outpatient care, partial hospitalization, emergency services, and consultation and education services. This made it possible for individuals with adjustment problems as well as those with severe emotional disorders to obtain free or low-cost mental health services. Approximately 600 community-based mental health centers could trace their origins to this act (Burger & Youkeles, 2000).

Many other acts were also passed during this decade. For instance, amendments to the 1964 NDEA expanded the training of counselors to include counselors from elementary school through junior college. In fact, by 1967 nearly 20,000 school counselors were trained as a result of this act (Tolbert, 1982). In addition, a number of acts such as the Manpower Development and Training Act, Job Corps, Elementary and Secondary Education Act, Head Start, and the Work Incentive Program provided various job opportunities for counselors. Other key legislative initiatives such as the Civil Rights Act, Economic Opportunity Act, and Voting Rights Act helped to reshape attitudes in the country toward social ideals and community service with one result being a more accepting attitude toward the counseling profession. Clearly, the 1960s was the decade of expansion, acceptance, and diversification of the counseling profession largely as the result of legislative actions.

With this expansion and diversification came an increased urgency for professionalism in the field. One outgrowth of this was the emergence of ethical standards of practice. We therefore saw the development of APGA's first guidelines for ethical behavior in 1961. The 1960s also saw a flurry of activity around the need for accreditation standards of counseling programs (Lloyd, 1992; Sweeney, 1992). A series of meetings throughout the country were the precursors to the development, in 1981, of the Council for Accreditation of Counseling and Related Programs (CACREP). Finally, the 1960s saw the continued expansion of APGA with increased membership, the formation of what are now the Association for Assessment in Counseling (AAC, 1965), the National Employment Counseling Association (NECA, 1966), and the recommendation in 1964 by APGA to have state branches (ACA, 1995b).

The 1970s: Continued Proliferation of the Counseling Field

During the 1970s a number of events occurred that increased the need for counselors in a variety of settings. For instance, the 1975 Supreme Court decision in Donaldson *v.* O'Connor led to the deinstitutionalization of tens of thousands of state mental hospital patients who had been hospitalized against their will (see Box 2.3). This case concluded

BOX 2.3

Donaldson *v.* O'Connor

Kenneth Donaldson, who had been committed to a state mental hospital in Florida and confined against his will for 15 years, sued the hospital superintendent, Dr. J. B. O'Connor, and his staff for intentionally and maliciously depriving him of his constitutional right to liberty. Donaldson, who had been hospitalized against his will for "paranoid schizophrenia," said he was not mentally ill, and even if he was, stated that the hospital had not provided him adequate treatment.

Over the 15 years of confinement, Donaldson, who was not in danger of harming himself or others, had frequently asked for his release, and had relatives who stated they would attend to him if he was released. Despite this, the hospital refused to release him, stating that he was still mentally ill. The Supreme Court unanimously upheld lower court decisions stating that the hospital could not hold him against his will if he was not in danger of harming himself or others (Swenson, 1997). This decision, along with the increased use and discovery of new psychotropic medications, led to the large-scale release of hundreds of thousands of individuals across the country who had been confined to mental hospitals against their will and who were not a danger to themselves or others.

that individuals who were not in danger of harming themselves or others could not be held against their will. With the release of individuals from the hospitals came an increased need for community mental health counselors.

Thus, in 1975 Congress passed an expansion of the original Community Mental Health Centers Act and expanded from five to twelve the number and type of mandated services that mental health centers needed to provide. They included:

- Short-term inpatient services.
- Outpatient services.
- Partial hospitalization (day treatment).
- Emergency services.
- Consultation and education.
- Special services for children
- Special services for the elderly.
- Preinstitutional court screening.
- Follow-up care for mental hospitals.
- Transitional care from mental hospitals.
- Alcoholism services.
- Drug abuse services.

The 1970s also saw the passage of legislation for individuals with disabilities. These laws resulted in the need to hire highly trained rehabilitation counselors and expanded the role of school counselors. For instance, the Rehabilitation Act of 1973 assured vocational rehabilitation services and counseling for employable adults who had severe physical or mental disabilities that interfered with their ability to obtain and/or maintain a job. The Education for All Handicapped Children Act of 1975 (PL94-142) assured the right to an education within the least restrictive environment for all children identified as having a disability that interferes with learning. PL94-142 resulted in school counselors increasingly becoming an integral part of the team that would determine the disposition of students with disabilities.

This decade also saw a major shift in the training of counseling students. The influence of the humanistic movement had fully taken hold by the 1970s, and a number of individuals began to develop what became known as "microcounseling skills training" (Carkhuff, 1969; Egan, 1975; Ivey & Gluckstein, 1974). The teaching of these microcounseling skills was based on many of the skills deemed critical by Carl Rogers and other humanistic psychologists. These packaged ways of training counselors showed that basic counseling skills such as attending behaviors, listening, and empathic understanding could be learned in a relatively short amount of time and that the practice of such skills would have a positive impact on the counseling relationship (Neukrug, 1980).

The 1970s was also the decade of increased professionalization in the field. For instance, the early 1970s saw the Association of Counselor Educators and Supervisors (ACES) provide drafts of standards for master's level counseling programs. National credentialing became a reality when certification was offered for the first time by the Council for Rehabilitation Education (CORE) in 1973 and by the National Academy for Certified Mental Health Counselors (NACMHC) in 1979 (Sweeney, 1991). Finally, state licensure had its beginnings when, in 1976, Virginia became the first state to offer licensing for counselors.

The legislative actions of the 1970s brought with them an increased diversification of the counseling field, resulting in large numbers of counselors settling into the mental health, rehabilitation, higher education, and school counseling specialty areas. One result of this diversification was the burgeoning membership in APGA, which reached 40,000, and the founding of a number of divisions of ACA (then called APGA) including the Association for Multicultural Counseling and Development (AMCD, 1972), the Association for Spiritual, Ethical, and Religious Values in Counseling (ASERVIC, 1974), the Association for Specialists in Group Work (ASGW, 1973), the International Association of Addictions and Offender Counselors (IAAOC, 1972), and the American Mental Health Counselors Association (AMHCA,1978) (ACA, 1995b; Goodyear, 1984).

The 1980s–2000: Recent Changes in the Field

The 1980s and 1990s saw a continued expansion and diversification of the field of counseling as well as a settling-in phase of our profession. Counselors could now be found in almost any mental health setting, while expanded services were offered in colleges and schools. We also saw counselors expand into areas where minimal mental health services had been provided in the past, including substance abuse agencies, agencies that work with older persons, and business and industry. With the profession clearly having come of age, it became increasingly evident that there was an urgent need for the standardization of training and the credentialing of counselors. Therefore, in 1981 the Council for Accreditation of Counseling and Related Educational Programs (CACREP) was formed to further delineate standards for the profession. Today, CACREP accredits master's programs in community counseling, school counseling, college counseling, mental health counseling, career counseling, gerontological counseling, student affairs, and marriage, couple, and family counseling/therapy (see Chapter 3 for a detailed discussion of CACREP).

The 1980s and 1990s saw a phenomenal increase in the types of credentials being offered and the numbers of individuals becoming certified or licensed. In 1981 APGA established the National Board for Certified Counselors (NBCC), which offers a national standardized test for counselors. Today, NBCC has certified over 31,000 individuals as

National Certified Counselors (NCCs) and offers subspecialty certifications in clinical mental health counseling, school counseling, addictions counseling, and as an approved clinical supervisor (ACS) (NBCC, 2001). In addition, the International Association of Marriage and Family Counselors (IAMFC), a division of ACA, now offers certification for family therapists through the National Academy for Certified Family Therapists (NACFT). Finally, today, 46 states and the District of Columbia have passed state licensing laws for counselors, and today states have credentialed over 140,000 credentialed counselors (Neukrug, Milliken, & Walden, 2001) (see Chapter 3 for a detailed discussion of credentialing).

Probably one of the greatest changes in the field of counseling during the 1980s and 1990s was the increased focus on multicultural counseling (Claiborn, 1991a). This was partly due to CACREP's requirement that multicultural counseling should be infused into the curricula of all accredited graduate programs as well as the ever-increasing volumes of work being published in the field of multicultural counseling. The knowledge and skills needed to work with diverse populations became readily attainable for all students in the field of counseling.

The 1990s also saw an increased emphasis on the importance of ethical and professional issues in counseling. Whereas prior to 1980 few counseling texts discussed ethical issues, today almost all do. In addition, ethical concerns have increasingly been addressed from a variety of perspectives including supervision, teaching, and counseling (Gibson & Pope, 1993). Also, in 1995 ACA revised its Code of Ethics and added Standards of Practice, which represent the "minimal behavioral statements of the Code of Ethics" (ACA, 1995a, p. 20). Finally, as with multicultural counseling, the increased emphasis that CACREP placed on such codes became another force pushing ethical and professional issues to the forefront.

There is little doubt that the changes that took place during the 1980s and 1990s were reflected in changes in the professional association. In 1983 APGA changed its name to the American Association for Counseling and Development (AACD), and in 1992 the association again underwent another name change to the more streamlined American Counseling Association (ACA). The 1980s and 1990s saw the founding of a number of new divisions and a new affiliate of ACA, including the Association for Counselors and Educators in Government (ACEG, 1994), the Association for Adult Development and Aging (AADA, 1986), the International Association of Marriage and Family Counselors (IAMFC, 1989), the American College Counseling Association (ACCA, 1991), the Association for Gay, Lesbian and Bisexual Issues in Counseling (AGLBIC, 1997), and the affiliate organization, Counselors for Social Justice (CSJ). Membership in ACA soared and by 2000 was over 55,000 members, with AMHCA and ASCA representing the two largest divisions. At that point, ACA had 17 divisions and 1 affiliate, representing the differing specialty areas in counseling, with close to 500 counselor training programs in the country (Hollis & Dodson, 2000).

2000 and On: The New Millennium

As we moved into the 21st century, some issues from the 1980s and 1990s continued to be important. In 1992 the American College Personnel Association (ACPA), one of ACA's founding divisions, disaffiliated from the association. Also, in the latter part of the 1990s the boards of the two largest ACA divisions, AMHCA and ASCA, both threatened disaffiliation from ACA. Although ASCA and AMHCA have not disaffiliated, both organizations have become increasingly independent. It now seems clear that after nearly a century of pulling together to create a unified force within one association, some divisions are now asserting that their numbers are large enough and their differences too great to continue to justify this unification. The new century may bring some interesting changes to the nature of the counseling profession.

Other issues from the last century will also continue to be important. For instance, there is little doubt that an increasing number of counselor education programs will become CACREP accredited. Similarly, we will no doubt see increased numbers of individuals becoming nationally certified and licensed. Also, as litigation of malpractice spreads, ethical and professional issues will continue to be highlighted (Neukrug, Milliken, & Walden, 2001; Swenson, 1997). In addition, it is clear that as we move deeper into the new century the increased national attention to multiculturalism will be paralleled by a continued and even greater focus on multicultural issues within the counseling profession. Even as you read this text, there is a renewed effort to assure that the ethical guidelines adequately address multicultural issues; and cross-cultural issues in the training of counselors are increasingly being highlighted. There is little doubt that the way we train counselors, our understanding of the counseling process, and even the way we understand the world will be affected by trends in multiculturalism in the new millennium.

The new millennium has brought with it a renewed emphasis on understanding counselor training. Whereas in the past counselor training seems to have been from a "cookbook" orientation, in recent years some researchers have advocated the importance of understanding the developmental needs of trainees (McAuliffe & Eriksen, 2000). Whereas some counselors-in-training enter a graduate program already embodying many characteristics needed for working effectively with clients (e.g., being empathic, accepting, and caring and having good mental health), others may not show those characteristics. A developmental perspective on counselor education assumes that the positive qualities associated with working effectively with clients are a function of age, experience, and exposure of the trainee, and that different teaching methods should be applied to individuals at different developmental levels. If research in this area continues to be borne out, it may dramatically affect the training of counselors in the future (McAuliffe et al., 1998; McAuliffe et al., 2000; Neukrug & McAuliffe, 1993).

Do We Have to Memorize All Those Names? A Devleopmental Perspective

There's a lot of information in this chapter, and a student of mine recently came into my office and complained about having to memorize the names of "picayune" individuals from the counseling profession's past. "What does this have to do with me being an effective counselor?" he argued. Admittedly somewhat put on the defensive, I tried to explain the importance of knowledge building on knowledge, and that these individuals have given us a base of understanding that has affected the profession today. I believe that this explanation makes a justifiable argument concerning the need to learn such names. However, one thing I did not discuss with him was the concept of "roots." Most of us would agree that our past is important in our development. Our experiences, whether negative or positive, relate strongly to the essence of who we are today. And so it is in the life of a profession. We are what we are because of our past. Be it positive or negative, we have become what we are because of our history, and perhaps as importantly, we will become what we will become as a function of our past. We are a profession in process—a living entity that unravels through time. Yes, we could decide to forget our past, not look at our roots, and attempt to move forward. However, I believe that unconsciously our roots will still be directing us. Why not have consciousness, understand from whence we came, and attempt to make smart, conscious choices about the future? Let's not repress what our past has been; let's be open to understanding it and to forging a new and better future for ourselves and our profession. Such understanding takes courage and work. It is not easy taking a hard look at one's self, and it is damned difficult memorizing all those names (see Table 2.1).

Multicultural Issues: Learning from the Past, Moving toward the Future

Although the counseling profession's history includes adaptability to changing circumstances, some have criticized how slowly it has moved toward making substantive changes in how counselors work with clients who are culturally diverse (Hartung, 1996). Some reasons for this may include (1) the profession's not taking diversity issues seriously, (2) the reluctance of counselors to look at their underlying belief systems related to cross-cultural issues, (3) the reluctance of researchers to take a critical look at multicultural issues because of denial of the critical nature of this issue, and (4) fears of being viewed as being politically incorrect if specific research was not seen as supportive of current multicultural trends (Weinrach & Thomas, 1996).

Today, much attention is placed on sensitizing counselors toward multicultural issues. There is now a professional organizational specifically oriented toward diversity issues (AMCD). There are workshops on diversity at most regional and national conferences. Counseling programs are increasingly infusing multicultural issues into their programs, and the literature increasingly speaks to issues of diversity. However, if we are to make the critical changes necessary to be a profession that truly embraces diversity, we must all be willing to examine our own biases, develop new approaches to working with all clients, increasingly stress multiculturalism in counselor education programs and at conferences, and expand and be willing to take a critical view of the research on multicultural counseling. Our history tells us that we have moved slowly on the crucial issue of multicultural counseling; but perhaps more critical is whether we will learn from this history.

Ethical, Professional, and Legal Issues: Changing over Time

With the development of the ACA Ethical Guidelines in 1961, the counseling profession made a commitment to the conscientious and principled use of counseling approaches. As with all forward-thinking professional associations, since 1961 the guidelines have been revised. Changes in ethical guidelines often reflect changes in the society. For instance, as a result of AIDS and other new communicable diseases, a section has been added to the most recent Ethical Standards that addresses how counselors should handle their responsibility to client confidentiality if they learn that a client is endangering another person

TABLE 2.1

Summary of Important Historical Events Related to the Field of Counseling

3000 B.C.E. Ancient Egypt	"Psychological" writings found on papyrus.
400 B.C.E Hippocrates	First "modern-day" reflections on the human condition.
350 B.C.E. Plato	Believed introspection and reflection to be the road to knowledge.
350 B.C.E. Aristotle	Considered by many to be "first psychologist"—studied objectivity and reason.
250 Plotinus	Believed in dualism—the concept that the soul is separate from the body.
400 Augustine	Examined the meaning of consciousness and self-examination.
1250 Thomas Aquinas	Examined the meaning of consciousness and self-examination.
1468 Sanchez de Arevalo	Wrote first job classification system in *Mirror of Men's Lives*.
1500s Elizabethan Poor Laws	Established legislation for the Church to help the destitute in England.
1650 Descartes	Believed that knowledge and truth come through deductive reasoning.
1700 John Locke	Believed the mind is a blank slate and that experience generates ideas.
1800 James Mill	Believed the mind is a blank slate and that experience generates ideas.
1800 Philippe Pinel	Founder of the field of psychiatry. Viewed insanity from a scientific perspective.
1800 Benjamin Rush	Founder of American psychiatry. Advocated for human treatment of mentally ill.
1800 Anton Mesmer	Discovered first uses of hypnosis.
1800s Charity Organization Societies	Volunteers who would offer assistance to the poor and destitute.
1850 Jean Martin Charcot	Examined the use of hypnosis in the understanding of physical disorders.
1850 Dorothea Dix	Advocated "moral treatment" for the mentally ill. Helped establish 41 "modern" mental hospitals.
1875 Wilhelm Wundt	First "experimental psychologist."
1875 Sir Francis Galton	Early experimental psychologist.
1890s Sigmund Freud	Developed theory of psychoanalysis.
1890s G. Stanley Hall	Founded the APA, early American experimental psychologist.
1890s James Cattell	Early American experimental psychologist.
1890s to mid-1900s John Dewey	Educational reformer who advocated for humanistic teaching methods.
1896 Alfred Binet	Developed first individual intelligence test for the French Ministry of Public Education.
1899 Jane Addams	Established Hull House in Chicago.
1900 Emil Kraepelin	Developed one of the first classifications of mental diseases.
1900 Pierre Janet	Saw a relationship between certain psychological states and organic disorders.
1900 Ivan Pavlov	Developed one of the first behavioral models of learning.
1900 William James	Advocated the philosophy of "Philosophical Pragmatism" and subjective reality as it relates to science.
1906 Eli Weaver	Developed vocational guidance in New York City schools.
1907 Jesse Davis	Developed one of the first guidance curriculums in Grand Rapids, Michigan, schools.
1908 Anna Reed	Established vocational guidance in Seattle school system.
1908 Frank Parsons	Founder of vocational guidance movement. Developed first comprehensive approach to vocational guidance.

(continued)

TABLE 2.1 *(continued)*

Summary of Important Historical Events Related to the Field of Counseling

1908 Clifford Beers	Former Yale student institutionalized for schizophrenia wrote *A Mind That Found Itself* and advocated for humane treatment of the mentally ill.
1913 NVGA	National Vocational Guidance Association formed. Distant forerunner of ACA.
1917 Army Alpha Test	First large-scale use of test of ability developed.
1917 Woodworth Personal Data Sheet	One of first structured personality tests developed.
1927 Strong Interest Inventory	One of first interest inventories to assist in the career counseling process.
1930 E. G. Williamson	Developed comprehensive theories of counseling initially used for vocational guidance. Called "Minnesota Point of View, or "trait and factor approach."
1932 John Brewer	Suggested guidance be seen in total educational context.
1932 Wagner O'Day Act	Established U. S. Employment Service.
1921 American Psychiatric Association	American Psychiatric Association took current name. Originally founded in 1844.
1940s Carl Rogers	Developed nondirective approach to counseling. Advocate of humanistic counseling and education.
1940s Division 17 of APA	Formally becomes part of APA.
1945 AAMFT	AAMFT is officially formed.
1950s Virginia Satir	One of first social workers to stress contextual or systems thinking.
1952 APGA	American Personnel and Guidance Association formed out of four associations. Forerunner of ACA.
1955 NASW	National Association of Social Workers founded from merger of seven associations.
1958 NDEA	National Defense Education Act allocated funds for training institutes for secondary school counselors. Later expanded to lower levels.
1961 Ethical Codes	APGA develops guidelines for ethical behavior.
1963 Community Mental Health Centers Act	Federal law funded establishment of community mental health centers nationally.
1965 Great Society Initiatives	Numerous laws passed under President Johnson's administration greatly affected the development of social service agencies nationally.
1973 Rehabilitation Act	Ensured access to vocational rehabilitation services for adults. Increased need for trained rehabilitation counselors.
1973 CORE	Council for Rehabilitation Education offers first credentialing for counselors.
1975 PL94-142	Education of All Handicapped Children Act. Right to education within least restrictive environments. Extends need for school counselors.
1975 Donaldson *v.* O'Connor	Supreme Court decision that led to deinstitutionalization of mental hospital patients.
1979 NACMHC	National Academy for Certified Mental Health Counselors offers national certification.
1981 CACREP	Councils for Accreditation of Counseling and Related Programs was founded. Established accreditation standards for counseling programs.
1981 NBCC	National Board for Certified Counselors offers generic certification for counselors and eventually offers subspecialty certification in career, gerontological, addictions, and clinical mental health counseling.
1983 AACD	APGA becomes the American Association for Counseling and Development (AACD).
1992 ACA	AACD becomes the American Counseling Association.

through unsafe sexual practices (see ACA Ethical Standard B.1.d. in Appendix B). And today, ACA is calling all of its members to review the ethics code to consider whether or not it is cross-culturally biased (ACA, 2001b)

As the values of our profession evolve and society changes, our ethical standards will continue to be revised to reflect new viewpoints. Prior ethical standards and laws tell us something about where we have been as a profession and as a country. Current standards and laws reflect the current thinking and values of our profession and country, and challenges to guidelines reflect the current struggles we have and point us in the direction of the future. Counselors need to be knowledgeable of the past, aware of the present, and speculative about the future if they are to feel thoroughly involved with the profession.

The Counselor in Process: Looking Back, Looking Ahead, and Paradigm Shifts

Upon looking back in our history, we can see the paradigm shift that took place near the turn of the last century that led to the creation of our field. By looking at the midpart of the 20th century we can see the next paradigm shift, which led to the expansion of the profession as well as the shift toward a humanistic emphasis. But perhaps most significantly, by examining our history we are able to look forward. History is our grounding for the future, for only if we know from whence we came can we know where we are going. Look from whence we came, look at the current trends in the field, and you decide: Are we on the verge of another paradigm shift? If yes, are we prepared for what might take place?

Summary

This chapter examined the history of counseling from its early beginnings to current-day practices. We learned that the human condition has been pondered for thousands of years and that the historical roots of the counseling profession can be traced back to early philosophers. We discovered that the helping professions of social work, psychology, and psychiatry had different beginnings from those of counseling, and that all these professions have, over the years, moved toward many of the same goals and objectives.

More specifically, in this chapter we examined the historical roots of the field of social work and saw how social work's emphasis on systems and advocacy has influenced the counseling profession. We also saw how social work's emphasis on "in-the-field" experiences has had a great impact on counselor education training and its recent trends toward increasing practicum and internship hours. We saw that many of the philosophical roots of modern-day counseling theories arose from the early beginnings of psychology. We examined how laboratory science and research techniques have become important tools for counselors as they research the efficacy of programs they develop and of specific counseling techniques they use. We also examined how tests used by many counselors today had their origins in the early days of testing as originated by psychologists. Finally, we saw how the field of psychiatry has offered us ways of understanding and classifying mental health problems, and how crucial it is for counselors to have an understanding of the possible organic nature of some mental health problems.

Besides being influenced by other professions, we examined the unique history of the counseling profession. With its early focus in vocational counseling, we saw how, over the years, the counseling profession has moved from the somewhat moralistic, directive approach of vocational guidance to the humanistic approach it adopted starting in the 1940s. We examined how the profession expanded and diversified in the latter part of the 20th century and how a number of legislative actions during this part of the century greatly influenced the direction and expansion of the profession. We explored how the development of ACA paralleled the expansion and diversification of the profession during the 20th century. We also saw how professionalization of the counseling field increased over the years with such things as the creation of ethical standards, an increase in the types and numbers of individuals becoming credentialed, and the establishment of accreditation standards for counseling programs.

As we moved into the next millennium, we highlighted a number of issues that will continue to be important to the counseling profession. These included an increased number of CACREP accredited institutions, more credentialed counselors, an increased focus on ethical and professional issues, and more scrutiny to multicultural issues. We highlighted the fact that how we address ethical issues and multicultural issues is a reflection of what is occurring in society and the values inherent in our professional association. Finally, we noted that the counseling profession is at a precipice and that we might see increased independence of the divisions of ACA.

This chapter ended with a brief discussion of the importance of understanding our past as it pertains to our future directions. We noted that we can close our eyes, forget the past, and move in unknown ways toward the future, or have knowledge of our past and make conscious, hopefully wise decisions as we move further into the 21st century. Why not keep our eyes open?

INFOTRAC and Other Information Resources (e.g., ERIC and PsycINFO)

Note: When relevant, key words are in quotation marks.

1. Take one or more historical event(s) from this chapter that is particularly interesting to you and research it in more detail.
2. Examine how ethical guidelines have changed as a function of the values of the time period.

CHAPTER 3

Standards in the Profession: Ethics, Accreditation, and Credentialing

It was 1976, and I was working at a mental health center as an outpatient therapist seeing a client who was known to have made up to 50 somewhat serious suicide attempts. I'll never forget that, at the end of one session, she looked at me and said, "I'm going to kill myself," and walked out. I immediately ran to get my supervisor, who said, "Get in my car," and the next thing I knew we were in a car chase after my client. We caught up to her, just about forced her into coming back to the center, and hospitalized her against her will. As we were doing all of this, I was wondering about the ethics of having a car chase and bringing her back to the center. I also thought about the legal ramifications if we had not done anything and risked a potential suicide, to say nothing of our moral obligation!

After receiving my doctorate in counselor education, I became a faculty member at a small college in New Hampshire. I took the national counselor certification exam and became a national certified counselor. A few years later I applied for licensure as a psychologist in New Hampshire and nearby Massachusetts. Both state licensing boards gave me a hard time, saying my degree was in counseling, not psychology, and not from a school accredited by the American Psychological Association. Eventually, they did license me (which would probably be unlikely today). A few years later I moved to Virginia, where the psychology licensing board told me I could not get licensed as a psychologist and suggested that I get licensed as a Licensed Professional Counselor (LPC). How odd, I think, that different states view my same background in different ways.

I teach at a state university in a CACREP-accredited program. Because the program is CACREP accredited, students can take the National Certification Exam (NCE) as they near their graduation date, prior to actually graduating. Students who have graduated from a non-CACREP accredited university must wait until they graduate before taking the exam and must complete 3000 hours of supervised experience within three years before they can be certified. Clearly, students from a CACREP-accredited program are at an advantage.

The examples above reflect some of the struggles and oddities related to three standards in the profession that will be examined in this chapter: the development and use of ethical codes and the legal issues that affect them, the history and current status of accreditation in the profession, and the state of credentialing. The development of standards is a symbol that a profession has matured and has taken a serious look at where it has been, where it is, and where it wants to go. As standards evolve, professions can reflect upon, revise, and sometimes even eliminate their standards. Despite the helping professions having been in existence for over 100 years, the development of standards is relatively new and reflects the fact that the helping professions have only recently moved into the establishment phase of their existence (Bradley, 1991). Let's examine how professional standards in the helping profession have been established and the impact they currently have on the delivery of counseling services today.

Ethics

Defining Values, Ethics, Morality, and Their Relationship to the Law

I discover that Julie, my 16-year-old daughter, is sexually promiscuous. I therefore decide that if she is going to continue with such behavior, she no longer can live in my household. I explain to her that our religious beliefs view her behavior as immoral, that the ethical code we live by demands that she stop such behavior, and that because she is dating a man who is 20, she is acting illegally.

Well, thank God, I don't really have a 16-year-old daughter yet. However, this vignette speaks to a number of critical issues we will examine in this chapter. The fact that I believe my 16-year-old daughter is "promiscuous" is a value I hold. Would I have used the same term if it were my 16-year-old son? What is promiscuity? Is dating a number of men being promiscuous? What about having sex with a man, or two men, or more? Or having sex with a member of your same sex; is this promiscuous? The beliefs I adhere to are based on my values and are closely tied to how I view morality. To make things even more complicated, if Julie is 16 and having sex with a 20-year-old, there is a likelihood that a law is being broken.

What if a counselor were seeing my 16-year-old daughter? With which values and moral questions might the counselor struggle, and are there ethical obligations to which the counselor must abide? Also, are there legal implications for the counselor? If a law is being broken, does the counselor have to respond in some manner? And what is the legal obligation of the counselor to the parents of this "child"?

Whereas morality is generally concerned with how we conduct ourselves, the term *ethics* is usually used to describe the process of examining moral behavior (Barry, 1982; Gladding, Remley, & Huber, 2001; Mowrer, 1967; Sieber, 1992). Morality is often based on the consensus values of a group such as a religious sect, societal beliefs, or the beliefs of professional groups. Codes of ethics are generally used by professional groups to describe morally "correct" behavior within the context of that professional group (Swenson, 1997). Therefore, what might be unethical behavior for a minister might be ethical behavior for a counselor. For instance, by relying on the interpretation of religious writings of a minister's sect, the minister might oppose abortion. On the other hand, relying on the ethical guidelines that assert a client's right to self-determination, a counselor might support a client's decision to have an abortion.

As each of us has different values, based on our personal sense of morality, these values sometimes will come in conflict with our professional ethics (e.g., our ethical obligation might be to listen to a woman who is leaning toward having an abortion, while our personal values may want to oppose such an option). Clearly, understanding our values, our own sense of what is right and wrong, and our professional ethics can at times be quite an undertaking. And to make things even more confounding, sometimes the law will contradict our values, our sense of morality, and/or our professional ethics.

> *The study of ethics provides guidance for professionals, aid in stating professionals' responsibilities to society, provides society with reassurance, and helps professionals maintain their integrity and freedom from outside regulation. When legislatures pass laws requiring conduct incompatible with ethical codes, professional associations first try to change the laws. If that fails they modify the ethical codes to fit the new laws.* (Swenson, 1997, p. 58)

Finally, despite the fact that ethical standards guide our behavior, the perceptions of what is and what is not ethical can vary greatly. In a survey of 1024 counselors with a return rate of 59%, Gibson and Pope (1993) found some interesting perceptions of various ethical situations. Sending out an instrument that asked counselors to rate whether or not 88 potential counselor situations were ethical, they found a great deal of disparity on a number of items (see Table 3.1).

The Development of and Need for Ethical Codes

The establishment of ethical guidelines is relatively new to the helping professions. For instance, the American Psychological Association (APA) first published its code of ethics in 1953, the American Counseling Association (ACA) developed its ethical guidelines in 1961, and the National Association of Social Workers (NASW) established its guidelines in 1960. Because ethical standards are to some degree a mirror of change in society, the associations' guidelines have undergone a number of major revisions over the years to reflect society's ever-changing values (see ACA, 1995a; APA, 2001b; NASW, 1999).

In the development and revision of ethical guidelines, deciding what might be considered ethically correct behavior is most likely a difficult task. For instance, those who view themselves as "ethical relativists" believe that moral rules are "preferences predominant in particular cultures" (Brace, 1992, p. 18), and, therefore, they believe that ethical judgments might vary from culture to culture or even setting to setting. These individuals might argue that a set of ethical guidelines such as a code should be based on "consensus values" (Bergin, 1985). Others believe that ethical judgments should be based on a set of "universal truths" with which most rational people would agree (Gert, 1988). Such universal truths, or principles, might include the following: not killing, not causing pain in another, and not depriving another of freedom. Individuals who adhere to this orientation would argue that ethical guidelines should be based, at least in part, on these universal principles.

Those charged with the formation of ethical guidelines often wrestle with which societal and professional values the guidelines should reflect and whether these values should be grounded in universal principles and/or consensus values. Despite examining many different values, it is interesting to note that the ethical guidelines of the three major helping professions of counseling, psychology, and social work all share similar values

TABLE 3.1

What Is Ethically Correct Behavior?

ITEM	PERCENTAGE*	ITEM	PERCENTAGE*
1. Becoming social friends with a former client	59	46. Using a lawsuit to collect fees from client	67
2. Charging no fee for counseling	79	47. Becoming sexually involved with former client	23
3. Providing counseling to one of your friends	30	48. Avoiding certain clients for fear of being sued	64
4. Advertising in newspapers or similar media	83	49. Seeing a colleague's client without consulting him or her	9
5. Not disclosing to a client the purpose of testing	3	50. Lending money to a client	17
6. Filing an ethics complaint against a colleague	96	51. Providing counseling to one of your employees	40
7. Telling a client you are angry at him or her	83	52. Having clients address you by your first name	95
8. Using computerized test interpretation services	96	53. Sending holiday greeting cards to your clients	81
9. Hugging a client	86	54. Kissing a client	16
10. Terminating counseling if the client cannot pay	48	55. Engaging in erotic activity with a client	0
11. Accepting services from a client in lieu of fee	53	56. Giving a gift worth at least $50 to a client	9
12. Seeing a minor client without parental consent	44	57. Accepting a client's invitation to a party	34
13. Having clients take tests (e.g., MMPI) at home	26	58. Engaging in sex with a clinical supervisee	2
14. Altering diagnosis to meet insurance criteria	6	59. Going to a client's special event (e.g., wedding)	86
15. Telling client, "I'm sexually attracted to you"	17	60. Getting paid to refer clients to someone	8
16. Refusing to let clients read their chart notes	49	61. Going into business with a client	9
17. Using a collection agency to collect late fees	81	62. Engaging in sexual contact with a client	0
18. Breaking confidentiality if client is homicidal	95	63. Utilizing involuntary hospitalization	80
19. Performing work for a contingency fee	53	64. Selling goods to clients	16
20. Using self-disclosure as counseling technique	92	65. Giving personal advice on radio, TV, etc.	64
21. Inviting clients to an office open house	54	66. Advertising accurately your counseling techniques	90
22. Accepting a client's gift worth at least $50	21	67. Unintentionally disclosing confidential data	13
23. Working when too distressed to be effective	7	68. Allowing a client to disrobe	2
24. Accepting only male or only female clients	64	69. Borrowing from a client	3
25. Not allowing client access to testing report	24	70. Discussing a client by name with friends	1
26. Raising fee during the course of counseling	46	71. Providing services outside areas of competence	3
27. Breaking confidentiality if a client is suicidal	95	72. Signing for hours a supervisee has not earned	1
28. Not allowing clients access to raw test data	71	73. Treating homosexuality per se as pathological	14
29. Allowing clients to run up a large unpaid bill	38	74. Counseling while under the influence of alcohol	1
30. Accepting goods (rather than money) as payment	63	75. Engaging in sexual fantasy about a client	38
31. Using sexual surrogates with clients	17	76. Accepting a gift worth less than $5 from a client	70
32. Breaking confidentiality to report child abuse	96	77. Offering or accepting a handshake from a client	99
33. Inviting clients to a party or social event	21	78. Disrobing in the presence of a client	0
34. Addressing client by his or her first name	97	79. Charging for missed appointments	85
35. Tape recording without client consent	1	80. Going into business with a former client	46
36. Earning a fee that is a percentage of client's salary	55	81. Directly soliciting a person to be a client	25
37. Asking favors (e.g., a ride home) from clients	26	82. Being sexually attracted to a client	63
38. Charging *all* clients the same fee	72	83. Helping a client file a complaint about a colleague	68
39. Accepting client's decision to commit suicide	18	84. Not disclosing your fee structure to a client	4
40. Not prescreening group members	18	85. Not telling a client of the limits of confidentiality	4
41. Telling clients that their values are incorrect	22	86. Disclosing client's name to a class you're teaching	0
42. Telling clients your disappointment in them	66	87. Using agency affiliation to recruit private clients	24
43. Discussing clients without names with friends	22	88. Joining partnership that makes clear your specialty	98
44. Providing counseling to student or supervisee	44		
45. Giving gifts to those who refer clients to you	20		

*Percentage = The percentage of counselors thinking the item is ethical.

SOURCE: From "The Ethics of Counseling: A National Survey of Certified Counselors," by W. T. Gibson and K. S. Pope, *Journal of Counseling and Development*, *71*(3), 330–336.

while serving a number of other general purposes (Corey et al., 1998; Mabe & Rollin, 1986; Loewenberg & Dolgoff, 2000; VanZandt, 1990):

- They protect consumers and further the professional standing of the organization.
- They are a statement about the maturity and professional identity of a profession.
- They guide professionals toward certain types of behaviors that reflect the underlying values considered to be desirable in the profession.
- They offer a framework in the sometimes difficult ethical decision-making process.
- They can be offered as one measure of defense if the professional is sued for malpractice.

Although ethical guidelines can be of considerable assistance in a professional's ethical decision-making process, there are limitations to the use of such a code (Mabe & Rollins, 1986):

- There are many issues that cannot be handled in the context of a code.
- There are some difficulties with enforcing the code, or at least the public may believe that enforcement committees are not tough enough on their peers.
- There is often no way to bring the interests of the client, patient, or research participant systematically into the code construction process.
- There are parallel forums in which the issues in the code may be addressed, with the results sometimes at odds with the findings of the code (e.g., in the courts).
- There are possible conflicts associated with codes: between two codes, between the practitioner's values and code requirements, between the code and ordinary morality, between the code and institutional practice, and between requirements within a single code.
- There is a limited range of topics covered in the code, and because a code approach is usually reactive to issues already developed elsewhere, the requirement of consensus prevents the code from addressing new issues and problems at the cutting edge (pp. 294–295).

Although there are positive and negative aspects to ethical guidelines, the professional associations clearly feel the development of such codes has been crucial to the professionalization of the mental health fields.

Codes of Ethics in the Helping Professions

ACA's Ethical Standards: A Brief Overview

The ethical standards of ACA have undergone a number of revisions since their adoption in 1961. Besides changes within the code itself, the current ethical standards of ACA have an added section called Standards of Practice that further delineates the code as well as a section on the policies for responding to requests on interpretation of the code and a section on procedures for processing complaints. ACA's ethical code includes eight sections, briefly summarized below (ACA, 1995a) (please see Appendix B for the full code).

SECTION A: THE COUNSELING RELATIONSHIP Highlighting important issues within the counseling relationship, this section stresses that the primary responsibility of counselors is toward the welfare of their client, the need for counselors to respect diversity, the importance for counselors to properly inform clients of procedures (informed consent), the necessity of avoiding dual relationships (as when a client is also your coworker), the importance of properly screening and protecting clients who participate in group counseling, issues related to fees for service, termination issues, and the use of computers in counseling.

SECTION B: CONFIDENTIALITY Section B examines the limits of and exceptions to confidentiality; the nature of confidentiality with families, groups, and minors; the confidentiality of records; the importance of confidentiality in research; and the need for confidentiality when a counselor is in a consultative role.

SECTION C: PROFESSIONAL RESPONSIBILITY This standard discusses the importance of practicing within one's professional competence, accurately advertising one's abilities and credentials, not discriminating against people, not engaging in sexual harassment, accurately reporting information to third parties (e.g., insurance companies, courts), being accurate and careful when using the media (e.g., radio talk shows), not making unjustifiable treatment claims, respecting professionals in related fields, assuring the public can distinguish personal from professional statements, and how to assist a client who seeks you out who is already in an existing professional helping relationship.

SECTION D: RELATIONSHIPS WITH OTHER PROFESSIONALS Section D examines what to do if one's employer/employee relationship is not ideal, the importance of being evaluated by one's agency, the importance of acting in a competent fashion and of maintaining high levels of professional service and conduct, the significance of not overtly or covertly supporting discrimination on the job, and various ethical issues related to being an effective consultant.

SECTION E. EVALUATION, ASSESSMENT, AND INTERPRETATION This section highlights the importance of understanding test statistics, choosing good assessment instruments, assuring proper test-taking conditions, understanding cultural bias in testing, accurately scoring and interpreting test material, securing tests, and properly diagnosing clients as a result of testing.

SECTION F: TEACHING, TRAINING, AND SUPERVISION Section F examines important issues concerning admission of students to counseling programs, boundaries between faculty and students, evaluation of students, the importance of offering varying theoretical views when teaching counseling, offering proper credit to students when they assist in research, and the role of self-growth experiences and personal counseling for students.

SECTION G: RESEARCH AND PUBLICATION A wide range of ethical areas is discussed in this section, including the proper use of human subjects in research, precautions to be taken to avoid injury to subjects, the proper reporting and publishing of research results, and the importance of informed consent, voluntary participation, and confidentiality in research.

SECTION H: RESOLVING ETHICAL ISSUES This final section of the ethical code explains the proper steps to take in the reporting and resolution of suspected ethical violations.

Related Ethical Codes and Standards

In addition to the ethical guidelines as presented by ACA, a number of the divisions and affiliated groups of ACA have established ethical guidelines. In general, these guidelines are not intended to replace the ethical code of ACA but assist in clarifying the unique circumstances of counselors in varying settings (Herlihy & Remley, 1995). Highlighting just a few of these, we find ethical codes for school counselors (ASCA, 1998), mental health counselors (AMHCA, 2000), rehabilitation counselors (CRCC, 2000), nationally certified counselors (NBCC, 1997), counseling supervisors (ACES, 1993), group counselors (ASGW, 1998a, b), and marriage and family counselors (IAMFC, 2001).

Besides ACA and its divisions, all of the related mental health fields have ethical codes. Thus we find ethical guidelines for psychologists (APA, 2001b), social workers (NASW, 1999), marriage and family therapists (AAMFT, 2001b), psychiatrists (APA, 1981), and human service professionals (NOHSE, 1995). Although there is certainly much in common among the various ethical standards, differences do exist, and a conscientious professional will have some knowledge of these varying ethical guidelines. However, it is important to have a clear sense of one's professional affiliation and be particularly familiar with that association's guidelines when making difficult ethical decisions.

Resolving Ethical Dilemmas

Decision-Making Models

In view of the practical limitations of ethical guidelines noted earlier, and in search of a more flexible and comprehensive approach to resolving ethical dilemmas, models of ethical decision making have been devised (Cottone & Claus, 2000; Welfel, 1998). For instance, Corey and associates (1998) developed a seven step practical, problem-solving model that consists of: (1) identifying the problem, (2) identifying the potential issues involved, (3) reviewing the relevant ethical guidelines, (4) obtaining consultation, (5) considering possible and probable courses of action, (6) enumerating the consequences of various decisions, and (7) deciding on the best course of action.

Whereas Corey's model emphasizes pragmatism, other models stress the role of moral principles in this ethical decision making. For instance, Kitchener (1984) describes the role of five moral principles in the making of ethical decisions that include promoting the *autonomy* of the client (e.g., independence, self-determination, freedom of choice); the *beneficence* of society (promoting the good of others); the *nonmaleficence* of people (avoidance of harm toward others); *justice* or fairness to all (providing equal and fair treatment to all people), and *fidelity* of the counseling relationship (loyalty, commitment, and faithfulness). The counselor who employs this model will not necessarily decline the use of codes but will refer to them while using these moral principles in his or her decision-making process.

When faced with thorny ethical decisions, Rest (1984) suggests following a critical decision-making path that includes making an interpretation about the situation, gauging and selecting the moral principles that underlie the decision to be made (e.g., a person should not murder), and acting on the basis of the selected moral principle(s). At each stage in the model, Rest has pinpointed potential counselor difficulties in employing this way of making ethical decisions: (1) The counselor may misinterpret or fail to see the need for moral action; (2) the counselor may be incapable of making a principled moral

BOX 3.1

Critiques of Ethical Decision-Making Models

As useful as models of decision making might prove, they are not immune to criticism. Stress on autonomy, for example, has been called into question by writers on female psychology and by some who take a multicultural perspective when they note that autonomy does not figure into the ethical development of some women and minorities the way it does with white males (Belenky, Clinchy, Goldberger, & Tarule, 1997; Gilligan, 1982; Ivey, 1993).

In a similar way, some authors have asserted that ethical decision making is not based on universal principles, but on culture-bound values (Atkinson, Morten, & Sue, 1998; Jereb, 1982; Majors & Nikelly, 1983). Therefore, minority counselors might view ethical dilemmas from differing perspectives than do majority counselors. For instance, Gooley (1992) notes that many white Americans see moral and immoral behavior as dichotomous, whereas black Americans "adhere to a unity of opposites" when considering moral questions (p. 114). Therefore, when using decision-making models for some ethical dilemmas, one might find most majority counselors would come to a different decision than most counselors from a specific minority group.

In critiquing "moral" models of ethical decision making (e.g., Kitchener & Rest, 1990), Jordan and Meara (1990) assert that principles alone are insufficient to explain ethical decisions as they do not emphasize the person behind the principle; that is, learning a principle is not enough if the character of the person is not capable of acting on the principle. Or put more simply, I might "know" the "right" way to act, but I might not live that way. Finally, others assert that such models do not fully take into account the developmental level of the counselor (Neukrug, Lovell, & Parker, 1996). In other words, counselors respond differently based on their personal developmental maturity, and decision-making models pay little attention to this fact.

judgment in the face of a complex dilemma; (3) the counselor may be unable to plan a course of action; and (4) the counselor may lack the will to act. (See Box 3.1.)

Ethical decision-making models are one method of assisting the counselor when confronted with difficult ethical dilemmas, and they can give the counselor a running start when used in conjunction with a firm knowledge of the ethical guidelines. However, even one who has mastery of decision-making models and of the ethical guidelines may not make the wisest decision if he or she is not a seasoned professional.

A Developmental Perspective

> *John, a 55-year-old gay man, is seriously depressed and feels that he has no reason to continue living. Although he has been seeing you, his counselor, for several months, his outlook on life has not changed, and he is determined to end what he considers to be an "empty existence" before death overtakes him. John's partner of 15 years, Jim, died of AIDS two years ago after suffering prolonged pain and anguish. Although John himself has lived with HIV for over ten years, he has recently been diagnosed with AIDS, and the reality of his own mortality has become apparent. John, whose parents died when he was six, has no surviving relatives nor any close friends. He and Jim had isolated themselves from others, and in order to safeguard their privacy, severed all social ties years ago. As a self-employed writer who has chosen a solitary lifestyle, John has no support system and is not interested in trying to develop one now. He tells you that he has lived long enough and has accomplished most of what he wished to do in life. He is now ready*

to die and wants only to get it over with as quickly and painlessly as possible. He asks you to help him decide upon the most efficient means of achieving this goal. As his counselor, what should you do?

As in the case above, professional helpers are confronted routinely by stressful, ambiguous, and complex ethical dilemmas (Corey et al., 1998; May & Sowa, 1992; Welfel & Lipsitz, 1983). For guidance, helpers can turn to the codes of ethical standards and to the decision-making models already discussed. However, as helpful as codes and decision-making models may be, evidence suggests that the ability to make wise ethical decisions may well be influenced by the counselor's level of ethical, moral, and cognitive development (Hayes, 1994; Magolda & Porterfield, 1988; Neukrug et al., 1996; Neukrug & McAuliffe, 1993; Van Hoose & Paradise, 1979; Welfel & Lipsitz, 1983).

In most ethical, moral, and/or cognitive developmental models, lower-level thought characteristically tends toward dualism, rigidity, oversimplification, stereotyping, self-protectiveness, and authoritarianism, while higher-level thought is more flexible, complex, nondogmatic, and more sensitive to the context in which a decision is being made (Cottone, 2001; Kohlberg, 1984; McAuliffe et al., 2000; Pascarella & Terenzini, 1991). Although not all adults (or counselors) reach the higher levels of this development (Lovell, 1999a), these models suggest that, if afforded the right opportunities, most adults can reach the higher levels. Interestingly, this development seems to be universal across cultures (Snarey, 1985).

Counselors at the lower levels are rigid and dualistic about ethical decision making, often "want the answer," and are likely to adhere rigidly to a clearly written ethical code. Counselors at these levels of development might regard ethical codes as the singular authority, with any further soul searching deemed a needless exercise in over-complicating matters. On the other hand, counselors at higher levels of development, although fully aware of their ethical guidelines, may require less rigid adherence to such guidelines and are more apt to use such codes as a tool in a deeply reflective decision-making process (Neukrug et al., 1996). Although both types of counselors may use decision-making models, given the same ethical dilemma, the manner in which they employ them could be strikingly different.

The distinctions between lower- and higher-level thought can be elucidated by considering how two different counselors, Donna and Rita, might respond to the ethical dilemma posed earlier in the case of John. Both counselors are convinced that John has both the motivation and means to end his life; however, the processes they employ in coming to their conclusion, and in this case the eventual decisions they arrive at, differ markedly.

Perceiving the severity of the situation, Donna refers to ACA's Code of Ethics and Standards of Practice (1995a) and decides that she must intervene to save her client's life. She knows that not to do so would be in violation of the ethical codes, because the guidelines state that it is her responsibility to "prevent clear and imminent danger to the client or others . . ." (ACA, 1995a, Standard B.1.c). In addition, she recognizes that legal action could be taken against her if a suicide occurred. Besides, examining Kitchener's decision-making model, she knows that for the good of society (beneficence), John must not kill himself because he would not be following the law, and society would fall apart if everyone were lawless; that it is important that she does all she can to prevent him from emotionally harming others as would occur if he were to commit suicide (nonmaleficence); that he must be in a better state of mind to make a rational decision (autonomy);

that many people in life have to undergo very difficult ordeals, and why should he be an exception (fairness); and that she has been committed to the counseling relationship, and to his life, and so should he (fidelity). Donna therefore concludes that she has no choice. Against his wishes, she has John committed to a psychiatric facility.

Rita also understands the seriousness of John's condition but resolves the dilemma differently. She reviews the ethical guidelines and is quickly reminded that the code advises a counselor to take action when clients endanger themselves or others and that they equally emphasize the need to respect the privacy of the client and the client's freedom to choose his or her goals in counseling (ACA, 1995a). She ponders the apparently conflicting advice found in the guidelines. She reflects and considers Kitchener's model. Knowing that John does not want to live, maybe she should allow him to choose death (autonomy). However, she wonders whether John is capable of making such a decision in his deteriorated physical and mental state. She then considers whether killing oneself is in best the interest of society (beneficence). She also considers who would be emotionally harmed if he did choose suicide and who would be harmed if he was prevented from killing himself (nonmaleficence). In a quandary, she thinks more and reflects on her sessions with him. She wonders what is fair and just in this situation (fairness). She considers how loyal he has been to the counseling relationship and how committed she has been to helping him (fidelity). She consults with others, particularly those who might have differing views than hers. Finally, after reflecting on a variety of different scenarios, Rita makes her decision. She hopes she has made the best decision.

Donna's decision making exemplifies dualistic thinking that relies on external authority to distinguish between right and wrong. She reflects little, comes to decisions quickly, and does not value consultation and differing opinions. In contrast, Rita's relativistic ethical reasoning is characterized by introspection, a willingness to consider fully a variety of variables, and the determination that after deliberate and exhaustive review, she will have to come up with some decision to resolve this complex situation.

It is important to highlight the fact that counselors who are at varying stages developmentally could come to the same decisions. This model assumes that what decision is made is not as crucial as how the individual comes by that decision. Donna's decision is based on little reflection, a rigid adherence to rules and regulations, little understanding of the contextual world of the client, and a reliance on outside authority (the code). Rita's decision is made with introspection, openness, reflection, a deep understanding of the client, and a desire to examine opposing points of view. In many ways Rita has a more difficult time in the decision-making process because she has examined varying viewpoints and may always have some doubt about her decision. Donna, on the other hand, is so convinced that her decision is correct that she may never question herself.

Final Thoughts on Resolving Ethical Dilemmas

Developmental theory suggests that the counselor's general skill at making ethical decisions tends to increase over time as the helper learns to reason in ethically reflective ways (Pelsma & Borgers, 1986; Tennyson & Strom, 1986; Van Hoose, 1980). It is hoped that over time the counselor will not need to have "the answer" but instead will make reflective ethical decisions that show self-understanding, a grasp of ethical guidelines, and an understanding of ethical decision-making models. Although the counselor may not always be confident about having made the best decision, he or she will be secure in having made a deeply reasoned decision.

Ethical Complaints and Violations

Ethical Problem Areas for Counselors

Although it is difficult to assess the types and actual numbers of lawsuits being filed against counselors, we do have a sense of the types and numbers of complaints being made against licensed professional counselors. A study by Neukrug, Milliken, and Walden (2001) revealed that for one year, 2325 complaints were made to state licensing boards against credentialed counselors, resulting in 1018 investigations. Of these, 241 actions were taken, ranging from having one's credentials revoked or suspended to being reprimanded, requiring supervision, being fined, or some other punishment (e.g., community service).

Of the 1018 complaints identified, 24% were for inappropriate dual relationships; 17% for incompetence in the facilitation of a counseling relationship; 8% for practicing without a license or other misrepresentation of qualifications; 7% for having sexual relationship with a client; 5% for breach of confidentiality; 4% for inappropriate fee assessment; 1% for failure to inform clients about goals, techniques, rules, and limitations of the counseling relationship; and 1% for failure to report abuse. Another 33% of the complaints were identified in the "other" category.

It is important to note that whether these complaints were adjudicated in a court of law is not known. Also, the complaints probably do not mirror the ethical complaints made against counselors who do not work in private practice (e.g., school or agency counselors), as many of the issues are not prevalent in these other settings (e.g., insurance reimbursement issues). It is commonly believed that the ethical dilemmas that most frequently plague school counselors revolve around issues of confidentiality, reporting of abuse, and the transmission of particular values (e.g., sex education or problem pregnancy counseling) (Huey, 1988). Some other apparently high-risk areas for all counselors include failure to diagnose or treat adequately, inadequate referrals, breaches of contract, slander and libel, birth control and abortion counseling, and wrongful commitment (Swenson, 1997).

In addition to complaints reported to state licensing boards, complaints are also reported to ethics committees of state professional associations and to the ethics committee of the American Counseling Association, although these are far fewer in number than complaints made to state licensing boards. However, it is interesting to note that of 621 informal inquiries made to the ACA Ethics Committee, the vast majority concerned confidentiality and a large number were about the counseling relationship (e.g., dual relationships, counseling techniques, the client–counselor interaction), and professional responsibility (Brown & Espina, 2000). A smaller number concerned relationships with other professionals, assessment, teaching, and supervision.

Reporting Ethical Violations

There are a few avenues that a consumer or fellow counselor can take when reporting suspected ethical violations. If the complaint is being made against a counselor who is a member of ACA or was a member of ACA when the alleged ethical violation was made, then the ACA Ethics Committee can have jurisdiction over the complaint. In these cases, complainants are always encouraged to have first gone directly to the counselor. However, if this is not done, or if no resolution is found in this manner, complainants need to place the alleged violation in writing to the Ethics Committee. The accused member has 60 days to respond to the complaint in writing and can request a face-to-face formal hearing before the Ethics Committee. If the accused member is found to have violated the ACA code of ethics, the ACA Ethics Committee can sanction the counselor by requiring remediation as determined by the Committee, suspending the member from ACA, or expelling the member from ACA (1995a).

State branches of ACA will often have similar procedures to those of the national group for dealing with ethical complaints. In addition, state licensing boards have generally developed procedures for dealing with ethical complaints. Neukrug and associates (2001) noted that of the complaints made against licensed professional counselors who were found to be in violation of ethical practices, 36% had their licenses revoked, 19% had their license suspended, 5% were sent letters of reprimand, 4% were required to receive supervision, and 1% were assessed a fine. Another 35% had some other action taken against them (e.g., community service, further education, or voluntary surrender of license).

Legal Issues Related to Ethical Violations

Civil and Criminal Liability

Because suspension or expulsion from a professional group is sometimes considered too mild a punishment, complainants will sometimes bring a civil suit. If there is a possible criminal act, they may also go to the authorities in hopes that a criminal case will be brought against the counselor. Whereas "criminal liability is the responsibility under the law for a violation of federal or state criminal statute, civil liability is the responsibility one has for a violation of a legal duty to another" (personal communication, Helman Brook, Esq., April 26, 2002). As has been widely publicized as a result of the O. J. Simpson lawsuits, the burden of proof in a criminal case is quite different than in a civil case. In a criminal matter, the burden is on the state to prove guilt "beyond a reasonable doubt." In a civil matter, the burden is on the plaintiff to prove the case by a "preponderance of the evidence." To highlight these differences, imagine the scale of justice. In a criminal case the scale needs to sharply drop to one side to show guilt, while in a civil case the scale need tilt only slightly for the complainant to win a judgment (personal communication, Carole Borstein, Esq., June 1, 2002).

Generally, in the case of malpractice, civil suits are brought against counselors, although counselors could be charged in both civil and criminal courts. For example, if a counselor had sex with a client in violation of a state statute, a prosecuting attorney could file charges against that counselor in criminal court, and the client could also bring a case against the counselor in civil court. Anybody can sue anybody for anything in a civil suit, although outlandish cases are generally quickly dismissed, and some states now penalize an individual for arbitrary suits.

The Role of Ethical Codes in Lawsuits

Although ethical guidelines are not legal documents, whether a counselor is involved in a criminal or civil suit, a professional association's code of ethics can be an important piece of evidence. For instance, a counselor would have a difficult time defending having had sex with a client because the ethical guidelines clearly assert that sex with a client is inappropriate behavior. However, cases are often not clear cut. For example, a counselor has sex with a former client she had seen three years earlier. The former client feels abused, brings the case to a prosecutor who determines that the statute is unclear about when a client stops being a client, and decides to file criminal charges against the counselor. The counselor then brings the most recent version of the ACA ethical guidelines to court, which state that "Counselors do not engage in sexual intimacies with former clients within a minimum of two years after terminating the counseling relationship" (ACA, 1995a, Standard A.7.b.). Although not a legal document, this statement could potentially help the counselor's cause. On the other hand, the prosecutor would undoubtedly retort with the following statement also found in the ethical guidelines: "Counselors who engage in such relationship after two years following termination have the responsibility to thoroughly examine and document that such relations did not have an exploitative nature . . ." (ACA, 1995a, Standard A.7.b.). Finally, because ethical guidelines are not legal documents, they are likely to hold more weight in a civil court than in a criminal court, because the burden of proof is less in a civil case.

Malpractice Insurance and Counseling

> *Regardless of how careful counselors are . . . malpractice lawsuits can still occur.*
> (Gladding, 2000, p. 69)

In today's litigious society, this simple statement by Gladding speaks an unhappy truth. Remember, anyone can be sued by anybody. Certainly, this does not mean a counselor will lose a frivolous suit. However, if a counselor found him- or herself in the dubious position of not having malpractice insurance and losing a civil suit, that counselor may be haunted by the monetary settlement for the rest of his or her life. There is little question that, in today's world, malpractice insurance is almost a necessity. Although most schools and agencies generally purchase an umbrella malpractice insurance policy, it is still prudent to own additional insurance protection. And, if you do work in a setting that has purchased a malpractice policy, review it carefully, study its monetary limits, and examine any possible exclusions to the policy. For instance, are you covered if you work after hours? What if your employer lets you run a workshop for your own personal profit at the agency on the weekend? Are you still covered?

Although colleges and universities almost always carry malpractice insurance for students doing practicum and internship, again it is always best to check and see if the school does indeed have a policy and the monetary limits of such a policy. The ACA (2001c) professional liability insurance program offers malpractice insurance for rates as low as $15 for students and between $272 and $507 for self-employed counselors, depending on whether one is purchasing $200,000 or $2,000,000.

Corey and associates (1998) give an exhaustive list of ways in which a person can avoid being sued for malpractice in either civil or criminal court. For instance, they note that counselors should:

- Have a clear definition of fees.
- Keep good records.
- Preserve appropriate confidentiality.
- Avoid searches of students.
- Avoid dual relationships, especially having sex with a client.
- Consult with colleagues when need be.
- Whenever possible, obtain permission from a client to consult with others.
- Use informed-consent procedures.
- Have a sound theoretical approach.
- Know how to assess clients who are a danger to themselves and others.
- Maintain their competence.

- Have clear, well-documented treatment plans.
- Report suspected abuse, as required by law.
- Not barter for services.
- Not abandon their client (e.g., avoid long absences).
- Refer and transfer clients wisely.
- Be aware of potential legal problems when discussing abortion and birth control.
- Treat their clients with respect.
- Avoid power relationships with clients.
- Maintain malpractice insurance.

Accreditation

The History and Development of Professional Preparation Standards

> *Regardless of what degree or training model you ultimately seek, you want to assure that you receive competent training by a recognized academic institution that offers a legitimate degree certificate. Professionals in psychology and related fields often have responsibilities that impact heavily on the lives of other's, many of whom are exceptionally vulnerable. Shoddy or inept training could lead you, even inadvertently, to harm or wrong people.*
>
> *Unfortunately, the United States is cluttered with bogus "institutions of higher learning" that issue master's and doctor's "degrees" that are not worth the paper they are printed on and that can even get you into legal trouble if you attempt to proffer them as legitimate credentials. These outfits are unconcerned with ethical standards or with whom they might hurt, and simply prey on people who are looking for shortcuts.* (Keith-Spiegel, 1991, p. 55)

Although written over 10 years ago, these words, unfortunately, still hold truth today. One mechanism of thwarting poor training is through accreditation of programs, which can be traced back to the early part of the 20th century in the field of social work and to the mid-1940s in the field of psychology (Morales & Sheafor, 1997; Sheridan, Matarazzo, & Nelson, 1995). Few then realized that today there would literally be hundreds of accredited programs offering graduate training in counseling, social work, marital and family therapy, and psychology. Although starting a little later than the fields of psychology and social work, within the last 25 years the counseling field has made great leaps in its efforts toward accreditation.

The Council for Accreditation of Counseling and Related Educational Programs (CACREP): A Short History

> *The acronym CACREP is a mouthful to say. . . . In fact, without the Council for Accreditation of Counseling and Related Educational Programs, counseling would be far less credible as a profession compared to other human service fields that have such an agency.* (Sweeney, 1992, p. 667)

Although the concept of having standards for counselor education programs can be traced back to the 1940s (Sweeney, 1992), it was not until the 1960s that these ideas began to take form with the adoption of training standards for elementary school counselors, secondary school counselors, and student personnel workers in higher education (Altekruse & Wittmer, 1991). Soon, ACES began to examine the possibility of merging these various standards into one document entitled the Standards for the Preparation of Counselors and Other Personnel Service Specialists (Altekruse & Wittmer, 1991; Sweeney, 1995). Although the Standards were being unofficially used as early as 1973, it was not until 1979 that APGA (now ACA) officially adopted them, and in 1981 APGA created CACREP, a freestanding incorporated legal body that would oversee the accrediting process (Brooks & Gerstein, 1990). Adoption of the CACREP standards started slowly, and they have gone through a number of revisions before their most recent form, which went into effect in January of 2001. Today they are considered to be the standard bearer to which all programs should strive (CACREP, 2001).

Considering the vast number of changes that most programs have to make and the amount of time that it takes to implement such changes, it is a tribute to CACREP that currently 150 of the approximately 500 counseling programs nationally are CACREP accredited (CACREP, 2000). In addition, all evidence seems to indicate that most of the remaining programs will eventually become CACREP accredited (Smaby & D'Andrea, 1995). Considering the positive points of accreditation, perhaps this is not unexpected (Altekruse & Wittmer, 1991; Schmidt, 1999):

- Students who graduate from accredited programs study from a common curriculum, are generally more knowledgeable about core counseling issues, and usually participate in more intensive and longer field work experiences.
- Accreditation often becomes the standard by which credentialing bodies determine who is eligible to become certified or licensed.
- Accreditation bodies offer the impetus for setting and maintaining high standards.
- Accreditation almost always results in improved programs.
- Administrators and legislators are often more willing to provide money to maintain the high standards of accredited programs than to less rigorous nonaccredited programs.
- Those who graduate from accredited programs generally have better job opportunities.
- Accredited programs will often attract better faculty.
- Accredited programs will often attract better students.

Although some have argued that the accreditation process can limit creativity, is too costly, dictates the type of faculty, may not be related to program quality, and "locks the profession into its present state of development" (Thomas, 1991, p. 203; Weinrach, 1991), it is clear that CACREP is here to stay.

A Quick Overview of the CACREP Standards

Today, CACREP offers standards for the doctoral degree in counselor education and for the master's degree in community counseling, school counseling, college counseling, mental health counseling, career counseling, gerontological counseling, student affairs, and marriage, couple, and family counseling/therapy. With the exception of mental health counseling, which requires a 60-semester-hour master's degree, each program area requires a minimum of 48 semester hour credits for the master's degree.

For all master's programs seeking CACREP accreditation, curriculum requirements include course work in the areas of professional orientation, helping relationships, group work, social and cultural foundations, career and lifestyle development, appraisal, research and evaluation, and human growth and development. Also, each program area requires specialty course work within the program area emphasis. In the area of clinical instruction, field work experiences, which include a 100-hour practicum and a 600-hour internship, are required of all students. The standards also delineate a variety of requirements listed within six sections: the Institution, Program Objectives and Curriculum, Clinical Instruction, Faculty and Staff, Organization and Administration, and Evaluations in the Program. The standards leave some room for flexibility, are broad in scope, and offer specific guidelines within each of the six areas.

In order to become CACREP accredited, programs need to meet the requirements within each of the six sections of the program standards. To meet the accreditation standards, most programs find that they need to undertake at least moderate changes. Following the changes, and often while they are being made, a self-study report is written that spells out how the program meets each of the sections of the program standards. This report is then sent along with an application to the CACREP office, which has independent readers review the report. If the report is accepted, then a CACREP team is appointed to visit and review the program and make a final recommendation for or against accreditation.

The CACREP accreditation process tends to be long and arduous. Despite this fact, or perhaps because of it, CACREP has become a major force in the preparation of highly trained mental health professionals and will no doubt continue to have an impact on the counseling field.

Other Accreditation Bodies

A number of other accreditation bodies set standards in related fields. For instance, in the field of rehabilitation counseling, the accreditation of programs has been overseen by the Council on Rehabilitation Education (CORE, 2001). Although CORE and CACREP have much in common, the field of rehabilitation counseling has remained separate from other counseling specialty areas. In another related field, we find a number of pastoral counseling programs being accredited by the American Association of Pastoral Counselors (AAPC, 2001).

In the field of psychology, the American Psychological Association currently sets standards for doctoral-level programs in counseling and clinical psychology (APA, 2001c). The Council on Social Work Education (htpp//www.cswe.org) is responsible for the accreditation of both undergraduate and graduate social work programs, while the AAMFT's Commission on Accreditation for Marital and Family Therapy Education (COAMFTE) is the accrediting body for marriage and family therapy programs. Although somewhat in conflict with CACREP's accreditation of marriage and family therapy counseling programs, this commission has accredited 79 marriage and family therapy programs (COAMFTE, 2001).

Credentialing

One method of assuring that professionals in the field are competent is through accreditation. Another means is through credentialing. Although credentialing in the mental health professions is a relatively new phenomenon, regulating occupations began as far back as the 13th century when the Holy Roman Empire set requirements for the practice of medicine (Hosie, 1991). However, it was not until the 1900s that credentialing became common, and it was not until the 1970s that credentialing in the counseling field first started to become a reality. Today, credentialing cuts across many professions and can be found in many different forms. Usually, credentialing offers many benefits to the profession, the consumer, and the counselor (Bloom, 1997; Remley, 1991). Some of these include:

- *Increased professionalization*. Credentialing increases the status of the members of a profession and clearly identifies who those members are.
- *Parity*. Credentialing helps counselors achieve parity in professional status, salary, insurance reimbursement, and other areas with closely related mental health professions.
- *Delimiting the field*. The process of passing legislation to enable counselors to obtain credentials assists the profession in clearly defining who we are and where we are going.
- *Protection of the public*. Credentials help identify to the public those individuals who have the appropriate training and skills to do counseling.

Although credentialing takes many forms, the three most common forms of credentialing include registration, certification, and licensure.

Registration, Certification, and Licensure Defined

Registration

Registration is the simplest form of credentialing and involves a listing of the members of a particular professional group (Sweeney, 1991). Registration, which is generally regulated by each state, implies that each registered individual has acquired minimal competence, such as a college degree and/or apprenticeship in his or her particular professional area. Registration of professional groups usually implies that there is little or no regulation of that group. Generally registration involves a modest fee. Today few states provide registration for counselors, instead opting for the more rigid credentialing standards of certification and/or licensure.

Certification

Certification is more rigorous than registration and involves the formal recognition that an individual within a professional group has met certain predetermined standards of professionalism (Forrest & Stone, 1991). Although more rigorous than registration, certification is less demanding than licensure. Certification is often seen as a protection of a title; that is, it attests to a person's attainment of a certain level of competence. In contrast, licensure tends to protect the title and define the practice of a professional; that is, it not only attests to a certain level of competence but defines what a person can do and where he or she can do it. A yearly fee must usually be paid to maintain certification.

Certification can be offered by state or national boards. Until recently most states have certified school personnel (e.g., teachers, school counselors, school psychologists), which means that certain requirements are needed for a person to become certified in a specific area. For instance, the requirement in most states for school counselor certification is a master's degree in school counseling from a program accredited by the State

Board of Education. Besides state certification processes, national certification bodies, such as the National Board of Certified Counselors, also exist (NBCC, 2001). Although national certification implies that a certain level of competence in a professional field has been achieved, unless a state legislates that national certification will be used at the state level, such certification carries little or no legal clout. Finally, certification may also require ongoing continuing education for an individual to maintain his or her credential.

Licensure

The most rigorous form of credentialing is licensing. Generally regulated by states, licensure denotes that the licensed individual has met rigorous standards and that individuals without licenses cannot practice in that particular professional arena. Whereas certification protects the title only, licensure generally defines the scope of what an individual can and cannot do. For instance, in Virginia the counselor licensing law not only defines the requirements one needs to become licensed but also defines what is meant by counseling, who can do it, the limits of confidentiality and privileged communication (see Chapter 4), legal regulations related to suspected violations of the law (e.g., child abuse), and other various restrictions and regulations (Regulations Governing the Practice of Professional Counseling, 2000).

In terms of the day-to-day professional functioning, the most important aspect of counselor licensure has become the fact that in most states licensure carries with it legislation that mandates third-party reimbursement privileges. Such legislation requires insurance companies to reimburse licensed individuals for counseling and psychotherapy. As with certification, licensure generally involves a yearly fee, and often continuing education requirements are mandated.

Credentialing in Related Helping Professions

> *It is recognized that there is competition for clients among professionals providing mental health services and that there is also concern about the degree of preparation and expertise of a number of professions to deliver those services.*
> (Garcia, 1990, p. 495)

Master's Degree Social Work Credentialing

Today, close to one-half of the 155,000 members of NASW are ACSWs. Also, a social worker who works in the schools can become a Certified School Social Worker (CSSW). In addition to these certifications and others open to social workers, each of the 50 states offers credentialing for social workers, with the vast majority offering licensure (ASWB, 2000).

Doctoral Level Credentialing as a Psychologist

The first push for credentialing of doctoral level psychologists came during the 1950s (Cummings, 1990). Today, every state offers licensure for doctoral level psychologists, and many states now offer hospital privileges for licensed psychologists. Such privileges afford psychologists the right to treat those who have been hospitalized with serious mental illness. Not surprisingly, psychologists have recently sought, so far with little success, to gain the right to prescribe prescriptions for emotional disorders (Foxhall, 2000).

Marriage and Family Therapy Credentialing

Today, almost half the states in the country have enacted credentialing laws for marriage and family therapists. In some cases, state marriage and family licensure boards are independent and generally have followed the guidlines set by the AAMFT. In other cases, such marriage and family licensure has been subsumed under the counseling board or the boards of other related mental health professions. Finally, the International Association of Marriage and Family Counselors (IAMFC), a division of ACA, has developed a certification process for family therapists that is offered through the National Academy for Certified Family Therapists (NCFT) (Smith, Carlson, Stevens-Smith, & Dennison, 1995, NACFT, 2001).

Credentialing as a Psychiatrist

Because licensure is not specialty specific, individuals are licensed as physicians, not pediatric physicians, psychiatrists, surgeons, and so forth. Therefore, a physician who obtains a license within a state theoretically can practice in any area of medicine. However, because hospitals need to hire board-certified physicians to maintain their accreditation, almost all physicians today are board certified in a specialty area (B. Britton, M.A., personal communication, March 9, 2002).

Credentialing as a Psychiatric Nurse

Psychiatric nurses can have an associate's, bachelor's, or master's degree and can be certified or board certified. Certification can be in a number of areas, including a generalist certification in psychiatric nursing, a certification in child and adolescent psychiatric nursing, and a nurse practitioner certification in adult or family psychology. In many states, psychiatric nurses can receive third-party reimbursement and have gained prescription privileges.

Credentialing for Counselors

Although the first credentialing of counselors can be traced back to the certification of school counselors in the 1940s (Bradley, 1995), counselor credentialing in the form of certification and licensure did not take off until the 1970s. Below is a brief examination of some of the certification and licensure gains within the past 30 years.

Certified Rehabilitation Counselors

In 1974, the field of rehabilitation counseling became one of the first counseling specialty areas to obtain certification for its members through the Commission on Rehabilitation Counselor Certification (CRCC, 2001; Livingston, 1979). This certification has certified over 30,000 rehabilitation counselors since its inception.

National Counselor Certification

In 1981, APGA established the National Board for Certified Counselors (NBCC), which offers the National Counselor Exam for Licensure and Examination (NCE). The test covers the content required by CACREP for accreditation of counseling programs (NBCC, 2001). Today, more than 31,000 counselors have become Nationally Certified Counselors (NCCs). Students who have graduated from a CACREP-approved program may take the

NCE prior to graduation from their program and, assuming they have passed it, are certified upon graduation. Those who have not graduated from a CACREP-approved program may take the NCE immediately following graduation; however, they receive their NCC only after they have successfully completed a minimum of two years of post-master's experience with 100 hours of supervision and 3000 hours of work experience. Finally, 40 states have adopted the NCE as part of their credentialing, usually licensure, process.

Specialty Certifications in Counseling

In 1979, the National Academy of Certified Clinical Mental Health Counselors (NACCMHC) became one of the first boards to certify counselors. In 1993, NACCMHC merged with NBCC and became a subspecialty certification of NCC. In addition to the clinical mental health certification, NBCC offers subspecialty certifications in addictions counseling, school counseling, and as an approved clinical supervisor (ACS). Finally, as noted earlier, the International Association of Marriage and Family Counselors has developed a process of national certification for marriage and family counselors. This process, which is currently separate from NBCC, is new, and its future is not clear.

In the past 20 years, the certification process has done much for the professionalization of the counseling field. Although the spread of licensing laws has led some to question the relevance of NBCC (Weinrach & Thomas, 1993), the NCC and the specialty certifications still seem an important credential. Signifying competence in our field, the NCC and the specialty certifications demonstrate a unifying force within the profession that links all specialties. Similar to physicians, where one is first a physician and secondarily a cardiologist, pediatrician, psychiatrist, or so forth, a counselor is first a counselor and secondarily a school counselor, community agency counselor, college student personnel counselor, or so forth.

> *The profession and practice of counseling will be strengthened if all counselors have a minimum foundation of counseling knowledge and competencies and build accepted specializations on that foundation.* (Pate, 1995, p. 181)

Counselor Licensure

The movement toward professional counselor licensure began slowly in the 1960s but picked up steam in 1976 when Virginia became the first state to pass a licensing law for counselors. Today, 46 states and the District of Columbia offer licensing (see ACA, 2001d). Although the NCE, discussed earlier, is used by many states for the licensure exam, remember that licensure is more involved than certification and may include taking the exam, sometimes additional course work, usually a minimum of two years of post-master's-degree supervision, and sometimes additional requirements.

Over the years the number of states that have credentialed counselors has quickly risen, and today there are over 140,000 counselors credentialed by 46 states and the District of Columbia (Neukrug, Milliken, & Walden, 2001). It appears that it will be a relatively short time before all the states will have a credentialing process.

Lobbying for Credentialing and Counseling-Related Issues

Political action committees, lobbyists, offering free lunches to legislators—certainly these are not the realm of counselors, or are they? Today, the lobbying and the grassroot efforts that counseling associations take to introduce and/or defeat legislation have become crucial to the survival of the profession. If there ever is a national health bill passed, and licensed professional counselors are not included as third-party providers for mental health services, the counselor as private practitioner might no longer exist. If counselors hadn't lobbied for the establishment of elementary and middle school counselors, they would not be in existence today. Counselors are constantly being challenged to show their worth—challenged to be accountable. In today's world, the public wants to see proof that the counselor's role is necessary. Lobbyists and our grassroot efforts help to show the importance of counseling. Credentialing helps to show the public that we are expert at what we do. Who pays for these efforts? We do! A portion of our professional association membership fees goes to pay for lobbyists and legislative days in which counselors get together to learn about the hottest political issues affecting them and devise plans to tackle these concerns. When you do *not* join your professional association you reap the benefits for which others are paying!

Multicultural Issues: How Our Standards Address Multicultural Counseling

Multicultural counseling is the hot topic in the counseling profession today. It is not surprising, therefore, that all of the standards discussed in this chapter are now addressing this important area.

Changes in ACA's Ethical Standards

Although some have attacked the last revision of the ACA ethical standards as continuing to favor Euro-American values while paying lip service to multiculturalism (ACA, 2001b; Pedersen, 1996a), it is clear that they go further than previous codes in addressing issues of multicultural counseling. For instance, the preamble states the importance of embracing issues of diversity, and multicultural issues are addressed throughout the code. For example, under Section A.2.: The Counseling Relationship: Respecting Diversity, the code states:

> *a. Nondiscrimination. Counselors do not condone or engage in discrimination based on age, color, culture, disability, ethnic group, gender, race, religion, sexual orientation, marital status, or socioeconomic status.*
>
> *b. Respecting differences. Counselors will actively attempt to understand the diverse cultural backgrounds of the clients with whom they work. This includes, but is not limited to, learning how the counselor's own cultural/ethnic/racial identity impacts her/his values and beliefs about the counseling process.*

The ethical guidelines also note that counselors should not participate in discrimination in hiring, promotion, and training or discriminate against clients, students, or supervisees. Also, the guidelines address issues of bias in the administration and interpretation of tests. In addition, the standards speak to the importance of diversity in the training and retention of students. Finally, there is currently a call by ACA to re-examine the guidelines to assure that they address multicultural issues.

Credentialing

Today, almost all credentialing processes require knowledge of multicultural issues in counseling. For instance, knowledge of social and cultural issues is one of the eight content areas covered in the NBCC exam, and state licensing boards and state boards of education invariably require knowledge of social and cultural issues in order to obtain a license or certification.

Accreditation

The CACREP standards of accreditation of counseling programs require knowledge of social and cultural issues in counseling as one of their eight curriculum content areas. This knowledge can be infused throughout the program and/or offered in a separate course in multicultural counseling.

Multicultural Counseling Competencies

The Association of Multicultural Counseling and Development has developed a set of multicultural counseling competencies that represent minimum standards needed by counselors to work effectively with diverse clients. Although not mandatory, these standards delineate attitudes and beliefs, knowledge, and skills in three areas: (1) counselor awareness of his or her own assumptions, values, and biases; (2) the world view of the culturally different client; and (3) intervention strategies and techniques (Arredondo et al., 1996) (see www.counseling.org/multi_diversity/competencies.htm).

Ethical, Professional, and Legal Issues

Unified Ethical Standards?

Herlihy and Remley (1995) note that out of the ACA divisions, seven have developed their own sets of ethical guidelines. They state that the proliferation of so many codes leads to difficulties in enforcing the codes and confusion for the consumer and professionals. For instance, counselors become confused as to whether to adhere to a specialty code, the ACA code, or both. And complainants are unclear about which ethical code governing body should be contacted when there is a problem. In an attempt to delineate some of the problems that result from a multitude of codes, ACA developed a lengthier, more complex code of ethics in 1995 that attempted to take into account ethical concerns of all specialty areas (ACA, 1995a; see Appendix B). Their hope is that some of the specialty areas will dissolve their codes in an attempt to have one unified code. We'll have to see what happens.

Counseling Online: Is It Ethical?

It's here. When counseling online first started people questioned it, wondered about whether it was ethical or legal, and debated about how to offer it. The Internet has become so popular that it was inevitable that eventually we would see counseling being done online. So, being that counseling online is a reality, ACA decided it was crucial to develop Ethical Standards for Internet Online Counseling (ACA, 1999). Take a look at them to see if you think it's feasible and ethical.

Promoting Professionalism

> *. . . professionalism is generally defined as internalized attitudes, perspectives, and personal commitment to the standards, ideals, and identity of a profession.*
> (Spruill & Benshoff, 1996, p.468)

Standards in our profession are a mark of our commitment to professionalism. However, standards are not enough to promote professionalism; it takes dedication on the part of the counselor. How does one make such a commitment? There are numerous ways, such as:

- Joining and becoming active in your professional associations.
- Acquiring certifications and/or licenses.
- Attending conferences and continuing education workshops.
- Advocating for legislative initiatives.
- Being a mentor to others.
- Respecting the need for ongoing supervision and the responsibility to supervise others.
- Abiding by the ethical guidelines or actively seeking change in them when disagreeing with portions.
- Embodying the personal characteristics that transmit to others that you are a professional.

The Counselor in Process: A Lifelong Commitment to Professionalism

Embracing a professional lifestyle does not end once one finishes graduate school, obtains a job, becomes licensed, has ten years of experience, or becomes a "master" therapist. It is a lifelong commitment to a way of being, a way that says you are constantly striving to make yourself a better person and a more effective counselor, committed to professional activities. Our profession has come a long way since the turn of the last century, yet 100 years from now our successors will probably look back and say, "How naive they were." We must be ever vigilant to improve ourselves and ultimately our profession.

Summary

This chapter examined three standards in the profession: ethics, accreditation, and credentialing. Noting that these standards are a reflection of the maturity of a professional group, each standard was examined in detail.

In the realm of ethics, we considered what is meant by moral beliefs and values and how these could conflict with our professional ethics. We also examined the relationship of law to ethics. The relative newness of ethical guidelines in the helping professions was noted, along with the pros and cons of having such codes. We spent some time examining the ethical code of ACA and noted that related professional associations also have ethical guidelines. Examining different models of ethical decision making, we explored how codes can be helpful in making ethical decisions and how such a decision-making process is probably mediated by the developmental level of the decision maker.

Noting the close relationship between ethical and legal issues, we highlighted the fact that poor ethical decision making is an invitation for civil or criminal action to be taken against the counselor. We distinguished between these two types of lawsuits and then showed the types of ethical complaints most likely to result in a lawsuit or disciplinary action being taken against a counselor. This was followed by an explanation of how to properly file an ethical complaint and the importance of having malpractice insurance if legal action is taken as a result of an ethical complaint.

The second standard discussed in this chapter was that of accreditation. A brief history of accreditation in the helping professions was noted, followed by the history, development, and implementation of the CACREP standards. Some benefits of accreditation were highlighted, and a short outline of the CACREP standards was presented. Accreditation bodies in closely related fields were noted. Highlighting that graduating from an accredited institution often makes it easier to become certified or licensed, we moved into a discussion concerning credentialing.

The last section of the chapter emphasized the benefits of credentialing and described the differences among registration, certification, and licensure. A brief overview of credentialing in related helping professions was offered, followed by the status of licensing and certification in the counseling profession. It was noted that a large number of counselors have obtained national certification, and most states in the country now have a licensing process in place. The importance of joining your professional associations was stressed, particularly in light of the lobbying efforts that the associations support.

Within this chapter we noted that multicultural issues are infused throughout our ethical standards. We showed how CACREP has included social and cultural issues as a major content area to be addressed when designing curricula for graduate programs. We also noted that all aspects of credentialing now include knowledge of social and cultural issues, and we told you about the multicultural competencies that many have suggested graduate programs should follow.

We noted that the proliferation of ethical codes is a recent ethical concern in the field and highlighted the fact that this could be a disservice to both the consumer and counselor. We noted that the new ACA code of ethics has attempted to incorporate ethical guidelines from all specialty areas with the hope that others will dissolve their codes in favor of ACA's.

As we concluded this chapter, we discussed the importance of a lifelong commitment to professional attitudes and behaviors. Specifically we suggested that counselors join and become active in their professional associations, acquire credentials, attend professional activities, advocate for legislative initiatives, mentor others, supervise and be supervised, address ethical concerns, and embody a professional attitude.

INFOTRAC and Other Information Resources (e.g., ERIC and PsycINFO)

Note: When relevant, key words are in quotation marks.

1. Compare and contrast different "ethical decision making models."
2. Compare the state of "credentialing" among the varying professional associations.
3. Review the current state of "accreditation" of counseling programs. How do they compare to related professional associations?

SECTION II

The Helping Relationship I: Theories and Skills

Overview

This section provides an orientation to some of the theories and skills used in individual counseling. Chapter 4 describes four broad conceptual orientations and some select theories associated with them, including the psychodynamic approach, existential and humanistic therapies, behavioral counseling, and cognitive therapy. Near the end of the chapter I will discuss two current theoretical trends: integrative approaches (eclecticism), and brief and solution-focused therapies. Chapter 5 examines some of the basic skills necessary for a successful counseling relationship, many of which are common to all of the theoretical approaches we use. In this chapter I will also discuss case conceptualization as well as the stages of the counseling relationship and highlight some of the skills associated with the stages.

As you read through Chapter 4, consider the similarities and differences among theories. Think about whether or not it is feasible to combine theories. Later, as you examine the many skills in Chapter 5, reflect back on the theories and consider which skills might be more applicable with the varying theories you have studied.

CHAPTER 4

Individual Approaches to Counseling

I've attended counseling a lot. My first counselor was able to hear the deepest parts of my being. He helped me work through some entrenched pains and hurts. He helped me look at myself and open myself up to my feelings. He was an existential–humanist.

My next therapist challenged me. He would ask me to close my eyes; get in touch with my thoughts, feelings, and sensations; and discuss them. He would point out inconsistencies, such as noticing that I would smile when I was angry. He would challenge me to go deeper into myself. He was a Gestalt therapist.

The third therapist I saw used to sit on his chair and listen to me, rarely responding. I would accuse him of being a psychoanalyst; he wouldn't say anything. I rarely, if ever, received feedback. I think he *was* a psychoanalyst, or at least psychodynamically oriented.

My next therapist was a good listener and would point out the choices I had in my life. He would try to understand what was important to me and helped me to redefine myself through the choices I made. He was a very well known existentialist therapist.

I saw a behaviorist for a short while. He helped me work on some very focused issues. He took a long history, and then we got down to work. I kind of liked it.

Recently, I saw a constructivist. He helped me understand how I make meaning out of the world. He did this by assisting me in identifying the thoughts I have and by helping me see the intricate ways that my thinking defines my being. This was interesting, but change sure seems difficult.

I've been in counseling a lot. I've seen male therapists, female therapists, short therapists, tall therapists, bad therapists, and good therapists. I think counseling has helped me become a better person. I know it has deepened me. I know it has helped me become a better counselor.

This chapter will examine four broad conceptual orientations of counseling and the theories associated with them. Under the psychodynamic approach, I will review Freudian psychoanalysis, Jungian analytic psychology, Adlerian therapy, and Mahler's object relations therapy. In the arena of existential and humanistic therapies, I will present person-centered counseling, existential therapy, and Gestalt therapy. In the area of behavioral counseling, I will give an overview of the generic practice of behavior therapy and review Lazarus's multimodal therapy and Glasser's reality therapy. Finally, in the area of cognitive therapy, I will review Ellis's rational emotive-behavior therapy, the cognitive therapy approach of Beck, and the constructivist approach of Mahoney. Also in this chapter I will present two recent trends in the practice of counseling and psychotherapy, eclecticism or integrative approaches, and brief-treatment approaches.

Why Have a Theory of Counseling?

. . . In theory-driven science, an unending cycle of discovery and testing creates and evolves theories of ever increasing scope that can guide counseling practice. (Strong, 1991, p. 204)

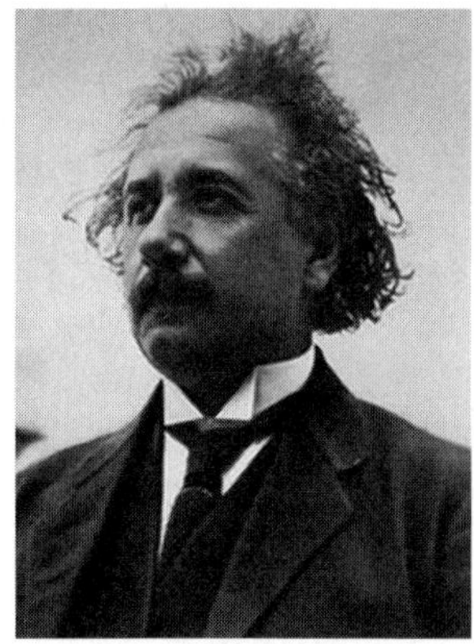

Albert Einstein

A former professor of mine would refer to the discovery of new knowledge as the virgin branch on a tree. Past knowledge leads to new discoveries, and new discoveries are only the result of all that has come before. So it was with the discovery that the earth was round; and with Einstein's theory of relativity; and so it will be when a cure for AIDS is found or a new counseling theory is developed. New knowledge is based on sound scientific hunches, connected to all of what has come before and only later accepted as scientific proof. As noted in Chapter 2, knowledge periodically leads to paradigm shifts. Such shifts occur infrequently and mark a change in the perception of scientific knowledge. Using our tree analogy, a paradigm shift represents a bud of the tree giving birth to a new branch. These shifts in our understanding of knowledge radically change perceptions of reality (see Box 4.1).

In the arena of counseling theories, it was not until Freud put forth his theory of psychoanalysis that the first comprehensive theory of psychotherapy was formulated. Freud's theory created a shift in thinking—it brought forth a new way of understanding the person. However, his theory was not developed in a vacuum; it evolved because others before him had pondered similar questions. Over the years we have learned that we can discard some of Freud's theory, accept other aspects of it, and continue to examine the rest. Whether it's psychoanalysis or New-Age therapy, theory offers us a framework in which we can research and ultimately examine which aspects of the theory may be valid.

A counseling theory offers us a comprehensive system of doing counseling and assists us in understanding our client, in the application of techniques, and in predicting client change. In addition, by examining what we say to our clients, we are able to evaluate whether we are acting congruently with our theory. Theories are heuristic; that is, they are researchable and testable and ultimately allow us to discard those aspects shown to be ineffective. Even more significantly, having a counseling theory tells the world that we are not haphazard in how we apply our knowledge (Brammer et al., 1993) because to "function without theory is to operate without placing events in some order and thus to function meaninglessly" (Hansen et al., 1994, p. 9).

Probably the most important aspect of any theory is its view of human nature, which is critical to the formation of the theory's template. Typically, the view of human nature each theorist holds takes into account the effects of biology, genetics, and environment on the personality development of the individual. So, if I believe that an

BOX 4.1

Chaos and Superstring Theory: Paradigm Shifts?

Our linear, cause-and-effect understanding of the world is being challenged these days by two theories: chaos theory and superstring theory. Read the excerpts below and consider how our perceptions of the world might change if these two theories are shown to have validity.

> Chaos theory: *That even an eensy change in input can make certain kinds of supposedly simple dynamic systems—e.g., weather, heart function, the stock market—go haywire. Therefore, since eensy changes in input are unavoidable, such systems have to be considered inherently unpredictable, that is, a certain amount of chaos is built into them. . . . [T]here's order lurking beneath the disorder; chaotic behavior itself follows simple rules and forms recognizable patterns.*

> Superstring theory: *The universe is composed, not of subatomic particles . . . but of tiny strings tied together at the ends to form loops. These strings exist in a ten-dimensional universe, which sometime before the Big Bang, cracked into two pieces, a four-dimensional universe (ours; that's three dimensions plus time) and a six-dimensional universe that [is] so small we haven't been able to see it. What physicists have been thinking of as subatomic particles are actually vibrations of the strings, like notes played on a violin.*
> (Jones & Wilson, 1995, p. 508)

individual's behavior is determined by genetics, my theory will reflect this notion. On the other hand, if my belief is that the environment holds the key to personality formation, then my theory would reflect this. Prior to reviewing the theories in this chapter, you may want to reflect on your view of human nature and personality formation. Then, read the chapter and consider which of the theories best aligns with your beliefs.

Well over a hundred years have passed since the development of psychoanalysis, and today there are more than 450 types of psychotherapy (Gabbard, 1995a). However, it is generally agreed that, based on the views of human nature of these 450 types, most of them can be categorized into four or five conceptual orientations. This chapter is organized to provide information on the psychodynamic, existential–humanistic, behavioral, and cognitive conceptual orientations to counseling and psychotherapy and offers an overview of a few of the theories associated with each. More specifically, the theories of psychoanalysis, person-centered counseling, modern-day behaviorism, and rational emotive behavior therapy, which are respectively associated with each orientation, will be presented with a moderate amount of detail, while two or three other theories within each orientation will be presented in brief form. The theories included were chosen due to their influence on the field, their popularity, and perhaps to some degree because of my own biases. As you read through these theories, examine what aspects you think would be particularly useful when working with clients. Then read the section on integrative approaches, sometimes called eclecticism, and consider how you might integrate some of your favorite aspects of the varying theories into your own unique approach. An integrative approach is used by many counselors today, as is the relatively new approach of brief therapy, which we will examine near the end of the chapter.

Four Conceptual Orientations to Counseling and Psychotherapy and the Theories Aligned with Them

Psychodynamic Approaches

Early Beginnings and the View of Human Nature

Beginning with Freud's theory of psychoanalysis in the late 1800s, many approaches to counseling and psychotherapy have been developed over the years that can be considered psychodynamic in nature. Freud (1856–1939), who developed quite a following early in the 20th century, dominated the psychodynamic field for almost half a century. However, because Freud tolerated little divergence from his viewpoints, many of his disciples eventually split from his rigidly held views and developed their own related theories.

Psychodynamic theories hold that an individual's personality is constructed through a complex interaction of an individual's drives with his or her early experiences. An individual's behaviors are therefore a result of early childhood patterning and are often unconscious. In other words, we have needs and desires that drive our behavior; and, based on our interactions with others during early childhood, we learn distinctive ways of satisfying these drives. Psychodynamic theorists believe that often individuals continue to meet their needs in the manner that they did when they were younger. Psychodynamic theories lean toward determinism, as they generally believe that early patterning is difficult and sometimes impossible to change.

In addition to Freud's theory of psychoanalysis, some of the many other psychodynamic approaches that have been developed include the theories of the neo-Freudians such as Alfred Adler, Carl Jung, Harry Stack Sullivan, Otto Rank, and Wilhelm Reich, and the object-relations theorists such as Melanie Klein, Heinz Kohut, and Margaret Mahler. Although they depart significantly from Freud's theory, all psychodynamic approaches focus on how drives and other factors motivate the client, how the past is instrumental in personality formation, how we consciously and unconsciously affect behavior, and how these forces combine in complex ways to shape and to some degree determine the individual's personality (Goldenson, 1984). On the other hand, some of the major differences among these theories are listed in Table 4.1.

This section will offer an overview of psychoanalysis and then examine in brief the neo-Freudian approaches of Carl Jung and Alfred Adler. Finally, the object-relations approach of Margaret Mahler will be discussed.

Psychoanalysis

As the first comprehensive psychotherapeutic approach, psychoanalysis dramatically changed the view of mental health and mental illness in the Western world. Freud, who was trained as a physician, to a large degree believed in biological determinism, or the notion that instincts and drives greatly affect behavior. However, Freud's explanation for personality formation was much more complex than just the notion of biology causing behavior, for Freud also believed that parenting styles within the first five years of life interact in a complex fashion with instincts and developmental stages to produce one's personality. Freud believed that we were born with specific instincts that pressed on us as we passed through what he called the psychosexual stages of development. Eventually the

TABLE 4.1

Comparison of Psychoanalysts, Neo-Freudians, and Object-Relations Theorists

PSYCHOANALYSTS	NEO-FREUDIANS	OBJECT-RELATIONS THEORISTS
Emphasize unconscious. Emphasize instinctual drives. Emphasize the influence of early development in personality formation. Instincts and early development determine behavior. Early development determines later development. Highly deterministic.	Emphasize conscious and unconscious with conscious taking priority. De-emphasize instincts. The individual is driven by social and/or interpersonal factors. Emphasize sociocultural and interpersonal factors as crucial to personality development. Behavior affected mostly by cultural and social factors. Early development is often but not always key to later development. Somewhat deterministic.	Emphasize conscious and unconscious with unconscious taking priority. Emphasize the ability to control instincts through consciousness. Early interpersonal factors are crucial to personality formation. Early interpersonal experiences affect behavior (instincts can be mediated by ego functioning). Early development is key but does not necessarily determine later development. Moderately deterministic.

structure of personality, which consisted of the id, ego, and superego, would be formed through a dynamic interaction of instincts, developmental changes, and early childhood experiences. Freud felt that it was necessary for the person to develop defense mechanisms to deal with the natural anxiety inherent in living as well as neurotic anxiety that resulted from faulty parenting and internal conflicts among one's id, ego, and superego.

INSTINCTS Freud believed that there were life instincts and death instincts. Life instincts included all of one's life-supporting drives, including hunger, thirst, and sexual energy. Sometimes called the libido, the life instinct directs behavior toward life-supporting activities and ultimately the continuation of the species. Death instincts, on the other hand, are humankind's tendency toward destruction and self-annihilation. Freud believed that the organism held remnants of the first living matter, which had a tendency to move toward an inanimate state (Nye, 2000). He postulated that the evolutionary process maintained this tendency and resulted in the individual's tendency to project self-destructive feelings outward. The death instinct also helped to explain suicidal behavior. Look around us, Freud said, and you see aggression running rampant, wars, hurtful behaviors toward one another, potentially lethal sexual acting-out behavior, and other evidence of self-destruction; isn't it obvious that we are at least partly motivated by a destructive drive!

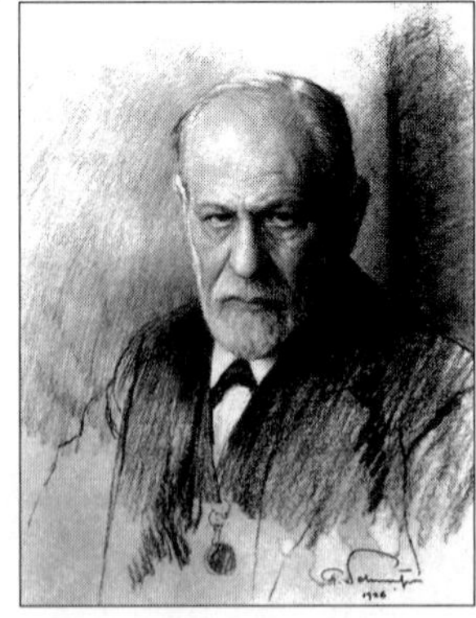
Sigmund Freud

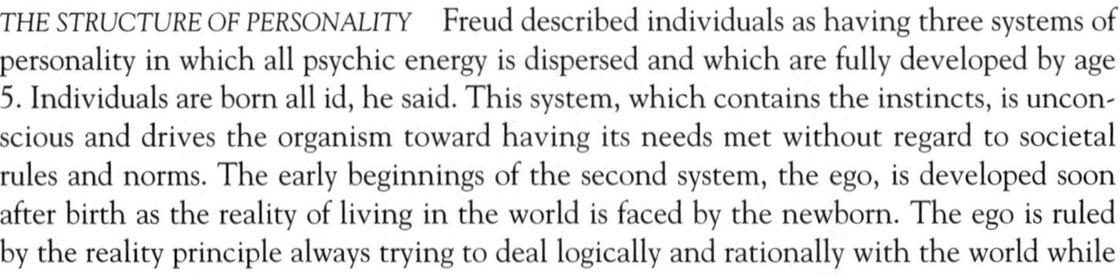
THE STRUCTURE OF PERSONALITY Freud described individuals as having three systems of personality in which all psychic energy is dispersed and which are fully developed by age 5. Individuals are born all id, he said. This system, which contains the instincts, is unconscious and drives the organism toward having its needs met without regard to societal rules and norms. The early beginnings of the second system, the ego, is developed soon after birth as the reality of living in the world is faced by the newborn. The ego is ruled by the reality principle always trying to deal logically and rationally with the world while

BOX 4.2

The Hidden Nature of Man (and Woman)

The film entitled *The Hidden Nature of Man* (1970) depicts the id, ego, and superego in an interesting way. A young man, interested in a woman, is having lunch with her. His ego is represented by him sitting at the table as he tells her how pretty she looks. His id and superego stand behind him and exert pressure on the ego (the young woman only hears the ego talking). The id, dressed in red, is saying "I want, I want! Warm. Breasts." The superego, dressed in white, is saying, "Honor thy mother. Be a good boy." The young man makes suggestive remarks concerning them going back to her apartment, and ultimately, the young woman notes that her roommate is away and suggests they go back to her apartment. Thus, we see the complex interaction of the id, ego, and superego. Clearly, what is not shown in this film is the woman's id and superego!

attempting to control the id. The last system, the superego, includes one's conscience and moral code. It also inhibits the id and attempts to supersede the rational behavior of the ego with moralistic behavior (see Box 4.2).

PSYCHOSEXUAL STAGES OF DEVELOPMENT Freud stated that the way energy is dispersed to the id, ego, and superego is a function of how children are parented during the first five years of life. He believed that parenting through what he described as the oral, anal, and phallic stages of development dictates later behavior. Later stages of development, called the latency and genital stages, affect personality development little, he said, but behaviors in these stages are reflective of what was learned in the first three stages. Although called psychosexual stages, Freud's reference to children's sexuality was described as "the experience associated with the child's discovery of his or her own body and the meaning of that experience to the child's parents" (Baker, 1985, p. 27). As you read the brief descriptions of the stages below, imagine how differing parenting styles can affect personality development as the child's erogenous zones shift from one part of his or her body to another.

Oral stage. During this stage, occurring between birth and 1½ years of age, the infant's erogenous zone is the mouth, and pleasure is received through sucking and eating. Withholding of the breast and/or bottle and food can greatly affect the child's sense of self and sense of trust and security in the world.

Anal stage. Obtaining control over bowel movements is a major task of this stage, which occurs between ages 1½ and 3. Pleasure is received through this control, and children begin to learn that they can control their bodies as well as their environment. How parents deal with toilet training and the broader experience of the child's sense that he or she can control the world is crucial during this stage (think of the "terrible twos" when the child is attempting to get his or her way and control the world).

Phallic stage. Experiencing pleasurable genital sensations is a major realization during this stage, which occurs between ages 3 and 5. Children in this stage will self-stimulate and have a fascination with bodily functions. They can be particularly affected by the moral imperatives of their parents.

Latency stage. Little occurs with children during this stage, between the ages of 5 and puberty, and there is a holding pattern as the child readies for adulthood.

Genital stage. Resulting patterns of behavior from the oral, anal, and phallic stages become evident as the young adult and adult exhibit behavior, consciously and unconsciously.

EGO-DEFENSE MECHANISMS Freud postulated that ongoing pressure exists on the developing child to express the raw impulses that originated in the id. However, the child quickly learns that expression of these impulses is disapproved of by parents, and he or she eventually learns to internalize the parents' code of behavior within the superego. However, being instinctual, the impulses continue to exist and press on the organism. Due to concerns about their parents' reaction to the expression of impulses, children may have fears of "annihilation, rejection, abandonment, isolation, engulfment, castration, loss of self-control, and impaired self-definition or identity" (Baker, 1985, p. 26). To manage these fears, children and adults create defense mechanisms. For instance, consider a child in the phallic stage stimulating himself. Seeing the child masturbate, the parent slaps his hand and says, "Don't do that." The child subsequently unconsciously fears annihilation and castration by his parent and develops a defense mechanism to deal with the impulse to masturbate in the future (e.g., perhaps sublimating the desire by getting very involved in sports). Such defenses are an important and healthy response to these fears and only become dysfunctional when any one defense becomes excessive.

Although there are many defense mechanisms, some of the more common ones are *repression*, the pushing out of awareness of threatening or painful memories; *denial*, the distortion of reality in order to deny perceived threats to the person; *projection*, viewing others as having unacceptable qualities that the individual him- or herself has; *rationalization*, the explaining away of a bruised or hurt ego; *regression*, reverting to behavior from an earlier stage of development; *sublimation*, channeling impulses into socially accepted forms of behavior; *identification*, identifying with groups or others in an effort to improve one's sense of self-worth; *compensation*, exaggerating certain positive traits in an effort to mask weaker traits; and *reaction formation*, replacing a perceived negative feeling with a positive one.

TECHNIQUES Traditional psychoanalysis is a long-term intensive process in which the therapist attempts to make the unconscious conscious, that is, to assist the client in understanding the intrapsychic forces that control and dictate his or her behavior. This is done through the use of a number of techniques, including:

Use of empathy. An important yet seldom discussed technique of psychoanalysis is the use of empathy and good listening skills. This allows the therapist to begin to build a relationship with the client while revealing little if anything about him- or herself. It also allows the therapist to set up the transference relationship.

Analysis of transference. A transference relationship occurs when the client sees in the therapist personality characteristics that are actually a projection of the client's personality. Projection of personality characteristics is facilitated by the therapist remaining aloof in the relationship, thus creating a blank wall on which the client projects. This is the reason analysts initially request clients to lie on the couch. Of course, such projection leads to a distortion by the client of the character of the therapist. Eventually, the therapist can interpret these distortions to the client, relate them back to the client's past relationships, and facilitate the client's uncovering of significant patterns in relationships that were crucial to the client's personality formation.

Free association. By encouraging the client to say whatever comes to mind without filtering, free association allows the client to uninhibitedly express his or her unconscious desires and repressed memories. This allows the therapist to understand patterns of past relationships and how they shaped the client's personality development.

Dream analysis. Freud believed that dreams were the "royal road to the unconscious." Therefore, analysts will examine both the manifest (obvious) content of dreams as well as the latent (hidden) meaning of dreams in an effort to understand unconscious desires and repressed memories.

Interpretation of resistance. Freud believed that clients would develop defense mechanisms and begin to resist treatment as important issues began to bubble up to the surface. Therefore, resistance is a sign to the analyst that the client is attempting to avoid an important issue. With careful timing, such resistance can be interpreted to the client and then explored.

THE THERAPEUTIC RELATIONSHIP Traditional psychoanalysis is a long-term, in-depth process in which the client may meet with a therapist three or more times a week for five or more years. In an effort to build the transference relationship, the counselor remains aloof from the client. Whereas empathy and listening skills are crucial to the beginning of therapy, interpretation and analysis become key techniques later in the relationship. As therapy continues, and as issues are resolved, the therapist will begin to be seen by the client in a more objective and realistic manner. Late in the therapeutic process, as anonymity becomes less important, the therapist may feel free to reveal small aspects of him- or herself. Ultimately, the relationship ends when the client has gained increased knowledge and awareness of underlying dynamics and how this gets expressed through his or her patterns and symptoms, and when the client has made some changes based on these insights.

SYNOPSIS Psychoanalysis is an in-depth therapy that assists clients in making the unconscious conscious. Seen as a pessimistic theory by many, psychoanalysis proposes that our personality is determined through a complex interaction between our instincts and our early experiences. However, with intensive therapy, we can gain insight and become a little more conscious of our personality construction. Today, it is the rare individual who can participate in traditional psychoanalysis, as it is very lengthy and costly. And, although much of the theory has not been borne out through research, many of the paradigms have been adapted by other counseling approaches and can even be found throughout our culture. Can you imagine not having the word "unconscious" in our vocabulary, or not having the belief that early experiences and drives affect our behavior? Clearly, Freud greatly affected all of our views of the world.

Jung's Analytical Psychology

A colleague of Freud, Carl Jung (1875–1961) was initially trained in the psychoanalytical tradition. However, as he developed he became disheartened by psychoanalysis, describing it "as a psychology of neurotic states of mind, definitely one-sided . . . not a psychology of the healthy mind, and this is a symptom of its morbidity . . ." (Jung, 1975, p. 227). Jung departed from Freud over his pessimistic, deterministic view of human nature, as well as some of his views on childhood sexuality. Instead, Jung optimistically believed that we could become conscious of unconscious forces and gradually integrate such knowledge into a healthier way of living.

> *For my part, I prefer to look at man in the light of what in him is healthy and sound, and to free the sick man from just that kind of psychology which colours every page Freud has written.* (Jung, 1975, p. 227)

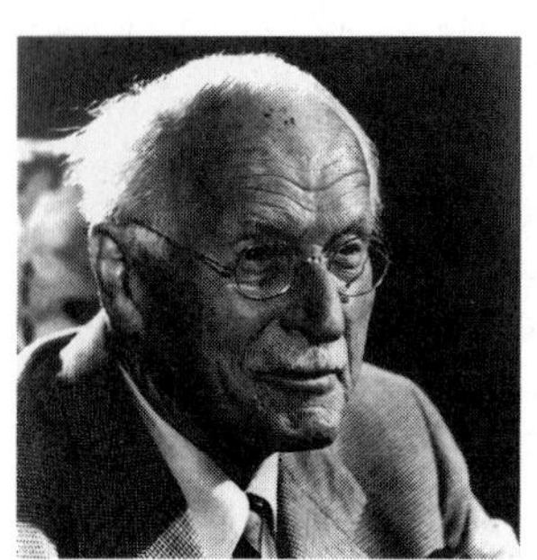

Carl Jung

Jung believed in a personal unconscious and a collective unconscious. The personal unconscious differed from person to person and one could become "conscious of almost anything" within the personal unconscious (Jung, 1968, p. 48). On the other hand, almost mystical in its nature, the collective unconscious is a depository of ancient experiences—an entity from the early beginnings of civilization that has been passed down to each of us.

> *The deepest we can reach in our exploration of the unconscious mind is the layer where man is no longer a distinct individual, but where his mind widens out and merges into the mind of mankind, not the conscious mind, but the unconscious mind of mankind, where we are all the same. . . . On this collective level we are no longer separate individuals, we are all one.* (Jung, 1968, p. 46)

The collective unconscious is both positive and negative and is revealed through archetypes. The archetypes include the persona, or the mask we wear in public life; the anima and animus, which represent the feminine and masculine characteristics that all of us have; and the shadow, which represents the darkest, most hidden, and scariest parts of ourselves.

Jung believed that the role of therapy is to raise consciousness about our unconscious and how it is exhibited through our archetypes. Awareness of all parts of ourselves, including our dark side, is the first step to integration and self-acceptance. Like Freud, Jung believed that our unconscious could be accessed through dreams and free association, as well as what Jung called active imagination. The information gained from these three methods of analysis holds symbols that are a source of hidden meanings and can assist a client in understanding his or her archetypes.

Adlerian Therapy

Like Jung, Alfred Adler (1870–1937) was originally trained in the psychoanalytic tradition and became Freud's colleague. However, discouragement over some of Freud's basic tenets led Alder to develop his own theory. Although Adler also believed that early childhood experiences greatly affected later personality development, he postulated that such experiences were mediated much more by social urges than by sexual or aggressive instincts. And, although Adler believed in an unconscious, he felt that consciousness drove individual behavior much more than unconsciousness. In addition, Adler believed it was not *what* happened in the past that influenced behavior, but the *memory* and *interpretation* of what happened.

Adler posited that we all develop styles of life that seek to compensate for innate feelings of inferiority. These styles of life are based on our perceptions of our past, particularly how we perceived ourselves within our family constellation. Feelings of inferiority motivate us as we seek to overcome them and as we strive for feelings of superiority and completeness. As with feelings of inferiority, Adler felt that all individuals had a striving for superiority, defined as a desire to achieve and do well in life. Adler believed that we are often victims of faulty assumptions about our lives that are based on false or inaccurate perceptions of the past and that end up affecting the choices we make in life. However, as opposed to Freud, Adler felt that through the therapeutic process individuals could understand their lifestyles and faulty assumptions and make dramatic changes.

Described as one of the first humanists (Corey, 2000a), Adler believed that people can change, create the future, make meaning in life, and be goal directed and not necessarily directed by past events. In fact, his concept of "encouragement" has been seen as a skill that embodies humanistic philosophy and can be used in brief treatment modalities. This skill includes showing empathy, communicating respect and confidence, focusing on strengths, helping clients combat faulty assumptions, and focusing on goals (Watts & Pietrzak, 2000). He also felt that success in life could be gauged by an individual's degree of social interest, or sense of connectedness to others and to a worldwide community (Adler, 1959). Although applied in many different counseling settings, Adler's approach has been particularly adopted by many school counselors because of its heavy emphasis on family constellation, birth order, and education (Dinkmeyer, 1982a, 1982b; Dinkmeyer, Dinkmeyer, & Sperry, 1987; Dreikurs, 1953).

Mahler's Object-Relations Approach

Margaret Mahler (1971) subscribed to the object-relations approach to therapy, which believes the crucial element in personality formation is the way in which the infant and young child separate and individuate from the primary caregiver within the first few years of life. This approach, which has recently gained in popularity, does not place as much emphasis on the id as a depository of sexual and aggressive instincts as did traditional psychoanalysts. Instead, object-relations theorists view such impulses as "appetites." This implies that at times we may have a desire to aggress or be sexual, but we are not pressure cookers, having to release such energy if appropriate outlets are not found. We are not, in other words, driven by these so-called instincts.

De-emphasizing the psychosexual stages of Freud, Mahler and other object-relations theorists feel that reality is inextricably connected with how one separates from the primary caregiver.

> *. . . the most important transitory step in the adaptation to reality . . . [is the one] in which the mother is gradually left outside the omnipotent orbit of the self.*
> (Mahler, 1952, as cited by Sugarman, 1986, p. 55)

Such individuation, say object-relations therapists, occurs through a maturational process within the first few years of life (Todd & Bohart, 1999). In Mahler's approach, this process occurs through four stages: normal infantile autism (birth to 1 month), symbiosis (2 to 3 months), separation/individuation (4 to 14 months), rapprochement (14 to 24 months), and consolidation of individuality or constancy of self (24 to 36 months).

Mahler, like many object-relations theorists, also believed that the infant needs to separate self-object experiences into good and bad (Alford, 1989; Klein, 1975; Kohut, 1984; Weininger, 1992). This defense mechanism, known as splitting, allows the very young child, who does not yet have the capacity to see individuals as complex, to split the person (the object!) into either "all good" or "all bad" (e.g., the 2-year-old who is angry at her parent one moment, and dependent and loving the next). Some individuals carry this splitting into adulthood, thus seeing the world in terms of good or bad, or having an "us and them" mentality (e.g., terrorists who see the world dualistically). Such a person is also likely to have difficulty in relationships as he or she flip-flops—one moment loving, the next moment hating. In actuality, this splitting is seen as a projection of the individual's early unresolved experiences with primary caretakers, who at various times were perceived by the young child as good or evil. One major challenge for the client (and people in general) is to gain the capacity to integrate bad and good images of others and thus maintain a more complex view of people.

Because object-relations therapies maintain many of the tenets of traditional analysis, their approach to therapy can be seen as a long-term, in-depth, analytical process that attempts to have the person understand early experiences in terms of separation and individuation. This is accomplished by having the therapist use empathy and interpretation as the client slowly relives early childhood conflicts with parents. Eventually, the client is able to integrate a new parental model and becomes individuated. In essence, the therapist becomes the healthy parent the client never had (Masterson, 1981).

Existential-Humanistic Approaches

Early Beginnings and View of Human Nature

At the turn of the 20th century, existential philosophy, with its emphasis on how people make meaning, became the popular philosophy in the Western world. Philosophers such as Kierkegaard, Tillich, Sartre, Camus, and others wrote about the struggle of life and how people construct meaning in their lives. Many of these existential philosophies criticized the psychoanalytic method for its deterministic view (e.g., Sartre, 1962). With the rise of Nazi Germany, many European philosophers and psychotherapists who held existential views of humankind emigrated to the United States. Their existential views were quickly taken up by many American psychotherapists who were looking for a more optimistic, less deterministic, and more humane way of working with clients.

In contrast to the deterministic view of psychoanalysis, existential-humanistic approaches believe in free will, that individuals either consciously or unconsciously create their existence and, if afforded the right circumstances, can recreate their existence—in other words, change. Most existential-humanistic approaches believe that there is an inborn tendency for individuals to self-actualize to fulfill their potential if they are afforded an environment conducive to growth (Maslow, 1968, 1970).

Existential-humanistic approaches take a phenomenological perspective as they stress the subjective reality of the client. In addition, these approaches de-emphasize the role of the unconscious while consciousness and awareness are stressed. Existential-humanists believe that anxiety is a natural part of living as well as a message about a person's existence. Every choice we make, including choosing not to choose, is a decision concerning how we live out our existence and is reflected in how we feel about ourselves and how we treat others. Therefore, existential-humanistic therapists do not try to "fix" or remediate one's feelings of anxiety, but instead attempt to help the client make meaning out of the anxiety he or she is experiencing. Deeply opposed to the reductionistic, nonpersonal tradition of psychoanalysis and early behavior therapy, existential-humanistic therapy stresses the personal qualities of the professional and how the therapist uses himself or herself in the relationship to affect change.

Although many modern-day approaches to counseling and psychotherapy have borrowed concepts from the existential-humanistic schools, a few in particular have taken on prominence in the field. The person-centered approach of Carl Rogers has probably most affected the art of psychotherapy, and we will explore this approach in some detail. We will also take a brief look at a school of therapy sometimes called "existential therapy," which is a conglomeration of a number of existentially based therapies such as those by Viktor Frankl (1963), Rollo May (May, Angel, & Ellenberger, 1958), and Dugald Arbuckle (1975). Finally, we will also take a brief look at Gestalt therapy, originally founded by Fritz Perls. Gestalt therapy was very popular in this country for many years and tends to offer a unique view of how existential and humanistic philosophies can be applied.

Person-Centered Counseling

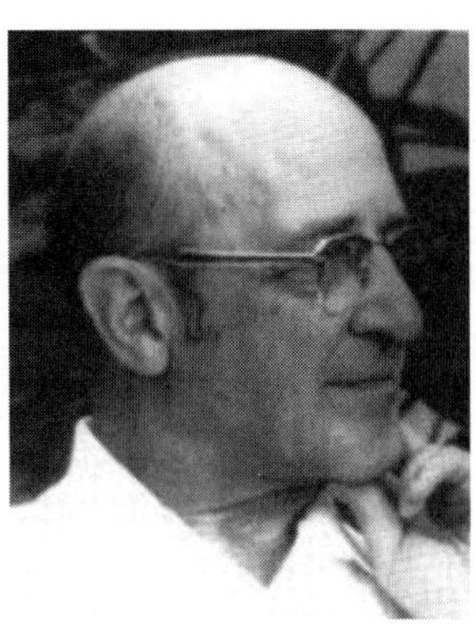

Carl Rogers

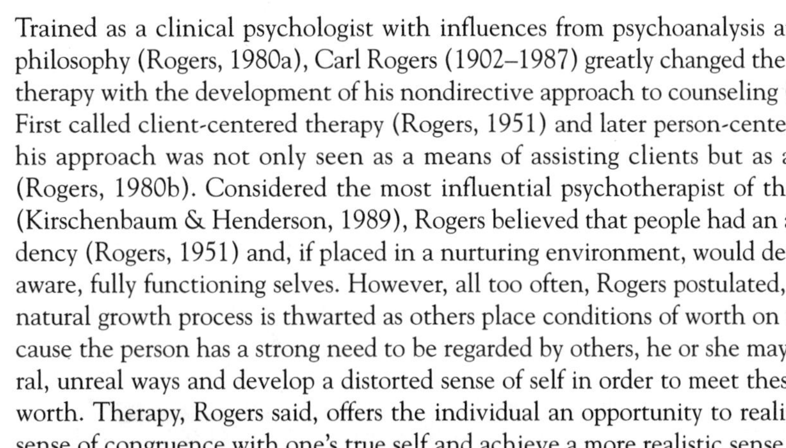

Trained as a clinical psychologist with influences from psychoanalysis and educational philosophy (Rogers, 1980a), Carl Rogers (1902–1987) greatly changed the face of psychotherapy with the development of his nondirective approach to counseling (Rogers, 1942). First called client-centered therapy (Rogers, 1951) and later person-centered counseling, his approach was not only seen as a means of assisting clients but as a way of living (Rogers, 1980b). Considered the most influential psychotherapist of the 20th century (Kirschenbaum & Henderson, 1989), Rogers believed that people had an actualizing tendency (Rogers, 1951) and, if placed in a nurturing environment, would develop into fully aware, fully functioning selves. However, all too often, Rogers postulated, an individual's natural growth process is thwarted as others place conditions of worth on the person. Because the person has a strong need to be regarded by others, he or she may act in unnatural, unreal ways and develop a distorted sense of self in order to meet these conditions of worth. Therapy, Rogers said, offers the individual an opportunity to realize an increased sense of congruence with one's true self and achieve a more realistic sense of what Rogers called the ideal self, or the self we strive to be (Rogers, 1959).

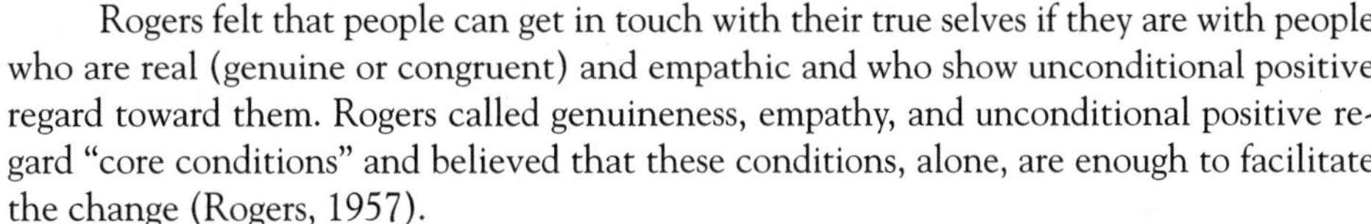

Rogers felt that people can get in touch with their true selves if they are with people who are real (genuine or congruent) and empathic and who show unconditional positive regard toward them. Rogers called genuineness, empathy, and unconditional positive regard "core conditions" and believed that these conditions, alone, are enough to facilitate the change (Rogers, 1957).

Because Rogers felt that the attributes of empathy, congruence, and unconditional positive regard were important in all interpersonal relationships, he spent much time later in his life advocating for social change and helping people understand differences among themselves (Kirschenbaum & Henderson, 1989). Working with such people as Protestants and Catholics in Northern Ireland, blacks and whites in South Africa, and individuals in what was then the Soviet Union, he attempted to get people who held widely disparate philosophical points of view to hear one another and form close, long-lasting relationships (see Box 4.3).

BOX 4.3

I Guess No One Is Perfect, Not Even Dr. Rogers

In the late 1970s I went to hear Carl Rogers talk for my second time. I was excited—Rogers was my hero. There were thousands of people in the audience, and as he fielded questions, I shyly raised my hand. Suddenly, he was pointing to me. I stood up, and blurted something out, at which point he asked me to repeat myself. I again tried to formulate my question, and he said something like, "I can't understand what you're talking about." He moved onto another question. I was shattered, hurt, and felt like rolling up into a ball. And, he, yes Carl Rogers, had not been very caring to this young counselor. I then discovered that even our heroes are not perfect.

THE NECESSARY AND SUFFICIENT CONDITIONS Rogers believed that personality change would occur if the following necessary and sufficient conditions existed within the therapeutic framework:

- Two persons are in psychological contact.
- The first, whom we shall term the client, is in a state of incongruence, being vulnerable or anxious.
- The second person, whom we shall term the therapist, is congruent or integrated in the relationship.
- The therapist experiences unconditional positive regard for the client.
- The therapist experiences an empathic understanding of the client's internal frame of reference and endeavors to communicate this experience to the client.
- The communication to the client of the therapist's empathic understanding and unconditional positive regard is to a minimal degree achieved (Rogers, 1957, p. 96).

Rogers believed that if the counselor could offer these conditions to the client, the client would begin to open up and understand past pains and hurts that were caused by conditional relationships in the client's life. In fact, such a therapeutic relationship could help the client change behaviors and assist him or her in movement from a false self to a real self. Other results of therapy could include: increased openness to experience, more objective and realistic perceptions, improved psychological adjustment, increased congruence, increase in self-regard, movement from an external to an internal locus of control, more acceptance of others, better problem solving, and a more accurate perception of others (Rogers, 1959).

TECHNIQUES Rogers did not refer to his conditions as techniques, as he believed they were natural ways of being in the world. However, he did spend much time attempting to define these qualities.

Congruence or genuineness. Rogers believed that the counselor needs to be in touch with his or her feelings, regardless of what they may be. A counselor may have strongly negative or strongly positive feelings toward a client, or feelings may emerge within the counselor during a session that may be mysterious, threatening, or frightening (Rogers, 1957). In either case, the counselor needs to be in touch with and aware of these feelings. The level of self-disclosure that the therapist shows the client, however, may vary depending on the session and whether or not the feeling was persistent. Rogers noted that although he may have had negative feelings toward some clients during a session, almost invariably these feelings dissipated as the client opened up and unraveled his or her inner self. This is why he warned therapists against using excessive self-disclosure. However, at the same time, he felt it was important to be real in the relationship. Finding the balance between the counselor's awareness of his or her own feelings and the expression of those feelings in an effort to be real is one of the challenges facing the person-centered therapist.

Unconditional positive regard. Rogers believed that counseling relationships should be highlighted by a sense of acceptance, regardless of what feelings are expressed by the client. In other words, the counselor should not accept certain feelings and experiences of the client and deny others. This unconditional acceptance allows the client to feel safe within the relationship and to delve deeper into him- or herself. As the client begins to take steps toward understanding this deepening self, he or she will understand those aspects of self that are false and those that are real. In other words, the client will begin to see how he or she is living out a false life as the result of past conditions of worth that were placed upon him or her. Although Rogers states that unconditional positive regard should be present for the totality of a session, he admits that this is the ideal and suggests that all therapists must continually strive to achieve this state of being.

Empathic understanding. Perhaps the most researched and talked-about element of the counseling relationship, empathy or deep understanding of the client was Rogers's third crucial element to the helping relationship. Such understanding can be shown in a number of ways, including by accurately reflecting the meaning and affect of what the client expressed; by using a metaphor, analogy, or visual image in showing that he or she heard the client accurately; or by simply nodding his or her head or gently touching the client during the client's deepest moments of pain. Such acknowledgment of the client's predicament tells the client that the therapist experiences his or her world "as if it were [his or her] own, but without ever losing the 'as if' quality" (Rogers, 1957, p. 99). In other words, the therapist is "with" the client; "hears" the client; understands the client fully, totally; and is able to communicate such understanding to the client.

Over the years, Rogers's explanation of empathic listening has been interpreted and often packaged into what many of us now call "reflection of feelings," or parroting what the client said. In one of the last articles written by Carl Rogers, he voiced anger toward some of the ways his concept of empathic understanding had been interpreted. Noting in particular the use of the terms "reflection of feeling" and "parroting" of client statements, Rogers stated that he never meant the counselor to mimic what the client had said but to use all possible avenues to show the client that the counselor understood his or her way of making meaning out of the world.

> *From my point of view as therapist, I am not trying to "reflect feelings." I am trying to determine whether my understanding of the client's inner world is correct, whether I am seeing it as he or she is experiencing it at this moment. . . . Am I catching just the color and texture and flavor of the personal meaning you are experiencing right now?* (Rogers, 1986, p. 376)

Rogers noted that the best empathic responses to a client are those in which the therapist is able to "subceive" feelings beyond those of which the client is aware. As opposed to interpreting feelings that the therapist thinks the client might be having, subceiving feelings means that the therapist is sensing deep feelings from the client, feelings of which the client may not be aware. Only when the client agrees that he or she is experiencing these feelings is the therapist "on target" with his or her response.

THE THERAPEUTIC RELATIONSHIP As might be expected, Rogers viewed the therapeutic relationship as one in which the counselor is effectively able to embody and maintain the core conditions of empathy, genuineness, and unconditional positive regard. The ability of the counselor to do this is directly related to the client's experiencing of a caring, empathic relationship in which the client feels accepted. This kind of relationship allows the client to experience a deeper level of knowing about self, facilitates client movement toward a truer sense of self, and awakens the ability of the client to experience some of the many outcomes of therapy as noted earlier.

When originally developed, person-centered counseling was considered a short-term therapy, at least in comparison to the then widely popular psychodynamic methods. However, with recent changes in the health care system and the move toward brief treatment, what was traditionally considered short-term is now seen as long-term. Although the principles of person-centered counseling can be applied if you meet with a client one time or for five years, generally person-centered counseling lasts from a few months to a year or more. Probably the most important determining factors in the length of treatment are the level of incongruence in the client and the kind of issues the client is bringing to treatment. However, it should be noted that many counselors today have integrated the core skills used in person-centered counseling with many of the shorter-term approaches currently used.

SYNOPSIS Rogers developed a type of therapy that has affected counseling and psychotherapeutic practices perhaps more than any other. The attributes of congruence, unconditional positive regard, and empathy have become core conditions used by many therapists across differing disciplines. His humanistic philosophy has not only affected the ways in which therapists interact with clients but has also had an impact on human relationships around the world. Although this philosophy has been criticized by some as too simplistic, many therapists have difficulties embodying the qualities of empathy, genuineness, and unconditional positive regard. Through years of research, properly applied person-centered counseling has been shown to be effective with a wide range of clients.

Rogers's influence from the existential-humanistic framework is obvious. Believing that people can change, his theory is strongly antideterministic. Trusting the phenomenological world of the client, Rogers does not offer a preset objective or interpretive framework in attempting to understand and work with the client. Instead, Rogers suggests that the innate actualizing process of the client, if allowed to flourish through the use of his core conditions, will facilitate client movement through the change process. This positive, person-centered, nondirective approach, argued Rogers, could make beneficial and long-lasting changes for the client.

Gestalt Therapy

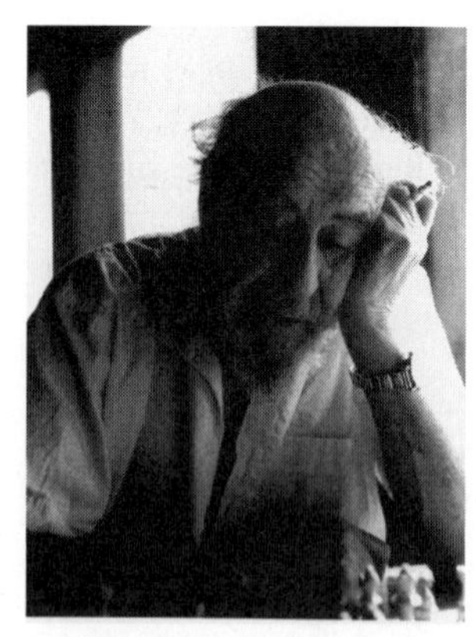

Fritz Perls

Developed by Fritz Perls (1969), this existential-humanistically based therapy shares some basic tenets with person-centered counseling but drastically differs in its implementation and use of techniques. Gestalt therapy is an antideterministic approach that aggressively proposes that individuals have the ability to change by becoming more aware of self. However, Gestalt therapists believe that individuals reach impasses in their lives, or get "stuck in their neurosis" and will spew "elephant shit" in order to maintain their neuroses. It is too scary, said Perls, to give up these neurotic patterns. This is why Gestalt therapists take an active, directive approach to the change process—an approach that confronts the client into awareness.

Taking on a strong phenomenological perspective by stating that awareness equals reality, the Gestalt therapist believes that one's current reality is often clouded by unfinished business from the past. It is therefore necessary to urge the client to experience the "now." Such awareness will help the client understand how he or she uses external supports to disguise his or her past hurts and pains. Such external supports might include the use of nonverbal behavior (imagine a person who unconsciously taps his foot when a potentially anxious subject is brought up), or intellectualizing (avoiding one's feelings by getting into one's head), or blaming others (rather than taking responsibility for her lack of studying, someone states that the midterm exam was unfair).

Because the Gestalt therapy approach assumes that individuals have a tendency to avoid unfinished business, Gestalt therapists have developed a number of techniques to confront the client into awareness (Passons, 1975; Zinker, 1978, 1994).

TECHNIQUES

Awareness exercises. With this technique the therapist asks the client to close his or her eyes and experience all the feelings, thoughts, and senses that are prevalent. This allows the client to quickly get in touch with hidden feelings or thoughts that are defended against when one uses the external world to avoid inner senses.

Use of "I" statements. Assuming that one of the most frequently used defenses by clients is the projection of issues onto people or things, the therapist will encourage clients to use "I" statements as frequently as possible. "This world sucks," becomes, "I suck, I don't take responsibility for my happiness."

The exaggeration technique. With this technique, the therapist asks the client to exaggerate a word, phrase, or nonverbal behavior that the therapist believes has some hidden meaning. For instance, a client who is slouched over might be asked to slouch more and to attach words to what it feels like to be so slouched. One client might say, "I feel as though the world is on my shoulders." Continued exploration by the therapist might find that the "world" represents demands the client feels placed upon him. Further exploration reveals how the client blames others for his inability to stop taking on tasks.

Empty chair technique. This popular Gestalt technique asks a client to imagine that a person or a part of the client's self is sitting in an empty chair. The therapist then helps to facilitate a dialogue between the client and this "other person" in order to uncover underlying issues within the client. For instance, a therapist might ask a client who feels as if she has the world on her shoulders to have a conversation with the world, eventually getting to the hidden meanings "the world" holds.

Playing the projection. When an individual has strong feelings about other persons or things, the therapist may ask the client to make an "I statement" about that person or thing. The assumption here is that the client's strong feelings about the "other" are really a projection of a strong feeling about self. Imagine a client who states that she doesn't trust men in relationships, saying "I don't trust myself in relationships with men."

Turning questions into statements about self. Gestalt therapists assume that all questions hide a statement about one's self. Therefore, the therapist asks the client to change questions into statements about self. Imagine a client asking "Why don't people care more about others?" stating "I feel that people don't care about me."

Other techniques. Assuming that individuals will often avoid responsibility, project onto others, and try to find ways of not dealing with hidden feelings, Gestalt therapists use a wide variety of other techniques to confront clients into awareness. For instance they encourage clients to "stay with the feeling," to play out different parts of their dreams, to make statements asserting that they take responsibility for their behaviors, and/or to act out the opposite behavior or symptom to which they seem to be exhibiting.

In summary, the Gestalt therapist is an active, directive therapist who has an existential-humanistic orientation and shares many similar goals with the person-centered therapist but who facilitates client growth in very different ways using a wide range of techniques.

Existential Therapy

A number of theorists belong to a school of therapy that relies directly on existential philosophy when working with clients. Such individuals as Dugald Arbuckle (1975), Rollo May (1950; May et al., 1958), and Viktor Frankl (1963) have greatly influenced this approach to psychotherapy. Corey (2000a) identifies six principles or underlying tenets that seem to be common among their approaches. They include:

1. *Capacity for self-awareness*. All people have the capacity for self-awareness.
2. *Freedom and responsibility*. All people have the ability to make some choices, regardless of their circumstances, and need to take responsibility for their actions as each choice a person makes will affect others.
3. *Striving for identity and relationships*. We have the ability to create our identity and to establish meaningful relationships with others.
4. *Search for meaning*. Part of the process of living naturally involves the search for meaning and purpose in life.
5. *Anxiety as a condition for living*. The nature of choice means that anxiety is a natural condition of living—we are always choosing to live life fully or to die.
6. *Awareness of death and nonbeing*. As we move through life toward our death, we have the capacity to become aware of the choices we make and how those choices affect our sense of selves and the lives of others.

Although there are no preset techniques that existential therapists use in applying the above principles, most existential therapists will stress the importance of the relationship between the therapist and the client, discuss the philosophy of existential psychotherapy and how it might apply to the individual's particular life circumstances, be authentic with the client, and view the therapeutic process as a shared journey. This shared journey is significant as it is only through a genuine relationship that change can occur. Therapy is not seen as a process of applying techniques but instead is viewed as a joint discussion concerning the meaning of life and how one can make constructive change to alter one's sense of fulfillment and meaningfulness. Therefore, inherent in existential therapy is the assumption that the client can change, has the ability for deepening self-awareness, and can build a meaningful and real relationship with the therapist that can have an impact on both the client's and the therapist's lives.

Although they have goals and underlying philosophy similar to the person-centered and Gestalt therapy approaches, existential therapists tend (1) to be more didactic than person-centered therapists in that they freely teach the existential concepts, (2) not to feel bound by Rogers's core conditions in assisting clients to explore their existence and ways of making meaning, (3) not to be as confrontational as the Gestalt therapists, and (4) to feel free to use any techniques that will raise the consciousness of the client concerning the basic existential principles.

Behavioral Approaches

Early Beginnings and View of Human Nature

Around the turn of the century, the Russian scientist Ivan Pavlov (1848–1936) found that a hungry dog that salivated when shown food would learn to salivate to a tone if that tone were repeatedly paired or associated with the food. In other words, eventually the dog would salivate when it heard the tone, regardless of whether food was present. Pavlov discovered what was later called classical conditioning. John Watson (1925; Watson & Raynor, 1920) and later Joseph Wolpe (1958) would eventually take these concepts and apply them in clinical settings.

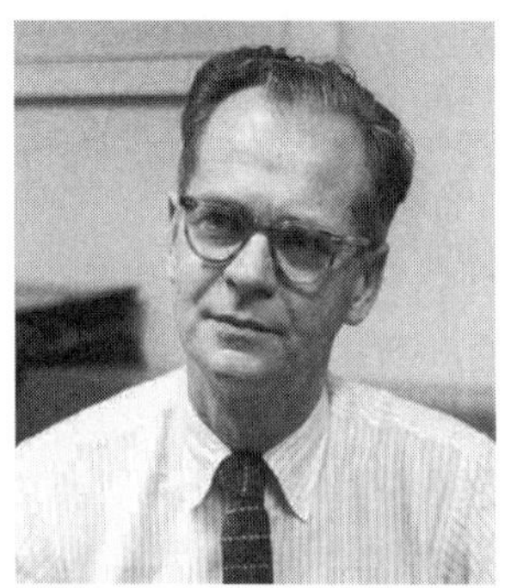

B. F. Skinner

During the 1930s the psychologist B. F. Skinner (1904–1990) showed that animals would learn specific behaviors if the behavior just emitted was reinforced (Nye, 1992, 2000; Skinner, 1938, 1971). His operant conditioning procedures demonstrated that positive reinforcement, the presentation of a stimulus that yields an increase in behavior, or negative reinforcement, the removal of a stimulus that yields an increase in behavior, can successfully change behavior. So proficient did Skinner become at changing behaviors in animals that during the Second World War he was able to positively reinforce pigeons so that they would steer gliders with explosives attached toward enemy targets (Skinner, 1960)! Despite great accuracy, the military decided not to use this pigeon-directed missile. As significant as the finding that positive reinforcement and negative reinforcement could change behavior was the discovery that punishment, the addition of an aversive stimulus following an unwanted behavior, was a very poor means of modifying behavior (Skinner, 1971).

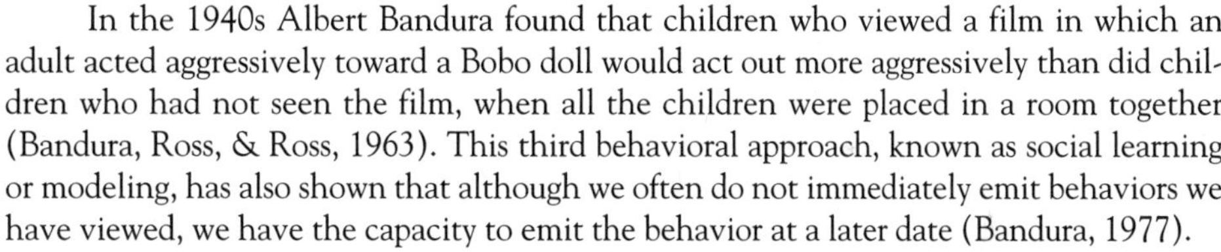

In the 1940s Albert Bandura found that children who viewed a film in which an adult acted aggressively toward a Bobo doll would act out more aggressively than did children who had not seen the film, when all the children were placed in a room together (Bandura, Ross, & Ross, 1963). This third behavioral approach, known as social learning or modeling, has also shown that although we often do not immediately emit behaviors we have viewed, we have the capacity to emit the behavior at a later date (Bandura, 1977).

The three behavioral approaches of classical conditioning, operant conditioning, and modeling share a common view of human nature and have been widely applied within the psychotherapeutic context. Generally, when working with clients, these three approaches are combined to afford the fullest treatment possible (Krumboltz, 1966b; Lazarus, 1971).

Behaviorism does not stress the unconscious and does not place emphasis on gaining insight into our early childhood experiences. Instead, this approach assumes that we have learned our current behaviors and can learn new behaviors by applying the principles of behaviorism. Therefore, by using classical conditioning, operant conditioning, or modeling in a scientific and empirical manner, we can explore with our clients the types of behaviors they wish to change and use these approaches to assist them in the change process. Although the past may have been important in conditioning our current behaviors, focusing on the past is not considered important in behavioral change.

In its early days, the behavioral approach was seen as a directive approach to working with clients in that the helpee's situation was examined and diagnosed, and strategies for behavior change were suggested and implemented by the therapist. However, the importance of establishing a relationship through such nondirective approaches as the use of empathy and modeling has taken on prominence recently (Spiegler, 1998). In addition, as opposed to early behaviorists who adhered strictly to their behavioral paradigms, it is now common to see behaviorists borrow techniques from other schools of therapy when working with clients. In fact, modern-day behaviorists rarely view the psychotherapeutic process in the rigid ways of the early behaviorists (Corey, 2000a). For instance, since the 1960s many behaviorists have included a cognitive component to behavior therapy approach (Beck, 1976; Ellis & Harper, 1997; Meichenbaum, 1977), and today many therapists use behavioral principles while working within a humanistic or even psychodynamic framework.

Today, many cognitive and behavior therapists identify themselves as cognitive-behaviorists. This chapter will separate the two for historical reasons and for clarity to the reader. Initially we will present in some detail a generic approach to modern-day behavior therapy that has been influenced by individuals such as Skinner, Wolpe, Krumboltz, Watson, and Lazarus. This will be followed by a brief description of two offshoots of behavior therapy, Lazarus's multimodal therapy and Glasser's reality therapy.

Modern-Day Behaviorism

Today many behavior therapists have adapted the theories of operant conditioning, classical conditioning, and modeling into one comprehensive behavioral process. Such an approach can be described through a series of stages.

THERAPEUTIC STAGES

Stage 1: Building the Relationship. During this stage, the major goal of the therapist is to build a strong relationship with the client and begin to clearly define the goals of therapy. Building the relationship can be done in many ways, and it is not unusual to find behavior therapists using empathy and listening skills, showing concern and positive regard, and discussing superficial issues in an effort to be friendly and build trust. As a supportive trusting relationship is developed, the therapist begins to explore specific problem areas the client would like to address.

Stage 2: Defining the problem and setting goals. During the second stage, it is particularly important that the counselor obtain accurate and broad-reaching information about the defined problem(s). The counselor must therefore secure adequate background information about the client and ask probing questions to reveal the true nature of the problem. A misdiagnosed problem sets the stage for the use of incorrect techniques. Once a problem is clearly identified, it is generally advisable to obtain a baseline on its frequency, duration, and intensity. This assists the client and therapist to fully understand the extent of the problem. After gathering all of this information, the client, in collaboration with the counselor, can begin to determine what issue to focus upon and set some tentative goals.

Stage 3: Choosing techniques. By drawing from social-learning theory, operant conditioning, and classical conditioning, therapists have a large array of techniques to assist the client through the change process. At this stage in the therapeutic process, the therapist must carefully pick techniques that closely match the goals delineated in Stage 2. Some of the more prevalent techniques included are discussed in the next section.

Stage 4: Assessment of success. Because a baseline of the intensity, frequency, and duration of the problem behavior is usually recorded, it is a relatively easy process to assess whether or not there is a lessening of the problem behavior. If no such progress is seen, it is important to reassess the problem and the techniques chosen (or recycle from step 2). If the problem was originally diagnosed accurately, and if appropriate techniques were chosen, the client should begin to see an amelioration of the problem.

Stage 5: Closure and follow-up. Reinforcement theory suggests that extinction of most behaviors will usually be followed by a resurgence of the targeted behavior (Nye, 1992, 2000). Therefore, it is important to remain with the client long enough to assure success and to prepare the client for a possible resurgence of the problem after therapy has ended. Therefore, many behaviorists build in follow-up sessions to the course of therapy. Of course, as in any therapy, it is important that the client experience a sense of closure when ending therapy.

TECHNIQUES Because the therapist attempts to make an objective analysis of the problem and choose techniques that will address specific issues, it is helpful to have a wide range of techniques at hand. Some of the more popular techniques used are noted below.

Modeling. Almost any behavior can be observed in the clinical setting and practiced by clients, first in the office and later on their own. Such behaviors as communication skills, empathic listening, paced eating, and study skills are just a few of the large number of behaviors than can be first viewed and later practiced by clients. Perhaps the skill most often taught and practiced within the therapeutic setting is assertiveness. Often demonstrated within a group setting, this behavior is viewed by a client and later practiced through role playing during the session.

Use of operant conditioning techniques. Following the establishment of a baseline, the counselor will work with the client to begin extinction of unwanted behaviors. Abruptly stopping a behavior is usually very difficult; therefore a process of slow extinction with positive reinforcement of new behaviors is often established (of course, some behaviors seem to usually work best if one goes "cold turkey," such as cigarette smoking). For instance, a weight loss program might have the client reinforce himself for a decrease in calories eaten (e.g., positive self-talk). In addition, the client's significant other could reinforce him for the gradual loss of weight (e.g., "You're looking really good!"). Also, the client might join a self-help weight reduction group for additional reinforcement. In addition, stimulus control could be introduced (e.g., only low-fat foods allowed in the home). Finally, other behaviors such as exercise or meditation might be introduced as a means of reinforcing a new lifestyle.

Relaxation exercises and systematic desensitization. Since an individual cannot experience anxious and calm feelings simultaneously, relaxation exercises are often taught to clients who are experiencing anxiety and/or fear. Although a number of relaxation techniques can be used, the classical relaxation procedure was developed by Jacobson (1938). In this method the client is progressively relaxed by focusing on each major muscle group in the body tightening and then feeling the muscle relax until the whole body is relaxed.

Relaxation training is also used as a component of the classical conditioning technique of systematic desensitization, where an individual pairs a fear response with the sense of relaxation. This method has been shown to be particularly successful when used for phobic behaviors. In working with clients using this technique, a hierarchy of fears is developed. For instance, imagine an individual who has a fear of elevators. A hierarchy might include (1) looking at an elevator, (2) standing in an elevator with the door held in the open position, (3) going up one flight in an elevator, (4) going up five flights in an elevator, (5) going up 20 flights in an elevator, (6) going up 50 flights in an elevator, (7) going up the Empire State Building. In the office, a counselor would start with the first level of the hierarchy, ask the client to close her eyes, do the relaxation exercise with the client, then ask her to imagine looking at the elevator. The client would be told to raise a finger as soon as she experienced any anxiety. When anxiety is felt, the counselor reestablishes the relaxing feeling and starts over. This technique takes time, sometimes as many as four or more sessions until the client completes the hierarchy. After completing the hierarchy in the office, the client can practice in real life. Nowadays, it is not uncommon for therapists to accompany clients while trying these behaviors.

Self-management techniques. Recently, teaching clients various behavioral techniques and having them develop and practice new behaviors on their own has become common. In this process it is important for clients (1) to select accurate and achievable goals and strategies, (2) to clearly understand the various behavioral techniques and the pitfalls that might be involved, (3) to do accurate self-monitoring, (4) to reassess the process if success is not achieved, (5) to follow through on the goals, and (6) to plan for future and expected setbacks.

Flooding and implosion techniques. Usually used in the treatment of phobias, flooding and implosion techniques involve having a client expose him- or herself to an intensive amount of the stimuli associated with the phobia. In flooding, the client either imagines being in the presence of the stimuli or actually places him- or herself "in vivo" to the stimuli (riding elevators in the Empire State Building for those who have an elevator phobia without desensitization!!!). Implosive techniques involve the use of exaggerated mental imagery that is in some abstract manner related to the phobia (e.g., imagine yourself in an elevator in the Empire State Building. You're going to the top floor. You get to floor 90 and one-half, and the elevator stops. You're stuck. And, you're in the elevator with your ex-spouse and a person who's hysterical!!!). Both techniques maximize anxiety with the expected result being an eventual state of relaxation because such intensive anxiety cannot be tolerated by the person for long periods of time. Eventually, the individual begins to feel calm with the stimuli. Obviously, such techniques should be used only by well-trained therapists.

THE THERAPEUTIC RELATIONSHIP Modern-day behavior therapy stresses the importance of a positive and caring relationship between the therapist and the client. This allows for trust and rapport to be built and affords the therapist a greater opportunity to accurately assess problem areas. In addition, it is important for the therapist to collaborate with the client and direct the client toward techniques that would best ameliorate any identified problems. The therapist also acts as an objective scientist who assists the client in assessing the frequency, duration, and intensity of the behavior(s) to be changed and who helps the client assess progress from an objective viewpoint. The client therefore experiences the therapist as a caring and humane person who can effectively listen, assess problems, teach the client about techniques, and direct the client toward treatment goals.

SYNOPSIS Behavior therapy was developed during the first half of the 20th century and is based on three types of behavioral paradigms: operant conditioning, classical conditioning, and modeling. Although behavior therapy was originally viewed as a scientific, re-

BOX 4.4

Can a Behaviorist Be a Humanist?

During the defense of my doctoral dissertation my advisor, who was a behaviorist, asked me if "a behaviorist can be a humanist." I went on to give what I thought at the time to be a rather esoteric response noting that the basic orientations of the approaches were philosophically different and therefore incompatible with one another. A few years later I had the opportunity to hear B. F. Skinner talk at a church in New Hampshire. Following his talk I went up to him and asked, "Can a behaviorist be a humanist?" Waiting a moment he turned to me, and with a deeply reflective look he said, "Well, I don't know about that, but he can surely be humane."

ductionistic, and a mostly sterile approach to counseling, today's behavioral therapist has integrated many humanistic methods into his or her approach. For instance, it is not unusual for the modern-day behaviorist to use empathy and develop a collaborative working relationship with the client. This allows the therapist to build trust and correctly identify targeted behaviors the client would like to change. After behaviors are identified, goals can be established and techniques chosen. The modern-day behaviorist has a myriad of techniques to choose from, and it is not uncommon for the behaviorist to start off working with the client within the office but later to work with a client in the field. Modern-day behaviorists act as humane, caring professionals and teachers of techniques who assist in directing clients toward treatment goals and a sense of fulfillment in life (see Box 4.4).

Multimodal Therapy

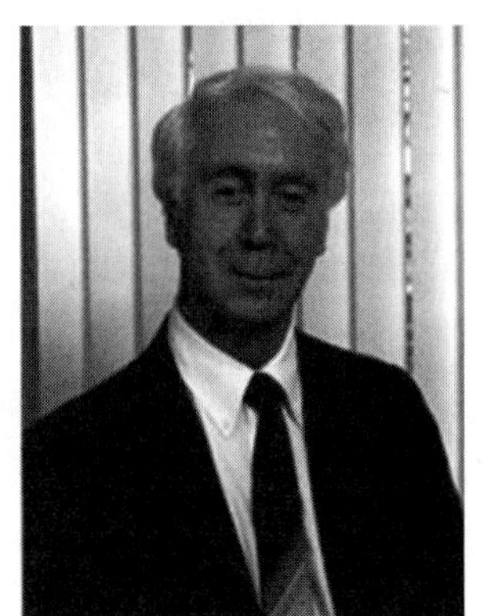

Arnold Lazarus

Feeling that behavior therapy had a limited range of techniques and strategies, Arnold Lazarus developed what he called multimodal therapy (Lazarus, 1976; Wolpe & Lazarus, 1966). Today, multimodal therapy employs a vast array of techniques and has been identified as a systematic eclectic approach by many (Lazarus, 1976; Lazarus & Beutler 1993; Mahalik, 1990). Because of Lazarus's attempts to clearly define the problem, set goals, identify techniques, and measure success, he seems in many ways to fit the modern-day definition of behaviorism. In addition, his theoretical leanings toward social learning theory and his lack of focus on "dynamic processes" point his theory more toward a behavioral orientation (Corsini & Wedding, 2000; Lazarus, 1986). However, as you will see, Lazarus's formulations have gone far beyond the more traditional work of the behavior therapist.

Lazarus's approach is based on a careful analysis of the client within seven modalities known by the acronym BASIC ID. In assessing a client's needs in therapy, Lazarus asks a client to develop his or her own modality profile by responding to questions in the following domains:

> *Behavior*. Make a list of those overt behaviors, such as acts, habits, gestures, responses, and reactions, that you want to increase and those that you would like to decrease. What would you like to start and stop doing?
>
> *Affect*. Write down your unwanted emotions, moods, and strong feelings (e.g., anxiety, guilt, anger, depression).
>
> *Sensation*. Make a list of any negative sensations related to your senses of touching, tasting, smelling, seeing, and hearing (e.g., tension, dizziness, pain, blushing, butterflies in stomach).

Imagery. Write down any bothersome recurring dreams and vivid memories and any negative features about your self-image. Make a list of any mental images or auditory images that may be troubling you.

Cognition. Make a list of any attitudes, values, opinions, and ideas that get in the way of your happiness. Include negative things you often say to yourself (e.g., "I am a failure").

Interpersonal relationships. Write down any bothersome interactions with other people (relatives, friends, lovers, employers, acquaintances). Any concerns you have about the way other people treat you should appear here.

Drugs/biology. Make a list of all drugs you are taking, whether prescribed by a doctor or not. Include any health problems, medical concerns, and illnesses that you have or have had (paraphrased and shortened from Lazarus, 1986).

Following a thorough analysis of the client's BASIC ID, straightforward treatment strategies and treatment goals are developed for each of the modalities. Although each modality will be addressed, some modalities will likely be stressed over others. Clearly, Lazarus's approach is pragmatic and can be adapted by any therapist who has an in-depth knowledge of treatment interventions and is able to match these effectively with clients' profiles.

Reality Therapy and Choice Theory

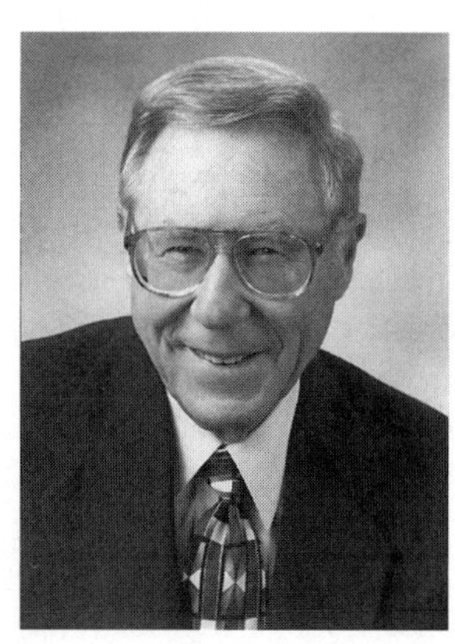

William Glasser

Reality therapy was developed in the 1950s by William Glasser, who borrowed concepts from existential therapy, behavior therapy, and, later, cognitive therapy (Glasser, 1961, 1965, 1994). Initially working with delinquent youths, Glasser believed that people are not victims of their past and can make choices in their lives to change their perceptions of themselves. In Glasser's more recent writings, he states that we have five inborn needs: belonging, power, freedom, fun, and survival. Glasser proposes that every behavior we exhibit is an attempt to have these needs met. However, Glasser also believes that sometimes we learn dysfunctional ways of getting these needs met, and these dysfunctional behaviors become the basis for how we perceive reality. He asserts that we continue to exhibit these behaviors, even if they are destructive, in order to maintain our view of the world. This feedback loop leads to Glasser's statement that, "Behavior is the control of our perceptions (BCP),"(Glasser, 1994). Through the counseling process Glasser believes that clients can be shown how they are creating their own reality through the behaviors they choose. Understanding that they create their own reality, clients can then be shown how to choose new behaviors which will ultimately affect how they view reality and how they feel; thus, the term *choice theory* (Glasser, 1999).

Glasser's theory is strongly antideterministic to the point that he believes that mental illness as well as most problems in life are an indication that a person has not yet found healthy ways of having his or her needs met. For example, Glasser believes that people depress themselves, anger themselves, make themselves psychotic, make themselves learning disabled, and so forth in a dysfunctional attempt to get their needs met (this is the only way they know). His goal is to assist clients in finding healthy behaviors that will meet their basic needs and eventually move them from a failure identity to a success identity.

For Glasser, the therapeutic process first involves creating a trusting environment. He does this by involving himself and being a friend to his clients. For instance, he might talk about common issues or activities a client enjoys. As the therapeutic process unravels, Glasser helps clients focus on what they are doing to continue their negative feelings and their failure identity. He gently challenges clients to take responsibility for their lives and encourages clients to identify the behaviors they want to modify. He believes that clients must devise a plan for change and that the counselor can assist the client in formulating this plan. Although Glasser believes a counselor should not accept excuses when clients do not follow through on their plans, he also strongly feels that counselors should make a commitment to clients and not give up on them. Clients who do not follow through need a reassessment of their plan and/or encouragement to keep trying.

Glasser's ideas have been applied to larger settings, such as schools and psychiatric hospitals. In these cases, involvement from the whole institution is crucial. The institution, says Glasser, must develop a set of behavioral rules, and all involved need to clearly understand and abide by them. Glasser states that noncompliance to rules should lead to specific natural consequences, as opposed to punishment, which Glasser frowns upon.

Glasser's theory is optimistic, action oriented, and forward moving, and it can be applied in many settings. Because many of the concepts are existentially and cognitively based, some could argue he should not be listed as a behavior therapist; however, because Glasser focuses on behavior as the key to change, I believe his theory has a home in the realm of behavior therapy.

Cognitive Approaches

Defining Cognitive Therapy and View of Human Nature

The early behaviorists paid little attention to the cognitions that might be mediating behaviors. In fact, Skinner (1972) stated that it is useless to look for internal causes of behavior, because they are only developed through external reinforcement contingencies:

> *. . . we have no direct access to states of mind, feelings, purposes, attitudes, opinions, or values. What we do is try to change the behavior from which we infer things of that sort, and we change it only by changing the environment. . . .* (p. 423)

However, since the 1960s cognitive psychotherapy has challenged this strict view of the radical behaviorists. Although most cognitive therapists believe that there is a complex interaction among thinking, feeling, and acting, as the name implies, their emphasis throughout the change process is how we think and make meaning in our world. This emphasis is not new:

> *. . . if you have right opinions, you will fare well; if they are false, you will fare ill. For to every man the cause of his acting is opinion. . . .* (Epictetus, c. 100 A.D.)

During the 1960s cognitive therapy became popularized by Albert Ellis (Ellis, 1962; Ellis & Harper, 1997). Not long after Ellis's views became known, a number of individuals joined the "cognitive revolution." For instance, Aaron Beck (1976), Donald Meichenbaum (1977), and Michael Mahoney (1974) offered new approaches in cognitive psychotherapy.

The traditional cognitive therapist believes the individual is born with the ability to think rationally or irrationally, with one's thinking processes becoming reinforced over the years, established and difficult to extinguish. Although feelings and behaviors may have an important role in the life of the individual, emphasis is placed on the thinking processes, with the belief that illogical thinking can be replaced by logical thinking in an almost surgical manner.

Recently, some cognitive therapists have moved toward a constructivist understanding of how people think and make meaning of the world (Mahoney, 1991, 1995a). Whereas the rationalist from the traditional schools views cognitive therapy as a logic-oriented process that involves replacing irrational thoughts with rational ones, the constructivist emphasizes how our construction of reality is based on a complex interaction between our thinking, acting, and feeling worlds, with each individual creating his or her own unique meaning-making system. And, whereas the rationalist uses common sense, logic, and rational thinking in an effort to change cognitions, the constructivist will use such techniques as story telling, metaphors and analogies, abstractions, unconscious suggestion, and other complex processes to assist the individual to adopt a new meaning-making system and a new view of the world that is more adaptive (Goncalves & Machado, 1998; Mahoney, 1995a; Neimeyer & Mahoney, 1995).

Although the traditional and constructivist approaches vary in some core ways, there is also much in common. Both are antideterministic in that they believe the individual can change. Both believe that one's current way of viewing the world is the key to making change, either in a logical, systematic way as with the traditionalists, or in a deeply self-reflective manner that analyzes meaning and offers a complex change process that relies mostly on abstract thinking (Neimeyer, 1995). Although both may not deny the concept of unconscious motivations, unconscious processes are not a core concept in therapy.

In this section I have chosen Ellis's rational emotive behavior therapy (REBT). Ellis, who is considered a traditionalist by most (Mahoney, 1995a) but a constructivist by himself (Ellis, 1988a, 1990, 1993), has greatly influenced the field of cognitive therapy. In addition, Beck's cognitive therapy (1976), which expanded on Ellis's ideas while offering some new directions for cognitive psychotherapy, will be discussed briefly as will the more recent constructivist notions of Mahoney (Mahoney, 1995b; Mahoney, Miller, & Arciero, 1995; Neimeyer & Mahoney, 1995).

Ellis's Rational Emotive Behavior Therapy

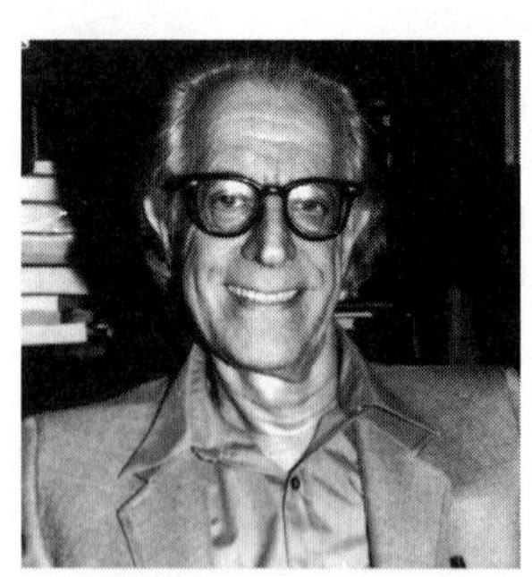

Albert Ellis

Ellis believes that humans create psychological disturbance by thinking illogically and by maintaining a set of irrational beliefs (Ellis, 1988a; Ellis & Harper, 1997). Individuals reindoctrinate themselves, says Ellis, with these illogical thoughts and irrational beliefs because our nature is to be highly influenced by others—others who themselves hold illogical beliefs:

> *Humans, in other words, are highly suggestible, impressionable, vulnerable, and gullible. And they are self-talking, self-indoctrinating, self-stimulating creatures. They need, of course, some environmental influences to develop into suggestible and self-propagandizing individuals, just as they need external stimulation in order to develop at all.* (Ellis, 1973, p. 34)

Ellis's therapy involves five basic steps. First, the therapist needs to convince the client that he or she is thinking irrationally. Second, the therapist needs to show the client how he or she is maintaining this illogical and irrational thinking. Third, the client needs to learn how to challenge his or her irrational beliefs. Fourth, the client needs to consider how specific irrational beliefs may be based on one or more of 11 generalized irrational beliefs that have become internalized (see Box 4.5). Fifth, the client needs to work on developing a more rational way of living in the world.

In order to assist the client in identifying illogical thoughts and irrational beliefs, Ellis has developed a number of techniques.

BOX 4.5

Underlying Irrational Beliefs

1. The idea that it is a dire necessity for an adult to be loved or approved by virtually every significant person in the community.
2. The idea that one should be thoroughly competent, adequate, and achieving in all possible respects if one is to consider oneself worthwhile.
3. The idea that human unhappiness is externally caused and that people have little or no ability to control their sorrows and disturbances.
4. The idea that one's past history is an all-important determinant of one's present behavior and that because something once strongly affected one's life, it should indefinitely have a similar effect.
5. The idea that there is invariably a right, precise, and perfect solution to human problems and that it is catastrophic if this perfect solution is not found.
6. The idea that if something is or may be dangerous or fearsome one should be terribly concerned about it and should keep dwelling on the possibility of its occurring.
7. The idea that certain people are bad, wicked, or villainous and that they should be severely blamed and punished for their villainy.
8. The idea that it is awful and catastrophic when things are not the way one would very much like them to be.
9. The idea that it is easier to avoid than to face certain life difficulties and self-responsibilities.
10. The idea that one should become quite upset over other people's problems and disturbances.
11. The idea that one should be dependent on others and need someone stronger than oneself on whom to rely. (Ellis, 1973, pp. 152–153, 242–243)

TECHNIQUES Although REBT originally focused mostly on cognitions (the "E" and "B" in REBT were added later), today there is more to this therapy than merely identifying irrational thoughts. In fact, Ellis freely admits that he will encourage clients to change their illogical thoughts in a number of ways, such as through the use of behavioral or emotive techniques. This is because Ellis believes there is an intimate relationship among one's thinking, feeling, and acting. The following is a sampling of the wide range of techniques that Ellis might use.

Using a technique called "uncovering the ABCs of personality formation," Ellis believed that it was not the activating event (A) that caused emotional consequences (C), but the belief (B) about the event. For instance, faced with a similar situation, the loss of a relationship, one person's belief system might lead her to feel suicidally depressed, while another person's belief system might lead her to feel fine about the breakup. Whereas one person might be making a catastrophe of the loss of a relationship and making self-statements (B) like, "I'm worthless," "I'm ugly," and "I'll never find another person like that person," a second person might be saying, "This is an opportunity for me to meet new people" and "The relationship sure did have its downside."

Within the therapeutic process Ellis encourages individuals to examine whether they are making rational or irrational self-statements. For instance, in the example above, although the loss of a relationship is a significant change in a person's life, there is no evidence that the individual is worthless or that she will never be involved with another person (irrational beliefs). In addition, the REBT counselor would encourage the client to examine deeper, underlying beliefs that may be related to her self-talk (see Box 4.5).

One role of the REBT therapist is to create a disputing intervention (D) for the irrational belief (B) that will effect (E) a new, and better, feeling (F). Therefore, counseling is an active, directive process in which the counselor helps the client identify irrational thinking and then assists the client in combating and challenging those irrational beliefs. In the example above, the client might start practicing by saying to herself such things as, "I'm worthwhile" and "I will find another relationship," in an active method of combating the ingrained self-deprecating negative thoughts. Thus, the disputing intervention is the client practicing self-talk (D), which effects (E) a new, more positive belief about self (B) and results in good feelings about self (F).

Ellis's other techniques include the following.

Cognitive homework. After clients leave the therapist's office, they can actively pursue cognitive restructuring by disputing irrational beliefs; identifying shoulds, musts, and the absolutist thinking that leads to such irrational beliefs; and continually working to reorganize their thinking to become less bound up and freer in life.

Bibliotherapy. By reading books that support Ellis's basic hypotheses and are specific to a client's problem, clients can continue to actively change their ways of thinking and acting and work on issues on their own.

Role-playing. Clients can try out new behaviors both in the therapist's office and on their own. This active process helps to challenge existing irrational beliefs and provides a beginning behavioral framework for change.

Shame-attacking exercises. Ellis suggested that to lessen the influence that people too often have on others, clients should do unconventional social things and practice being different. For instance, a person who is shy might go to a party and act outlandishly extroverted to the point where people avoid him. This allows individuals to shed the "shoulds" and "musts" and act in a more free-spirited fashion.

Imagery exercises. Ellis encourages people to imagine how they would like to be. Imaging, especially if followed by behavioral practice, can move an individual to new ways of being in the world.

Behavioral techniques. Ellis encourages using any behavioral technique that would facilitate client change. Such techniques as operant conditioning, modeling, assertiveness training, self-management, flooding, and implosion may be used in treatment.

Emotive techniques. Although often criticized for being too cognitive, Ellis is not immune to examining emotions. Despite not believing that catharsis is in and of itself curative, Ellis does believe it is important to examine one's emotions and understand feelings that may be a result of irrational thinking. Therefore, Ellis encourages clients to get in touch with their feelings in an effort to make a serious self-examination of their belief system.

THE THERAPEUTIC RELATIONSHIP REBT is an active, directive, and didactic approach to counseling. Ellis does not believe that the therapeutic relationship requires the necessary and sufficient conditions that Rogers advocated (see Box 4.6). What is important, states Ellis, is the client's belief in the philosophy of REBT, regardless of his or her feelings toward the therapist. Therefore, the therapeutic process involves a therapist who teaches the client about the ABCDs of thinking and encourages and confronts clients to actively

BOX 4.6

An Encounter with Albert Ellis

A few years after finishing my doctorate I considered doing a postdoctoral fellowship at the Rational Emotive Behavior Institute in New York City. I sent in my resume and was called for an interview. At first, I interviewed with one of the directors; then I was told I would have to do a role-play with "Al." I was brought in to see Al, who was sitting in a big comfortable arm chair. He proceeded to ask me to role-play a counselor. He was the client, presenting a male college student who had difficulty dating. I began to listen and respond with empathy, thinking that after hearing about the problem, I would move into an REBT style of response. After about three empathic responses in a row, Al said to me, something like, "Don't give me any of that Rogerian ____! I want to see a rational emotive counselor." I proceeded to give him what he wanted, thinking to myself, "He sure is serious about the unimportance of the 'necessary and sufficient conditions.' " I decided to not pursue the fellowship.

take on new ways of thinking and of living life. Ellis believes that the client must make the shift from being a victim of his or her own circumstances to being a person who can control his or her life and make active cognitive shifts and behavioral changes.

SYNOPSIS Albert Ellis has been a leader in developing and refining a rational approach to cognitive therapy. His approach assumes that individuals are capable of rational and irrational thinking and that irrational thinking, not events in one's life, causes negative emotional consequences. Based on this view, Ellis developed his ABCD theory of emotional disturbance in which A is the activating event and B the belief about the event that causes C, the emotional consequence. Once an individual identifies irrational beliefs, he or she can dispute (D) these beliefs and begin to live a less neurotic lifestyle. Ellis believes that the relationship between therapist and client is not as important as whether the client follows through with the techniques and understands the philosophy of REBT. Ellis has developed a number of cognitive, behavioral, and emotive techniques to assist an individual in moving from an irrational to a rational style of life.

Aaron Beck's Cognitive Therapy

Although similar in many ways to Ellis's theory, the underlying philosophy and some of the techniques of Beck's approach vary from that of Ellis. Although both Beck and Ellis work on the ways clients think, Beck disagrees with Ellis over the concept of irrational thinking, believing that this term is too loaded, too strong, and can potentially give the message to the client that he or she lives irrationally. Beck prefers to believe that problems in living are caused by cognitive structures. This disagreement over the term *irrational thinking* is representative of a broader difference between Beck and Ellis. Where Ellis teaches and directs, Beck collaborates and listens. Where Ellis persuades and cajoles, Beck softly probes into the client's cognitive world, and where Ellis disavows the importance of the conditions of empathy and unconditional positive regard, Beck states that for successful therapy to take place, a warm, nonjudgmental relationship is crucial (Beck, 1987). Overall, it is clear that Beck values the relationship and its impact on the change process much more than does Ellis.

After establishing a relationship, Beck assists the client in identifying hierarchical ways of thinking and perceiving that involve cognitive events, cognitive processing, and cognitive structures (Beck, 1972; Beck & Weishaar, 2000). Cognitive events are the never-ending stream of automatic thoughts that we all have but are often out of our consciousness. Getting in touch with our stream of thoughts can assist us in understanding the negative feelings that may be associated with a particular thought (Beck, 1976). Secondly, Beck encourages clients to understand their cognitive processes, which underlie the ways in which individuals process information. Such processes sometimes involve faulty thinking, which can lead to cognitive distortions and a false sense of reality. Examples of such distortions include dichotomous reasoning, where individuals tend to view the world in dualistic ways rather than seeing the world in a more complex fashion (e.g., "Republicans are right, Democrats wrong!"); personalization, where individuals assume that unrelated external events are somehow related to the individual (e.g., "My therapist was late for her session with me; she must not like me"); and overgeneralization, in which a person exaggerates the influence of an event based on little information ("I've had two clients not show for sessions this week, I must be doing something wrong"). The third part of the hierarchy is cognitive structures, which represent the schemata or floor plans that influence how each individual, with his or her own unique way of viewing the world, has made sense out of it. In essence, our cognitive structures mediate our cognitive processes (how we distort information), which in turn mediate our cognitive events (automatic thoughts).

Structures →	Processes →	Events
(Schema)	(Distortions)	(Automatic Thoughts)

Although each individual has his or her own unique set of structures, processes, and events, Beck believes that within diagnostic categories, one can find some similarities. Lynn and Garske (1985) note that, "The anxious individual processes information within a schema dominated by ideas of threat and danger. The depressed individual processes information within a schema of social rejection and failure" (p. 338). Beck believes that once a warm, caring relationship with the client is developed, the client and therapist can jointly reflect on the kinds of cognitive structures, processes, and events that are unique to the client. This process can be expedited if one has a clear sense of the client's diagnosis.

Mahoney's Constructivist Approach

> *From a Constructivist perspective, rationality is intrinsically relativistic, and, as such, it can only refer to contextually and historically situated efforts to attain meaning and coherence.* (Guidano, 1995, p. 93)

As noted earlier, some therapists have recently changed their focus from the rationalist tendencies of early cognitive therapists to the relatively new constructivist perspective to working with clients. Although usually placed within cognitive therapy conceptual framework, constructivist theory is often at odds with the more traditional, rational cognitive approaches of Ellis, and to a lesser degree, to that of Beck. Mahoney, who himself started out as a more traditional cognitive therapist, highlights some of the following concepts related to Constructivist notions of psychotherapy (Mahoney, 1995b; Mahoney et al., 1995; Neimeyer, 1995).

1. Constructivist theory challenges the assertion of objectivists that there is a single, authenticated, external reality.
2. Through the process of living and interacting with the environment, and as a function of our cognitive processes, people are continually creating and recreating their understanding of reality.

TABLE 4.2

Comparison of Rationalists and Constructivists Views

RATIONALISTS	CONSTRUCTIVIST
Humans are mostly rational beings who are beset by irrational thoughts. Thoughts can overpower feelings and behaviors.	Humans are complex with thoughts, feelings and behaviors being interdependent.
The thinking process obeys logical reasoning, which therefore means that illogical/irrational beliefs can be replaced by logical rational ones.	Thoughts are metaphors about our existence and how we make meaning. Understand a person's meaning-making system, and you stand a chance of assisting him or her in new and profound ways.
Psychotherapy involves understanding one's inner thoughts and replacing illogical thinking with logical/rational thinking that will lead to a mentally healthy individual.	Individual meaning making can be understood through the stories the person makes. Through a variety of psychotherapeutic techniques, new constructions of reality can be developed.

3. Deep underlying schemata, such things as unconscious processes and a person's sense of self and identity, are more difficult to change than surface structures.
4. There is a complex and inseparable interaction between one's thoughts, feelings, and actions.
5. We do not simply have thoughts and interpretations of the world; we are our thoughts and interpretations, constantly undergoing reconstruction as we interact with others in the world.

Comparing the more traditional rational approach with the constructivist approach, we find some major differences (Goncalves, 1995; Mahoney, 1995b; Mahoney et al., 1995) (see Table 4.2).

The goal of therapy for Mahoney and other constructivists would be to assist the client in understanding his or her unique ways of knowing and making sense out of the world and to help the client create new constructions that may work better for him or her. This would occur through a dialectical process in which the client shares his or her meaning-making system and the therapist attempts to understand and offer new ways for the client to make meaning or create a new reality. Partly, the therapist does this by attempting to understand how the client views significant past and present relationships. The narratives the client reveals about these relationships hold the meaning to the client's ways of knowing the world and to his or her unique cognitive structures. As meanings and deep structures become understood, the client may choose to change his or her ways of being in the world. The therapist can facilitate this process through a variety of techniques, including use of empathy, metaphor and analogy, hypnotherapy, traditional cognitive therapy, and any other techniques that may assist in revealing deeper structures and supporting the client through the change process.

Current Theoretical Trends

Integrative Approaches to Counseling (Eclecticism): From Chaos to Metatheory

The idea that a counselor might be able to combine two or more theoretical approaches when working with a client is not new (Lazarus & Beutler, 1993). In fact, studies show that between 39% and 70% of counselors and other mental health professionals identify themselves as "eclectic" (Jensen, Bergin, & Greaves, 1990; Neukrug, Milliken, & Shoemaker, 2001; Neukrug & Williams, 1993; Norcross, Prochaska, & Gallagher, 1989). Thus, it is important to determine how to combine theories effectively and to identify which approaches work best with which clients (Krumboltz, 1966a, b), especially in light of the fact that the efficacy of such practice has always been in question (Ginter, 1988; Kelly, 1991; Lazarus & Beutler, 1993; McBride & Martin, 1990; Nance & Myers, 1991; Simon, 1991).

Unfortunately, all too often a therapist who calls himself or herself "eclectic" is practicing a mishmash of techniques that have little or no underlying theoretical basis. This type of atheoretical eclecticism is counterintuitive and is considered by many to be "shooting from the hip" therapy. Eclecticism of this kind is not based on systematic research and is detrimental to the goals of our profession and, more importantly, to the successful treatment of clients. How then are counselors to make smart decisions if choosing an integrative approach to counseling? Although different models attempt to explain theoretical integration from somewhat disparate viewpoints (see Beutler, 1986; Gilliland, James, & Bowman, 1994; Howard, Nance, & Myers, 1986; Lazarus & Beutler, 1993; Mahalik, 1990; McBride and Martin, 1990; Prochaska & DiClemente, 1986), all of the models appear to address some common concerns that lead me to view theoretical integration as a developmental process that starts with chaos and ends with a commitment to a metatheory.

Stage 1: Chaos. Called syncretism by McBride and Martin (1990), this initial stage of developing an eclectic approach is atheoretical, sloppy, based on moment-to-moment subjective judgments of the counselor, and most likely hurtful to clients (Garfield, 1982; Patterson, 1985; Rychalk, 1985). Beginning counseling students who are just starting to understand counseling theory and are attempting to haphazardly combine theories may be at this chaos stage.

Stage 2: Coalescence. As theory is learned, most counselors begin to drift toward adherence to one approach. As they begin to feel comfortable with this approach, they may begin to integrate different techniques from other approaches into their primary approach.

Stage 3: Theoretical integration. During this stage, counselors have thoroughly learned one theory and are beginning to gain a thorough knowledge of one or more other theories. The knowledge that for many clients any of the theories may be equally effective presents the counselor with a dilemma: What theoretical perspective should I adhere to, and how might I combine two or more theoretical perspectives in a systematic fashion that will lead to the most effective treatment? Ultimately, the counselor is able to think through these important questions and develop a theoretical approach that can combine two or more theories.

Stage 4: Metatheory. As counselors develop a full appreciation of many theories, they begin to wonder about underlying commonalities and themes among the varying theories. This leads some counselors to develop their own or embrace an existing superordinate theory or metatheory (Beutler, 1986; McBride & Martin, 1990; Simon, 1991). For instance, a systems approach to counseling may take precedence over any one theoretical approach, and the counselor may integrate many theories within the systems approach. In evaluating one's metatheory, the following points should be addressed: (1) How are theories addressed within the metatheory? (2) How do client issues affect the treatment approach? (3) How is the therapeutic relationship developed? (4) What techniques are used, and how are they employed systematically? and (5) What causes change? (Mahalik, 1990)

If you are just beginning your journey as a counselor, you might expect to pass through these four stages as you begin to sort through the various theoretical approaches and develop your own unique style of counseling.

Brief and Solution-Focused Therapies

> *To many observers, it appears that interest in brief treatment has greatly increased over the past decade. Psychoanalytic, cognitive, interpersonal [e.g., Existential-humanistic], and behavioral clinicians, seemingly persuaded by theoretical factors, research findings, and/or the hard realities of third-party reimbursement pressures, have examined ways in which treatment can be made maximally effective in the shortest period of time.* (Budman & Gurman, 1988, p. ix)

A recent literature review of counseling and psychology journals reveals that between 1995 and 2001 more than 971 journal articles in some manner addressed the term *brief therapy* or *brief psychotherapy*, and one study showed that today 89% of all psychologists conduct some brief therapy (Levenson & Davidovitz, 2000). So, although various forms of brief treatment have been around for a number of years, there clearly has been an emphasis on brief treatment recently. It's interesting to note that what has been considered brief treatment in the past is now often considered longer-term therapy. For instance, person-centered counseling, which was originally seen as a brief treatment alternative to psychoanalytic therapy, is now considered by many to be a long-term treatment approach.

Pressure to offer brief treatment is coming from many places, such as health care organizations wanting counselors to limit sessions, schools viewing counseling as short-term, and agencies that have a limited number of therapists to work with a large number of clients. As a result, and with evidence that brief treatment may be as effective as longer-term therapy (Gingerich & Eisengart, 2000), brief treatment approaches seem an important and practical approach in today's world (Carlson & Sperry, 2000; Gelso, 1992; Koss & Butcher, 1986). Although brief treatment has its critics (e.g., Dryden & Feltham, 1992; Webb, 1999), it is clear that, for the near future, brief treatment approaches will be around.

Brief treatment has been defined by some as ranging from one to 20 sessions and by others as including as many as 50 sessions (Budman & Gurman, 1988; Dryden & Feltham, 1992). However, Budman and Gurman (1988) probably offer the most interesting definition when they note that "Brief treatment is therapy in which the time allotted to treatment is rationed" (pp. 5–6). Although all of the theoretical orientations we looked at in this chapter offer some form of brief treatment approach (Carlson & Sperry, 2000; Budman, 1981; Budman & Gurman, 1988), how the counselor feels about using a brief treatment approach seems more important to client outcomes than is theoretical approach chosen (Budman & Gurman, 1988) (see Table 4.3).

Garfield's Stage Model of Brief Therapy

Recently, there has been an emphasis on a cross-theoretical integrative model of brief treatment (see Garfield, 1998; Webb, 1999). One such model by Garfield (1998) suggests that all brief treatment approaches pass through four stages that include (1) building the relationship and assessing the problem; (2) developing a plan for the client, encouraging homework assignments, and working on the problem; (3) following through on treatment plans and reformulating the treatment plan based on new information and client feedback; and (4) termination, in which the client's feelings concerning progress are assessed,

TABLE 4.3

Comparative Dominant Values of the Long-Term and the Short-Term Therapist

LONG-TERM THERAPIST	SHORT-TERM THERAPIST
1. Seeks change in the basic character.	Prefers pragmatism, parsimony, and least radical intervention, and does not believe in notion of "cure."
2. Believes that significant psychological change is unlikely in everyday life.	Maintains an adult developmental perspective from which significant psychological change is viewed as inevitable.
3. Sees presenting problems as reflecting more basic pathology.	Emphasizes patient's strengths and resources; presenting problems are taken seriously (although not necessarily at face value).
4. Wants to "be there" as patient makes significant changes.	Accepts that many changes will occur "after therapy" and will not be observable to the therapist.
5. Sees therapy as having a "timeless" quality and is willing to wait for change.	Does not accept the timelessness of some models of therapy.
6. Unconsciously recognizes the fiscal convenience of maintaining long-term patients.	Fiscal issues often muted, either by the nature of the therapist's practice or by the organizational structure for reimbursement.
7. Views psychotherapy as almost always being useful.	Views psychotherapy as being sometimes useful and sometimes harmful.
8. Sees patient's being in therapy as the most important part of patient's life therapy.	Sees being in the world as more important than being in therapy.

SOURCE: Budman & Gurman, 1988, p. 11.

future plans discussed (e.g., follow-up, referral, ways of continuing progress), and closure accomplished.

Garfield also suggests that a number of common elements are present in all brief treatment approaches including: (1) the importance of a good therapeutic relationship; (2) a focus on interpretation, insight, and understanding; (3) some emotional release; (4) the confrontation of one's problem; (5) reinforcement of new behaviors; and (6) a gradual lessening of the seriousness of the problem. Some common techniques to all brief treatment approaches include listening and reflection, suggestion, providing information, confrontation, reassurance, homework assignments, modeling and role-playing, questioning, and self-disclosure. Of course, each therapist will use these techniques with his or her own special spin.

Solution-Focused "Brief" Therapy

One brief treatment approach that has received a lot of attention lately is solution-focused therapy (Gingerich & Eisengart, 2000). As opposed to many brief treatment approaches that tend to focus on the problem, solution-focused therapy suggests that the key element to brief treatment is to focus on the future (de Shazer, 1991; Hoyt, 2000; O'Hanlon & Weiner-Davis, 1989). In fact, these authors go so far as to suggest that focusing on the problem may actually be detrimental to finding a solution, as the problem is mired in power struggles among people involved with the problem and conjures up negative feelings.

Solution-focused therapists suggest that clients define what they want their future to look like and develop strategies that would help them get there. For instance, de Shazer

(1985, 1988) suggests the counselor ask the client to reflect on a "miracle question," which involves how the future would look if the client's problem(s) were miraculously solved. Then the therapist helps the client focus on creating a future that would reflect these changes. One can see how solution-focused therapy is in many ways an approach based in constructivism in that clients focus on reconstructing their meaning-making system (Hoyt, 2000).

Multicultural Issues

Counseling Approaches Are Eurocentric and Developed by Men

Let's start out by saying that just because a counseling approach has a Western perspective and was probably developed by a man does not in itself mean it's bad. However, we must look at how a Western and male perspective may hold certain biases (McFadden, 1999; Pedersen, 2000; Yutrzenka, 1995). For instance, such a perspective generally assumes that individuals are capable of change (pick yourself up by your bootstraps!), assumes that the self is more important than the community, de-emphasizes an individual's spirtuality, and stresses an internal locus of control. This may work for many, yet be antagonistic to some. Let's examine how the four conceptual orientations and brief treatment approaches examined in this chapter may hold bias.

Bias in Counseling Approaches

Psychodynamic Approach

Most forms of psychodynamic therapy are seen as long-term, thus the poor or even most of the middle class cannot afford to partake in it. These approaches place a heavy emphasis on the development of the self and de-emphasize the relationship of the self to the community. This approach assumes that, through the development of the self, the individual is the source of his or her neuroses and places little emphasis on how external conditions can be an ongoing source of problems.

Existential-Humanistic Approach

Existential-humanistic therapists believe clients create their own reality and are responsible for their existence; they emphasize self-disclosure and de-emphasize external influences. Thus, some Asian clients who believe that mental health is achieved by avoiding negative thoughts might be turned off by the emphasis this approach places on revealing deeper parts of self (Root, 1998). Also, some blacks who mistrust white counselors might be wary of the existential-humanist who believes this mistrust to be an internal creation, as opposed to an external truth (Poston, Craine, & Atkinson, 1991). In addition, because existential-humanistic therapists tend to be facilitators as opposed to problem solvers, some clients who might work well in a process that identifies problems and sets goals would be hampered by this model. Finally, clients who are faced with difficult life events that seem out of their control (e.g., racism, poor economic times) may feel helpless in the face of the existential therapist suggesting that the client is responsible for creating his or her reality.

Behavioral Approach

This approach places a large value on "rugged individualism." People can solve their problems if they follow the routine. Corey (2000a) states that the focus on the individual at the expense of the culture sometimes can be harmful for the cross-cultural client who places significance on the values of the larger culture. The behaviorist who stresses that the client must set goals for him- or herself without the realization of the importance of the larger community can lead some clients down a road of guilt and shame and to being ostracized by their communities.

Cognitive Approach

With cognitive therapy's emphasis on "irrational" or "unhealthy" ways of thinking, the culture-bound, unaware counselor may assume that a client is thinking irrationally when in fact this way of thinking is natural within the client's culture. For instance, whereas Albert Ellis stresses the importance of not believing that unhappiness is externally caused, some Hispanic cultures place a heavy emphasis on fatalism, "or the belief that some things are meant to happen regardless of the individual's intervention . . ." (Comas-Dias, 1993, p. 248).

Brief-Treatment Approaches

Like most of the other approaches, brief treatment approaches tend to view the problem as internal, while de-emphasizing the cultural context and stressing specific problem-solving activities (Steenbarger, 1993). Thus, like some of the approaches already discussed, brief treatment may isolate the culturally diverse client from his or her larger community and lead to feelings of depersonalization within the community.

Ethical, Professional, and Legal Issues

A number of ethical issues arise in reference to the counseling relationship. Although we cannot touch on all of these issues, we will attempt to highlight some of the more common ones. While reading this section, you are encouraged to review the Ethical Standards of the ACA (1995a) in Appendix A of the text.

Respecting the Welfare of the Client

One of the primary elements of the counseling relationship is respect for the welfare of the client (see Section A.1.a, Appendix A). This is done in many ways but includes promoting client growth and development, developing counseling plans collaboratively with clients, recognizing the importance of families in the lives of clients, and understanding the importance that careers play in a clients' lives.

Respecting Diversity

Counselors have a responsibility to not discriminate against clients of any culture and to respect differences of all cultural groups (see section A.2, Appendix A).

Clients' Rights

Clients have the right to be informed about all of the procedures of the counseling relationships and the risks involved. This includes information about the kinds of approaches to be used, billing arrangements, and the limitations of confidentiality (see section A.3., Appendix A).

Dual Relationships

Counselors attempt to avoid any dual relationships that may cause harm to the client. Some examples would include counseling friends, relatives, or coworkers. Counselors never have sexual relationships with clients (see section A.6., Appendix A).

Termination and Referral

When a client is no longer benefiting from the counseling relationship, the counselor has a responsibility to terminate the relationship and make appropriate referrals when necessary (see section A.11, Appendix A).

The Client's Right to Confidentiality

Clients have a right to expect that their conversations with counselors are private, except under specific circumstances that are explained to the client prior to the counseling relationship (see section B.1, Appendix A).

Exceptions to Confidentiality

Exceptions to confidentiality include the situation of a client in clear or imminent danger of harming him- or herself or of harming others. If a client might be in danger of harming another, the counselor has a duty to warn that person (see Box 4.7). Confidentiality can also be broken when the law demands that it should be, such as when a counselor is ordered by a judge to release his or her records to the court and the counselor has no legal footing not to do so (see section B.1.c.).

Privileged Communication versus Confidentiality

Privileged communication is a conversation conducted with someone that the law (state or federal statute) delineates as a person with whom conversations may be privileged (i.e., attorney–client, doctor–patient, therapist–patient, clergy–penitent, husband–wife, and the like). In the case of counselors, the goal of the law is to encourage the client to engage

BOX 4.7

The Tarasoff Case and Duty to Warn

A client named Prosenjit Poddar, who was being seen at the counseling center at the University of California at Berkeley, told his psychologist that as a result of his girlfriend's recent threats to break up with him and date other men, he intended to kill her. As a result, his psychologist informed his supervisor and the campus police of his client's threat, at which point the campus police detained him. The supervisor reprimanded the psychologist for breaking confidentiality; and, finding no reason to further detain Mr. Poddar, the campus police released him. Two months later he killed his girlfriend, Tatiana Tarasoff. Ms. Tarasoff's parents sued the university, the therapist, the supervisor, and the police, and won their suit against all but the police. The decision, which was seen as a model for "duty to warn," was interpreted by courts nationally to mean that a therapist must make all efforts to prevent danger to another or to self.

in conversations without fear that the counselor will reveal the contents of the conversation (e.g., in a court of law). The privilege belongs to the client and can only be waived by him or her (Attorney C. Borstein, personal communication, November 1, 2001; Swenson, 1997, p. 464). Counselors need to check the state where they work to see if they hold privilege. Generally, it is licensed professional counselors who have been given the right to privileged conversations, but there are exceptions, such as states that have given such a right to school counselors. Privilege communication should not be confused with confidentiality, which is the ethical obligation of the counselor to keep conversations confidential (Glosoff, Herlihy, & Spence, 2000).

The Counselor in Process: Embracing a Theory but Open to Change

For a few years after obtaining my master's degree, I remember dogmatically adhering to an existential-humanistic approach to my counseling style. I staunchly argued against a psychodynamic approach, even though I had minimal knowledge about this orientation. Although I was barely aware of it at that time, the views I had were at least partly based on some of my own unfinished issues.

As I have grown older, I have acquired a deep appreciation for all counseling approaches. I believe each of them offers us something. No doubt, as you have read through the various theories, you have identified more with some than others. Probably this is due to some personal style and perhaps some unfinished business of your own. Although I encourage you to practice and learn more about the theory or theories to which you feel an affinity, I also strongly suggest that you not get stuck in one approach; I hope that you gain some knowledge from all theories. As your professional life as a counselor proceeds, and as you read new research about differing theories, I hope that you remain open to changing your theoretical views and adapt your theory accordingly (see Spruill & Benshoff, 2000). Those who are closed to this ongoing process are stuck in one view of the helping relationship and are likely to hinder client growth.

Perhaps we can learn something from Hoyt (1995) when he suggests that counselors, like clients undergoing solution-focused therapy, might want the counselor to answer a "miracle" question:

> *Suppose tonight, while you're sleeping, a miracle occurs . . . and when you awaken you find you are helping clients in a more positive and effective way than before! How will you notice your practice has changed? What new skills will you be using?* (p. 8)

Summary

This chapter examined some of the major conceptual orientations related to theories of counseling and psychotherapy. By explaining the concept of paradigm shifts, we reviewed how past knowledge is crucial for an understanding of current knowledge. Relating this concept to counseling theories, we realized that such theories are our current best conception of what is effective in the counseling and psychotherapy process. We noted that by their very nature, theories are heuristic, or researchable and testable, and can be modified over time.

Focusing on psychodynamic, existential-humanistic, behavioral, and cognitive conceptual orientations, we highlighted each of their unique views of human nature and explored a few of the many counseling and psychotherapy theories most closely associated with them. More specifically, under the psychodynamic approach we examined Freudian psychoanalysis, Jungian analytic psychology, Adlerian therapy, and Mahler's object-relations therapy. In the arena of existential-humanistic therapies we explored person-centered counseling, developed by Rogers; existential therapy; and Gestalt therapy. By examining behavior therapy we saw that its origins were based on three major paradigms: operant conditioning, classical conditioning, and modeling; and within the behavioral orientation we specifically reviewed the generic practice of behavior therapy, Lazarus's multimodal therapy, and Glasser's reality therapy. Finally, in the area of cognitive therapy we reviewed the approach of Ellis's rational emotive behavior therapy, the cognitive therapy approach of Beck, and the constructivist approach of Mahoney.

Within this chapter we also explored two recent trends in counseling and psychotherapy, the adaptation by many therapists of an eclectic or integrative approach to therapy and the recent surge in the use of brief treatment. We highlighted a developmental process to an integrative approach to counseling with stages ranging from chaos, to coalescence, to theoretical integration, to adherence to a metatheory. We noted that although there are many forms of brief treatment, what might be most important is not the type of brief treatment, but whether or not the therapist is committed to brief treatment. We noted that Garfield believes that all forms of brief treatment contain common elements and techniques, and that they all should follow identifiable stages for treatment to be effective. We also suggested that another form of brief treatment, solution-focused approaches, tends to be future oriented and drawn from constructivist theory.

We examined in this chapter how most of the counseling theories used today have been developed from a European perspective that stresses individualism and the self and de-emphasizes the community and spirituality. We noted specific cultural biases inherent in the four conceptual approaches and in brief treatment approaches examined in this chapter.

In this chapter we also noted a number of ethical, professional, and legal issues that impinge on the counseling relationship, including respecting the welfare of the client, respecting diversity, client rights, dual relationships, termination and referral, and having the client give informed consent. We noted the importance of respecting the client's right to confidentiality and times when confidentiality can be breeched, such as when there is a duty to warn. Finally, we ended this chapter by stressing the importance of adhering to a counseling approach yet leaving ourselves open to new ideas and new ways of working with clients.

INFOTRAC and Other Information Resources (e.g., ERIC and PsycINFO)

Note: When relevant, key words are in quotation marks.

1. Delve more deeply into any one of the conceptual orientations discussed in the chapter ("psychodynamic," "existential," "behavioral," "cognitive," "brief").
2. Develop your own "integrative" ("eclectic") approach to counseling.
3. Research the "limits of confidentiality."

CHAPTER 5

Counseling Skills

The first time I counseled was at a drug crisis clinic in college. I had no training, but somehow I instinctively knew that it was probably best to listen and have a caring attitude. I had never had a course in counseling theories or counseling methods. I knew little about the correct way to respond to a drop-in at the center. Hopefully, I did more good than harm as I tried to help students who had overdosed or were "bumming."

In graduate school I learned the way to counsel. I became an ardent existential-humanist and believed that it was best to help people express their feelings. After obtaining a job at a crisis center, I began to practice my skills on my unsuspecting clients. Although my counseling approach had become somewhat focused, my old untrained self, which sometimes would get very advice oriented, periodically raised its ugly head.

Over the years I have had numerous jobs, obtained my doctorate, attended continuing education workshops, and read the professional journals. Experience, education, and reading have all helped me fine-tune my skills. Although there are some whom I believe to be natural counselors, I have come to suspect that one is not born with an ability to counsel, but must learn, as I have, how to apply counseling skills. In fact, even those with natural ability need training to become masters at what they do.

Much like riding a bicycle or putting on rollerblades for the first time, learning counseling skills at first feels awkward. However, you will find that the more you practice, the more natural and at ease you will feel. In my own life, I now approach the learning and refinement of my skills as a never-ending process.

This chapter will examine the importance of the counseling environment and some of the techniques that have been shown to be effective in working with clients. We will also explore one model of client case conceptualization, which is a method of organizing one's thinking around working on client problems. In addition we will identify six stages of counseling and review how the case conceptualization process can be understood in relationship to these stages. The chapter will also present important issues related to record keeping and the keeping of case notes.

The Counseling Environment

A client who walks into a counselor's office immediately encounters the world of the counselor as reflected in his or her work environment. Soon, this client will be asked to look at his or her own inner world. Although we have no control over the defensiveness the client brings to the session, through a careful assessment of the counseling environment we can reduce or eliminate any external irritation that might increase that defensiveness. Thus, that first experience of the counselor's environment is crucial to building an effective counseling relationship.

What creates the counseling environment? Three components are particularly important: the office itself, the use of nonverbal behaviors, and how the counselor presents him- or herself to the client. Let's take a look at how each of these important factors plays a role in the success or failure of the counseling relationship.

The Office

Whether in an agency, business, or school, doing counseling requires that you have a place to go where you can establish your relationship. Almost always, this will be your office. The counseling relationship requires the quiet, comfort, safety, and confidentiality that an office provides. Although school counselors and others may find that their job necessitates the building of relationships outside an office, ultimately the office allows one to deepen the relationship.

The arrangement of one's office can be crucial to eliciting positive attitudes from people (Pressly & Heesacker, 2001). How should the office be arranged? There is little question that it should be soundproofed, have soft lighting, be relatively uncluttered, have client records filed, be free from distractions such as the phone ringing or knocks on the door, and have comfortable seating. As we create our offices, each of us will try to find a balance between having our office reflect our taste and having it still be appealing to the vast majority of our clients (see Box 5.1).

Of course, no matter how you arrange your office, there will be some people who are offended by something. Thus, Scissons (1993) suggests that "[a]t the very least, [office] arrangements should not adversely impinge on the process or outcome" of counseling (p. 149). Of course, it may be that you will want to attract a certain clientele who would

BOX 5.1

What Should Your Office Look Like?

Review the items below and reflect on whether or not you think any of them would be offensive to you if you walked into a counseling office. Then think about the most liberal and the most conservative person you know and imagine how he or she might feel with each of the following:

- Feminist literature.
- A bear rug.
- Gay literature.
- A cluttered desk.
- Information on abortion.
- Religious artwork.
- A compulsively clean desk.
- An AIDS pin.
- A desk between you and your client.
- Information on female and male sexuality.

feel comfortable with a particular ambiance. For instance, a Christian counselor might include articles of a religious nature in his or her office, while a person dealing with mostly gay issues might include gay literature in his or her office.

How one dresses and the language one uses with clients are two more components of the office environment. Should you wear jeans at work? What about an expensive suit? Are your clothes revealing? What does your jewelry or hairstyle say about you? Do you call your client by his or her first name? Should you change your mode of language for the client, such as using less complex language for a client who is less educated? Ultimately, each counselor must determine the importance of these factors and how they will be addressed.

Nonverbal Behavior

> *. . . when humans communicate, as much as eighty percent of the meaning of their messages is derived from nonverbal language. The implication is disturbing. As far as communication is concerned, human beings spend most of their time studying the wrong thing.* (Thompson, 1973, p. 1)

The importance of our nonverbal interactions with clients is vastly underrated. In fact, nonverbal behavior seems largely out of a person's conscious control (Argyle, 1975; Wolfgang, 1985); is difficult to censor; and, as compared to verbal behavior, is often a more accurate representation of how the client and the counselor feel (Mehrabian, 1972). Posture or tone of voice that communicates, "Don't open up to me," will obviously affect clients in very different ways than the counselor who is nonverbally communicating, "I'm open to hearing what you have to say." We tell our clients that we are there for them through our body posture, our eye contact, and in the types of verbal responses we make.

Personal space is an additional nonverbal factor that affects the counseling relationship (Germain, 1981; Sommer, 1959). Mediated at least somewhat by culture, age, and gender, individuals vary greatly in their degree of comfort with personal space (Evans & Howard, 1973). Therefore, the counselor must allow for enough personal space so that the client feels comfortable, yet not so much that the client feels distant from the counselor. Although this will generally happen in very subtle ways, when necessary, the counselor should take the lead in respecting the client's need for personal space.

Touch is a final aspect of nonverbal behavior important to the counseling relationship. Touching at important moments is quite natural. For instance, when someone is expressing deep pain, it is not unusual for us to hold a hand or embrace a person while he or she sobs. Or, when a person is coming to or leaving a session, many of us may find it natural to place a hand on a shoulder or give a hug. However, in today's litigious society, touch has become a particularly delicate subject, and it is important for each of us to be sensitive to our clients' boundaries, our own boundaries, and limits as suggested by our professional ethics (Gabbard, 1995b). Some have become so touchy over this issue that a therapist in Massachusetts, branded "the hugging therapist," was fired from his job at a mental health agency because he hugged his clients too much. Brammer and MacDonald (1999) suggest that whether or not one has physical contact with a client should be based on (1) the helper's assessment of the helpee, (2) the helper's awareness of his or her own needs, (3) what is most likely to be helpful within the counseling relationship, and (4) risks that may be involved as a function of agency policy, customs, personal ethics, and the law.

Traditionally, counselors have been taught to lean forward, have good eye contact, speak in a voice that meets the client's affect, and rarely touch the client. However, research suggests that there are cross-cultural differences in the ways clients respond to the nonverbal behaviors of counselors (Morse & Ivey, 1996; Sue & Sue, 1999). Therefore, it is now suggested that counselors be acutely sensitive to client differences that may be a function of culture. Counselors must understand that some clients will expect to be looked at, while others will be offended by eye contact; that some clients will expect you to lean forward, while others will experience this as an intrusion; and that some clients will expect you to touch them, while others will see this as offensive. In respect to nonverbal behavior, effective counselors keep in mind what works for the many and are sensitive to what works for the few.

Counselor Qualities to Embrace/Counselor Qualities to Avoid

How we bring ourselves into the counseling relationship can positively or negatively affect the outcome of counseling. Therefore, the qualities highlighted in Chapter 1 are crucial to the establishment of an effective counseling relationship. They include empathy, genuineness, acceptance, open-mindedness, mindfulness, psychological adjustment, relationship building, and competence. The counselor who continually makes empathic failures is not hearing the client. The counselor who seems false, judgmental, and closed minded will create an atmosphere of defensiveness during the session. The counselor who is not mindful does not appear focused during the session. The impaired counselor's unfinished business will hinder client growth. The counselor who cannot build a relationship with his or her client will leave the client floundering, and the counselor who lacks the knowledge and skills to be competent can hardly be expected to be effective.

Not only must the counselor be able to demonstrate the personal characteristics that will nurture a healthy counseling relationship, but he or she must avoid attitudes and behaviors that will foster a destructive relationship. The many common attitudes that would be detrimental to a counseling relationship and need little explanation include: being critical of, disapproving of, disbelieving, scolding, threatening, discounting, ridiculing, punishing, and rejecting one's client (Benjamin, 1987). No doubt these attitudes and behaviors as well as others of a similar nature are to be avoided. Let's now take a look at some of the specific skills that will foster a productive counseling relationship.

Counseling Skills

Ask a room filled with therapists to agree on the time of day, and you're most likely to have a room filled with therapists arguing that it would be dependent on one's time zone and discussing the subjective nature of time. In the same way, to come to any consensus regarding what may be considered the most important skills to use within the counseling relationship would, to say the least, be difficult. However, I have attempted to categorize skills into five broad categories to which many therapists might agree. These include essential skills, commonly used skills, commonly used advanced skills, skills to use cautiously, and advanced and specialized skills. Certainly, regardless of what skills you use, the misuse or abuse of counseling skills can quickly have a deleterious effect on the outcome of counseling.

Foundational Skills

Regardless of the theoretical orientation to which you adhere, some skills are essential to establishing the relationship, building rapport and trust, setting a tone with the client, and beginning the client's process of self-examination. Although important throughout the counseling relationship, these skills are generally most crucial near the beginning of the relationship and should be continually revisited, especially when an impasse is reached. They include the ability to listen, show empathy, and use silence effectively.

Listening Skills

> *. . . First there is the hearing with the ear, which we all know; and the hearing with the non-ear, which is a state like that of a tranquil pond, a lake that is completely quiet and when you drop a stone into it, it makes little waves that disappear. I think that [insight] is the hearing with the non-ear, a state where there is absolute quietness of the mind; and when the question is put into the mind, the response is the wave, the little wave.* (Krishnamurti, cited in Jayakar, 1986, p. 325)

Webster defines *listen* as, "To give close attention in order to hear, to give ear; to hear and attend to." Although easy to define, this skill is perhaps the most difficult to implement, as Americans are rarely taught how to hear another person. In fact, ask an untrained adult to listen to another, and usually he or she ends up interrupting and giving advice. Summarizing some of the reasons it is important to be an effective listener, Scissons (1993) stresses that listening helps to build trust, convinces the client you understand him or her, encourages the client to reflect on what he or she has just said, ensures that you are on track with your understanding of the client, and is an effective way of collecting information from a client without the potentially negative side effects of using questions (see questions, pp. 122–124). Clearly, good listening is intimately related to client outcomes. A good listener (1) talks minimally, (2) concentrates on what is being said, (3) does not interrupt, (4) does not give advice, (5) gives and does not expect to get, (6) accurately hears the content of what the helpee is saying, (7) accurately hears the feelings of what the helpee is saying, (8) is able to communicate to the helpee that he or she has been heard (through head nods, "uh-huhs," or reflecting back to the client what the helper heard), (9) asks clarifying questions such as "I didn't hear all of that. Can you explain that in another way so I'm sure I understand you?" and (10) does not ask other kinds of questions.

BOX 5.2

Listen to Me

When I ask you to listen to me and you start giving me advice, you have not done what I asked.
When I ask you to listen to me and you begin to tell me why I shouldn't feel that way, you are trampling on my feelings.
When I ask you to listen to me and you feel you have to do something to solve my problem, you have failed me, strange as that may seem.
Listen: All that I ask is that you listen, not talk or do—just hear me.
When you do something for me that I can and need to do for myself, you contribute to my fear and inadequacy.
But when you accept as a simple fact that I do feel what I feel, no matter how irrational, then I can quit trying to convince you and get about this business of understanding what's behind these feelings.
So, please listen and just hear me.
And, if you want to talk, wait a minute for your turn—and I'll listen to you.

(Author Unknown)

HINDRANCES TO LISTENING Even when we know how to listen, a number of factors can prevent our ability to listen effectively. Some potential hindrances to listening include (1) having preconceived notions about the client that interfere with the counselor's ability to hear the client, (2) anticipating what the client is about to say and not actually hearing the client, (3) thinking about what you are going to say and therefore blocking what the client is saying, (4) having personal issues that interfere with your ability to listen, (5) having a strong emotional reaction to your client's content and therefore not being able to hear the client accurately, and (6) being distracted by such things as noises, temperature of the office, or hunger pains.

PREPARING TO LISTEN When you are ready to listen, the following practical suggestions should assist you in your ability to effectively hear a client (Egan, 1998; Ivey & Ivey, 1999).

1. Prior to meeting your client, calm yourself down: Meditate, pray, jog, or blow out air, but calm your inner self.
2. Maintain appropriate eye contact with the client (be sensitive to cultural differences).
3. Have an open body posture that invites the client to talk (be sensitive to cultural differences).
4. Be sensitive to the personal space between you and the client.
5. Clear your mind of extraneous thoughts that are not relevant to hearing the client (e.g., personal issues or interpretations of client behavior).
6. Concentrate on the client and be prepared to focus on the meaning and feeling of what the client is discussing.
7. Do not talk except to gently encourage the client to talk.
8. Listen.

Whereas basic listening is a crucial skill for counselors, empathic understanding, the next essential skill, takes listening to new depths.

Empathy and Deep Understanding: A Special Kind of Listening

Highlighted as one of the eight personal qualities to embrace in Chapter 1, empathy is also one of most important counseling skills to develop. The importance of listening to a person from a deep inner perspective was extolled by many early Greek philosophers and recognized for centuries for its healing qualities (Gompertz, 1960). During the 20th century Lipps (1935) is given the credit for coining the word *empathy* from the German word *Einfuhlung*, "to feel within," but probably the person who has had the greatest impact on our modern-day understanding and use of empathy is Carl Rogers.

> *The state of empathy, or being empathic, is to perceive the internal frame of reference of another with accuracy and with the emotional components and meanings which pertain thereto as if one were the person, but without ever losing the "as if" condition.* (Rogers, 1959, pp. 210–211)

The popularity of Rogers in the 1950s and 1960s naturally led to a number of operational definitions of empathy. For instance, Truax and Mitchell (1961) developed a nine-point rating scale to measure empathy, which was later revised by Carkhuff (1969)

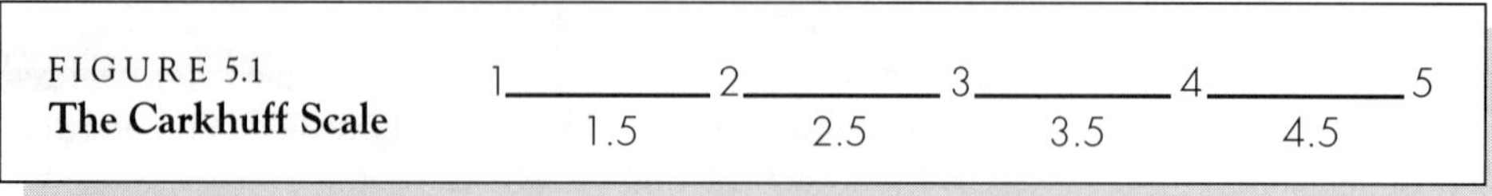

FIGURE 5.1
The Carkhuff Scale

into a five-point scale. A scale to measure empathy had important implications. For the first time, researchers could measure the empathic ability of counselors and determine whether there was a relationship between good empathic responses and client outcomes in therapy. Indeed, numerous research studies indicated that good empathic ability was related to progress in therapy (Carkhuff & Berenson, 1977; Lambert et al., 1986; Matarazzo & Patterson, 1986; Neukrug, 1980).

The Carkhuff scale became a mainstay of counselor training during the 1970s and 1980s, and although it is no longer used as extensively, the scale set the stage for similar microcounseling skills training methods in counselor education (Egan, 1998; Gazda, Asbury, Balzer, Childers, & Walters, 1977; Ivey & Ivey, 1999). The scale ranged from a low of 1.0 to a high of 5.0 with .5 increments. Any responses below a 3.0 were considered subtractive or nonempathic, while responses of 3.0 or higher were considered empathic, with responses over 3.0 called "additive" responses (see Figure 5.1). The original Carkhuff scale in its entirety is reproduced in Table 5.1. This scale dramatically changed counselor education as professors, students, and counselors could now assess one another's ability at making an empathic response.

As is obvious in Table 5.1, a "level 1" or "level 2" response in some ways detracts from what the person is saying (e.g., advice giving, not accurately reflecting feeling, not including content) with a "level 1" response being way off the mark and a "level 2" only slightly off. For instance, suppose a client said, "I've had it with my Dad, he never does

TABLE 5.1

Carkhuff's Accurate Empathy Scale	
Level 1	The verbal and behavioral expressions of the first person either *do not attend to* or *detract significantly from* the verbal and behavioral expressions of the second person(s) in that they communicate significantly less of the second person's feelings than the second person has communicated himself.
Level 2	While the first person responds to the expressed feelings of the second person(s), he does so in such a way that he *subtracts noticeable affect from the communications* of the second person.
Level 3	The expressions of the first person in response to the expressed feelings of the second person(s) are essentially *interchangeable* with those of the second person in that they express essentially the same affect and meaning.
Level 4	The responses of the first person add noticeably to the expressions of the second person(s) in such a way as to express feelings a level deeper than the second person was able to express himself.
Level 5	The first person's responses add significantly to the feeling and meaning of the expressions of the second person(s) in such a way as to (1)accurately express feelings levels below what the person himself was able to express or (2) in the event of ongoing, deep self-exploration on the second person's part, to be fully with him in his deepest moments.

SOURCE: Carkhuff, 1969, p. 121.

anything with me. He's always working, drinking, or playing with my little sister." A level 1 response might be, "Well, why don't you do something to change the situation, like tell him what an idiot he is," (advice giving and being judgmental). A level 2 response might be, "You seem to think your Dad spends too much time with your sister" (does not reflect feeling and misses content). On the other hand, a "level 3" response, such as "Well, it sounds as though you're pretty upset at your Dad for not spending time with you," accurately reflects the affect and meaning of the client.

"Level 4" and "level 5" responses reflect feelings and meaning beyond what the person is outwardly saying and add to the meaning of the person's outward expression. For instance, in the above example a level 4 response might be, "It sounds as though you're pretty angry at your Dad because he doesn't pay any attention to you" (expresses a new feeling, anger, which the client didn't outwardly state).

Level 5 responses are usually made in long-term therapeutic relationships by expert therapists. They express to the helpee a deep understanding of the pain he or she feels as well as a recognition of the complexity of the situation.

Usually, in the training of helpers it is recommended that they attempt to make level 3 responses, as a large body of evidence suggests that such responses can be learned in a relatively short amount of time and are beneficial to clients (Carkhuff, 1983; Neukrug, 1980, 1987). Effective empathic responses not only accurately reflect content and feelings but do so at a moment when the client can hear this reflection. For instance, you might sense a deep sadness or anger in a client and reflect this back to him or her. However, if the client is not ready to accept these feelings, then timing is off, and the response is considered subtractive.

Often, when first practicing empathic responding it is suggested that beginning counselors make a formula response, which generally starts with reflection of feeling followed by paraphrasing of content. Look at the example below:

Client: *I'm at my wit's end. I'm as depressed as ever. I keep trying to change my life and nothing works. I try communicating better, I change my job, I change my looks. I even take antidepressants, but nothing helps.*

Counselor: *You feel frustrated because you try making all of these changes and things are not any better.*

As counselors become more comfortable with formula responses, they can begin to use more natural conversational tones when making empathic responses. For instance, to the client above, a counselor might say:

Counselor: *Your frustration really shows—you've tried so many different things yet nothing seems to work. I can see your frustration and sadness in your eyes.*

Master therapists become very creative with empathic responding and will use metaphors, analogies, and self-disclosure in an attempt to tell the client he or she has been heard accurately (Neukrug, 1997):

Counselor: *It's kind of like you re rearranging deck chairs on the Titanic.*

Or

Counselor: *When you just told me what you're going through I felt my stomach twist and turn. I imagine this is how you must be feeling.*

As noted in Chapter 4, over the years, empathic responses have been sometimes confused with "active listening" or "reflection of feeling." Although Carl Rogers was instrumental in encouraging the use of empathy, he warned against the mechanistic, stilted, and wooden response to clients that is sometimes found when helpers practice reflection of feeling. Usually with practice, however, a helper's response to clients becomes more naturally empathic, as in some of the more advanced examples given above.

Silence

When is empty space facilitative and when does it become a bit much?

Silence is a powerful tool that can be used advantageously by the counselor for the growth of the client (Hutchins & Cole, 1997; Kleinke, 1994). It allows the client to reflect on what has been said and gives the counselor time to process the session and to formulate the next response. It shows the client that communication does not always have to be filled with words and that words can sometimes be used as a diversion from feelings. Silence is powerful. It will sometimes raise anxiety within the client, anxiety that on the one hand could push the client to talk further about a particular topic and on the other hand could cause a client to drop out of treatment.

A former professor of mine used to suggest waiting 30 seconds before making a response. During a counseling session, 30 seconds is a veeeeeeeeeeery loooonng tiiiiiiiiiiiiiiiiime. There have been times when I've had a student role-play a client and I've waited 30 seconds before responding. Trust me, this is a very long time. I would have difficulty waiting this much time during a counseling session. However, others may feel comfortable with this amount of silence. For instance, during these 30 seconds you could see my former professor thinking about the client's last statement, moving in his chair, and thinking about what he was to say next. This worked for him. Silence is powerful.

Finally, silence may be somewhat culturally determined. For instance, some research has found that the "pause time" for different cultures varies. Therefore, one's natural inclination to talk—to respond to another—will vary as a function of culture (Tafoya, 1996). As a counselor, you may want to consider your pause time to discover your comfort level with silence, and when working with clients you might consider a client's pause time. In fact, Tafoya notes that Native Americans have at times been labeled reticent and resistant to treatment when in fact they merely have long pause times. Treated by Native American therapists, they most likely would not have been labeled in this fashion.

Commonly Used Skills

The Purpose of Questions

What purposes do questions serve? Can you tell me more about the use of questions? Is a question a question or a statement about self? When should questions be questioned? Would you prefer the use of short or long questions? Why do you question questions? A question can come in many different forms, can't it? Would you prefer a question that gives you two options from which to choose, or would you like a question that offers you an open-ended type of response?

Questions can serve a multitude of purposes, including finding historical patterns, revealing underlying issues, gently challenging the client to change, or encouraging the client to deepen his or her self-exploration.

Types of Questions

OPEN VERSUS CLOSED QUESTIONS Open questions offer a client greater options in the kinds of responses he or she can make and are generally considered more facilitative than closed questions, which limit client response. For instance, one could ask the closed question, "Do you feel you had a good or bad childhood?" An even more limiting question would be, "What made your childhood so bad?" Instead, why not ask the open question, "What was your childhood like?" Although open questions are generally considered more effective than closed ones, there may be some times when you want to zero in on a couple of responses rather than leaving the question wide open.

DIRECT VERSUS INDIRECT QUESTIONS Benjamin (1987) notes that a question can be made even more open if it is asked indirectly. For instance, I could ask an open question directly: "What feelings did you have concerning your wife leaving you?" However, to make the question even more palatable, I might ask it in the following manner: "I would guess you must have had many feelings concerning your wife leaving?" In fact, this indirect question is more akin to making an empathic response.

Open questions that are indirect tend to sit well with clients. They're easier to hear, help the session flow, help to create a nonjudgmental open atmosphere, and are easily responded to by clients.

THE USE OF "WHY" QUESTIONS Why do you feel that way? Ever been asked that question? Feel defensive? In actuality, if one could honestly answer "why," the "why" question would be the most powerful question used in counseling. However, clients are in counseling to find the answer why; if they knew, they wouldn't be in your office. Because "why" questions tend to make a person feel defensive, it is generally recommended that counselors use other kinds of questions or empathic responses. I have found that after I've formed an alliance with a client, I might periodically slip in a soft "why" question and say something like, "Why do you think that is?" However, if I use this type of question at all during a session, I use it sparingly.

PROBLEMS WITH QUESTIONS Although questions can be helpful in uncovering patterns, inducing self-exploration, and in challenging the client to change, their overuse can create an authoritarian atmosphere where the client feels humiliated and dependent as he or she expects the counselor to come up with a solution for him or her (Benjamin, 1987; Byrne, 1995; Cormier & Cormier, 1998). In addition, a question is generally not as facilitative as an empathic response that empowers the client to discover answers on his or her own (Neukrug, 2002; Rogers, 1942). In fact, often an empathic response can be made in place of asking a question. For instance, suppose the client said the following:

Client: *You know, I can't stand talking about my parents' destructive attitude toward me and my siblings any longer.*

A counselor could respond with an open question, such as:

Counselor: *What is it about discussing your parents' destructive attitude that is so disturbing to you?*

However, probably a more effective response would be:

Counselor: *I hear how upset you get when you begin to talk about your parents' destructive attitude toward you and your siblings.*

Whereas the question is not a bad response, it changes, at least to a minor degree, the direction of the session. The empathic response affirms the client's feelings and yet allows the client to take the session where he or she would like. A counselor who views him- or herself as more directive than nondirective might choose the question over the empathic response. Generally, it is suggested that beginning counselors attempt to make reflective and empathic responses rather than questions.

Although much more can be discussed about the use of questions, suffice it to say that one should be careful whenever questions are used. Keeping this in mind, Benjamin (1987) suggests the following when asking questions:

- Are you aware that you are asking a question?
- Have you weighed carefully the desirability of asking specific questions and challenged their usage?
- Have you examined the types of questions available to you and the types of questions you personally tend to use?
- Have you considered alternatives to asking questions?
- Are you sensitive to the questions the interviewee is asking, whether he or she is asking them outright or not? And, most significantly,
- Will the question you are about to ask inhibit the flow of the interview?

Counselor Self-Disclosure

A former student of mine was in therapy with a psychiatrist, who, over time, increasingly began to disclose *his* problems to *her*. One day she heard that he had committed suicide. Following his death she revealed to me that she felt intense guilt that she hadn't saved his life. What a legacy to leave this student! Clearly, the psychiatrist's self-disclosure was unhealthy and unethical. However, under some circumstances, certain amounts of self-disclosure may facilitate a client's ability to open up and may also serve as a model of positive behaviors.

Although self-disclosure can be important and helpful for clients (Kleinke, 1994; Pennebaker, Colder, & Sharp, 1990; Pennebaker & Susman, 1988), as a counseling skill it is at best a mixed bag (Donley, Horan, & DeShong, 1990; Doster & Nesbitt, 1979). Kleinke (1994) identifies two types of self disclosure, content self-disclosure, when one reveals information about him- or herself; and process self-disclosure: when one reveals information about how the counselor is feeling toward the client in the moment.

CONTENT SELF-DISCLOSURE This kind of disclosure could have a number of positive results, including showing your client that you are "real," and thus creating a stronger alliance; developing deeper intimacy in the helping relationship, which ultimately could foster deeper client self-disclosure; and offering behavior your client can model. Sometimes clients may gently push counselors into content self-disclosure (see Box 5.3).

PROCESS SELF-DISCLOSURE Sometimes called "immediacy," process disclosure involves the counselor sharing his or her moment-to-moment experience of self in relation to the client (George & Cristiani, 1995). Such process comments could help a client see the type of impact he or she has on the therapist and, ultimately, on others in his or her life; help a client see how moment-to-moment communication can enhance relationships; and act as a model for a new kind of communication that can be generalized to important relationships in the client's life. Similar to the Rogerian concept of genuineness, process self-disclosure suggests that the counselor be real with his or her feelings toward the client.

BOX 5.3

Awkward Self-Disclosure with a Client

A former client of mine who was in a dysfunctional relationship with her boyfriend was struggling with feelings of attraction toward me. We had discussed these feelings and noted that perhaps they were being exaggerated as she contrasted her feelings toward an "idealized" me with her feelings toward her verbally abusive boyfriend. She was a runner, as I was, and during one session she informed me she was interested in going to Bermuda to run in an international race. I had already planned on running this race and was planning on going to Bermuda with the woman I was dating. I suddenly was faced with a number of dilemmas. Do I disclose my plans to go to Bermuda and reveal an intimate aspect of my life, or do I wait, and almost assuredly run into my client in Bermuda? Or I could decide to not go to Bermuda. I quickly assessed the situation, and it seemed obvious to me that I needed to reveal my plans to her. I believe it would have been a mistake for me to change my plans, yet I did not want to create an awkward situation for my client in Bermuda. Revealing as little information as possible about my life, I said to my client that I was planning on going to Bermuda with a woman friend. Having this information, my client eventually decided not to go.

> *. . . Certainly the aim is not for the therapist to express or talk out his own feelings, but primarily that he should not be deceiving the client as to himself. At times he may need to talk out some of his own feelings (either to the client, or to a colleague or supervisor). . . .* (Rogers, 1957, p. 98)

Warning counselors not to share transient feelings toward clients, Rogers (1957) pointed out that clients were rapidly changing as they shared deeper parts of themselves; and, as they changed, the counselor's feelings toward them would likely change. Instead of sharing moment-to-moment feelings, he suggested sharing persistent feelings, as these are more meaningful to the relationship (Rogers, 1970).

Regardless of the kind of self-disclosure made, it has been found that its effectiveness is closely related to the kinds of expectations clients have about the use of self-disclosure (Derlega, Lovell, & Chaikin, 1976; Neimeyer, Banikiotes, & Winum, 1979; Neimeyer & Fong, 1983). Therefore, the amount of the therapist's self-disclosure should be directly proportional to how much the client expects self-disclosure to be a part of the therapeutic process.

Self-disclosure needs to be done sparingly, at the right time, and only as a means for client growth not to satisfy our needs (Evans, Hearn, Uhlemann, & Ivey, 1998). A general rule of thumb is: If it feels good to self-disclose, don't. If it feels good, you're probably meeting more of your needs than the needs of your client. Finally, I agree with Kahn (1997) who states that,

> *I try not to make a foolish fetish out of not talking about myself. If a client, on the way out the door, asks in a friendly and casual way, "Where are you going on your vacation?" I tell where I'm going. If the client were then to probe, however ("Who are you going with? Are you married?") I would likely respond, "Ah . . . maybe we'd better talk about that next time."* (p. 150)

Modeling

Irrespective of the kind of theoretical orientation practiced, counselors will act as models for their clients *regardless of whether or not they want to be* (Brammer & MacDonald, 1999). We are constantly modeling for our clients. If we are empathic, then they may learn how to listen to loved ones more effectively. If we are assertive, they may learn how to positively confront someone in their lives. And, if we can show a client how to resolve conflict, then he or she will learn new ways of dealing with conflict in his or her life. Using modeling, counselors can be change agents in two ways, circuitously or intentionally.

CIRCUITOUS MODELING Circuitous modeling occurs when behaviors learned by a client are a by-product of the counseling relationship. In this case, the counselor does not purposefully set out to change client behaviors. However, behavior change does occur as the client takes in the "being" of the counselor. This occurs because it is common for a client to look up to a counselor, even idealize him or her, and when a model has perceived power, status, competence, and knowledge, that counselor's behaviors will often be perceived very powerfully by the client (Brammer & MacDonald, 1999).

The counselor who is a circuitous model tends to practice from a psychodynamic or existential/humanistic framework, and the very skills used in the practice of therapy are the skills the client will apply in his or her life. For instance, the person-centered counselor who uses empathy, unconditional positive regard, and genuineness is a model of these qualities, and ultimately the client will begin to apply these skills in his or her own relationships. Similarly, the psychodynamic therapist who uses empathy, interpretation, and inquisitiveness will model these behaviors for his or her clients.

INTENTIONAL MODELING Many therapists, especially those who use a cognitive and behavioral orientation, use modeling as an important tool in their arsenal of change methods. Modeling offers us a number of ways to have clients change targeted behavior (Perry & Furukawa, 1986). Three main ways that the counselor might use modeling intentionally are: (1) through the deliberate display of specific behaviors on the part of the helper (e.g., expressing empathy, being nonjudgmental, being assertive), (2) through the use of role-playing during the session (e.g., the counselor might role-play job interviewing techniques for the client), and (3) by teaching the client about modeling and encouraging him or her to find models outside the session to emulate (e.g., a person who has a fear of speaking to a large group might choose a speaker he or she admires and view the specifics of how that person makes a speech).

With intentional modeling, any targeted behaviors that the client wishes to acquire need to have a high probability for success. Also, because such modeling involves a two-part process that includes observing the targeted behavior and then practicing it, clients need not only to find appropriate models but also to practice the desired behavior within or outside of the session. For instance, an individual who has a fear of making speeches would first need a model to emulate. After observing this model, a hierarchy could be devised whereby the client would make a speech first to the therapist, then to some trusting friends, then to a small group, and so forth, perhaps asking for feedback along the way in order to sharpen his or her performance.

Commonly Used Advanced Skills

Confrontation: Challenge with Support

People generally define confrontation as some type of hostile challenge when attempting to overcome an obstacle. However, within the context of the counseling relationship, confrontation is generally thought of as a much softer challenge to the client's understanding of the world (Byrne, 1995). To be effective, this gentle challenge needs to be preceded by the building of a trusting and caring relationship, thus lessening the likelihood that any harm to the client will occur (Egan, 1998; Kleinke, 1994; M.E. Young, 1992). The use of good listening skills and empathy is generally considered to be the most effective way to develop a relationship that can successfully process a challenge and potentially change the client's perception of reality (McAuliffe et al., 2000). In short, confrontation requires accurate timing, tact, and gentility on the part of the counselor.

Hackney and Cormier (2001) remark that confrontation assists the client to see discrepancies among words, feelings, and/or behaviors. Three types of discrepancy they highlight include: (1) a discrepancy between a client's values and behavior (e.g., a client says she believes in honesty in relationships, yet won't express her anger toward her lover because she is afraid he will leave her), (2) a discrepancy between a client's feelings and behavior (e.g., a person who says he loves his wife deeply then tells the counselor about the affair he is having); and (3) a discrepancy between a client's verbal statements describing self (e.g., a client who states she wants to communicate more effectively but finds excuses for not doing so–"If only I had more time to work on my communication problems"). A fourth type of discrepancy might be a discrepancy between a client's verbal expression of feelings and the underlying feelings to which a client won't admit or of which he or she is not currently aware (e.g., a person who states she feels fine about her marriage and yet she seems to be holding back tears; you note this, and she begins to sob).

Following the building of a trusting and caring relationship, there are a number of ways a discrepancy can be confronted:

1. *You/but statements*. Such statements point out client incongruities by reflecting them back in a you/but framework (Hackney & Cormier, 2001). For instance, to a client who states he believes in honesty but is having an affair, the counselor might state:

   Counselor: *On the one hand you say that you believe in honesty, but you seem to be hiding a serious matter from your wife.*

BOX 5.4

Confronting Sally

Sally made close to $60,000 a year and was in a verbally abusive relationship. Even though she had no major bills, she insisted that she could not leave the relationship and live on a "meager" $60,000 dollars a year. Clearly, her verbal statement that she could not leave the relationship did not match the reality that one could live on this amount (certainly, most of us would be happy to live on this amount). After building a relationship using empathy, I gently challenged this perception. I did this by using many of the techniques above. Using "you/but" statements, I pointed out the obvious discrepancy between her salary and her perceived inability to live on her own. Also, I gently asked her to justify to me how she could feel this way. This assisted her to see that her logic did not hold up. Using higher level empathy I reflected back a deeper issue that I experienced her saying—that she felt as if she was a failure in the relationship and was scared to be alone (she was a recovering alcoholic and was concerned she would start drinking again if alone). I encouraged her to work on communication issues with her lover. At the same time I assisted her in reframing her situation so that she could believe that she could live on her own—if she chose eventually to do this. I did not use irony with her, as I felt it would be too disturbing for her. The result for this client was that she became a more assertive woman who improved her communication with her lover and could realistically see her choices about staying in the relationship or finding a place on her own.

2. *Asking the client to justify the discrepancy.* This kind of response has the counselor gently asking the client to explain to the counselor how he or she justifies the discrepancy. For example, in the above example the counselor might say:

   Counselor: *Based on your knowledge of who you are, tell me how you make sense of the fact that you say you are honest, and yet you are hiding an affair from your wife?*

3. *Reframing.* This way of highlighting the discrepancy challenges the client to view his or her situation differently by offering an alternative reality.

   Counselor: *What you're telling me is that in some cases honesty is not always the best way to go.*

4. *Using irony.* Using irony highlights the absurdity of the discrepancy and is more confrontational than the other techniques. This technique should be used carefully. For instance, in the above example, you might say:

   Counselor: *Well, I guess it's okay in this instance to be dishonest; after all, you are saving your wife from those painful feelings, aren't you?*

5. *Higher-level empathy.* Higher-level empathy, the final way of challenging a client's discrepancy, reflects to the client underlying, out-of-awareness feelings and conflicts, and challenges the client to expose deeper parts of him- or herself. For instance, in the above example:

   Counselor: *You must be feeling quite conflicted. On the one hand, you say you believe in honesty; on the other hand, you are hiding an affair. I guess I sense there is more to this story for you.*

Interpretation

A client offers details about his current lover. Later he shares details about his relationship with his parents. You hear similar themes and feelings running through these relationships and reveal your analysis to the client. The client nods his head in agreement. Is this interpretation or is this empathy? Although some may consider this interpretation (Benjamin, 1987; Cormier & Cormier, 1998), I consider this a high-level empathic response (above 3.0) for a number of reasons. First, it is a result of deep listening and concentration upon the part of the counselor. Second, it is based on a deep understanding of the client's framework of reality. Third, you have reflected back your understanding of the client's predicament without adding material from an external source, such as a counseling theory, that might suggest certain conclusions about your client. And finally, the client agrees with your assessment. You are on target with your response. This definition of empathy is a profound response to the client that reaches deep inside the client's soul and speaks to the imaginary line between facilitating and leading a client (Benjamin, 1987).

On the other hand, true interpretation is the analysis of a client's behaviors and meaning-making system from the perspective of the counselor, usually with a preset model of counseling and psychotherapy in mind that makes assumptions about how a person would react under certain circumstances. Psychoanalysis uses interpretation as a major therapeutic intervention. In this vein, psychoanalysts believe that our dreams hold symbols to unresolved conflicts from our psychosexual development and can provide the client with understanding of his or her development (Brill, 1960). For example, a dream about a goat being your pet in an immaculately clean apartment could represent an underlying need to rebel against a repressive upbringing, the goat representing the archetypal oppositional animal. Similarly, some cognitive therapists assume that individuals with specific diagnoses would be expected to have certain kinds of underlying cognitive structures, which can be explained (interpreted) to the client (Lynn & Garske, 1985). For example, it would be assumed that a person with an anxiety disorder has underlying cognitive beliefs that the world is a fearful and dangerous place. Whether we are psychodynamically oriented, cognitively oriented, or relying on some other theoretical approach, the timing of the interpretation is crucial, with the desired result being a deeper understanding of why the client responds the way he or she does, an understanding that may lead to client change.

When on target, interpretations can assist a client in making giant leaps in therapy. However, there are risks involved in using this technique. For instance, interpretation sets the therapist up as the "expert" and lessens the realness of the relationship (Kleinke, 1994). In addition, it lessens the here-and-now quality of the therapeutic relationship while increasing the amount of intellectualizing that occurs as both the counselor and client discuss the interpretive material (Safran & Segal, 1990). Finally, research does not show strong evidence that interpretation is related to successful client outcomes (Orlinsky & Howard, 1986). For these reasons Carl Rogers and others (e.g., Benjamin, 1987; Kahn, 1997) vehemently opposed the use of the interpretation.

> *. . . To me, an interpretation as to the cause of individual behavior can never be anything but a high-level guess. The only way it can carry weight is when an authority puts his experience behind it. But I do not want to get involved in this kind of authoritativeness. "I think it's because you feel inadequate as a man that you engage in this blustering behavior," is not the kind of statement I would ever make.* (Rogers, 1970, pp. 57–58)

Skills to Use Cautiously

Although the skills we are about to look at are frequently used with clients, many consider them questionable in their effectiveness for client outcomes. This is at least partially because these skills lead or direct the client, whereas the thrust of more traditional counseling skills is to facilitate a relationship that fosters client self-discovery. In point of fact, many would consider some of the skills we have already looked at to be leading and counselor-centered. Such skills as interpretation, confrontation, and some types of self-disclosure can be classified in this way because the counselor forms the response from his or her frame of reference as opposed to following the client's lead. However, these skills have at least some amount of long-standing acceptance, whereas the skills we are about to look at—encouragement, affirmation, and self-esteem building; offering alternatives, information giving, and offering advice—have not been so acclaimed. If used at all, the following skills should certainly be used tentatively and carefully.

Encouragement, Affirmation, and Self-Esteem Building

> *The need for supporting core self-esteem doesn't end in childhood. Adults still need "unconditional" love from family, friends, life partners, animals, perhaps even an all-forgiving deity. Love that says: "no matter how the world may judge you, I love you for yourself."* (Steinem, 1992, p. 66)

Although it is not usually considered a technique, it is the rare therapist who does not encourage and affirm clients. Fleeting statements such as "good job," or "I'm happy for you," or strong handshakes, warm hugs, and approving smiles are just a few of the ways in which we as therapists affirm and perhaps encourage our clients. Whether called reinforcement or a genuine response to our client's hard work, such relatively minor counselor responses may greatly affect our clients and perhaps not always in positive ways. In fact, some believe that the use of such responses may lead to the formation of a therapeutic relationship based on external validation (Benjamin, 1987). Therapists must reflect upon whether or not affirmations and subtle encouragement of client progress are assisting in the formation of a higher degree of self worth or if they may actually be fostering dependency and the continuation of a higher degree of externality. In my own practice, I attempt to find some balance between genuinely affirming a client and my concerns that I might be fostering a dependent relationship.

Offering Alternatives, Information Giving, and Advice Giving

Like affirmations, encouragement, and self-esteem building, the skills of information giving, offering advice, and offering alternatives are not typical responses offered by counselors because of their tendency to lead the client (Benjamin, 1987; Kleinke, 1994). In fact, as with previous skills noted, these skills may portray the therapist as an expert, encourage externality, and foster dependency. It is therefore not surprising that some research has shown that these types of responses are not particularly effective (Kleinke, 1994; Orlinsky & Howard, 1986). Despite this, there may be times when these responses are helpful, such as when a client and therapist have agreed upon a specific course of action and the client is wanting suggestions on how to move in that direction (e.g., a client who is committed to working on her social skills is advised by the therapist to join a local community group), or when it appears obvious that the actions of a client will be harmful to the client or others (Kleinke, 1994).

Although offering alternatives, information giving, and advice giving are similar in the sense that they all move the focus of the session from the client to the counselor, each has a different potential for being destructive to the counseling relationship.

Clearly, of the three possible leading responses, offering alternatives would be least likely to have destructive influences in the counseling relationship (see Figure 5.2). As we move toward advice giving, the counselor's responses become more value laden and more counselor centered (Doyle, 1992). Whether any of these responses are used should be based on a careful understanding of your client's needs and whether an alternative response could be more effective for the client. Finally, as Meichenbaum (cited in Kleinke, 1994) notes, when therapy is at its optimal, the timing of this kind of response should be such that the client is "one step ahead of . . . the advice that would otherwise" be offered (p. 87). Thus, the client in essence is gaining so much from counseling that he or she is coming up with solutions prior to the counselor suggesting them.

Advanced and Specialized Counseling Skills

We have examined in this chapter a number of basic skills that can be used by all counselors, whether they are beginning students or advanced master therapists. Although not within the purview of this text, there are many other skills that can be attained through additional training by an interested and astute therapist. Many of these skills are unique to specific counseling approaches. Mentioning just a few, they include such things as the use of metaphor, hypnosis, strategic skills, cognitive restructuring methods, narratives and

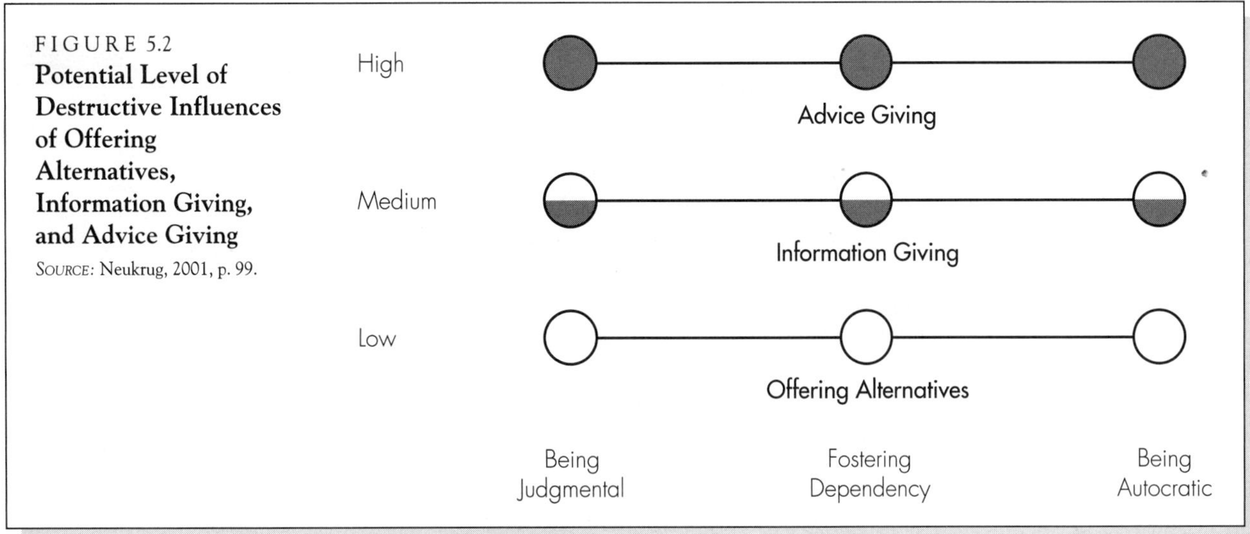

FIGURE 5.2
Potential Level of Destructive Influences of Offering Alternatives, Information Giving, and Advice Giving
SOURCE: Neukrug, 2001, p. 99.

storytelling, therapeutic touch, paradoxical intention, and visualization techniques (Rosenthal, 1997, 2001). Suffice it to say that use of these skills may often take training beyond the master's degree. Today, there are many institutes nationally and internationally that offer such advanced training. Such training can also be obtained through the attainment of an advanced degree, attendance of workshops at conferences, and good supervision.

Conceptualizing Client Problems: Case Conceptualization

Case conceptualization is a method that allows the counselor to understand a client's presenting problems and subsequently apply appropriate counseling skills and treatment strategies based on the counselor's theoretical orientation. Whereas experienced counselors develop their own systematic method of conceptualizing client problems, beginning counselors, who are often still struggling with their theoretical orientation, have a more difficult time conceptualizing client problems (Glidewell & Livert, 1992; Loganbill, Hardy, & Delworth, 1982; Martin, Slemon, Hiebert, Hallberg, & Cummings, 1989). One model of case conceptualization is Schwitzer's (1996, 1997) inverted pyramid heuristic (IPH).

IPH is a step-by-step method that can be used to identify and understand client concerns while offering a visual guide for counselors in how to organize client information; see connections among client concerns, symptoms, and behaviors; and consider different areas to focus on in counseling. The inverted pyramid method includes four steps in clinical problem formulation (see Figure 5.3). These include:

1. Broadly identifying symptomatic behavior.
2. Organizing client difficulties into logical groupings or constellations.
3. Tying symptom groups to deeper theoretical, interpretive, or causal references.
4. Narrowing these symptom groups to the client's most basic difficulties in development or adjustment based on one's theoretical orientation.

FIGURE 5.3
Inverted Pyramid Method of Case Conceptualization
SOURCE: Adapted from Schwitzer, 1976, p. 260.

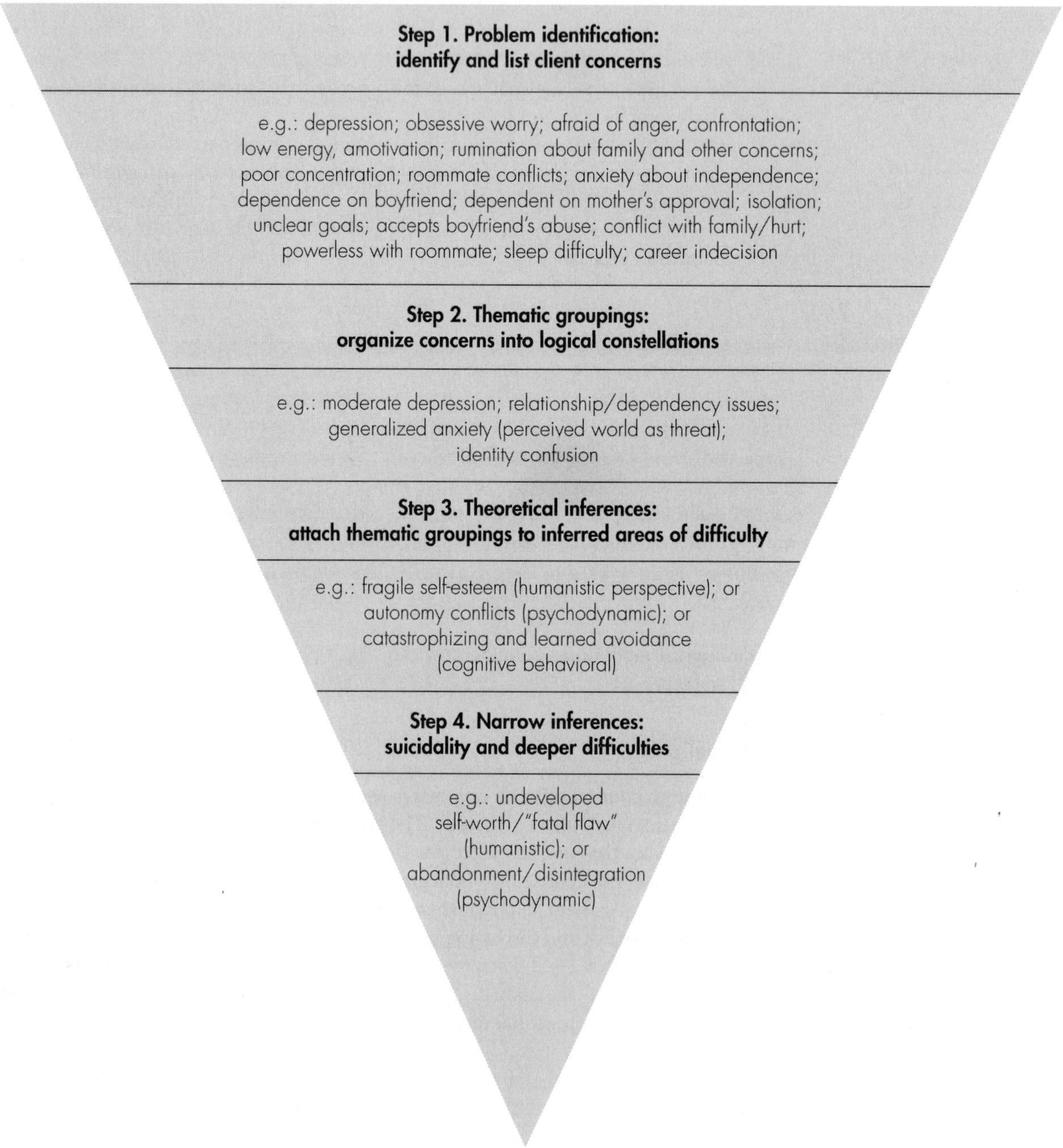

Step 1. Problem identification: identify and list client concerns

e.g.: depression; obsessive worry; afraid of anger, confrontation; low energy, amotivation; rumination about family and other concerns; poor concentration; roommate conflicts; anxiety about independence; dependence on boyfriend; dependent on mother's approval; isolation; unclear goals; accepts boyfriend's abuse; conflict with family/hurt; powerless with roommate; sleep difficulty; career indecision

Step 2. Thematic groupings: organize concerns into logical constellations

e.g.: moderate depression; relationship/dependency issues; generalized anxiety (perceived world as threat); identity confusion

Step 3. Theoretical inferences: attach thematic groupings to inferred areas of difficulty

e.g.: fragile self-esteem (humanistic perspective); or autonomy conflicts (psychodynamic); or catastrophizing and learned avoidance (cognitive behavioral)

Step 4. Narrow inferences: suicidality and deeper difficulties

e.g.: undeveloped self-worth/"fatal flaw" (humanistic); or abandonment/disintegration (psychodynamic)

Using this method, a beginning counselor would start at the top of the inverted pyramid and attempt to identify problem behaviors. Going down the inverted pyramid, the counselor would in Step 2 attempt to organize the information obtained in Step 1 into a few groups called "thematic groupings" (Schwitzer, 1996, p. 260). During Step 3 the groupings developed in the two previous steps are related to the counselor's theoretical perspective. In Step 4, inferences from Step 3 are further distilled into deeper difficulties in functioning or deeper personality traits, when present.

The pyramid offers a visual and cognitive map that assists us to consider horizontal choices (for example, addressing depressed mood versus a relationship problem in the topmost section of the diagram) and vertical decisions (for example, addressing career indecision, topmost section, versus underlying identity confusion or struggle for independence, third section down) in making treatment decisions. It is clear that decisions concerning treatment approaches can be greatly aided through the use of the case conceptualization process.

Stages of the Counseling Relationship

The application of counseling skills can vary considerably as a function of the counselor's job role, setting, and theoretical orientation. Despite these differences, there are many commonalties within the counseling relationship. For instance, all counselors have to address technical issues unique to the first session (e.g., meeting times, length of session, billing issues, and frequency of sessions). All counselors will face issues of trust. All counselors will need to identify client concerns, develop goals, and assist the client in working on the identified goals. And all counselors will have to deal with termination. These commonalities will be displayed in a series of stages of the counseling relationships through which all clients will pass. Let's identify each of these stages and examine how our conceptual model may be applied within them. Refer back to Figure 5.3 as you consider this material.

Stage 1: Rapport and Trust Building

Clients come to counseling with one major agenda, "Can I trust my counselor to discuss with him or her what I need to discuss?" The counselor, on the other hand, is dealing with a number of issues that are crucial to the development of an effective working relationship. For instance, the counselor is concerned about using basic skills to build trust in the relationship, assuring that the physical environment feels safe, informing the client about the counseling process, and discussing technical issues such as length of the sessions, credentials held, potential legal concerns, agency rules, payment issues, and limits to confidentiality (Brammer & McDonald, 1999; Scissons, 1993). Some have recently suggested the use of a written professional disclosure statement to cover many of these issues (see Box 5.5).

During the first stage, the development of a comfortable, trusting, and facilitative relationship can be accomplished through the use of listening skills, empathic understanding, cultural sensitivity, and a fair amount of good social skills (Hackney & Cormier, 2001). During these beginning sessions, I find it not unusual to discuss superficial items with clients or common interests in an effort to establish a camaraderie.

BOX 5.5

Professional Disclosure Statements

Recently, some have advocated the use of a professional disclosure statement that explains the counseling process, the counselor's theoretical orientation and credentials held, relevant agency rules, limits to confidentiality, legal issues, and other important information relative to the counseling relationship (Corey et al., 1998). Such a statement can be read and signed by the client prior to initiating counseling.

Despite this recent push toward written professional disclosure statements, the reality is that most counselors still rely on verbal professional disclosure statements, and many disregard this aspect of the counseling relationship. This may be a mistake as counselors are not protecting themselves fully in case of litigation and are not offering basic knowledge that each client deserves. Although clients such as an acutely psychotic person, someone who is intoxicated, or a very young child may have difficulty understanding a professional disclosure statement, all clients deserve basic respect by informing them *in the best way that we can and in the manner that they can best understand* the essentials of our work with them.

However, I always keep in mind that the one major purpose of counseling is to assist the client toward disclosure of self-identified problems. Therefore, I do not want to make the session too chatty.

As this stage continues, the counselor will begin to mentally identify and eventually delineate the issues presented by the client. This is the first step of our case conceptualization model. The counselor should review and evaluate the accuracy of this list with the client by reflecting back to the client those problems thought to be highlighted during this stage or by asking the client directly if the list is accurate.

Stage 2: Problem Identification

The building of a trusting relationship and the ability to do an assessment of client problems are signs that you are moving into the second stage where you and your client will validate your initial identification of the problem(s). It may be that what the client initially came to counseling for was masking other issues. Or additional issues may arise as you explore the client's situation—perhaps even issues of which the client was not fully aware. In either case, during these sessions you validate your original assessment and make appropriate changes as necessary. Validation of original concerns or reassessment and identification of new issues allow you to move into Step 2 of your conceptual model, the grouping of identified problems into broad themes.

Stage 3: Deepening Understanding and Goal Setting

Although your basic counseling skills are still important, because trust has been built in the earlier stages, other skills can now be added—skills that will allow you to understand your client in deeper ways. For instance, the client will now allow you to confront him or her, ask probing questions, and give advanced empathic responses. You can increasingly push the envelope and move into the inner world of the client. However, it is always crucial to maintain sensitivity to your client's needs and to maintain a supportive and nurturing base. Move too fast, and the client will rebuff your attempts to expose his or her inner world. Move at the right pace for the client, and the counseling relationship will deepen, and advanced skills based on your particular theoretical orientation can be used.

As you begin to understand your client in deeper and broader ways, you move into Step 3 of your conceptual model, where you begin to make inferences based on your theoretical orientation about underlying themes. These may be shared with your client, and at this point clients are likely to begin to work on some of these identified themes. If given enough time, with some clients you will move into Step 4 of your conceptual model. In this step, based on your theoretical orientation, you can now identify specific underlying themes that permeate the client's life and affect many aspects of his or her functioning.

Now that themes have been identified from Step 3 or Step 4 of your conceptual model, goals can be established based on these themes. The counselor, in collaboration with the client, can determine how the client would like to reach these goals. This will be based partly on the practicality of the relationship (e.g., the number of sessions available for counseling), the desires of the client (e.g., the client may want short-term counseling), and the theoretical orientation of the counselor. The result of this collaboration should be anything from an informal verbal goal agreement to a written contract that is signed by both the client and counselor.

Stage 4: Work

During the fourth stage, the client is beginning to work on the issues that were identified in stage 3 and agreed upon between the counselor and client. The counselor will use his or her counseling skills to facilitate progress, and, if necessary, the counselor and client may want to revisit and reevaluate some of the goals set.

The client in this stage is taking responsibility for and actively working on his or her identified issues and themes. For instance, if the counselor is humanistically oriented, the client is pushing him- or herself to work on identified existential-humanistic themes (e.g., issues related to self-esteem). If the counselor is cognitive/behavioral, the client will be actively working on changing cognitions and behaviors (e.g., self-statements like "I am worthless" are worked upon, and self-affirming behaviors are practiced). If the counselor is psychodynamic, the client will be exploring identified analytical themes in the session (e.g., what impact past overdependency on his or her mother has on current relationships). Advanced skills based on the counselor's theoretical orientation are used in this stage. As clients work through their issues, they become ready to terminate counseling.

Stage 5: Closure

The main issues of the closure stage are termination and the loss associated with it. As the client has successfully worked through some of his or her issues, it becomes increasingly clear that there is little reason for counseling to continue. Counseling is one of the few intimate relationships that is time-limited, which consequently means that clients (and counselors) will have to work through their feelings of loss (Ward, 1984).

When is a client ready to terminate a counseling relationship? Kleinke (1994) has found a number of reasons to consider termination, including (1) the reduction or elimination of symptoms; (2) the gaining of enough insight to deal with future recurring symptoms; (3) the resolution of transference issues; (4) the ability to work effectively, enjoy life, and play; and (5) having reached the point of diminishing returns in therapy (remaining issues may not be worth the effort and time).

Termination should be a gradual process in which the client and counselor have time to deal with the loss involved and discuss whether or not stated goals have been met. As with many issues that carry a heavy emotional burden, many clients will attempt to defend or resist against the termination process (Goodyear, 1981). This can happen in a number of ways:

1. The client may insist that he or she needs more time to work on the problem(s).
2. New issues may suddenly arise.
3. The client might start to miss sessions in an effort to avoid discussion of termination or even abruptly end therapy.
4. The client may suddenly become angry at the therapist in an effort to distance him- or herself.
5. The client might prematurely end therapy.

Because counselors also may find themselves resisting termination (Goodyear, 1981), it is important that they be vigilant about working through their own loss issues while, at the same time, being sensitive to the loss issues of their clients. Of course, consultation with colleagues and supervisors can be invaluable at this point in the therapeutic relationship.

Finally, successful termination is more likely if (1) clients discuss termination early, (2) goals are clear so clients know when counseling is near completion, (3) the counselor respects the client's desire to terminate yet feels free to discuss feelings that termination may be too soon, (4) the relationship remains professional (e.g., does not move into a friendship), (5) clients know they can return, (6) clients are able to review the success they had in counseling, and (7) clients can discuss feelings of loss around termination (Kleinke, 1994).

Stage 6: Follow-Up

We believe that patients can and should return as needed.
(Budman & Gurman, 1988, p. 20)

The end of counseling may not be the end. Clients may return with new issues, may want to revisit old issues, or may desire to delve deeper into themselves. In fact, it is not unusual for clients to return to the same counselor or seek out another counselor at some other date (Neukrug, Milliken, & Shoemaker, 2001; Neukrug & Williams, 1993).

Follow-up with clients can function as a check to see if clients would like to return for counseling or would like a referral to a different counselor. Follow-up also allows the counselor to assess if change has been maintained. Follow-up, usually done a few weeks to six months after counseling has been completed, enables the counselor to look at which techniques have been most successful, gives him or her the opportunity to reinforce past change, and is one way in which the counselor can evaluate services provided (Hutchins & Cole, 1997; Kleinke, 1994; Neukrug, 2000, 2002). Some counselors follow up by a phone call, others send a letter, and still others do a more elaborate survey of clients.

Theory, Skills, Stages, and Case Conceptualization: A Reciprocal Relationship

The application of our counseling skills deepens our relationship with our client and moves the client into the next counseling stage. Movement into the next stage necessitates the use of new skills and brings forth a deeper understanding of our client from our unique theoretical orientation. Concurrently, application of our case conceptualization model will facilitate our understanding of our client from our particular theoretical per-

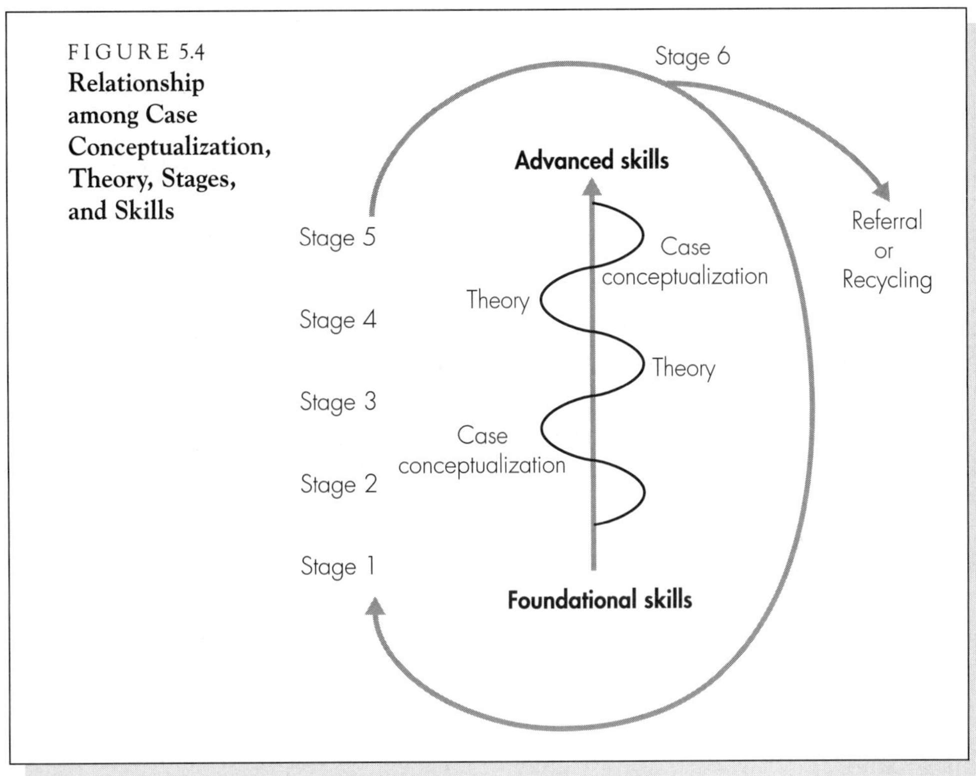

FIGURE 5.4
Relationship among Case Conceptualization, Theory, Stages, and Skills

spective. As we understand our client in new and deeper ways, we move into later stages of the counseling relationship that necessitate the use of new counseling skills. After the counseling relationship has ended, counselors should follow up, at which point they may find that the client wants to recycle through the stages of the relationship or be referred to a new counselor. Thus we see a deepening reciprocal relationship among the skills that we use, our case conceptualization model, our theoretical orientation, and the stages of the counseling relationship (see Figure 5.4).

Case Notes and Record Keeping

> *Problems associated with writing and reading mental health records are well worth our attention. . . . increasing numbers of people are writing and reading increasing numbers of mental health records for increasing number of purposes, and that trend is likely to continue.* (Reynolds, Mair, & Fischer, 1995, p. 1)

The Importance of Case Notes

With the increasing numbers of people reading and writing case notes, note taking has become particularly important in the life of the counselor. Regardless of the setting in which you work, there are numerous reasons why the writing of careful case notes has become so critical (Kleinke, 1994; Neukrug, 2000, 2002):

- They are a measure of our standard of care and subsequently can be used in court, if necessary, to show adequate client care.
- They assist in our understanding of whether or not our clients have made progress.
- They can be useful when we obtain supervision.
- They can help us pull together our thoughts when making a diagnosis.
- They can help us remember what our client said.
- They are needed by insurance companies, agencies, and schools to support the treatment we are providing to our clients.

Writing Your Case Notes

Today, there are many kinds of case report writing including daily case notes, intake summaries, quarterly summaries, summaries for insurance companies, summaries for students' individual education plans, summaries for vocational rehabilitation planning, summaries for referrals to other clinicians, and termination summaries. Although many settings require the counselor to write notes during or directly following a session, the frequency of writing more involved case summaries, such as quarterly or semiannual summaries, varies dramatically from setting to setting.

Although most agencies and educational settings require case notes, how they are recorded may vary. In an ideal world you would have a Dictaphone and an administrative assistant to type your notes. More than likely, however, you will be using a computer for your case notes or employing the tried-and-true fashion of writing them out (Tiedeman, 1983). Although laborious, writing notes out can help a counselor organize his or her thoughts about a client.

Because taking notes during a session can be distracting and, for some counselors, make it difficult to listen, many suggest waiting until after the session is finished to write notes. On the other hand, some counselors find that case note taking during the session helps them focus and adds to the ability to conceptualize client problems. Regardless of when you take notes, it is important to be objective and not to include speculation that has little basis in fact. Although the requirements for case note writing can vary dramatically, daily notes are generally less than a page long, whereas quarterly summaries are a few pages long. Although the kinds of headings may vary from setting to setting, some common headings include demographic information (e.g., DOB, address, phone, date of interview), reason for report, family background, other pertinent background information (e.g., health information, vocational history, history of adjustment issues/emotional problems/mental illness), mental status, assessment results, diagnosis, and summary, conclusions, and recommendations.

Security of Record Keeping

The security of your records is vital, as clients have the ethical and often legal right to have information they share with others kept confidential (Swenson, 1997). Therefore, it is critical that information obtained both verbally and in writing be kept confidential, secured, and not shared with others without client permission. Some exceptions to this are if you share client information with your supervisor, if the court subpoenas your records, and in some cases, if parents request information regarding their children. If you are going to share information with other agencies who might also be working with your

BOX 5.6

How Secure Are Records?

When I worked as an outpatient therapist at a mental health center, a client of another therapist had apparently obtained his records, which had been left "lying around." As his records tended to be written in psychological jargon, he was understandably quite upset by what he found. He therefore would periodically call the emergency services at night and read his records over the phone to the emergency worker while making fun of the language used in the records.

Another time, while taking a class in my doctoral program, we reviewed an assessment of an adolescent that had been done a number of years prior. Suddenly, one of the students in the class yelled out, "That's me!" Apparently, although there was no identifying names on the report, he recognized it as himself (he had been given a copy of the report previously).

client, it is essential that you obtain permission in writing from your client or your client's parent(s). This both assures your client's right to privacy and affords you legal protection.

Written client records need to be kept in secured places such as locked file cabinets. If records are kept on computers, then access to those files needs to be limited to you and possibly your supervisor. Clerical help should have explained to them the importance of confidentiality when working with records. In fact, it is now not unusual for agencies to have nonclinical staff who have access to client information sign statements acknowledging that they understand the importance of confidentiality and that they will not discuss client issues outside the office. Obviously, the importance of hiring nonclinical staff whom you can trust with client information is paramount.

Multicultural Issue: Applying Skills Cross-Culturally

It must be stressed that while the application of specific counseling skills discussed in this chapter may be beneficial to some clients, they may not be helpful and even may be harmful to the counseling relationship when used with other clients. This is particularly true in the cross-cultural counseling relationship. For instance, many Latin-American clients are comfortable with less personal space than other clients and may interpret counselor distance as aloofness; a Muslim may consider being touched by the left hand of a counselor as obscene, because the left hand is seen as unclean and used as an aid in the process of elimination, while the right hand is seen as clean and used for eating; and an African-American client may be put off by eye contact from a white counselor (Sue & Sue, 1999).

In a similar vein, some clients may feel defensive with the use of questions, while other clients may feel stonewalled because the counselor uses too much empathy. Some clients may feel as though they are being pushed to self-disclose—a quality viewed as weak in their culture—while other clients may feel offended that the counselor has not allowed them to talk more, as their culture tends to feel comfortable with the expression of feeling. And some cultures may be embarrassed with counselor self-disclosure, while for others, such disclosure may bring a counselor and client who are from two different cultures closer together.

Clearly, counselors need to have knowledge of the cultural background of the client and how a specific client's values, beliefs, and customs will play a part in the counseling relationship. At the same time, it must be remembered that each client is unique. For instance, although many Latin-American clients may be turned off by too much counselor–client personal space, some will not and may even feel more comfortable with less. Or an African-American client may be offended by the intentional lack of eye contact from his or her white counselor as a result of the counselor's false belief that African Americans would prefer less eye contact from white counselors.

Ethical, Professional, and Legal Issues

The Clients' Rights to Records

Although a gray area, clients probably have a legal right to view their records, and increasingly they have been exercising these rights in schools and agencies (Swenson, 1997; Wicks, 1977). Along these same lines, it has generally been assumed that parents have the right to view records of their children (Attorney C. Borstein, personal communication, June 1, 2001). In line with this, ACA's ethical standards state that clients should be provided access to their records if the client is competent and the material is not misleading or detrimental. Of course, specific local and state laws may vary, and each counselor should make him- or herself aware of how the laws apply.

In terms of federal law, the Freedom of Information Act of 1974 allows individuals access to any records maintained by a federal agency that contain personal information about the individual, and every state has followed along with similar laws governing state agencies (ACLU, 2001). Similarly, the Buckley Amendment of 1974, otherwise known as the Family Education Rights and Privacy Act (FERPA), assures parents the right to access their children's educational records (Committee on Government Operations, 1991). It has always been unclear as to whether this law applies to notes held by school counselors.

In a more practical vein, rarely does a client ask to view his or her records. However, if a client did make such a request, I would first explore with the client why he or she wants to see the records. Next, I would want to talk with the client about what is written in the records. If this was not satisfactory to the client, I would suggest that I might write a summary of the records. However, if a client steadfastly states a desire to view his or her records, I believe that this is his or her right.

Confidentiality of Records and Privileged Communication

A recent ruling appears to uphold the right to confidentiality of records if a licensed professional has privileged communication (Jaffee *v.* Redmond, 1996; see Box 5.7). In this case, the Supreme Court held the right of a licensed social worker to keep her case records confidential. Describing the social worker as a "therapist" and "psychotherapist," the ruling will likely protect all licensed therapists in federal courts and may affect all licensed therapists who have privileged communication (Remley, Herlihy, & Herlihy, 1997).

Despite this ruling, licensed counselors should continue to act cautiously, as the definition of privileged communication varies dramatically as a function of the state in which one is licensed and there are many exceptions to privilege (Glosoff et al., 2000) For instance, look below at how limiting the privileged communication statute is in Virginia.

BOX 5.7

Jaffee v. Redmond

Mary Lu Redmond, a police officer in a village near Chicago, responded to a "fight in progress" call at an apartment complex on June 27, 1991. At the scene, she shot and killed a man she believed was about to stab another man he was chasing. The family of the man she had killed sued Redmond, the police department, and the village, alleging that Officer Redmond had used excessive force in violation of the deceased's civil rights. When the plaintiff's lawyers learned that Redmond had sought and received counseling from a licensed social worker employed by the village, they sought to compel the social worker to turn over her case notes and records and testify at the trial.

Redmond and the social worker claimed that their communications were privileged under an Illinois statute. They both refused to reveal the substance of their counseling sessions even though the trial judge rejected their argument that the communications were privileged. The judge then instructed jurors that they could assume that the information withheld would have been unfavorable to the policewoman, and the jury awarded the plaintiffs $545,000. (Remley et al., 1997, p. 214)

After a series of appeals, the case was heard by the Supreme Court on February 26, 1996. The Court decided that the licensed therapist did indeed hold privilege and that the judge's instruction to the jury was therefore unwarranted.

It starts out by asserting privileged communication and ends by stating that the court, for almost any reason, can nullify such privilege:

> *. . . no duly licensed practitioner of any branch of the healing arts shall be required to testify in any civil action, . . . [except] when a court, in the exercise of sound discretion, deems such disclosure necessary to the proper administration of justice. . . .* (Code of Virginia, 1950)

The Counselor in Process: The Developmental Nature of Counseling Skills

When you first learn specific counseling skills, you may want to rigidly adhere to the techniques you are taught. I believe this is good, because the counselor who practices the skills again and again will learn them well. However, giving responses in a mechanistic manner can lead to a stiltedness in the helping relationship. Thus, one needs to try and find a balance between offering the "right" responses and being genuinely yourself in the relationship. Finding this balance is often not easy; yet, once you do, you will begin to feel more comfortable within the relationship, and you are likely to find your voice as a counselor.

As you continue through your career you will refine your skills, learn new skills, become more proficient at case conceptualization, and adjust and maybe even change your theoretical orientation. Slowly, you will become more grounded in your approach. It's as though you're continually finding yourself—rediscovering your voice and making it a little clearer. Carl Rogers used to say that as an individual goes through his or her self-discovery process, choices become clearer—almost as if one does not have a choice because his or her path in life becomes obvious (Rogers, 1989c). I believe a similar process occurs as we develop ourselves as counselors. Our skills, abilities, and who we are within the relationship become increasingly more refined and more focused. It's as if we have little choice in how we should act within the relationship—we become the master counselor.

Summary

This chapter examined the basic skills necessary for a successful counseling relationship and began with an overview of the importance of having an environment that can optimize the use of these basic skills. First, we examined the physical environment, including having a comfortable office that assures confidentiality and the importance of nonverbal behaviors with clients, especially when dealing with culturally diverse clients. We next talked about the importance of embracing the eight personal qualities highlighted in Chapter 1 in order to facilitate an effective counseling relationship while avoiding qualities likely to have a deleterious effect on the relationship.

Examining some foundational skills used in the counseling relationship, we first took a look at the use of silence, how to listen effectively, and how to make an empathic response. Empathic responding was highlighted as one crucial skill that could be taught in a systematic fashion. We next examined the more complex and advanced skills such as the use of questions, modeling, self-disclosure, confrontation, and interpretation. Later in the chapter we discussed the pluses and minuses of advice giving, offering alternatives, information giving, and affirmations. We particularly noted that such responses could be leading and can result in a dependent counseling relationship, if not used carefully. We ended this section by noting that, with advanced training, there are many advanced and specialized skills that a counselor can adopt.

Counseling skills are important to a successful counseling relationship; however, they become even more powerful when placed within the context of case conceptualization. Looking at one model of case conceptualization, we discussed how this process can assist the counselor in understanding symptomatic behaviors, feelings, and thoughts of the client and how it can help the counselor decide treatment planning and intervention strategies. We also showed how case conceptualization, counseling skills, and one's theoretical orientation can be applied across the stages of the counseling relationship. Defining six stages, we discussed the rapport and trust-building stage, the problem identification stage, the deepening-understanding and goal-setting stage, the work stage, the closure stage, and the follow-up stage, which could involve referral, recycling, and/or assessment of the counseling relationship.

Within this chapter we examined the importance of knowing the values, beliefs, and customs of clients from diverse backgrounds in the application of counseling skills. We highlighted the fact that in the cross-cultural counseling relationship some clients from diverse backgrounds may be turned off by what the counselor might consider to be common counseling skills. At the same time we encouraged counselors not to jump to conclusions about clients and assume that, because they have a specific cultural heritage, they will respond in a prescribed manner.

Near the end of this chapter we noted that ethical guidelines and laws generally protect clients' rights to their records. Such laws as the Freedom of Information Act and the Buckley Amendment (FERPA), as well as the ACA ethical guidelines, generally assure this right. We also noted that in the recent Jaffee *v.* Redmond Supreme Court decision, it was ruled that licensed therapists do have privileged communication. This decision is likely to have a positive impact on the right of all licensed therapists who have privileged communication. We warned, however, that currently full privilege is not offered in many states.

Finally, this chapter ended with a discussion that stressed the importance of continually developing one's counseling skills and ability at case conceptualization. These evolving skills and formulations allow the counselor to feel more capable about his or her ability and move the counselor toward ever-increasing self-assurance and effectiveness.

INFOTRAC and Other Information Resources (e.g., ERIC and PsycINFO)

Note: When relevant, key words are in quotation marks.

1. Research any "counseling technique" in this chapter that was particularly interesting to you.
2. Research the role of the "Jaffee" decision for all types of counselors.
3. Compare and contrast "privileged communication" with "confidentiality."

SECTION **III**

The Helping Relationship II: The Counselor Working in Systems

Overview

Section III takes a look at how the counselor works within systems. Each of these three chapters examines how knowledge of the complex interactions of systems is crucial to working effectively with families, groups, and when consulting or supervising.

Chapter 6 starts with an introduction to general systems theory, a model for understanding the ways all systems operate. This theory is basic to the content I will examine in all three chapters of this section. In Chapter 7, I remind the reader that groups, like families, follow the rules of general systems theory. I examine some advantages and disadvantages of group work compared to other forms of counseling, present a brief history of group counseling, and discuss the kinds of groups that are conducted by counselors. Chapter 8 will examine two important aspects of the helping relationship, consultation and supervision. I will note that knowledge of systems is important for both the consultant and the supervisor and define and offer different models of consultation and supervision.

As you read through these chapters consider how a contextual (systems) approach to the work of the counselor offers a different way of conceptualizing clients and adds a new dimension to the counseling relationship.

CHAPTER 6

Family Counseling

When I was in private practice, I received a call from a woman who wanted me to see her 12-year-old son; his grades in school had dropped dramatically, and he was having behavioral problems. Having had training in family counseling, I asked the whole family to come to the first session, rather than just seeing the boy. During the first session I obtained some basic information about the family. The boy was the older of two children; a sister was one year younger than he. The family was middle class, and there was no significant family history that could explain any problems. Both mom and dad had some difficulties in childhood, but nothing that one might not find in many families.

I decided to see the parents and the boy in family sessions. Although some family therapists would insist on seeing the whole family, I did not work like that. The parents saw no reason to have the daughter in the sessions, and I didn't want to resist their resistance. My style is to go with the family's wishes in order to build rapport. At a later date, if I felt the daughter should come in, I would request that of the family.

I saw the family, without the daughter, for approximately two months. Other than the school problems, there seemed to be no significant issues, at least any that I could get a handle on. I did, however, notice that most of the sessions were centered around the boy. Suddenly during one session the father blurted out, "I'm really depressed." Next thing I knew, he was talking about wanting to kill himself. Then the mother started saying she was bulimic, throwing up a few times a day; then she started alluding to having an affair.

As the parents continued to talk about *their* problems, I looked at the boy and saw that, for the first time, he was relaxed. It was becoming clear: The parents were using the boy to divert the pain of their own problems. I asked them to begin to look at their issues and lay off their son a little. Literally within the week, the boy's grades started to improve and his acting out ceased. Now the real work was to begin–helping the couple deal with their issues! *This* is family counseling.

This chapter is about family counseling. We will offer a brief history, define family therapy, and explain how families operate like many other living systems. We will attempt to define a healthy family and contrast that with a dysfunctional family. Most of the chapter will focus on the major theories of family counseling. The chapter will end with an examination of multicultural, ethical, professional, and legal issues related to family counseling.

Family Counseling: A Brief History

During the first half of the 20th century, counselors involved with child guidance in the United States began to see children and other family members concurrently, although not all together in the same room. This approach to counseling was unique; for the first time counselors were suggesting that problems in one family member affected the whole family. In 1942, individuals who practiced this approach to treatment formed the American Association of Marriage Counselors, which later became known as the American Association for Marriage and Family Therapy (AAMFT)(Everett, 1990; Foster & Gurman, 1985).

The 1950s saw a large push toward the treatment of the whole family, and a number of approaches to family counseling evolved. With the popularity of psychoanalysis during that time, it is not surprising that Nathan Ackerman (1958, 1966), a psychoanalyst, developed psychodynamic family therapy. At around the same time Murray Bowen (1976, 1978) developed what some would later call multigenerational family counseling. Meanwhile, a group in Palo Alto, California, that was studying communication theory was soon to produce a number of well-known family therapists and influence the creation of what later became known as the strategic and the communication schools of family therapy. Thus approaches were developed by Jay Haley (1973, 1976), Cloe Madanes (1981), the Milan Group (Palazzoli, Boscolo, Cecchin, & Prata, 1978), and Virginia Satir (1972a, 1972b). Salvadore Minuchin (1974, 1981) would also be somewhat influenced by communication theory, and his structural approach was particularly effective when working with poor families. With the concurrent spread of humanistic psychology during the 1950s and 1960s, it is not surprising that the experiential approach to family therapy, based on a mixture of humanistic philosophy and systems thinking, was to evolve around the same time. Carl Whitaker would come to be known as one of this group's main advocates (Napier & Whitaker, 1972, 1978; Whitaker, 1976). Finally, with the expansion of behavioral and cognitive approaches to individual therapy, we saw these philosophies applied within the family context.

Today, AAMFT and other family therapy associations, such as the International Association of Marriage and Family Counseling (IAMFC), a division of ACA, set separate curriculum standards and certification requirements in the field of family therapy (see Chapter 2; Smith et al., 1995; Stevens-Smith, Hinkle, & Stahmann, 1993). Although two competing associations, family therapy curricula and training are largely based on the theories of family therapy listed above.

With the popularity of family therapy increasing, in recent years new training methods have been developed (Getz & Protinsky; 1994; Gladding, 1994; Landis & Young, 1994; Smith, 1994; Spruill, 1994; West, Bubenzer, Pinsoneault, & Holeman, 1993). And, although more research needs to be completed, a review of the efficacy of family therapy has found the following (Carlson, 1993):

- Family treatment is more effective than no treatment.
- Marital and family therapy seems particularly effective for marital problems, sexual difficulties, and the treatment of aggressiveness and acting out in children.

- Marital and family therapy seems a particularly good treatment of choice for chemical dependency, many problems of childhood, depression, schizophrenia, family conflicts, and multiple personality disorder.
- Short-term family therapy seems at least as effective as long-term treatment.
- Usually, the more members involved in family counseling, the better the chances of positive results.
- One particular school of family counseling does not seem more effective than another.
- Regardless of the school of family therapy, therapist relationship skills seem a crucial factor in affording effective treatment.
- Although many clients will improve in family counseling, up to 10% may actually have a worsening of symptoms.

As the above implies, family therapy seems to be a viable alternative or addition to individual counseling. It also offers a different way of viewing clients as compared to individual counseling. Let's examine some of the basic tenets of family work and why at times it may be a more viable approach to individual counseling.

General Systems Theory

Living systems are processes that maintain a persistent structure over relatively long periods despite rapid exchange of their component parts with the surrounding world.

(Skynner, 1976, pp. 3–4)

The amoeba. The family. The universe. What do these seemingly dissimilar entities have to do with family therapy? Well, although knowledge of the amoeba and of the universe may seem like a far cry from helping us to understand the family, in actuality they all have something in common: They obey the rules of a system. The amoeba has a semipermeable boundary that allows it to take in nutrition from the environment. This delicate animal could not survive if its boundaries were so rigid that they prevented it from ingesting food or so permeable that they would not allow it to maintain and digest the food. As long as the amoeba is in balance, it will maintain its existence.

The universe is an exceedingly predictable place, and it has a certain cadence to it. It maintains a persistent structure over a long period of time. However, remove a star, planet, moon, or asteroid, and the system is shaken, momentarily disequilibrated as it moves to reconfigure itself. As long as the universe is in balance, it will maintain its existence.

Like the amoeba and the universe, what occurs in the family is predictable, because the family too has boundaries and structure that maintain themselves over long periods of time. As long as the family system is in balance, it will maintain its existence.

> *The concept of system thus treats people and events in terms of their interactions rather than their intrinsic characteristics. The most basic principle underlying the systems viewpoint has been understood for some time. An ancient astronomer once said, "Heaven is more than the stars alone. It is the stars and their movements."*
> (Baruth & Huber, 1984, p. 19)

General systems theory (Bertalanffy, 1934, 1968) was developed to explain the complex interactions of all types of systems including living systems, family systems, community systems, and solar systems. Each system is seen to have a boundary that allows it to maintain its structure while the system interacts with other systems around it. So the action of the amoeba, one of the smallest of all living systems, affects and is affected by surrounding suprasystems, while the universe, the largest of all systems, is made up of subsystems that have a predictable relationship to one another. Similarly, the action of subsystems in families will affect other subsystems (e.g., the parental subsystem will affect the child subsystem); family units will affect other families, and families make up communities that affect society, and so on.

Boundaries and Information Flow in Systems

A healthy system has fluid boundaries that allow new information to come into the system, be processed, and then incorporated into the system. When a system has rigid boundaries, information is not able to easily flow into or out of the system, and change becomes a difficult process. Alternatively, a system that has loose boundaries allows information to flow too easily into and out of the system, causing the individual components of the system to have difficulty maintaining a sense of identity and stability.

American culture allows for much variation in the permeability of various systems, but systems that have boundaries that are too loose or too rigid tend toward dysfunction. In the United States it is common for us to find families and community groups (e.g., some religious organizations) with a fairly rigid set of rules that maintain their functioning in relatively healthy ways. Alternatively, we may also find families and community groups that allow for a wide range of behaviors within a fairly loose system (e.g., encounter groups). Unfortunately, all too often we have seen the dysfunction that results from a system whose boundaries are too rigid or too loose (see Box 6.1).

BOX 6.1

Jim Jones and the Death of a Rigid System

During the 1950s and early 1960s, Jim Jones was a respected minister in Indiana. However, over the years he became increasingly paranoid and grandiose, believing he was Jesus. He moved his family to Brazil and later relocated to California where approximately 100 of his church followers from Indiana joined him. In California, he headed the "People's Church" and began to set rigid rules for church membership. Slowly, he became more dictatorial and continued to show evidence of paranoid delusions. Insisting that church members prove their love for him, he demanded sex with female church members, had members sign over their possessions, sometimes had members give their children over to him, and had members inform on those who went against his rules. In 1975, a reporter uncovered some of the tactics Jones was using and was about to write a revealing article about the church. Jones learned about this and, just prior to publication of the article, moved to Guyana, taking a few hundred of his followers with him. As concerns about some of the church practices reached the United States, California Congressperson Ryan and some of his aides went to Guyana to investigate the situation. Jones and his supporters killed Ryan and the aides and then ordered his followers to commit suicide. Hundreds killed themselves. Those who did not were murdered.

Jim Jones had developed a church with an extremely rigid set of rules. The writing of a revealing article as well as the congressperson flying into Guyana was a threat to the system. As with many rigid systems, attempts at change from the outside were seen as a potential lethal blow to the system. Jones dealt with the reporter's threat to the system by moving his congregation to Guyana. Then, rather than allow new information into the system, Jim Jones killed off the system, first killing the congressperson and then ordering the church members to commit suicide. The members had become so mired in the rules of the system that nearly 900 of them ended up committing suicide or being murdered (Axthelm, 1978).

Boundaries and Regulatory Mechanisms

Regardless of whether a system has fluid, rigid, or loose boundaries, the regulatory mechanism of the system maintains homeostasis, or the tendency of the system to maintain its unique way of interacting. The study of cybernetics, or control mechanisms in systems, has been used to explain this regulatory process. One type of cybernetic system of which we are all aware is a thermostat. As it becomes colder, the temperature drops, and the thermostat kicks in the heating system; as the temperature goes up, the thermostat shuts down the heat. This type of cybernetic system is called a negative feedback loop, because it keeps the irregularities within the system at a minimum. Positive feedback loops occur when one component in a system leads to a change in another component within the same system, which leads to a change in the first component, and so on. In spousal abuse you see a positive feedback loop when spouses egg each other on in a continual escalation of the fight until abuse occurs. Look at Box 6.2 for an example of a couple engaged in a positive feedback loop.

BOX 6.2

Joyce and Antonio: A Positive Feedback Loop

In the dialogue below, Joyce and Antonio are discussing going out to a play. As they realize that their expectations about the evening differ, they begin to get angry at one another. Eventually, there is an altercation at which point Antonio defuses the situation by leaving.

Joyce: *Are you going to the play with me tonight?*

Antonio: *Well, I was actually thinking I might go out with my friends. You know, I haven't really seen them for a while. Besides, I didn't really think that I committed myself to the play.*

Joyce: *Well, you did say you thought you would go with me.*

Antonio: *I don't remember saying that. I was thinking all along that I would go out with my buddies.*

Joyce: *I remember distinctly you telling me you would go. It's clear as day to me. You're either lying or have early dementia.*

Antonio: *Look, I don't want to get into a fight. You're always forcing me to get into a fight with you. I don't know why you egg me on like this. You must have a need to fight with me. I bet it has to do with the fact that you never felt loved by your father—you know, we've talked about that before.*

Joyce: *Not being loved by my father! Who are you kidding? The only one I don't feel loved by is you. At least my father was around. You just take off whenever you damn please! Half of the time you leave me with the kids, as if you have no responsibility around here. You just go out, get blasted and God knows what else.*

Antonio: *Look, I'm no slacker around here. You don't do a damn thing around this house. Look at it. It's a mess. I do plenty, and you can't even keep this house together. I work hard to fix this place up, and you can't even run a vacuum once in a while. You . . . it's disgusting!*

Joyce: *Don't call me disgusting!*

Antonio: *I didn't! I said IT'S disgusting—the house.*

Joyce: *No, I heard you, you were going to say I'm disgusting. I hate you! You and your drinking, you and your friends. You and those sluts you hang out with at work. I know what you're doing around my back!*

Antonio: *Screw you!*

Joyce: *Go to hell!* (Swings at him.)

Antonio: (Grabs her arm as she swings and throws her on the floor.)

Joyce: *You abusive bastard!*

Antonio: *Screw you . . . I'm getting out of here.* (Leaves the house.)

Joyce: (Sobs as Antonio leaves.)

Each family has its unique way of interacting, which includes negative and sometimes positive feedback loop systems. If you examine communication sequences in any family, you can begin to understand the unique boundaries, feedback loops, and homeostatic mechanisms involved.

Dysfunctional and Healthy Families

Divorce has ripple effects that touch not just the family involved, but our entire society. As the writer Pat Conroy observed when his own marriage broke up, "Each divorce is the death of a small civilization." When one family divorces, that divorce affects relatives, friends, neighbors, employers, teachers, clergy, and scores of strangers. (Wallerstein & Blakeslee, 1989, p. xxi)

Today, nearly 50% of marriages end in divorce. So great is the impact of divorce on the family that Wallerstein and Blakeslee (1989) found that in a five-year follow-up of children of divorce, a great majority of them were still negatively affected by it. They also found that the effects of divorce can have a major impact on the children as they grow into adulthood. From a systemic perspective, divorce is the systems response to stress that cannot be resolved. What is it that causes some families to maintain healthy ways of relating, while others seem to thrive on dysfunction, with the result often being the dissolution of the system? General systems theory helps provide us with some answers to this elusive question.

The Development of the Healthy Family

People in healthy families can talk to one another. They can share their feelings, are open about their concerns, are not particularly defensive, and have a clear sense of themselves and of others in the family. A healthy family has parents or guardians who are the main rule makers (a healthy family system can also have a single parent or guardian). Although rules will change from family to family, healthy families have a clear sense of hierarchy. This means that the parent(s) or guardian(s) are the main rule makers, and children, although possibly consulted in the rule making, are the recipients of those rules. Healthy families rely on negative feedback loops and don't have arguments that escalate into dysfunctional behaviors, such as spousal or child abuse.

A healthy family can deal with stressful situations. For example, when a couple has their first child, the husband–wife dyad faces a potential crisis as the rules in their family change in order to deal with the new family member. As children age, families will continually face developmental crises that again necessitate change in family rules. The unhealthy family will not deal with these changes effectively, and pain will resonate throughout the family (Minuchin, 1974; Satir, 1967). However, the healthy family will communicate in ways that will allow the family to support one another as the various family members go through changes. In addition, the healthy family will allow information from the outside world to visit the family, as it decides whether to adapt itself to this new information or to reject it and maintain its past level of functioning.

All families live with stress, and in our society with lots of it, but families that come into treatment have much more than their share. (Napier & Whitaker, 1978, p. 81)

Dysfunctional Families

All husbands and wives bring unfinished business to their marriage, which invariably will have an impact on their relationship. The more serious their issues, the more likely they will affect their marriage and, from a systems perspective, affect the family. A wife who was sexually molested as a child and has not worked through her pain will bring this unfinished business into the relationship. For instance, she might develop mistrust toward men and therefore unconsciously choose a man who is distant (and safe). Perhaps he is a workaholic. Alternatively, a man who has difficulty with intimacy might unconsciously pick a wife who allows him to be distant (and safe). Perhaps she was sexually molested and distrusts men. As the relationship unravels, the issues that each spouse brings to the marriage will get played out either on one another or on the children. The husband may become stressed at work and take this out on his wife and/or children. The wife may crave more intimacy, become discontent with the marriage, and take this out on her husband and/or children. Is it surprising that there are so many affairs and divorces?

When spouses are discontent with one another, and when they directly or indirectly take out this unhappiness on a child, that child is said to be scapegoated. Some families will unconsciously not allow a child to become a scapegoat, and one of the spouses may take on this role. In either case, when a family member is scapegoated, he or she often becomes the identified patient (I. P.), or the member who has the problem. In actuality, the whole family has the problem. When a child acts out in the family, in school, or in the community, it is often the result of that child being the member carrying the pain for the family.

Why is someone in a family scapegoated? Usually because it has become too painful for the couple to look at their issues. Rather than be open with one another or seek marital counseling to spill out their issues, they scapegoat a child or themselves (see Box 6.3).

In an effort to deal with dysfunctional families, a number of models of family therapy have been developed. Although each approach has a somewhat different orientation to working with the family, they all rely to some degree on the basic concepts of the system.

Models of Family Therapy

A family who enters family counseling is admitting to some level of dysfunction. Family counselors, in one fashion or another, will examine the family through a systems perspective and, as Barker (1998) suggests, are likely to borrow most of the following ideas from general systems theory:

1. Families (and other social groups) are systems having properties which are more than the sum of the properties of their parts.
2. The operation of such systems is governed by certain general rules.
3. Every system has a boundary, the properties of which are important in understanding how the system works.
4. The boundaries are semipermeable; that is to say, some things can pass through them while others cannot. Moreover, it is sometimes found that certain material can pass one way but not the other.
5. Family systems tend to reach relatively, but not totally, steady states [homeostasis]. Growth and evolution are possible, indeed usual. Change can occur, or be stimulated in various ways.

BOX 6.3

Pain in the Family

Psychotherapy, particularly marital psychotherapy, threatens to "uncover" the anxious turmoil in the marriage. "If we seek help as a couple," the partners say silently to themselves, "it will all come out." The anger, the bitterness, the hurt, the sense of self-blame that each carries—this will be the harvest of the opening up to each other. "Maybe it will destroy what we have" is their fear. They dread not only losing the stability of the marriage, but damaging their fragile self-images. Rather than risk their painful and tenuous security, they suppress the possibility of working on their marriage together. "Too dangerous," seems to be the final judgment, although at most this is only a hazily conscious decision. (Napier & Whitaker, 1978, p. 148)

6. Communication and feedback mechanisms between the parts of the system are important in the functioning of the system [*cybernetics*: positive and negative feedback loops].
7. Events such as the behavior of individuals in the family are better understood as examples of *circular causality*, rather than on the basis of *linear causality*.
8. Family systems, like other open systems, appear to be purposeful.
9. Systems are made up of *subsystems* and themselves are parts of *suprasystems*. (pp. 27–28)

As we explore a number of models of family therapy, you will find that there are many commonalities. The following is a sampling of some of the more prevalent family therapy approaches used today.

Structural Family Therapy

Although many family therapists consider themselves in the structural school, certainly the most well known is Salvadore Minuchin (1974, 1981). Minuchin (1974) states that all families have interactional and transactional *rules* that are maintained by the kinds of *boundaries* in the family as noted through the *structure and hierarchy* that exists. He goes on to note that all families will experience *stress*, which is handled differently by each family and is a function of the existing rules, boundaries, and structure and hierarchy in the family. In order to make change in families, structural family therapists must *join* with the family, map the family, and provide interventions for *restructuring*.

Rules

Universal rules are related to the power hierarchy in families; and, although they might change to some degree from culture to culture, all cultures appear to have a basic hierarchy with parents or guardians on a higher level of authority than children. Idiosyncratic rules are those unique to a family. For instance, a family might have a rule that whenever there is tension in the couple's relationship, the youngest child is yelled at for doing something wrong. In actuality, in this case the child has been scapegoated in an effort to diffuse tension between the couple. There are an infinite number of idiosyncratic rules, and they usually happen in an automatic, unconscious manner.

Boundaries

It is important for structural family therapists to determine how fluid the boundaries are between subsystems. Rigid boundaries lead to disengaged family members, while boundaries that are too permeable lead to family members who are enmeshed. For instance, a child subsystem that has a very permeable boundary with the parental susbsystem is said to be enmeshed. This leads to a loss of identity for all family members (e.g., a family with no doors on the rooms, where emotionality is shared among all members—when one person feels upset, all feel upset). On the other hand, a parental subsystem that has rigid boundaries is said to be disengaged from the child subsystem. This can lead to chaos in the family (e.g., parents who do not communicate effective parenting skills let their children run wild). The goal of the therapist in this case would be to help establish semipermeable boundaries between subsystems.

Structure and Hierarchy

The family structure maintains the homeostasis in the family, and family members will implicitly or explicitly attempt to sabotage any attempt at disequilibrizing the system. For instance, if through therapy there is an attempt to change the mode of communication so that the youngest child is not scapegoated, the family might drop out of therapy.

In understanding families, Minuchin states that it is particularly important to map the family structure. This map describes the executive subsystem—who is in charge under what circumstances—and the sibling subsystem—how siblings interact. It also examines whether or not boundaries are crossed between subsystems. For instance, a child may be inappropriately placed in an executive subsystem, thus causing confusion and conflict within the family (e.g., oldest son takes charge of the family while parents look on). Or, an older child may appropriately be placed in an executive subsystem for a limited time period (e.g., when a single mother is working).

Stress

Minuchin (1974) states that families respond differentially to stress based on the inherent health of the system. He lists four types of stress that are important to identify when working with families:

1. *Stressful contact of one member with extrafamilial forces* (e.g., difficulty at work)
2. *Stressful contact of the whole family with extrafamilial forces* (e.g., a natural disaster such as a hurricane)
3. *Stress at transitional or developmental points in the family* (e.g., puberty, midlife crises, retirement aging) (see Chapter 9)
4. *Idiosyncratic (situational) stress* (e.g., unexpected illness) (see Box 6.4)

Although there are different causes of stress, each family will tend to handle stress as a function of the strength of its boundaries. For instance, a family with fluid boundaries, clearly defined subsystems and suprasystems, little scapegoating, and healthy hierarchical structure (e.g., people know who's in charge and when they're in charge) will be able to effectively communicate and find positive ways to deal with stress. On the other hand, a family who is unclear about who is in charge, either enmeshed or disengaged, and whose members tend to blame others rather than take responsibility, will have a difficult time communicating and dealing with stress.

BOX 6.4

A Situational Family Crisis

When I was between the ages of 8 and 13, I had a heart disorder called pericarditis. This was a somewhat debilitating illness that enlarged my heart, caused me much chest pain, and left me periodically bedridden with a resulting mild depression. Although not considered extremely serious, this illness certainly affected my life in a major way. However, it also affected my parents lives and the lives of my siblings.

Although my illness potentially could have been a threat to the homeostasis in the family, it became clear that the family was healthy enough to deal effectively with this situation. As my parents' marriage was solid, the added stress did not dramatically affect their relationship. In addition, they were able to maintain the functioning of the family in a relatively normal way. This normalization of family patterns during a period of stress speaks highly of the health in the family.

Joining

Minuchin believes that change in the family can only occur if the therapist is able to "join" with the family. Joining is when the counselor is accepted by the family and wins their confidence. Joining can be done in many ways such as through empathy, being friendly, or sharing common stories with the family.

Joining the family allows the counselor to understand the family's rules, boundaries, structure and hierarchy, and stress. It is only then that the counselor can begin to restructure the family.

Restructuring

Restructuring the family occurs after the counselor has joined the family and mapped its structure. It involves creating healthier boundaries and changing structure and hierarchy in order to help the family deal with stress and function in a healthier manner. Restructuring can occur in numerous ways. Box 6.5 describes the restructuring of one family.

By using many of the basic concepts of general systems theory, Minuchin offers a practical, straightforward way of understanding families and making family interventions. Although many of these concepts are also used in the next school of family therapy, strategic family therapy, there they are applied in quite a different manner.

Strategic Family Therapy

During the 1950s a number of individuals gathered in Palo Alto, California, to consider and eventually write about the process of communication (Bateson, Jackson, Haley, & Weakland, 1956; Watzlawick, Beavin, & Jackson, 1967; Watzlawick, Weakland, & Fisch, 1974). These individuals, and later others such as Virginia Satir (1967), were to become major players in the field of family therapy. Although all schools of family therapy have to some degree used the concepts developed at Palo Alto, strategic family therapists and communication family therapists have applied these concepts more directly than others. Let's first examine strategic family therapy. Some important beliefs underlying the approach include (Watzlawick et al., 1967, 1974):

BOX 6.5

An Example of Family Restructuring

Mom and Dad have three children aged 15, 12, and 1. Since the birth of their new child, the two oldest children have been fighting constantly and having problems at school. The husband and wife seem depressed. Assessing the situation, you find that the whole family is dealing with transitional and idiosyncratic stress. The baby was not planned, and the family is stretched financially. The therapist notes that the family hierarchy has changed, that the spousal subsystem is showing depression, and that the parental subsystem is not able to maintain control over the two older children. The therapist wants to strengthen the spousal and parental subsystems. The current map of the family is:

Dad
———

Mom and Infant }

Child ✵ Child
(15) (12)

Legend

} = Cutoff

——— = Rigid boundary

✵ = Conflict

- - - - = Permeable boundary

↘ ↕ = Temporarily in other subsystem

Therefore, the following is prescribed:

1. Have the oldest child take a certification course in babysitting to assist with child care.
2. Ask the grandmother to assist with child care to relieve some pressure on Mom.
3. Have Dad take on some of the responsibilities related to the problems with the oldest children. He must meet with the teachers and school counselors.
4. Suggest that Mom, who now has assistance with child care, take on a part-time job to relieve some of the economic stress (she has always worked in the past).
5. Establish one evening a week where the grandmother or oldest child will watch the other two children so parents can go out.

The goal is to reestablish the spousal subsystem while strengthening the parental subsystem. The grandmother and oldest child will periodically take on a position of power in the family, with their power being time limited. The extra money and reduction of stress for Mom will result in reduced stress in the family. The family eventually looks like the following:

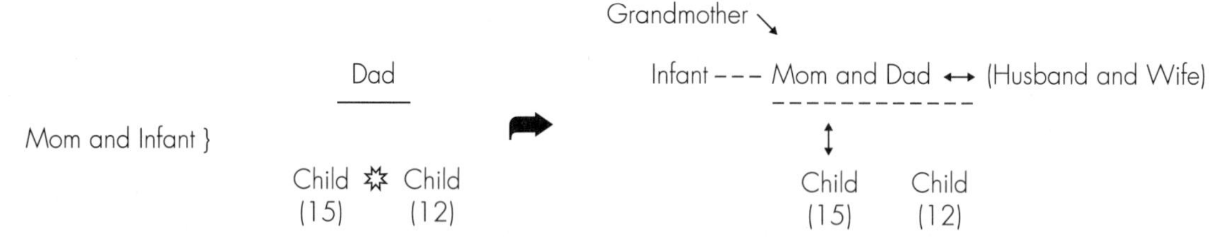

1. "Normal" or "abnormal" is a contextual phenomenon, not an objective state of being.
2. The unconscious is not an important factor in working with individuals; instead, what is important are the current behaviors people are exhibiting.

3. The whys are not as important as what is going on between people.
4. Behaviors tell a story about communication between people and are often more a sign of what's going on than the actual words that are communicated.
5. One cannot *not* communicate. Not saying anything is a communication about communication.
6. A message sent is not necessarily the message received. A person might send one message, but a different message might be heard.
7. Communication has two ways of expression: digitally, or the exact meaning of the words, and analogically, or the meaning about the meaning, often expressed nonverbally. For example, a person may be angry and say "I love you" in an angry tone. The digital message "I love you" is at odds with the analogic message.
8. Communication makes a statement about the content of the conversation and about the relationship one is in. In other words, each statement a person makes is an expression about the relationship.
9. A series of communications gives important meaning about the relationship (a husband might always discuss issues with a flat affect to his wife; this continual flat message may be more important than the actual words he says).
10. Any intervention made within the system, be it with one or more of the family members, will reverberate throughout the system.

The steps involved in strategic therapy are based on an understanding of communication and systems theory; and, because unconscious motivations play little if any role in this type of therapy, the approach is relatively pragmatic. Relative to the therapeutic process, the strategic approach is not particularly concerned with feelings (although the therapist wants the client to end up having good feelings!). This approach is based on how individuals communicate to one another, how communication sequences can be changed to help people feel better, and how power is dispersed in the family. Power for the strategic therapist is defined in some very nontraditional ways:

> *Power tactics are those maneuvers a person uses to give himself influence and control over his social world and to make that world more predictable. Defined thus broadly, a man has power if he can order someone to behave in a certain way, but he also has power if he can provoke someone to behave that way. One man can order others to lift and carry him while another might achieve the same end by collapsing.* (Haley, 1986, p. 53)

The therapist most associated with the strategic approach has been Jay Haley (1973, 1976), although others like Cloe Madanes and the Milan Associates have also become well known. Haley was greatly affected by Milton Erickson, a legend as a therapist because of his uncanny ability to induce change in clients. In Haley's 1976 book, *Problem-Solving Therapy*, he describes four stages of the first interview that set the stage for the change process. Although unique to the way Haley implements strategic therapy, it gives you a sense of the manner in which all strategic family therapists work.

Haley's Stages of Strategic Therapy

1. *The social stage*. During this stage the therapist invites the whole family to counseling and asks each member to introduce him- or herself. At this point the therapist can observe where family members sit, interactions among family members, and the overall mood of the family. The therapist at this point should not

share his or her observations with the family, and all formulations about the family should be tentative.

2. *The problem stage*. During the problem stage, each family member is asked to describe his or her perceptions of the problem. The therapist should carefully listen to each person's perception of the problem, which may be defined differently by varying family members. Interactions among family members should be carefully observed, and therapist interpretations about the problem should not be shared.
3. *The interaction stage*. The interaction stage is highlighted by the therapist's attempt to get the family to interact during the session in the same manner they might at home. This process assists the therapist in viewing how the family is organized around the problem.
4. *Goal-setting stage*. During this stage the family is asked to be clear about what they would like to change, and, in collaboration with the therapist, a problem is agreed upon. This problem is important and needs to be addressed; however, it also tells us something about how the family communicates and the hierarchies in the family (Foster & Gurman, 1985; Haley, 1973; Haley, 1976). Therefore, how the therapist addresses the problem may vary, based on an assessment of the structure and communication sequences in the family. Haley addresses problems in families through the method of directives.

Directives

> *It is important to emphasize that directives can be given directly or they can be given in a conversation implicitly by vocal intonation, body movement, and well-timed silence. Everything done in therapy can be seen as a directive.*
> (Haley, 1976, p. 50)

If enough progress has been made, directives can be made at the end of the first session, although sometimes it may take two or three sessions before directives are suggested. Haley (1976) identifies two types of directives: "(1) telling people what to do when the therapist wants them to do it, and (2) telling them what to do when the therapist does not want them to do it because the therapist wants them to change by rebelling" (p. 52).

In the first case, a therapist can either give good advice or give a directive that changes the structure of the family. Haley admits that advice, even good advice, is rarely followed by families. Therefore, he suggests giving directives in which the family wants to participate; directives that will address both the presenting problem and also broader problems inherent in the family organization and communication sequencing. The therapist generally does not reveal to the family his or her agenda of restructuring family dynamics, as this is not generally found to expedite change. For instance, parents might identify a problem as their daughter's use of drugs. However, in therapy it soon becomes clear that the family isolates and cuts off the daughter from the rest of the family. The therapist could give good advice, such as suggesting to the daughter that she take a drug education class. However, this would most likely be a wasteful suggestion because it is not likely to be followed by the rebellious daughter. Therefore, in this case it would be useful to offer a directive that deals with the drug use and the family organization—a directive in which all would participate. For example, the therapist might ask the family to include the daughter in as many family activities as possible in an effort to assure that she is not doing drugs. The parents will appreciate this directive as it is dealing with the problem, and the daughter will appreciate it as she is finally being included in the family.

The second type of directive, called a paradoxical directive, is when clients are asked to do something opposite of what might seem logical with the expectation that the directive is likely to fail, and that this failure will lead to success in therapy. If clients actually do follow the directive, success is also assured. For instance, a family has a child who is constantly angry and screaming. The therapist might reframe the situation by stating that this child is actually quite healthy in that he is expressing his feelings. The therapist suggests that listening to the child's feelings is not likely to be helpful because the child needs to release his healthy anger. Probably, the therapist suggests, it would be helpful instead to encourage the child to scream more. Parents who rebel against this suggestion end up listening to the child. On the other hand, parents who go with the suggestion are now compliant clients who have reframed the problem into a healthy one and are encouraged for being such good clients during the next session.

Another technique to induce change of this kind is through the use of metaphor. Look at how Haley (1976) uses metaphor to deal with a couple's uncomfortable feelings about talking directly to their son about his being adopted:

> *[The therapist] talked to the boy about "adopting" a dog who had a problem of being frightened. . . . When the boy said the family might have to get rid of the dog if he became ill and cost doctor bills [the boy had been ill], the therapist insisted that once adopted the family was committed to the dog and would have to keep him and pay his doctor bills no matter what. Various concerns the boy might have had about himself as well as the parents' concerns about him were discussed in metaphoric terms in relation to the proposed adoption of the puppy.* (p. 65)

Course of Treatment

Strategic therapy tends to be a short-term approach to counseling, because it focuses almost exclusively on presenting problems, does not spend time dealing with intrapsychic processes, and uses directives to facilitate the change process. Usually, directives can be made within the first few sessions with follow-up and revision to the original directives sometimes lasting a few more sessions.

Clearly, to be a strategic therapist takes a lot of training and confidence in one's ability to suggest effective directives. It is interesting to watch some of the more well-known strategic therapists work. Criticized as manipulative by some, they do not appear manipulative in practice. In fact, their directives, even ones with hidden agendas, appear to come from a real and caring place for these master therapists.

Communication Family Therapy

> *All of the ingredients in a family that count are changeable and correctable—individual self-worth, communication, system, and rules—at any point in time.*
> (Satir, 1972a, p. xi)

Virginia Satir, a systems communication theorist and a humanist, is considered to have been one of the foremost family therapists of the 20th century. After having been a family therapist for a number of years, Satir was invited to work with the Palo Alto group on communication theory (Satir, 1972b). However, the humanistic psychology movement was to also influence her, and she came to believe that individuals had a positive growth force and that by actualizing one's physical, emotional, spiritual, and behavioral resources one could reach one's potential. Thus, although Satir's communication approach has many of the same basic elements as Haley's strategic approach, it clearly shows the influence of the humanistic revolution in counseling.

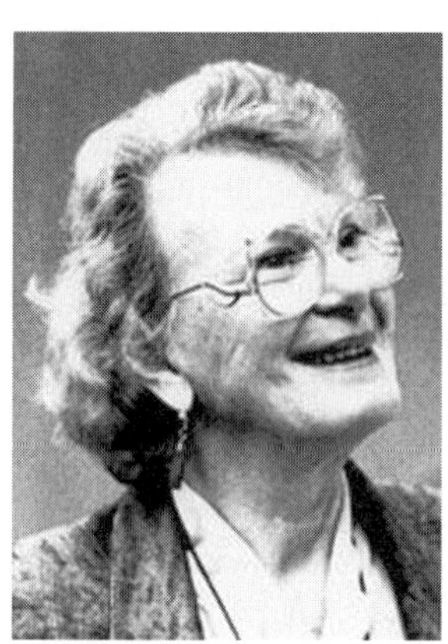

Virginia Satir

Satir believed that a primary survival triad exists that includes parents and the child, with each child's sense of well-being and self-esteem the result of this triad. Low self-esteem eventually leads individuals to take on one of four unhealthy universal communication patterns: (1) the placater, who appeases people so others won't get angry at him or her; (2) the blamer, who accuses others in an effort to diffuse hurt; (3) the computer, who acts cool, calm, and collected in an attempt to deal with the world as if nothing could hurt him or her, and (4) the distracter, who goes off on tangents in an effort to treat threats as if they do not exist (Satir, 1972a). On the other hand, Satir also believed that children who had healthy parenting would grow into adults who were congruent–in sync with their feelings, thoughts, and behaviors—and could thus communicate clearly with others.

Believing that communication and behavioral patterns are a result of complex interactions among family members and the legacy from past generations, Satir felt it was important to obtain graphic information about important past events in one's family. Thus, she would often have families complete a family life fact chronology, which is a history of important events within the extended family. Similar to a genogram, the family life fact chronology could be analyzed and reflected upon by all involved in therapy. Additionally, Satir was one of the first therapists to use family sculpting in an effort to bring forth blocked and unexpressed emotions (Piercy, Sprenkle, & Wetchler, 1996). This experiential work involves each family member taking a physical position that nonverbally represents how that member interacts with the rest of the family. For instance, a child who is withdrawing might stand near a door as if she were about to leave the room; a mother trying to control her son might stand over him with her finger pointed at him, and a father who is detached through drinking might sit at a table with a make-believe glass of beer in his hand.

Combining humanistic and communication theories, Satir believed that a family therapist should be caring and respectful, believe in the ability of the family to heal, actively encourage the family to change, be spontaneous, and act as "a facilitator, a resource person, an observer, a detective, and a model for effective communication" (Becvar & Becvar, 2000, p. 227). By creating a trusting atmosphere that encouraged the letting down of defenses, Satir hoped to open up communication patterns, look at past hurts, and help clients learn how to be more effective and open communicators.

Ultimately, through the process of family therapy and self-enhancement (Satir, 1972a), Satir hoped that couples and families could have a mature relationship in which each person could:

1. Be responsible for oneself and have a strong sense of self.
2. Make decisions based on an accurate perception of self, others, and the social context.
3. Be able to make wise choices for which a person takes full responsibility.
4. Be in touch with one's feelings.
5. Be clear in one's communication.

6. Be able to accept others for who they are.
7. See differences in others' as an opportunity to learn, not as a threat. (adapted from Satir, 1967, p. 91)

Multigenerational Family Therapy

Family counselors who take on a multigenerational approach to family therapy focus on how behavioral patterns and personality traits from prior generations have been passed down in families. Therefore, many multigenerational family counselors may encourage bringing in parents, grandparents, and perhaps even cousins, uncles, and aunts.

Although multigenerational family counselors focus on intergenerational conflicts, the way they go about this may differ. For instance, Ivan Boszormenyi-Nagy (1973, 1987) believes that families are relational systems in which loyalties, a sense of indebtedness, and ways of relating are passed down from generation to generation. Couples enter relationships with a ledger of indebtedness and entitlements based on their family of origin and what was passed down to that family. A couple who enter a relationship with an imbalanced ledger will invariably attempt to balance the ledger with each other. This is almost always unsuccessful, as the imbalance is a result of unfinished business from the family of origin, not from the spouse. For instance, one who felt unloved by his mother might attempt to settle up his account with her by trying to have his wife shower him with love. However, because this is unfinished business with the mother, the husband will continue to feel a sense of emptiness, even if the wife fulfills this request. Boszormenyi-Nagy believes that it is crucial for all family members to gain the capacity to hear one another, communicate with one another, and have the ability to understand their interpersonal connectedness to the current family as well as their family of origin.

> *When each generation is helped to face the nature of the current relationships, exploring the real nature of the commitments and responsibility that flow from such involvements, an increased reciprocal understanding and mutual compassion between the generations results. The grandchildren, in particular, benefit from this reconciliation between the generations; they are helped to be freed of scapegoated or parentified roles and they have a hope for age appropriate gratifications plus a model for reconciling their conflicts with their parents.* (Friedman, 1989, p. 405)

Another multigenerational family therapist, Murray Bowen, believed that previous generations could dramatically affect one's ability to develop a healthy ego. He considered the ultimate goal of family therapy to be the differentiation of self, which included differentiation of self from others and the differentiation of one's emotional processes from one's intellectual processes (Bowen, 1976, 1978). He believed that there was a nuclear family emotional system made up of all family members (living, dead, absent, and present), which continued to have an emotional impact upon the system. Such an emotional system, said Bowen, is reflective of the level of differentiation in the family, and is called the undifferentiated ego mass. Thus, previous generations could continue to have an influence on current family dynamics. Bowen used the genogram to examine in detail the family's functioning over a number of generations. Although the basic genogram includes such items as dates of birth and death, names, and major relationships along with breakups or divorces, usually the therapist will also ask the family to include such things as where various members are from, who might be scapegoated and/or an identified patient, mental illness and physical diseases, affairs, abortions, and stillbirths (see Figure 6.1).

FIGURE 6.1
Hannah Virginia Williams Neukrug's Abbreviated Genogram

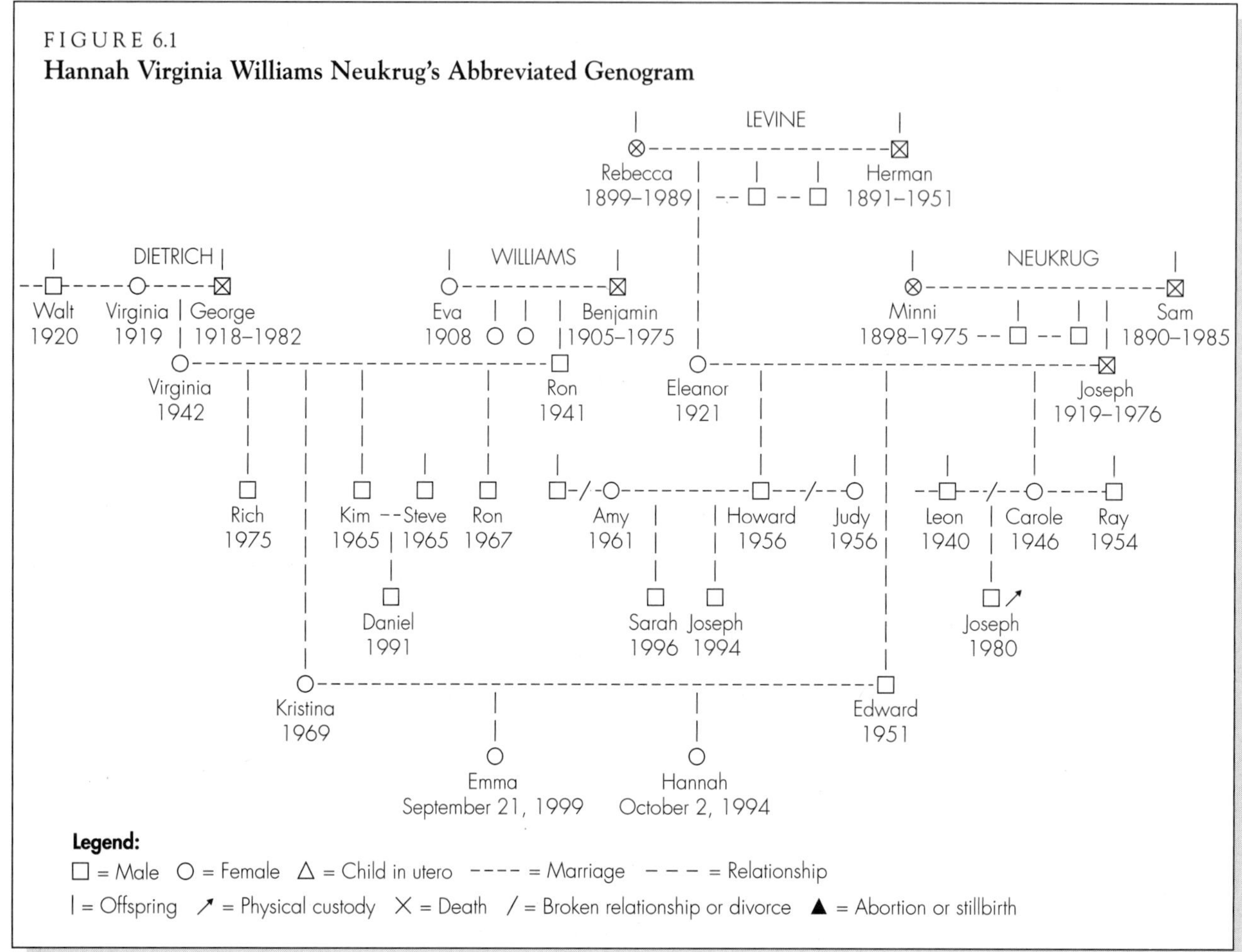

Bowen believed that individuals find others of similar psychological health with whom to form significant relationships. Therefore, an undifferentiated person will find a person with a similar level of undifferentiation, each hoping he or she will find completeness in the other. What initially seems like a perfect fit usually ends up as a major disappointment and often divorce. When undifferentiated parents do not deal with their issues, which by their very nature are frequent, a family projection process occurs in which parents unconsciously triangulate their children or project their own issues onto the children. The purpose of this projection is to reduce stress within the parental relationship while maintaining each spouse's level of undifferentiation. This allows the couple to continue to avoid their issues. An unhealthy relationship obviously leads to problems with child rearing, and ultimately the child grows into an undifferentiated self, thus continuing the cycle. This process could continue ad infinitum.

From a Bowenian perspective, therapists should be detached and take on the role of teachers and consultants, helping their clients to understand family dynamics and systems theory from an intellectual framework. Bowen mostly worked with couples, generally did not include the children in the process, and emotionality was kept at a minimum during the sessions by having the clients talk to and through the therapist. Bowen's goal was to help family members see themselves as they truly are (and were) and to begin to move toward differentiation of self.

Experiential Family Therapy

As the name implies, experiential family therapy stresses the experience of self, of each other, and of the therapist within the family therapy milieu. Based mostly on humanistic and existential psychology, this type of therapy has a positive view of human nature, believes that the individual (and the family) has a natural growth tendency, and relies on the relationship between the therapist and the family to induce change. The most well-known experiential family therapist is Carl Whitaker, who has prided himself in his lack of a theoretical approach (Whitaker, 1976):

> *I have a theory that theories are destructive and I know that intuition is destructive.* (1976, p. 154)

Despite this bold statement, it is clear that when working with families, Whitaker conceptualizes families from a systems perspective:

> *The major problem we see in the individual approaches is they fail to take into account the powerful interdependence between family members. . . . The "symptom" is merely a front for the family's larger stress.*
> (Napier & Whitaker, 1978, pp. 270–271)

In fact, if you read any of Whitaker's writings, it becomes quite clear that there are a number of underlying theoretical assumptions and that his approach is strongly influenced by humanistic psychology with a touch of psychodynamic theory. For instance, Whitaker believes that counselors should:

1. Respect each family member's self-actualizing process.
2. Respect the family's ability to unravel itself if placed in a trusting environment.
3. Create an atmosphere of oneness and nondefensiveness in order to make it difficult for the family to flee into defensive patterns.
4. Assist families in resolving the pain and anger that brings them to therapy.
5. Assist families in looking at their ghosts from the past.
6. Be powerful enough to "invade the family" (Whitaker, 1976, p. 163) in order to be part of the family and assist in breaking roles that have become solidified over time.
7. Have an "I–Thou" relationship with cotherapists and the family. This real relationship models openness, the ability to have a useful dialogue, and the expression of feeling. "Why should the family expose their tender underbelly if the therapist plays coy and self-protective?" (Whitaker, 1976, p. 164).
8. Not offer any particular framework or preconceived way in which the family should operate in an effort to have the family develop their own structure.
9. Model playfulness, craziness, and genuineness, in an effort to get family members to loosen up and be themselves and ultimately push them toward individuation.
10. Assist families in establishing a generation gap, or boundaries between parents and children.

Whitaker believes that the therapeutic process happens in stages. At first, the family is defensive and closed to the therapist. As the therapist invades and then joins with the family, they begin to see him or her as a genuine person and begin to open up. At this point, inner hurts and conflicts, often from the past, begin to emerge. The therapist now facilitates the family members' exploration of these hurts and helps the family see how they have affected each member within the family. At this point in the therapeutic process, family members begin to work on their own problems and move toward individuation. Napier and Whitaker (1978) note that this is often when family therapy seems more like a number of individual sessions occurring at the same time:

> *At the end of therapy the family should have resolved their major relationship conflicts, and the individuals should really be individuals in a psychological sense.* (Napier & Whitaker, 1978, p. 274)

Whitaker believes it is usually wise to have a cotherapist, as this will allow counselors to model the I–Thou relationship while also allowing each therapist the ability to consult with the other about the family, usually in front of the family (Napier & Whitaker, 1978). Also, because of the sheer numbers of people involved in family therapy, cotherapy enables counselors to pay more attention to the various family members as individuals. Cotherapists will often be perceived as the "parents" of the family, allowing families to make analogies to their families of origin. However, cotherapists can also be perceived in a variety of other roles, allowing family members to project their issues onto them (Napier & Whitaker, 1972):

> *Carl can be a very big-breasted, tender mother at times and a stern, tough grandfather at others, and I myself don't make a bad rebellious adolescent at times. It's a lot more complicated than the simplistic way in which we often identify personality with biology.* (Napier & Whitaker, 1978, p. 92)

Carl Whitaker in action is a master at work. He is witty, bright, reflective, real, strong, and willing to take risks. He says he has no theory, yet you see a consistency in his work, a consistency in the way he presents himself to the family that allows the family to grow, learn, deal with painful issues, dialogue, and ultimately change.

Psychodynamic Family Therapy

Family therapy from a psychodynamic perspective attempts to merge many of the concepts from systemic thinking with psychodynamic theory. For instance, when viewing psychoanalysis contextually, family dynamics is seen as a reflection of each family member's personality development through the psychosexual stages. The major difference for psychodynamically oriented family therapists from traditional individually oriented psychodynamic therapists is that the family therapist places great emphasis on how the client projects his or her internal world onto the family and the subsequent interactional processes that take place, whereas the individually oriented therapist focuses solely on the internal world of the client (Becvar & Becvar, 2000).

Nathan Ackerman (1958, 1966) and Robin Skynner (1981) are two well-known psychodynamically oriented family therapists. Like Ackerman and Skynner, most psychodynamically oriented therapists have generally been trained in traditional psychoanalysis methods but have decided to take on a systems perspective in working with clients. Most converts to this approach have found that this combination offers a broader perspective that allows for direct involvement with the cast of characters. Such *in vivo* sessions seem to speed up the usual slow process of most psychodynamically oriented individual approaches.

For the psychodynamic family therapist, there is generally an emphasis on how effective parents were in assisting their children through the developmental stages (Foster & Gurman, 1985). Because of this underlying assumption, unresolved issues through the developmental stages are thought to be reflected in the family in unconscious ways. Therefore, psychodynamic family therapy has as its major goal "to free family members of unconscious restrictions so that they'll be able to interact with one another as whole, healthy persons" (Nichols & Schwartz, 2001, p. 213).

Although strategies and techniques for the psychodynamically oriented therapist will vary, the major thrust is to have the couple or family explore their interactions and begin to understand how their behaviors result from unresolved conflicts from childhood. These conflicts may be multigenerational, in the sense that the parents pass on their conflicts to their children. It is therefore not uncommon to find psychodynamically oriented therapists encouraging their clients to go home and deal with unresolved issues and even to encourage grandparents or other extended family members to come in for a session.

Behavioral Family Therapy

Much like individual approaches to behavior therapy, behavioral family therapy is oriented toward symptom relief and does not focus on intrapsychic processes, underlying issues, or the unconscious. This approach tends to be highly structured and focuses on specific behaviors and techniques. As in individual behavior therapy, the family behavior therapist has at his or her disposal a wide array of techniques taken directly from operant conditioning, classical conditioning, and social-learning theory or modeling. Also as in individual behavioral therapy, there has been a trend toward the inclusion of cognitive therapy as an aspect of behavioral family therapy (Bussod & Jacobson, 1986; Piercy et al., 1996). Behavioral family therapists who adhere to a cognitive–behavioral approach believe that mediating cognitions can greatly affect family members and therefore should be addressed in treatment. For instance, when a parent continually puts a child down, this child begins to make negative self-statements concerning his or her self-worth. Therefore, in addition to behavioral change for the parents, many behavioral family therapists believe that the child's automatic thoughts also need to be addressed.

Whereas many traditional behavioral therapists have viewed problem behaviors in a linear, cause-and-effect fashion, most behavioral family therapists integrate systems theory with behavioral theory and view problem behaviors as the result of a number of feedback loops in which the dysfunctional behavior becomes reinforced from a number of different sources, including the family (Barker, 1981; Birchler & Spinks, 1980; Spinks & Birchler, 1982; Wahler, 1976). Because the behavioral family therapist is dealing with the family and not just one individual, it is particularly important in this approach to identify symptoms and target behaviors that the whole family will agree are important to change and to understand how various behaviors are reinforced in the system:

> *Learning theory may have been developed by observing white rats in laboratory mazes, but applying learning theory to families is quite a different matter. In behavioral family therapy it's important not to make simplistic assumptions about what may be rewarding and what may be punishing. Instead, it's critical to examine the interpersonal consequences of behavior. The therapist must find out what is reinforcing for each person and each family, rather than assume that certain things are universally rewarding. . . . For example, a child might throw tantrums, whine, or drop things at various times, but all of these may be reinforced by parental attention.* (Nichols & Schwartz, 2001, p. 278)

Although many different models of behavioral family therapy have been described, Foster and Gurman (1985) have identified a number of characteristics that seem common among these approaches:

- The importance of building a working relationship.
- Viewing therapy as an active approach that elicits the collaboration of the family.
- Believing that basic behavioral principles can be applied in a systems framework.
- Viewing therapy as brief and time-limited.
- Focusing on specific behaviors that will be targeted in treatment.
- Stressing the increase of positive behaviors over the elimination of negative behaviors.
- Teaching clients the relationship among events in their lives, behaviors, and consequences (e.g., negative or positive feelings).
- Setting goals that are clear, realistic, concrete, and measurable.
- Understanding the developmental nature of marriage and families.
- Actively teaching and supervising the change process within the family.

Whereas some family therapists believe it is always important to include the whole family in treatment, regardless of the problem (Napier & Whitaker, 1978; Satir, 1967), behavioral family therapists take into account what the presenting problem is and tend to include only those members who seem to be directly related to the change process (Foster & Gurman, 1985). For instance, if a child is having behavior problems at home and correction of the problem involves only parenting skills training, then there may be no need to include the child. Similarly, if a couple is having marital problems, although their problems will be spilling over to the children, the correction of the problem may not be directly involved with the children, and therefore they may not have to be included. In this process it is most important for the behavior family therapist to make a good assessment of the problem in an effort to determine correct treatment strategies and decide who in the family should be included in therapy (Becvar & Becvar, 2000; Foster & Gurman, 1985; Nichols & Schwartz, 2001; Piercy et al., 1996).

Multicultural Issues: Points to Consider When Working with Minority Families

Family therapists must exercise caution before using norms that stem from the majority cultural matrix in assessing the attitudes, beliefs, and transactional patterns of those whose cultural patterns differ from theirs. Beyond an appreciation of individual cultural influences, the family therapist must pay attention to what is unique about living as an ethnic minority–the language barriers, the cultural shock, the prejudice and discrimination, the feelings of powerlessness, the suspicion of institutions, the hopelessness, the rage. (Goldenberg & Goldenberg, 2000, p. 53)

Regardless of the family therapy approach being applied, when working with families from diverse cultures, a number of issues should be taken into account (Ho, 1987; McGoldrick, Pearce, & Giordano, 1996; Sue & Sue, 1999):

- Racism, poverty, and lower-class status are widespread for many minorities and can dramatically affect how families feel about themselves and their relationship to the counselor.
- Many minority families are bicultural, and all families face issues surrounding conflicting value systems between their culture of origin, and the larger culture.
- Language differences may cause problems of miscommunication and even misdiagnosis for clients in families.
- Many families have world-view differences with the counselor that could include such things as how they relate to time, how they interact with one another and with others, their relationship with nature, and other customs unique to the family's cultural background.
- The counselor's values, biases, and assumptions about families might interfere with the counseling process.
- Counselors should know appropriate intervention strategies with culturally diverse families that would "maximize success and minimize cultural oppression" (Sue & Sue, 1999, p. 108).

In short, the astute cross-cultural family counselor needs to understand family dynamics and know how his or her biases can affect families, the unique cultural styles of the families with whom he or she works, and specific techniques that would work best with families from culturally diverse backgrounds.

Ethical, Professional, and Legal Issues

Ethical Concerns

There are many unique ethical concerns related to the practice of family counseling, all of which cannot be covered in this short section. However, some issues that stand out include the following (Gladding, Remley, & Huber, 2001; Green & Hansen, 1986; Welfel, 1998).

Withholding Treatment

Because some family counselors insist on seeing the whole family, withholding treatment if one or more members balk at coming into therapy is not unusual. Although most ethical guidelines state that counselors cannot refuse services unless other arrangements are made for the client, a counselor can justify withholding treatment if he or she believes counseling will succeed only if the whole family is present. However, if such a position is taken, a family counselor should be able to defend this position from both a pragmatic and theoretical perspective.

Informed Consent

It is the counselor's ethical obligation to assure that knowledge about the counseling process be given to all clients, and all must willingly agree to participate in such a relationship prior to initiating the counseling relationship. Thus, each family member present must understand the nature of counseling, what might be expected of him or her, and any risks that might occur as a result of counseling.

Confidentiality

Family counseling offers some unique challenges to the ethical obligation one has for confidentiality. For instance, if a family member is seen individually and reveals information he or she does not wish discussed with the family, yet the counselor thinks this information is critical to the resolution of family issues, should the counselor break confidentiality? Is the client the individual or the family? Confidentiality also becomes problematic in that one cannot assure that each family member will honor it. Often dealing with such touchy issues that don't always have clear-cut answers requires a wise and sensitive counselor. Having clear ground rules before counseling begins can also help avoid these problems.

Dual Relationships

At times, a family counselor may begin to see an individual member of a family and only at a later date see the whole family. This can be a difficult switch to make, and the family therapist must consider if he or she will be able to develop an alliance with the whole family after having built a relationship with the individual family member.

Professional Issues

Individual or Family Therapy?

When should a member of a family be referred to individual counseling as opposed to the whole family being referred for family counseling? Although some therapists might suggest it is always appropriate to refer the whole family for counseling (Napier & Whitaker, 1978; Satir, 1967), most therapists today agree that it is often a matter of making a wise decision based on a careful assessment of the situation. For instance, a child who comes from an extremely dysfunctional family may be better off seeing a therapist individually, because working with the whole family may be seen as an extremely long process whereas individual counseling may give some immediate relief for the child. Or it may be prudent to refer a spouse for individual counseling to work on her unfinished business while the family undergoes family treatment. This might accelerate the treatment process for everyone.

My own bias for determining individual or family counseling is based on how much the presenting problem seems to be reverberating throughout the family. When the problems in the family seem to be seriously affecting all family members, I would suggest seeing the whole family. However, if a family member is experiencing a large amount of pain, and he or she is attempting not to let this spill into the family (it always spills over to some degree), then I might opt for individual counseling.

Professional Associations

AAMFT, IAMFC—which professional association should you join? Although there are many more similarities than differences between these two associations, IAMFC and AAMFT do suggest different graduate curricula, have different codes of ethics, support slightly different clinical and supervisory experience for licensing, and at times endorse different licensing initiatives. The professional family counselor should investigate both associations to see which seems to have the best fit. Then again, why not join both?

Accreditation and Credentialing

Today, two groups accredit marriage and family graduate therapy programs: the Commission on Accreditation for Marital and Family Therapy Education (CAMFTE), which is associated with AAMFT; and CACREP, which has a specialty accreditation in marriage and family counseling and is affiliated with ACA (Everett, 1990).

In 1987 the Association of Marital and Family Therapy Regulatory Boards (AMFTRB) was established by AAMFT to address licensure and certification issues; today, over one-half of the states have licensing laws that cover marriage and family counselors. Rather than following the guidelines of AMFTRB, some state licensure boards, such as the one in Virginia, have attempted to subsume the marriage and family credential under the counseling board or other related mental health licensing boards. In addition to licensing, the IAMFC has recently developed a certification process for family therapists offered through the National Academy for Certified Family Therapists (Smith et al., 1995).

Legal Concerns

Testifying against a Family Member

Because family counselors often work with families who are considering divorce, struggling with custody issues, or embroiled in a potential legal battle, each family counselor needs to be aware that a family member could ask, or subpoena, the counselor to testify in court. For instance, during divorce proceedings or in an effort to gain child custody, one spouse might ask the family counselor to testify against the other based on information gained during a session. Family counselors need to be aware of the limits of confidentiality in situations like this and the local and state laws that might affect their ability to testify.

Insurance Fraud

With cutbacks in the number of sessions allowable for mental health services, and with some insurance companies not paying for family counseling, some family therapists will list one family member as their patient, and when his or her insurance benefits run out, list a second family member, and so on. Unfortunately, in many cases this practice is illegal. With insurance fraud being one of the most often-made complaints against licensed therapists (Neukrug, Herlihy, & Healy, 1992; Neukrug, Milliken, & Walden, 2001), family counselors need to be aware of the idiosyncratic rules of insurance companies as well as state laws that might restrict this practice.

The Counselor in Process: Understanding Our Client's Family, Understanding Our Family

Most family counselors did not start out as family counselors (Ferber, Mendelsohn, & Napier, 1972). Most start out individually oriented and are slowly exposed to the broader perspective that family therapy has to offer. Eventually, however, the effective counselor does not view the client in isolation, unaffected by the systems in which he or she interacts. Instead this counselor sees the person as being an intricate part of a complex world. A wise counselor understands that the individual has a dramatic impact on the life of a family, and the family greatly affects the individual. Although many counselors will not choose a family therapy approach as their primary mode, the effective counselor will undoubtedly take into account the family from which the client came, the family with which the client now lives, and the broader community and society with which we all must contend.

Awareness of a client's contextual world, however, is not enough. The effective family counselor has also examined his or her own family of origin. The counselor who has avoided a family self-examination risks having his or her issues interfere with the effective treatment of clients and families. Although we can never fully know our family as they were, we can continually strive to know ourselves as we become.

Summary

This chapter examined the complex interactions of systems. First we examined general systems theory, which states that all systems have boundaries that are rigid, permeable, or loose and regulatory mechanisms that maintain the unique homeostasis of the system. We noted that the study of cybernetics, or control mechanisms in systems, has been used to explain this regulatory process and includes positive and negative feedback loops. In healthy systems, change occurs by permitting information to flow into the system and allowing this information to be evaluated and responded to, whereas dysfunctional systems have boundaries that are either too rigid or too permeable, resulting in poor information flow.

In families, we noted, the kinds of communication that occur are reflective of either rigid or loose boundaries and the hierarchy that exists in the family. Whether dysfunctional or healthy, in an effort to maintain the family structure, family members will exert covert or overt influence on one another and others (e.g., the therapist) to maintain the unique homeostasis of the system. We suggested that all spouses bring their unfinished business to the family, but that healthy spouses can openly work through their issues, whereas spouses who are undifferentiated will allow their issues to fester. Couples who cannot work through their issues will have poor communication, create families with rigid or loose boundaries, have power struggles, and scapegoat one another or the children in the family.

In this chapter we stated that family therapy techniques became popular in the 1950s with their focus on addressing dysfunctional family systems. We highlighted the fact that all family therapy approaches take into account the unique properties of systems, although some apply these concepts more than others. Some of the approaches examined in this chapter were strategic family therapy used by Jay Haley, Cloe Madanes, and the Milan Associates; communication family therapy, which was made popular by Virginia Satir; structural family therapy, which was popularized by Salvadore Minuchin; multigenerational family therapy, as practiced by Murray Bowen and Ivan Boszormenyi-Nagy; experiential family therapy, as shown by Augustus Napier and Carl Whitaker; psychodynamic family therapy, such as that offered by Nathan Ackerman and Robin Skynner; and behavioral family therapy.

This chapter also examined issues related to multicultural counseling within a family context. It was stressed that family counselors need to understand their own values and biases and the unique world view of the families with whom they work and be able to apply appropriate intervention strategies as a function of the family's cultural background.

In addition, it was stressed that family counselors should be aware of how issues of racism, poverty, class, and language affect the family and family counseling.

Some of the unique ethical concerns we discussed included the ethics of withholding treatment to some family members in order to see the whole family, the importance of having all family members give informed consent, problems with guaranteeing confidentiality in family counseling, and the difficulty of switching a client from individual to family counseling or from family to individual counseling.

Two legal concerns that we discussed included testifying against a family member as a result of information gained during family counseling sessions and insurance fraud, such as when family counselors inappropriately bill for individual sessions of family members. We also reviewed such professional issues as the importance of determining when individual counseling may be preferred over family counseling, which professional association to join, and the status of accreditation, licensing, and certification of marriage and family counselors.

Finally, within this chapter we examined the importance of continually knowing ourselves in reference to our families of origin and the impact that could potentially have on our understanding of and our interactions with our clients.

INFOTRAC and Other Information Resources (e.g., ERIC and PsycINFO)

Note: When relevant, key words are in quotation marks.

1. Research any of the family therapy approaches discussed in this chapter in more detail.
2. Examine issues related to "ethics in marriage therapy" or "ethics in family therapy."
3. Examine typical issues related to "family transitions" and "family development."

CHAPTER 7

Group Work

I decided I wanted to have a group counseling experience. It was 1975, and I had recently finished my master's degree and started a job at a mental health center. I found a therapist I trusted who was putting together a group with another therapist. There were eight of us, four men, four women—oh yeah, and the two therapists, that makes ten. But the therapists didn't really count as real people! Meeting once a week, it took a while to build trust. However, within a couple of months it seemed as though things really took off. We began to share deeper parts of ourselves. I heard people reveal things about themselves they had never mentioned to anyone else. I saw transformations take place as members began to work through their unfinished business. I saw the leaders, a man and a woman, model shared group leadership skills and openly work through their own conflicts in front of us.

After we had been meeting for about a year, the leaders suggested having a marathon group that would last from a Friday evening to late Sunday afternoon. I had always heard about such groups and was apprehensive about meeting for such an intensive amount of time. But at the same time I was excited about what lay ahead for me. The weekend was incredible, as people really got into their stuff.

The group continued for a year longer. It was painful to say goodbye, but necessary. We were finished, at least for now. We had done our work and now were ready to move on in life. We laughed, we cried, we hugged. For a while, some of us continued to maintain contact; others did not. Over time, I lost contact with everyone in the group. I wonder now what those other seven people are doing. Oh yeah, and the two therapists also.

That group experience was crucial for me. It helped me work through unfinished business. It showed me how effective group counseling could be. Watching the therapists taught me how to run groups. And it gave me an appreciation of the group process as the unique unfolding of a group that must be nurtured along if it is to blossom.

Since that time I have participated in other groups and have run a number of groups. I had a brief flirtation with EST, a very large (250 people) marathon group with a confrontational focus; I joined a leaderless men's support group; I visited some AA groups; I ran a weight-loss group; I ran a group as part of a graduate group counseling class (which has some ethical complications); I ran a support group for individuals who had been hospitalized for a psychotic disorder; and I ran guidance groups for high school students.

Groups come in all shapes and sizes. They last for different lengths of time. They have different numbers of people in them, and they focus on different things. Groups can seem so different, yet they all share many common elements. Groups! This chapter will examine groups—how they are different and how they are the same.

We will begin the chapter by explaining groups from a systemic perspective and then discuss the purpose of group counseling. We will then review how groups evolved during the 20th century. We will explore the differences among self-help groups, task groups, counseling groups, therapy groups, and psychoeducational groups and look at how theory is applied to group work.

We will examine the stages of group development and discuss group leadership skills, particularly as they relate to these stages. Finally, we will take a look at some important multicultural, ethical, professional, and legal issues related to group work.

Groups: A Systemic Perspective

A group is a living system, as is the cell of the body, the human organism, and society as a whole. . . . Looking at the therapy group as a system, it clearly contains many systems, including suprasystems and subsystems. . . . Certainly systems theory gives us a tool for approaching the complexity of the therapy group. (Lonergan, 1994, pp. 200–201)

Groups, like families, can be viewed from a systemic perspective in which individuals in the group can be understood by examining the dynamic interaction of its members and how that interaction results in specific communication patterns, power dynamics, hierarchies, and the system's unique homeostasis (Durkin, 1972; Gazda, 1989).

The effective group leader is able to work with the unique issues that the individual brings to the group and at the same time understand how system dynamics are a reflection of how these issues get played out in the group. Thus the group leader must be able to focus in like a laser beam on each group member and pull back as if he or she is viewing the whole group through a wide-angle lens. In a sense, the effective group leader must see him- or herself as an individual counselor and a systems expert.

Why Have Groups?

Groups are becoming increasingly popular and used by every type of mental health professional. In fact, it is now common to find many counselors having 20% of their clinical work in group activities (Partin, 1993). But why should a counselor choose a group over other treatment methods? Table 7.1 summarizes some of the advantages and disadvantages of group work (Jacobs, Masson, & Harvill, 2002).

Because group counseling has advantages and disadvantages as compared to individual and family counseling, it becomes the counselor's responsibility to assess the needs of the client and decide which treatment approach would be most beneficial. Sometimes group work can be offered as an adjunct to other forms of counseling, while at other times it may be appropriate to offer one specific form of therapy. Sometimes, if individual or family counseling is not available to the client, despite the fact that it might be deemed the most appropriate form of treatment, group work can be a viable alternative.

TABLE 7.1

Advantages and Disadvantages of Group Work

ADVANTAGES	DISADVANTAGES
1. *More efficient:* More clients can be seen in a shorter amount of time.	1. *Less focused time:* As compared to individual counseling, each group member generally has less focused time with the counselor.
2. *Economical:* Group work almost always costs less than individual counseling.	2. *Less intensity with leader:* Group counseling generally does not offer the same amount of intense one-on-one time with the group leader that is found in individual counseling.
3. *Sense of belonging:* Groups offer contact with other people on a deeply personal level.	3. *More intimidation:* Some individuals are intimidated by the group setting.
4. *General support:* Groups can offer foundational support for many clients.	4. *Fear of disclosure:* Some clients will not reveal deeply personal matters in a group setting.
5. *Microcosm of society:* Groups mimic society. Therefore one can obtain feedback about self and can test new behaviors prior to trying them in the "real" world.	5. *Therapeutic effectiveness:* Some problems may be more effectively dealt with in a family or individual setting.
6. *Support for commitment to change:* Groups provide an atmosphere where members will support one another as they define goals and follow through on new behaviors.	6. *Increased time commitment:* Generally, clients have to commit more time to group counseling than other forms of counseling–time they may not have.
7. *Vicarious learning:* Through modeling, group members can learn from one another and from the leader.	7. *Lack of flexibility:* One can generally change the meeting times of individual sessions more easily than group sessions.
8. *Systemic understanding:* Groups provide information to members about how they react in systems, information that can often be related to family of origin issues	8. *Lack of assurance on confidentiality:* Leaders cannot assure group members that everyone will keep information confidential.

Although groups are often a realistic treatment alternative, their availability as a therapeutic option is relatively new. In fact, due to the rather rapid rise in popularity of modern-day group work, some consider the training of group therapists to be lagging behind its demand and more important than ever (Bernard, 2000; Kottler, 1994). The following section will review how group work has developed and particularly focus on its relatively recent increase in popularity.

The History of Group Counseling

It has often been said that what happens in a group is a microcosm of society (Yalom, 1995); that is, the kinds of values and behaviors that we find in groups are reflective of those we find in society. Perhaps, then, it is not surprising that the types of groups we have seen over the past century have reflected the values prevalent at the times they were developed. Let's take a closer look at how some of these groups evolved.

Early History

Gladding (1999) notes that prior to 1900 the purpose of group treatment was to assist individuals in very "functional and pragmatic ways" (p. 3). This often revolved around helping people with daily living skills and arose out of the social group work movement, where individuals like Jane Addams organized group discussions that often had moralistic overtones and centered on such things as personal hygiene, moral behavior, nutrition, and self-determination (Pottick, 1988). Using groups as their vehicle, social reformers like Addams were particularly concerned with community organizing as an effort to assist the poor (Garvin, 1981).

At the turn of the last century, a number of parallel movements began to discover the power of groups. For instance, schools began to offer vocational and moral guidance in group settings. Although they were often preachy in their nature, and despite the fact that there was little opportunity for group members to discuss personal matters in reflective ways, these group guidance activities acknowledged the importance of groups. At around the same time, Dr. Joseph Henry Pratt became one of the first to practice group treatment with patients. Meeting with about 30 tuberculosis patients weekly, he would start out with a lecture, which eventually led to patients revealing their personal stories and offering encouragement to one another. With little if any group theory available at that time, Pratt followed what his predecessors did and practiced a little moral guidance by using persuasion and reeducation (Andrews, 1995; Pinney, 1970).

At the beginning of the 20th century a number of psychoanalytical principles such as primal urges, instincts, and parental influences were used to explain group dynamics (Andrews, 1995; Anthony, 1972; Lonergan, 1994). For instance, some believed that the tendency for group behavior represented a herd instinct where people sought out others for survival purpose. Others believed a mob instinct could emerge from group activities, where the natural aggressiveness of people would come out, and still others believed that one could find in groups a recapitulation of early family patterns and that group members would often blindly give their power over to the group leader (their parent). Although Freud even wrote a book on groups, *Group Psychology and the Analysis of the Ego* (1975/1922), his attachment to individual therapy prevented him from taking his ideas one step further, to develop and practice a broad-reaching theory of group therapy.

In 1914 J. L. Moreno, who was the originator of psychodrama and the individual given credit for coining the term *group psychotherapy*, wrote one of the first papers on that subject (Fox, 1987). Although not considered formal group counseling, psychodrama focused on individuals acting out their experiences in front of an audience. This form of therapy emphasized role playing, here-and-now interaction, expression of feeling, and feedback from the audience (the group) and is considered by some the forerunner of group counseling (Gladding, 1999).

The 1920s and 1930s saw the spread of Adlerian therapy, with its emphasis on birth order and the importance of social connectedness. Considered by some to have influenced both the family therapy movement and the group counseling movement, Adler and his colleagues practiced an early form of family group counseling as they worked with prisoners and groups of children in child guidance clinics (Gazda, 1989; Gladding, 1999). However, their techniques were far from what would be considered group or family therapy today. At around the same time, the spread of psychotherapeutic theory and sociological concepts concerning group interactions led to some of the first non-psychoanalytically oriented counseling and therapy groups (Gladding, 1999). During this period we saw the beginnings of some of the first associations for group work.

The 1930s saw an increase in group guidance activities in the schools. Mostly performed by homeroom teachers, these guidance activities focused on "helping to establish relationships, determining student needs and abilities, and developing proper attitudes" (Vander Kolk, 1990, p. 5). Continuing into the 1950s, these guidance activities were the forerunner of school group guidance activities of today.

The Emergence of Modern-Day Groups

The 1940s saw the emergence of the modern group movement. In 1947 Kurt Lewin and other nationally known theorists developed the National Training Laboratory (NTL) to examine group dynamics, or the intricate ways in which people in groups tend to interact (Capuzzi & Gross, 1998; Shaffer & Galinsky, 1974). NTL has always focused on the structural nature of groups and tends to be more didactic and cognitive than viscerally oriented. As it did when it first began, NTL continues today to train individuals in understanding communication in groups, group process, and how these relate to organizational goals. Therefore, NTL has been particularly attractive to business and industry.

It was also during this decade that Carl Rogers brought together therapists to discuss the problems they might encounter in working with returning GIs from World War II. He soon found that, for a good number of these therapists, self-disclosure within the group setting resulted in a deepening of expression of feeling and, in many instances, an uncovering of new awareness concerning themselves. Thus began the encounter group movement (Rogers, 1970). Few then would realize the far-reaching effects that the encounter and humanistic psychology movements were soon to have on American society.

Groups Become Faddish

The 1960s: Vietnam, the War on Poverty, the civil rights movement, assassinations of our heroes. The country was in upheaval, and this chaos was perhaps society's way of saying, "Free us." Free us from racism. Free us from war. Free us from poverty, and let us be free to love. Led by the encounter group movement, groups were soon to reflect this need for freedom and love. One outgrowth of this movement was the development of Esalen in Big Sur, California, by Michael Murphy. Murphy, who became involved in the encounter group movement, moved to an ashram in India for a year and a half and subsequently came back and established Esalen. A description of Esalen, written approximately 30 years ago by Murphy's guru, is still applicable today:

> *This was a very interesting experimental community, attempting to combine the ideal of self-realization and technology, drawing upon Eastern spirituality and Western thought. The emphasis was on the transformation of your personal life into the divine nature in our language, trying to evoke higher spiritual possibilities out of all your life.* (Gusataitis, cited in Verny, 1974, p. 10)

It was not unusual to find Carl Rogers, Abraham Maslow, and famous philosophers like Paul Tillich at Esalen. Esalen, and similar institutes that began to follow its model, were to attract therapists from around the world, some of whom would eventually become famous in their own right. Fritz Perls, for instance, started doing workshops at Esalen, and his notoriety there, along with his soon-to-be published books, were to make him a well-known figure. At Esalen, Perls began to put some of his Gestalt therapy ideas into a group framework. Others also applied their theories to the groups at Esalen. Individuals like Bill Schutz, a Harvard faculty member and originally an NTL devotee, were to develop group physical-contact games and group imagery exercises that had an emphasis on self-awareness:

> *Schutz will suggest to one or all members of the group simultaneously that they take a trip through their bodies. They are to enter their bodies by whatever orifice they wish. . . . I recall one lady who entered her body through her vagina and within*

a few seconds turned into a rat chewing away at herself. Naturally, when she came back from this nightmare it provided us with a lot of material with which to investigate her sexual identity, sexual relations, and related problems.
(Verny, 1974, p. 17)

Esalen and the encounter group movement in general had a distinct focus on feelings, and this eventually led to the formation of a number of different types of affect-oriented groups. Some of the more popular types included marathon groups, where individuals might spend 48 hours intensely sharing feelings and experiences; confrontational groups, like the ones modeled after Synanon, a drug and alcohol rehab where it was common for group members to attack one another verbally in an effort to break down defenses; Gestalt and sensitivity groups, which stressed the expression of feelings in order to get to deeper issues; and nude encounter groups. This ever-expanding push to express feelings and get in touch with oneself stretched traditional values and lured group members to deal with deep-seated issues. However, such groups were not always positive for all involved. With increasingly larger numbers of groups being run by untrained individuals, and with some people reporting negative results from their experiences, the American Psychological Association in 1973 published Guidelines for Psychologists Conducting Growth Groups, which limited what a professional could do in groups (Gladding, 1999).

The 1960s and 1970s also saw the spread of texts on the theory and practice of group counseling. In addition, at this time professional associations began to establish divisions for members interested in group work. One such association, the Association for Specialists in Group Work (ASGW), was formed in 1973 and is now one of the larger divisions of ACA.

Recent Trends

As groups became more commonplace, helping professionals began to use group counseling as an alternative or additional treatment to individual counseling. Group courses became more prevalent in training programs to the point where it is now unusual for a helping professional not to have course work and field experience in group work. Whereas the past 25 years have seen a decline in some of the more outrageous groups of the 1960s and 1970s, during this period there has been a rise in group counseling and therapy run by well-trained and experienced counselors.

In recent years the focus of professionally run counseling groups has changed. Whereas the typical counseling group used to be an ongoing, heterogeneous group of individuals who sought increased self-awareness and personality change, today, common-theme groups with a specialized focus (e.g., eating disorders) and time-limited, brief-counseling groups (usually fewer than 20 sessions) have become increasingly popular (Andrews, 1995). In addition, in recent years there has been a steady rise in the popularity of self-help groups. These grassroots groups have supported millions of Americans who have struggled with a variety of problems. Whereas the therapist of 25 years ago would rarely refer a client to a self-help group as an adjunct to counseling, the therapist of today who does not refer to a self-help group in certain instances (e.g., alcoholism, eating disorders) may be acting unethically (Riordan & Walsh, 1994).

With the continued popularity of group work, ASGW has developed Best Practice Guidelines as well as Professional Standards for the Training of Group Workers. The Best Practice Guidelines are "intended to clarify the application of the ACA Code of Ethics and Standards of Practice to the field of group work" (ASGW, 1998a). The training standards define the knowledge, skills, and experiences necessary for the training of group leaders and delineate four specialty areas: task groups, psychoeducational groups, counseling groups, and psychotherapy groups (ASGW, 2000). Today, it is reassuring to know that almost all counseling programs require knowledge and practice in group work and that, for CACREP-accredited programs, compliance to the ASGW training standards has been particularly high (Merta, Johnson, & McNeil, 1995; Wilson, Conyne, & Ward, 1994).

Defining Modern-Day Groups

Today, most groups can be placed into one of five categories: self-help groups, task groups, psychoeducational groups, counseling groups, and therapy groups, with most counselors being involved in psychoeducational, counseling, and therapy groups. Although these groups are different in many ways, they all are affected by group dynamics and have a unique group process (Trotzer, 1999).

The term *group dynamics* refers to the ongoing interactions and interrelationships among the group members and between the leader and group members. These interactions are a function of conscious and unconscious forces and are influenced by such things as the structure of the group, the theoretical orientation of the leader, the unique personalities of the leader and the members, and a myriad of other influences such as drives, needs, gender, age, power issues, culture, and other known and unknown factors (Amaranto, 1972; Gazda, 1989; Gladding, 1999). The term *group process* refers to the changes that occur in a group as a function of the developmental stages through which the group will pass (see pp. 184–192). Group process can be affected by the dynamics in the group but is ongoing and positive if the group is led effectively.

Following are brief descriptions of self-help groups, task groups, psychoeducational groups, counseling groups, and therapy groups.

Self-Help Groups

Although self-help groups have been around for more than 50 years, their growth has been phenomenal over the past 20 years. From Alcoholics Anonymous (AA), to codependency groups, to eating disorder and diet groups, to men's and women's groups, to groups for the chronically mentally ill, the kinds of self-help groups that have emerged seem endless. Self-help groups tend to espouse a particular philosophy or way of being in the world. Their purpose is the education, affirmation, and enhancement of existing strengths of the group member (Andrews, 1995). Generally there is a nonpaid volunteer leader who focuses the discussion and assists in defining the rules of the group. However, sometimes there may be no leader at all. Self-help groups are generally free or have a nominal fee and can be facilitated by a trained layperson or mental health professional. (See Box 7.1)

Self-help groups are not in-depth psychotherapy groups and hardly ever require a vast amount of member self-disclosure. In fact, because self-help groups tend to be open groups, their composition is constantly changing, and this can hinder the building of group cohesion, a critical element for in-depth work. Usually individuals in self-help groups are encouraged to share only the amount that feels comfortable. Some self-help groups even discourage intense self-disclosure, as that would be seen as more appropriate for individual or group counseling. Self-help groups have had limited evaluation and their effectiveness is unclear (Andrews, 1995; Yeaton, 1994). However, many people swear by them.

With self-help groups, the number of group members, length of meeting times, and atmosphere of the group setting can vary considerably. Some groups might have 200

BOX 7.1

A Men's Self-help Group

For one and one-half years, I was a participant in a men's support group established by ten men. The purpose of the group was to have a supportive group of men with whom we could share our feelings, thoughts, and concerns around a wide range of issues, particularly issues that were relevant to men. The group was leaderless, although we all periodically would take a leadership role. For one and one-half years, we shared some of our most intimate details about such issues as divorces and marriages, our sexuality, our families of origin, and relationship concerns. But perhaps most important, not having a female present enabled us to share in a way that we probably would not have shared otherwise. Although I did not remain in the group, the group continued for seven years with most of its original members.

members, while others might be limited to just a few people. Some groups might meet in the basement of a church, while others might meet in the comfort of the office of a therapist who has loaned the group space. Some self-help groups may be ongoing, others may be time limited; some might demand confidentiality, while others will not.

Although self-help groups are not generally led by counselors, they have become an increasingly important referral source and are often used as an adjunct to counseling. For these reasons, it has become increasingly important for counselors to be aware of the types of self-help groups in their communities.

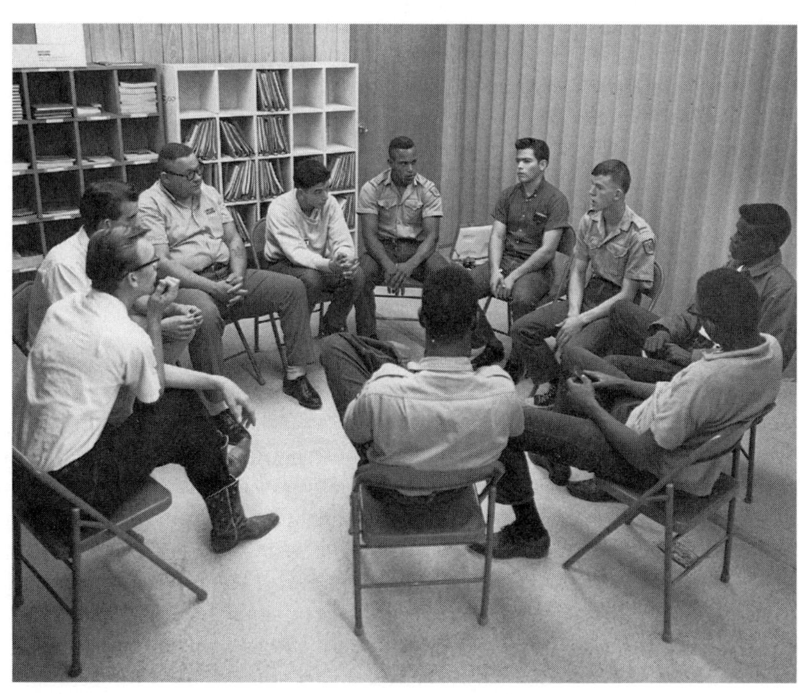

BOX 7.2

A Task Group at a Bank

Ed has been approached by the vice-president of the local bank because of bickering going on between various bank managers. The conflict seems to have affected their ability to work effectively. Ed decides to meet with the managers for four small group meetings and analyze some of their interactions. During the first meeting, Ed does some basic rapport building and asks the managers to define the problem. The next two meetings are spent doing role play problem-solving activities, selected by Ed. He watches the group carefully as they go through the problem-solving process. He is particularly aware of issues of control, hierarchies, and boundaries, especially in relationship to sexism and gender differences, prejudice and cross-cultural style differences, ageism and age style differences, and personal style differences. During the last meeting he shares what he has seen; and, based on his feedback, he asks the group to develop some problem-solving techniques to work through their interpersonal issues. He tells the group that he will come back in a month to see if they have followed through on their ideas.

Task Groups

Task groups emphasize conscious behaviors and focus on how group dynamics affect the successful completion of a product (Gladding, 1999). The National Training Laboratory (NTL) was the first systematic effort to understand the dynamics of groups in business and industry, and much of the knowledge learned from NTL is today applied to our understanding of task groups (Gazda, 1989). Task group specialists

> *. . . assist groups such as task forces, committees, planning groups, community organizations, discussion groups, study circles, learning groups, and other similar groups to correct or develop their functioning. The focus is on the application of group dynamics principles and processes to improve practice and the accomplishment of identified work goals.* (ASGW, 1992, p. 13)

Task groups specialists will often enter an organization and attempt to analyze and diagnose problems and work with the members to change the dynamics of work groups and the organization (Gazda, 1989). Many times difficulties within these organizations are related to problems in differing values and social norms that affect the dynamics of a task group. Such differences among employees can lead to problems in communication, feelings of dissatisfaction at work, low motivation, low productivity, gender issues (e.g., sexual harassment), cross-cultural problems, and so forth. (See Box 7.2.)

Psychoeducational Groups

Psychoeducational groups (sometimes called guidance groups) attempt to increase self-understanding, promote personal and interpersonal growth, and prevent future problems through the dissemination of mental health education in a group setting (ASGW, 2000; Capuzzi & Gross, 1998). A few examples of the many topics that psychoeducational groups have focused upon include sex education, conflict resolution, AIDS awareness, career awareness, communication skills, diversity issues, chemical dependence, stress management, and lifestyle adjustment.

Today, the term *psychoeducational groups* is often used instead of *guidance groups* because the latter term has held negative connotations in that such groups have been misconstrued as being highly advice oriented and as having a moral imperative (Kottler,

BOX 7.3

A Psychoeducational Group in the Schools (Classroom Guidance)

Jawanda is an elementary school counselor. Her school system requires her to do classroom guidance activities four times a year in each class. Each classroom guidance group is followed by four group sessions run by the teacher of the class who is coached by the school counselor. Some of the classroom guidance activities she does are "how to handle a bully," "friendship," and "drug awareness." Jawanda spends approximately one hour in the class, which is split between a presentation, a series of preset questions that she has for the students, and time for discussion and processing at the end of the group. The students seem to particularly enjoy the discussion aspect of the guidance program and become quite active in sharing their experiences and views.

1994). Although psychoeducational groups had their origins in the schools, today such preventive and educational groups can be found in many additional settings, such as business and industry, community centers, and community agencies. The psychoeducational group specialist

> *. . . seeks to use the group medium to educate group participants who are presently unaffected about a potential threat (such as AIDS), a developmental life event (such as a transition point), or how to cope with an immediate life crisis (such as suicide of a loved one), with the goal of preventing an array of educational and psychological disturbances from occurring.* (ASGW, 1992, p. 13)

Psychoeducational groups always have a designated, well-trained group leader and have as their purpose the preventive education and support of the group member. Leaders will usually offer a didactic presentation and generally there is not much client self-disclosure, although there may be an opportunity for discussion or limited amounts of personal sharing. Such groups may be ongoing or can occur on a one-time basis. Psychoeducational groups can vary dramatically in size and the number of times they meet, although they are generally short term, sometimes meeting only once. As with self-help groups, there is little or no charge to participants. (See Box 7.3.)

Counseling Groups

As with individual counseling and therapy, many people differentiate between group counseling and group therapy (Capuzzi & Gross, 1998; Gazda, 1989; Gladding, 1999). Usually, group counseling is focused on prevention, self-enhancement, increased insight, self-actualization, and conscious as opposed to unconscious motivations. Clients in group counseling may be struggling with adjustment problems in life such as the breakup of relationships, deaths, and job transitions. They generally are not dealing with severe pathology or a debilitating psychological problem. The group counseling specialist

> *. . . seeks to help group participants to resolve the usual, yet often difficult, problems of living through interpersonal support and problem solving. An additional goal is to help participants to develop their existing interpersonal problem-solving competencies that they may be better able to handle future problems of a similar nature. . . .* (ASGW, 1992, p. 13)

Group counseling tends to be shorter in duration than group therapy but longer than psychoeducational groups. The group leader needs to be well trained in group process and group dynamics. As in group therapy, group counseling is a small-group experience, usually involving four to twelve members. Recently, common-theme groups and brief counseling groups have gained in popularity (Andrews, 1995).

Common-Theme Counseling Groups

Common-theme counseling groups are specialized groups that focus on one theme and tend to be short term and action oriented. As with counseling groups in general, they tend to have between four and twelve members. Unlike self-help groups that may also have a specialized theme, common-theme groups tend to have continuity of group members and are led by trained professionals who use psychotherapeutic techniques to assist members in their psychological growth. Examples of some common-theme counseling groups include eating disorder groups, bereavement groups, chronic fatigue syndrome groups, and divorce groups.

Brief Counseling Groups

Brief counseling groups are time-limited common-theme groups. Although most groups meet for fewer than 20 sessions (Toseland & Siporin, 1986), because brief therapy groups are developed around a specified and limited number of group sessions, they tend to be more successful than groups that haphazardly meet for a limited number of sessions. These groups are focused, structured, and action oriented (Andrews, 1995). With recent cutbacks in mental health benefits across the country, these kinds of therapeutic experiences allow a counselor to see more individuals in a shorter amount of time with what appears to be a relatively high success rate.

Group Therapy

In contrast to counseling groups that tend to be preventive in nature and wellness oriented, group therapy typically focuses upon remediation of severe pathology and personality reconstruction. (See Box 7. 4.) Individuals who participate in therapy groups may suffer from severe emotional conflicts, deep-seated problems, neurotic and deviant behaviors, and severe problems that would need long-term treatment. The group therapy specialist

> *. . . seeks to help individual group members to remediate their in-depth psychological problems. Because the depth and extent of the psychological disturbance is significant, the goal is to aid each individual to reconstruct major personality dimensions.* (ASGW, 1992, p. 13)

As with group counseling, the group therapy leader needs to be well trained in group dynamics and group process and able to handle clients who might have extreme emotional responses to a group meeting. In addition, as with group counseling, group therapy has a limited number of members, and continuity of membership is crucial for the development of the group process.

Despite the fact that most authors differentiate counseling groups from therapy groups, there are many similarities. For instance, both counseling and therapy groups have designated highly trained leaders. Generally, there are between four and twelve group members, and usually such groups meet for a minimum of eight sessions; some may continue on an ongoing basis. Most counseling and therapy groups meet at least once a week for one to three hours, and confidentiality of the group is particularly crucial. Although leadership styles may vary, usually there is some expectation on the part of the leader that members will have the opportunity to freely express their feelings and eventually to work on change.

BOX 7.4

A Therapy Group

The group discussed at the beginning of the chapter, in which I participated for two years, I consider to have been a therapy group, although some might call it group counseling (see Figure 7.1). Often, there is a fine line between the two. Although I would not consider any member of the group as having had serious pathology, it was clear that many of us were dealing with major issues in our lives. There was a great push in the group for self-disclosure, insight, and change, and much of the time in the group was spent talking about past issues and uncovering conflicts, as group members attempted to work through unfinished business.

FIGURE 7.1
Comparison of Groups: Psychoeducational Groups, Counseling Groups, Therapy Groups

EMPHASIS OF VARYING GROUPS	(GUIDANCE) PSYCHOEDUCATIONAL	COUNSELING	PSYCHOTHERAPY
HIGH	Wellness and prevention		Insight and change
↕	Education	Group process	Past
		Group dynamics	Group process
			Group dynamics
			Pathology/severe distress
↕			Unconscious motivation
		Insight	Self-disclosure of members
		Self-disclosure of members	
↕		Change	
		Wellness and prevention	
MEDIUM	Insight		
↕	Group process	Past	
	Group dynamics	Unconscious motivation	
	Self-disclosure of members	Pathology/severe distress	
		Education	Wellness and prevention
↕			
	Pathology/severe distress		Education
	Change		
↕	Past		
	Unconscious motivation		
LOW			
	PSYCHOEDUCATIONAL (GUIDANCE) GROUPS	COUNSELING GROUPS	THERAPY GROUPS

Comparing Psychoeducational, Counseling, and Therapy Groups

Today, counselors can be found running all kinds of groups in a wide range of settings. Although all of the groups discussed are important, most counselors today are involved in conducting psychoeducational, counseling, and therapy groups, with task-group specialists generally being doctoral-level organizational development specialists. Therefore, Figure 7.1 compares the major differences that can be found between psychoeducational, counseling, and therapy groups.

The Use of Theory in Group Work

Theory is as important in group counseling as it is in individual counseling. As Corey and Corey (2002) point out, "leading a group without having an explicit theoretical rationale is like flying a plane without a flight plan—although you may eventually get there, you're equally likely to run out of gas" (p. 11). As in individual counseling, theory in reference to group counseling (1) gives us a comprehensive system of doing counseling, (2) assists us in understanding our client, (3) helps us in deciding which techniques to apply, (4) is useful in predicting the course of treatment, and (5) is researchable and thus can provide us information about its efficacy. If applied to group work, a theoretical model chosen should be an extension of the group leader's personality, for a theory discordant with one's view of human nature will feel awkward and be applied poorly.

Although the vast majority of theories of counseling and psychotherapy were initially developed for individual counseling, most have been applied to group work, with each having advantages and disadvantages when applied to a group setting (Gladding, 1999). The following are examples of the use of group counseling as applied by four counseling theories, one from each of the four conceptual orientations we examined in Chapter 4: psychodynamic, existential–humanistic, behavioral, and cognitive. More specifically, we will briefly review psychoanalysis group therapy, person-centered group counseling, behavioral group therapy, and rational emotive behavior group therapy.

Psychoanalytic Group Therapy

Psychoanalytic group therapy tends to stress many of the same issues of individual psychoanalysis, including the past, unconscious motivations, insight and self-examination, intrapsychic processes, and issues of transference and resistance (Wolf, Schwartz, McCarty, & Goldberg, 1972). In group psychoanalytic therapy, it is assumed that group members will unconsciously reenact family-of-origin issues within the group. The group therefore offers members a rich opportunity to work on past issues that affect current functioning. This occurs through the transference process where group members distort the personality of other group members and react to them as if they were significant persons from their past. The therapist or other group members can subsequently interpret this distortion in an effort to help the client understand past relationships. As Corey (2000b) so succinctly states, this kind of group "focuses on re-creating, analyzing, discussing, and interpreting past experiences and working through defenses and resistances . . ." (p. 147).

Some of the advantages to group analytic therapy over individual therapy include:

1. The sheer number of individuals in a group allow more opportunity to re-create past family issues through transference.

2. There is an increased opportunity for feedback concerning defenses and resistances.
3. There is less chance of extreme dependency on the therapist, because some of the authority is dispersed among other group members.
4. Seeing others work through similar issues helps to reduce defensiveness.
5. Observing other members working through resistances can be an encouragement to the client to do so as well.

Although the basic techniques used in individual analysis are also used in group analytic therapy, some adjustments are made for the group dynamics. For instance, in a process called "going around," all group members participate in free association in which they are encouraged to willingly share all their thoughts and feelings spontaneously in the group (Wolf & Schwartz, 1972). This allows members to quickly move beyond their defenses and helps to create group cohesion as members all share deeply personal issues. This sharing can later be interpreted by members and/or the group leader:

> *It quickly became clear that the encouragement to express associations, thoughts, and feelings freely led to much interaction of a highly charged quality. . . . In the course of working through, the patients were encouraged to choose more reasonable alternatives in reality.* (Wolf & Schwartz, 1972, p. 42)

Other psychoanalytic techniques are also easily used in the group setting. When using dream analysis, group members have the opportunity to offer possible interpretations to the dream. Sometimes these meanings may be on target; other times they are projections of the member's own issues, which also can be worked on. Transference can be directed at the leader or the members of the group, and both the leader and the group members can interpret this transference. Finally, resistance may occur within a member or with the whole group (e.g., attempting to accuse the leader of poor group skills), and this too can be interpreted by the group leader or by other members.

When psychoanalytic group therapy was originated, groups generally met three times a week for about one and a half hours, and group members could often be found discussing issues on their own in mini-sessions subsequent to the group (Wolf & Schwartz, 1972). With psychoanalytic theory not holding the same prominence it held in the past, and with cutbacks on mental health coverage by insurance companies, it is rare to find a purely psychoanalytic group any longer. However, it is common today to find many group leaders who have a neo-Freudian outlook and who meet once or sometimes twice a week.

Although most groups today are not psychoanalytically oriented, many groups borrow some of the tenets and techniques of psychoanalytic group therapy. For instance, the analysis of dreams, discussion of resistances and transference issues, and acknowledgment of the unconscious are commonly discussed in groups of many orientations.

Behavioral Group Therapy

Behaviorism entered the group therapy arena a little later than some of the other approaches and began to become more popular during the 1970s. As might be expected, many of the techniques used in individual behavioral therapy can be applied to behavioral group therapy. Therefore, the basic learning principals of operant conditioning, classical conditioning, and social learning or modeling have all been applied in the group setting. A few of the techniques that have been widely used in behavioral group therapy include reinforcement contingencies, relaxation training, systematic desensitization, assertiveness training, modeling, and behavior rehearsal (Corey, 2000b; Gladding, 1999).

Clients of behavioral group therapy experience a similar counseling process as do those who participate in individual behavior therapy, with the added benefit of having group members offer assistance through the change process. Initially, the group leader has to carefully assure that group cohesion is formed by building a trusting relationship with all the group members. Next, the problem has to be clearly defined. Based on problem identification, goals are specified and appropriate techniques are chosen. Evaluating the success of those techniques and working on termination and follow-up issues are the final stages of this process (Corey, 2000b).

There are many advantages to behavioral work within a group setting. First, the establishment of group cohesion early in the process allows each group member to receive feedback concerning problem identification and strategies for change from other group members. Also, because relationships are formed, the leader will encourage the group to reinforce the changes made by the members. A group member can also rehearse new behaviors in the group prior to trying them in the real world. Also, group members can act as models for other group members, thereby offering more opportunity to learn from others. Finally, coaching of new behaviors can be offered by the group leader or by group members. In this case, the coach will often sit behind the group member and offer continual feedback concerning a specific behavior being practiced in front of the group.

Leaders of behavioral groups are active and directive as they assist clients in working on behavioral goals and assist the group in learning how to respond to one another. Leaders of behavioral groups stress current behavior and consciousness and downplay intrapsychic processes.

As with individual behavior therapy, there are few pure behavior group therapists today. Many find a fit with cognitive therapy, thus practicing cognitive–behavior group therapy. Although stressing behavioral principles, some behavior group therapists will discuss issues of transference, resistance, insight, and self-reflection in the group. This may become particularly important when examining group dynamics and group process. For instance, a group member who is threatening to leave the group can have this behavior interpreted as resistance to the group process as a result of an underlying fear of change. It should be remembered, however, that the main focus of behavioral group therapy is on defining the problem and working on established goals.

Rational Emotive Behavior Group Therapy

As in individual therapy, the rational emotive behavior group therapist is directive, active, and confrontational as he or she attempts to get group members to challenge their ways of thinking and to internalize a rational philosophy of living (Corey, 2000b).

Because the REBT group leader does not place particular importance on building a warm relationship, little if any time is spent on rapport building. In fact, some REBT therapists view a warm or approving relationship as potentially damaging to the therapeutic process, as it can slow down group progress and prevent the REBT group therapist from getting to business (Capuzzi & Gross, 1998). However, as in individual counseling, the therapist does attempt to accept all members unconditionally, regardless of their tendency to think irrationally.

REBT group therapy can occur through a series of steps, with one of the first functions of the leader being to teach group members about REBT philosophy and challenge them to adopt this new way of thinking and living in the world. Some REBT group leaders will prime members prior to the beginning of the group by having them read relevant books and other printed materials. After members learn about REBT philosophy, they are taught how to confront their current ways of thinking and will be encouraged to challenge other group members' irrational thinking processes. As members begin to examine their illogical thinking processes and learn the ABCDs of REBT therapy (see Chapter 4), they will be encouraged to take on new behaviors that are in sync with a rational philosophy of living. Many of the techniques of REBT therapy taught in individual counseling are applied to group therapy. Therefore, it is common to see REBT group leaders using emotive techniques, behavioral techniques, imagery exercises, shame-attacking exercises, role-playing, bibliotherapy, and cognitive homework (see Chapter 4).

Group REBT has some advantages over individual REBT counseling. For instance, in group REBT members are able to (1) challenge one another to think and act differently, (2) practice new ways of acting in front of each other, (3) obtain reinforcement from one another for taking on a more rational way of living, and (4) encourage one another to continue to dispute irrational beliefs and take on new behaviors after initial changes have been made (Capuzzi & Gross, 1998; Corey, 2000b).

REBT group therapy is one cognitive approach to working with groups. Other cognitive approaches, such as those developed by Beck and by Meichenbaum, can also be applied to groups and will have their own unique take on group work (Corey, 2000b).

Person-Centered Group Counseling

As with the other approaches we have examined thus far, person-centered group counseling uses the basic premises of person-centered counseling and applies it in a group setting. Thus, the person-centered group counselor relies on the qualities of empathic understanding, genuineness, and unconditional positive regard to guide the group process (see Chapter 4).

Person-centered group counselors are not concerned about unconscious motivations, instincts, transference, or spending an inordinate amount of time working on past issues. However, person-centered group counselors do believe that increased self-awareness and insight will be achieved through this approach. They believe that the core conditions of empathy, genuineness, and unconditional positive regard are necessary and sufficient to the effectiveness of group counseling. If applied properly, they say, there will be a tendency for the group to move toward health and wholeness.

After leading many groups, Rogers (1970) noted that the same process generally transpired in groups. This process could be described in a series of steps in which clients (1) initially mill around and resist personal expression; (2) begin to share past feelings and negative feelings—feelings that are relatively safe to express; (3) slowly express personally meaningful feelings, deeper parts of self, and feelings about one another in the group; (4) begin to accept all parts of self and find a healing capacity within; (5) are increasingly able to hear feedback about self and let down their facades; (6) become healers themselves and begin to assist others inside and outside of the group; (7) are able to encounter another person fully in an "I–Thou" relationship; and (8) begin to look and act differently inside and outside the group.

This approach to group counseling is nondirective and worked effectively for Carl Rogers as he traveled the world running groups for people in conflict with one another, such as Catholics and Protestants in Northern Ireland. However, the total lack of directiveness, as portrayed by Rogers, is difficult for many therapists. Other existential–humanistic approaches, such as Gestalt therapy and existential therapy, tend to be more directive and have many of the same goals and ideals of the person-centered approach.

The Group Process

A group process occurs for all groups regardless of the leader's theoretical orientation. How the leader prepares the group can affect this process, which includes the following stages: the pregroup stage, the initial stage, the transition stage, the work stage, and the closure stage.

Preparing for the Group

Prior to starting a group, there are a number of practical issues that the effective group leader should consider in order to build the most conducive climate for the group. Climate can be affected by the characteristics of the members recruited for the group, whether the group is closed or open, the size of the group, the duration and frequency of meetings, and the atmosphere of the place in which the group meets (Andrews, 1995; Corey & Corey, 2002; Garvin, 1981; Posthuma, 1988).

Getting Members

What if I ran a group and nobody came? Believe me, this is a question that has been considered by many counselors who are considering running a group. There are a number of ways that members can be obtained, including: advertising; seeking referrals from colleagues; seeking referrals from appropriate sources (e.g., teachers, academic advising offices, physicians); placing signs, if appropriate (e.g., a sign in a residence hall); and referring appropriate clients from one's own caseload. Besides getting clients, the leader needs to be clear on whom he or she wants in the group. How and where I get my clients can be greatly affected by whom the leader wants in the group.

Group Composition

The composition of a counseling or therapy group can be a crucial factor in its success. Most significantly, leaders need to decide whether the group will be homogeneous or heterogenous. In considering this important factor, leaders will reflect on the following factors: age, sex, level of functioning, problem focus, and diagnosis of the members. Although research concerning the composition of groups is mixed, group leaders need to carefully consider all of the potential problems and advantages that might affect the particular group they will be running (Garvin, 1981; Posthuma, 1988).

Closed or Open Group

Groups that do not allow new members to join are called closed groups. Cohesion can generally occur more quickly in closed groups. Sometimes group leaders will decide to have a modified closed group, where the leader will replace a member as other members leave. This is particularly useful when running small groups, especially if there is an expectation of members leaving the group at some point. Open groups have members freely joining or leaving. AA is an example of an open group.

Size of Groups

For counseling and therapy groups, the ideal size ranges from five to twelve members. Some counselors feel comfortable with smaller numbers, others with larger numbers. Factors that should be considered when determining the size of the group include whether or not there is a coleader, the length of time that the group meets, and the focus of the group. For psychoeducational groups, the group can be large, but not so large that individuals would feel as though they could not ask a question or partake in a limited discussion on the topic.

Duration of Meetings

Groups can generally run from 30 minutes to 3 hours long, with the most common length being 1½ hours (Andrews, 1995). Factors to consider when deciding the length of group sessions include: the amount of time available (e.g., school counselors usually have limited time), the focus of the group, the energy level of the leader, the energy level of the participants, and whether or not there is a coleader.

Frequency of Meetings

Some groups meet daily, others monthly. Issues to consider in determining frequency include focus of the problem, availability of space, needs of clients, ability to pay, availability of clients, and the availability of the group leader(s).

Securing an Appropriate Space

As in individual counseling, groups should be led in a comfortable, confidential, safe environment, which has few if any distractions (Posthuma, 1988). Because of the multiple members in groups, this is not always an easy task. For instance, some groups, such as psychoeducational groups in the schools, are often conducted in the classroom, and another space would be difficult to find.

The Stages of Group Development

The development of a group has been shown to occur in predictable stages (Corey & Corey, 2002; Gladding, 1999; Tuckman & Jensen, 1977; Vander Kolk, 1990; Ward, 1982; Yalom, 1995). Although experts in group work differ on the terms they use to identify these stages, the characteristics of the stages are fairly consistent. Passage through all of the stages generally occurs only in counseling and therapy groups and not in self-help groups, task groups, and psychoeducational groups. Counseling and therapy groups have the continuity of membership and the length of time to stimulate the unveiling of personalities and the development of interpersonal relationships necessary for the full development of the group process. On the other hand, whereas self-help and psychoeducational groups might exhibit properties of one or more of the stages, their structure is such that they are not likely to pass through all of the stages.

Following are typical stages through which members might pass, as identified by a number of authors (Corey & Corey, 2002; Vander Kolk, 1990; Yalom, 1995).

The Pregroup Stage (Forming a Group)

> *Counselors screen prospective group counseling/therapy participants. To the extent possible, counselors select members whose needs and goals are compatible with goals of the group, who will not impede the group process, and whose well being will not be jeopardized by the group experience.* (ACA, 1995a, Section A.9)

As the above quote suggests, the group leader needs to find an effective method of prescreening potential group members. Some group leaders will have a pregroup meeting with all potential members. Other leaders provide potential members with thorough written or even videotaped knowledge of the expectations of the group in an effort to have them screen themselves out. However, probably the most effective and common method is the individual interview. Couch (1995) notes that the interview can assist in identifying needs, expectations, and commitment of the potential group member; challenging myths and misconceptions of the potential member; conveying and procuring information to the potential member; and screening out (or in) potential members.

The Initial Stage

The beginning stage of the group is often highlighted by anxiety, apprehension, and, for many group members, a desire to get started. During this stage group members are adapting to the rules and goals of the group and are wondering whether or not they can trust the other group members. Because of this initial apprehension and lack of trust, group members will often avoid talking about in-depth feelings, and discussions are relatively safe. Therefore, it is common for conversations to be superficial, for members to have a focus on others as opposed to a self-focus, and for discussions to revolve around past feelings as opposed to current feelings (Corey & Corey, 2002). Other ways that members exhibit early resistance are by being silent, laughing, talking excessively, monopolizing, intellectualizing, and generalizing (Higgs, 1992).

During this initial stage, group members are often self-conscious, worried about how others might view them, and concerned about whether they will be accepted. The major task for the group leader in this stage is to define the ground rules and to build a level of trust that will allow group members to begin to drop their defenses (Clark, 1992). If the leader is successful, group cohesion will begin to build by the end of this stage.

In the pursuit of trust and group cohesion, the leader must be able to set limits, assure that members abide by the ground rules, and simultaneously show empathy and unconditional positive regard. Structure, empathy, and positive regard enable group members to feel psychologically safe, which is the first step toward greater openness. Leaders need to be genuine and only slightly self-disclosing. This is sometimes a difficult balance, but, ultimately, the leader's purpose is to focus on group members, not self. Finally, Vander Kolk (1990) suggests that during this stage a balance between comfort and anxiety should be found. Comfort helps members feel safe, and a little bit of anxiety can be motivating.

From a systems perspective, group leaders need to be aware that in these early stages of the group, one or more group members may be scapegoated. Scapegoating keeps the attention and any pressure to self-disclose off the person(s) doing the scapegoating.

The Transition Stage

During the opening phase of the transition stage, group members are beginning to feel comfortable with the technical issues and ground rules of the group. However, anxiety is still felt as trust and safety issues continue. Issues of control, power, and authority become increasingly important in this stage as members position themselves within the system (Corey & Corey, 2002; Vander Kolk, 1990; Yalom, 1995). What are members trying to accomplish by positioning themselves? Ultimately, they are attempting to be the same person in the group as in the rest of their lives:

> *Given enough time, group members will begin to be themselves: they will interact with the group members as they interact with others in their social sphere, will create in the group the same interpersonal universe they have always inhabited.* (Yalom, 1995, p. 28)

As members attempt to find their place in the group, they are likely to experience anxiety, fear, and a myriad of other feelings. At this point in the group process members may begin projecting onto the group leader and struggling with transference issues (Kivlighan et al., 1994). A dance occurs in the group as members attempt to settle into the group process and simultaneously deal with all the feelings they are having. Attacking and scapegoating are common at this point, as members are fearful of taking ownership of their strong and sometimes confusing feelings and thus blame others for their discomfort. Although empathy and positive regard continue to be important in this stage, it is also vital that the leader actively prevent a member from being scapegoated or attacked as a result of the group instability. Failure to do so could prevent the group from progressing any further, as members become bogged down with conflict and fail to build cohesion.

As this stage continues, trust is slowly built, resistances diminish, and members begin to settle into their roles and feel safe enough to delve into self and to share personal concerns. Members are now transitioning to a place where they can demonstrate the ability to take ownership of their feelings, have a self- rather than other-focus, talk in the here and now, and not blame others for their problems (Higgs, 1992). It is at this point in the stage that the need for the leader to protect members dramatically decreases as members stop blaming others and stop acting out. Near the end of this stage, group members more clearly identify the goals they would like to achieve. Although goals were probably identified earlier by most group members, defensiveness and lack of clarity of self may have distorted the clients' perceptions of which issues to work on.

From a systems perspective, it is interesting to compare this stage to family counseling. Families come in with a system that has evolved over a number of years. Issues of control, power, and authority have already been decided. Therefore, the purpose of family therapy is to understand the family in order to devise strategies to change the system to lead to healthier functioning for all. Groups, on the other hand, are working to build a system (Matthews, 1992), and it is the responsibility of the leader to assure that strategies are used to develop a healthy functioning system. Ultimately, the goal for families and groups is the same: to develop a system that has open channels of communications, allows for the sharing of feelings, and rebuffs abuses of power that leave people feeling unsafe and victimized. When families and groups arrive at this place, they are ready to work.

The Work Stage

As members gain the capacity to take ownership for their feelings and life predicaments, a deepening of trust and a sense of cohesion emerges within the group. Members are now able to give and hear feedback, focus on identified problems, and take an active role in the change process. For instance, they may attempt new ways of communicating, acting, or expressing feelings. During this stage, conflict lessens; but, when it does occur, it is handled very differently than previously. Members now can talk through conflict and take ownership of their own part in it.

As this stage continues, members will begin to identify and work on behaviors they would like to change. As members accomplish their goals, they gain in self-esteem as they receive positive feedback from other members and acquire a sense of accomplishment for the work they have done. As members meet their goals, they are near the completion of the group process.

From a systems perspective, during this stage, the group has developed its own unique homeostasis; however, it is important that the group leader prohibit members from becoming too comfortable in their styles of relating, as this can prevent change and growth. Leaders can best facilitate movement during this stage through the use of a variety of advanced counseling skills such as support and confrontation, higher-level empathy, probing questions, and interpretation.

The Closure Stage

The last stage of the group process is highlighted by an increased sense of accomplishment, high self-esteem, and the beginning awareness that the group process is near completion. Saying good-bye can be a difficult process for many, and it is important that the leader facilitate this process in a direct yet gentle fashion. Often this is done by the leader encouraging members to share what they have learned about themselves and about one another and by having them express their feelings about one another and the upcoming termination of the group. Using empathy, the leader will often summarize the changes that have taken place and focus on the separation process. This important final stage in the group process allows members to feel a sense of completion and wholeness about what they have experienced.

It is important during this stage to assure that those who need to, or would like to, have an opportunity to follow up in counseling. Therefore, referrals are often necessary. In addition, other members may need to develop a method of assuring the continuation of changed behaviors. Members might decide to meet periodically on their own in a kind of ongoing support group, or there might be periodic planned meetings with the group leader that focus on reinforcement of changed behaviors. Some members might have periodic check-ins with the group leader on an individual basis.

Finally, to assess if the group has been beneficial, many leaders will complete an evaluation of the group. This is often suggested during the final group. A follow-up evaluation may also be completed a few months later to determine if change has been substantive and continual.

Group Leadership Styles

The group process noted above defines general stages through which most counseling and therapy groups will pass, regardless of the leader's theoretical orientation. However, the theoretical orientation of the group leader will affect the kinds of techniques that are used throughout the stages and can be a factor in determining the length of time in the various stages. For instance, a cognitive–behavioral group that places less emphasis on the relationship and greater importance on working on behavioral goals will spend less time in the first stage, building cohesion and trust, and more time in the work stage. This kind of group relies less on the sharing of deep personal feelings and more on identifying behavioral strategies.

Although leadership styles will vary based on the leader's theoretical orientation (Corey, 2000b; Gladding, 1999), all leaders need to be aware of basic group theory and process to facilitate groups appropriately (Brown, 1992). Therefore, knowledge of systems, familiarity with membership roles, awareness of group stages of development, having a theoretical orientation, and adeptness at basic as well as advanced counseling techniques are crucial. Good leaders are aware of the composition of their group and have adjusted their style to the needs of the group. A good leader will be strong without being authoritarian and knowledgeable about the rules and technical issues, yet flexible in the ways they are implemented. He or she is able to facilitate the interactions of group members as they pass through the stages of group development. Such a leader feels comfortable working with a vast array of member behaviors and is able to set the stage for the group to unravel in a natural way.

Multicultural Issues

Principles for Diversity-Competent Group Workers

In an effort to assure that individuals who do group work are appropriately knowledgeable about multicultural issues, the ASGW developed and endorsed Principles for Diversity-Competent Group Workers (Haley-Banez, Brown, & Molina, 1999). These principles speak to the knowledge, skills, and attitudes and beliefs that all diversity-competent group workers should have when working with clients. All professionals who practice group work should be knowledgeable about this document, which is attainable at the ASGW Web site (see www.counseling.org and go to ASGW link).

The Group as a Microcosm of Society

Because a group is a microcosm of society, prejudices that occur in everyday life are likely to raise their ugly heads within a group. Therefore, a group that is culturally diverse offers the potential for clients to work through unconscious and deep-seated feelings of racism and prejudice that may be directed to group members but are in actuality a projection of underlying prejudices. Counselors, therefore, have the opportunity to help heal some of our deeply held prejudices by considering, along with other factors, the cultural background of clients when deciding group membership. By actively seeking out diversity in group membership, counselors are likely to set the stage for group members to work on their prejudices.

Cultural Differences between a Group Member and the Group Leader

Because a group experience can be very powerful, and because anger is often projected onto the group leader early on, there is an opportunity, if a group leader is from a culturally different background from the members, to assist members in understanding deep-seated prejudices they may project onto the group leader. A skilled group leader can assist members both in examining their anger, which is a natural part of the group process, and in understanding feelings of prejudice they may have.

Ethical, Professional, and Legal Issues

Ethical Issues

The ethical code of ACA applies to group work as well as individual counseling. A counselor should be aware of the code, paying particular attention to the issues of informed consent and confidentiality when conducting a group.

Informed Consent

Informed consent becomes a particularly important concern in group work because a number of issues are at play that are generally not found in other forms of counseling. At the very minimum, when giving informed consent, group members should know (1) the credentials of the group leader, (2) the general therapeutic style of the group leader, (3) the goals of the group, (4) the general ground rules associated with the group, (5) expectations about self-disclosure on the part of the leader and potential members, (6) whether members are free to withdraw from the group at any time and the responsibility they may have to the other group members when terminating, (7) the limits of confidentiality, and (8) any psychological risks that may arise as a function of the group experience (Corey, 2000b; Corey & Corey, 2002).

Confidentiality

As in all forms of counseling, the group leader must assure group members that the leader will keep all shared material confidential and notify them of any limits to confidentiality, such as harm to self or harm to others. However, what the group leader cannot do is assure that other members of the group will keep information confidential (see "Legal Issue," below). The leader should stress the importance of confidentiality but also make group members aware of the possible limitations of confidentiality.

Professional Issues

Group versus Individual Counseling

When does one refer a client to group counseling as an alternative or adjunct to individual counseling? With the most current research indicating that group counseling is as effective as individual counseling, some suggest that group work should always be considered an alternative to individual treatment (Faith, Wong, & Carpenter, 1995; Tillitski, 1990; Toseland & Siporin, 1986). Although there is no easy method of determining when to use group or individual counseling, a few guidelines might help. For instance, it might be smart to refer to group counseling when:

- A client cannot afford the cost of individual counseling.
- The benefits for a client of individual counseling have gotten so meager that an alternative treatment might offer a new perspective.
- A client's issues are related to interpersonal functioning, and a group might facilitate working through these issues in a real-to-life manner.
- A client needs the extra social support that a group might offer.
- A client wants to test new behaviors in a system that will support him or her while simultaneously receiving realistic feedback about the new behaviors.

- The experiences of others who are working through similar issues can dramatically improve the client's functioning (e.g., alcoholism or depression).

Professional Associations

Although a number of professional associations focus on group issues, the major professional association for counselors interested in group work is ASGW, a division of ACA (see Web link via www.counseling.org). Its purpose is

> *. . . to establish standards for professional and ethical practice; to support research and the dissemination of knowledge; and to provide professional leadership in the field of group work. In addition, the Association shall seek to extend counseling through the use of group process; to provide a forum for examining innovative and developing concepts in group work; to foster diversity and dignity in our groups; and to be models of effective group practice.* (ASGW, 1998c)

A few of the many benefits of ASGW includes:

- Best Practice Guidelines to augment the ACA ethical guidelines.
- Professional Standards for the Training of Group Worker.
- The Principles of Diversity-Competent Group Workers.
- Publishing of a newsletter and of the *Journal for Specialists in Group Work*.
- Sponsoring the development of national group work leader certification.
- The sponsoring of workshops and conferences specific to group issues.
- The opportunity to be mentored and learn about supervisory practices relative to group work.

Legal Issue: Confidentiality and the Third-Party Rule

Most legal issues that would apply to individual counseling also apply to group counseling, with one possible exception: confidentiality of member information. Although group members might justifiably expect that other group members and the leader would respect their right to confidentiality, the legal system generally does not view information revealed to more than one person as confidential (in the legal system this is called the third-party rule) (Swenson, 1997). Thus, if a group member were to break confidentiality, such as reveal information about the group in a court of law, the court might then deem it desirable, and possible, to obtain information from other group members. In addition, if the leader does not hold privileged communication status, he or she can also be forced to reveal information said in the group.

The Counselor in Process: Allowing Groups to Unravel Naturally

Push a group, and it will push back. The members will resist, protest, confront, and perhaps even leave. A group needs to naturally unravel as the counselor slowly facilitates the development of the group process. The counselor's challenge in running groups is to be able to facilitate a client through the stages of group counseling without pushing the client out of therapy. This delicate balance is not always easily achieved. Perhaps hearing the words of Carl Rogers over 30 years ago can remind us that groups need to move at their own pace:

> *. . . Often there is consternation, anxiety, and irritation. . . . Only gradually does it become evident that the major aim of nearly every member is to find ways of relating to other members of the group and to himself. Then as they gradually, tentatively, and fearfully explore their feelings and attitudes toward one another and toward themselves, it becomes increasingly evident that what they have first presented are facades, masks. Only cautiously do the real feelings and real person emerge. . . . Little by little, a sense of genuine communication builds up. . . .* (Rogers, 1970, p. 8)

Summary

This chapter began by noting that, like families, groups follow the rules of general systems theory, and we then highlighted that group work offers some advantages over other forms of counseling. We discussed how group work has changed over the 20th century from its early moralistic and preaching orientation, to a rigid psychoanalytic focus, to encounter and training groups that arose in the 1940s. Today, most groups can be classified as one of five types: self-help groups, task groups, psychoeducational groups, counseling groups, and therapy groups. We also noted that common-theme groups and brief-therapy groups, which are types of counseling groups, have in recent years become very popular.

In this chapter we discussed the importance that theory has in group counseling and noted that a group leader tends to embrace a theory that is an extension of his or her personality. We examined one theory from each of four conceptual orientations: psychodynamic, behavioral, cognitive, and existential–humanistic. We stated that regardless of the theory chosen, all groups will be affected by group dynamics and reflect group process. We noted that the group process can be affected by how we prepare for the group, including such issues as examining characteristics of potential group members, whether the group is closed or open, the size of the group, the duration and frequency of meetings, and the atmosphere of the place in which the group meets. We then reviewed the five stages of group development: pregroup, initial, transition, work, and closure. We noted that passage through all these stages generally occurs only in counseling and therapy groups and not in self-help groups, task groups, and psychoeducational groups. We noted that the leadership style of the group counselor is crucial in building group cohesion and in facilitating the successful passage of the group through the various stages of group development.

In examining multicultural issues related to group work, we noted that recently ASGW developed Principles for Diversity-Competent Group Workers, which can assist in the cross-cultural training of group workers. We also noted that the group is a microcosm of society and thus offers us a rich opportunity to examine how we relate to many different types of people. Thus, if the group is culturally diverse, and/or if the leader is culturally different, the group member has a unique opportunity to safely examine his or her biases and prejudices as they play themselves out in this multicultural setting.

We noted that most ethical and legal concerns found in individual counseling are also issues in group work. However, we did highlight two ethical and legal concerns that differ. For instance, we highlighted the increased importance of informed consent in group work due to the increased risks involved. In addition, we stated that in group counseling confidentiality is much less assured and indeed cannot be guaranteed through our legal system.

As we neared the end of the chapter, we discussed some professional issues related to group work. First, we gave some guidelines for when one might choose group work over individual counseling. Then we discussed the activities of ASGW, noting that it provides us with The Best Practice Guidelines, the Professional Standards for the Training of Group Workers, the Principles of Diversity-Competent Group Workers, a journal, sponsoring of workshops and conferences, and many other member benefits. Finally, we concluded the chapter with a brief discussion of the importance of allowing groups to unravel naturally.

INFOTRAC and Other Information Resources (e.g., ERIC and PsycINFO)

Note: When relevant, key words are in quotation marks.

1. Examine issues related to "trust and group" counseling.
2. Review methods of "preparation and group" counseling.
3. Examine a special population of your choice, relative to group counseling (e.g., "group and children," "group and elderly," etc.)
4. Research "multicultural and group" issues.

CHAPTER 8

Consultation and Supervision

The principal of an elementary school asked me to spend a morning with a third-grade class. He wanted to discuss with me the students' feelings about having had a developmentally delayed young man, who was quadriplegic, mainstreamed into their classroom for six weeks. This was consultation.

Because I was concerned that a client of mine might be emotionally and/or learning disabled, I gave him a series of psychological and educational tests. I subsequently met with a colleague of mine to assist me in reviewing some of the results. This too was consultation.

Administrators from a local social service agency asked a colleague of mine to meet with them concerning communication problems at their agency. Following the meeting, they hired him to come to the agency and make an assessment of problems and suggest strategies for change. This was consultation also.

Our counseling program invited a counselor educator, who had expertise with the CACREP standards, to meet with our counselors and review the program's strengths and weaknesses before we applied for CACREP accreditation. This was consultation.

During my counseling career I have had numerous supervisors. For instance, when I worked as a therapist at a mental health center, I would meet weekly with my supervisor to discuss my cases. Also, while in private practice, our group hired a local psychologist to meet weekly with us for supervision. And, another time, while in private practice, I would pay a master therapist for biweekly supervision meetings. This was supervision, a special kind of consultation.

The examples above show that consultation and supervision have become a crucial aspect of every counseling specialty area, with most counseling programs now including consultation and supervision as a major part of their course work and field experiences (Borders, 1994a; Brown, Spano, & Schulte, 1988; Kurpius & Fuqua, 1993a, b; Werner & Tyler, 1993; West & Idol, 1993; Westbrook et al., 1993). This may be partly the result of the most recent CACREP standards requiring that consultation and supervision be an integral part of counselor training. Despite this inclusion, consultation is one of the most misunderstood components of all counselor training (Brown, 1993), while supervisory practices are still establishing themselves in the field (Borders & Cashwell, 1992; Borders & Fong, 1994; Prieto, 1996).

This chapter will examine the current status of consultation and supervision. Although supervision may be seen as a type of consultation, there are enough differences between the two to justify discussing them separately. Therefore, the chapter will first focus on consultation and later on supervision.

Consultation

Defining Consultation

In 1978 Kurpius and Robinson noted that "there is no one, broad, universally accepted definition of consultation" (p. 321). Unfortunately, some might say that this is still true today, as it seems evident that the field is still struggling to find its voice. For instance, today approaches to consultation vary, with theoretical orientations still very much developing, ethical guidelines not fully addressing the consulting relationship, and the place of consultation in the counseling field still being challenged (Brown, 1993; Newman, 1993). With this in mind, probably most would agree with the following uncomplicated definition of consultation: "[consultation is] me and you talking about him or her with the purpose of some change" (Fall, 1995, p. 151).

More specifically, consultation has been defined as a person or persons (the consultant) being contracted by another person (the consultee) to deliver direct service to a person, group, organization, or community in an effort to assist the individual or system in working through difficulties (Dougherty, 1990). But the definition I like best is the one from the 1988 ethical guidelines of ACA, which states that consultation is

> *. . . a voluntary relationship between a professional helper and help-needing individual, group, or social unit in which the consultant is providing help to the client(s) in defining and solving a work-related problem or potential problem with a client or client system.* (Section E)

Although I might personally quibble with the term *work-related problem,* as I believe consultants may be called in by individuals not involved in a work situation (e.g., a retirement community may call in a consultant to deal with interpersonal issues of the elderly), this definition seems to get to the core of what consultation is.

Consultation involves a triadic relationship in which the focus of the consultant and consultee is a third party, which can be an individual or a system. Because it involves scrutinizing a third party, consultants often increase self-understanding of those with whom they come in contact. However, it is important to remember that although consultation can be therapeutic, it is not therapy. Consultation is *not* a one-to-one intense counseling experience.

Consultation occurs in agencies, schools, businesses, and wherever there exists a consultee who would like to improve a problematic situation or would like to examine new ways for producing positive change. Although a consultant may work solely with one person in an organization, a group within the organization, or the whole organization, modern-day consultation tends to hold a systemic, contextual, and developmental perspective (Kurpius & Fuqua, 1993c). This is why consultation is included in the section on systems. Let's take a look at how this field has developed over the years and its relatively recent systemic focus.

A Brief History of Consultation

The Beginning

The decades of the 1940s and 1950s are considered by many to be the beginning of modern-day consultation methods (Kurpius & Robinson, 1978). At that time, a consultee, who was generally a supervisor or administrator of an organization, would invite a consultant to his or her setting with the expectation that the consultant, "the expert," would solve an existing problem. Once the consultant came to the agency, the consultee and consultant would have little contact, and the consultant was pretty much left to his or her own devices to solve the problem. This became known as the direct-service approach to consultation (Kurpius & Robinson, 1978).

> ***Example.*** *A principal finds that many parents are complaining about not being able to understand the test scores of their children. The principal asks an expert on assessment to come in and take care of this situation. The consultant decides to run a workshop for parents and designates the counselor to do future workshops for parents. He goes over the test material with the counselor to assure that she is adequately prepared. The principal remains uninvolved.*

By the end of the 1950s the consultee would generally be included in on the consultation process along with the staff. This would help to assure that if similar issues arose in the future, the consultee would have the training to deal with the problem.

> ***Example.*** *After finding a number of insurance forms returned for misdiagnosis, and believing that some clients may have been placed on the wrong medication due to similar errors, the clinical director of an agency asks a consultant to come in and teach the staff about the* Diagnostic and Statistical Manual (DSM-IV-TR). *The clinical director sits in on the workshops to also gain the knowledge and avoid future problems.*

Soon, a new twist on consultation evolved where the consultant was hired as a trainer who "had expert knowledge and skills for problem solving" (Kurpius & Robinson, 1978, p. 322). Here, the consultant's purpose would be to define problem areas and to educate staff in these problem areas.

> ***Example.*** *At a college counseling center, there is infighting among the staff and poor morale. The director has attempted to bring the staff together to discuss the problem, but there is little progress. A consultant is called in and, following some investigation, finds that the staff is polarized along ethnic and gender lines. The consultant makes recommendations to the staff, and the director of the agency agrees to have the consultant/trainer teach the staff, including the director, about some of the new research on the impact of gender, ethnicity, culture, age, and power on group dynamics. Discussion concerning the dynamics at the agency ensues, and the staff begin to share their feelings. The trainer uses her expertise in group dynamics to facilitate change and develop new, healthier coalitions.*

The Expansion of Models of Consultation

As we moved into the 1970s a number of consultation models evolved from the previous ones, and some new ones developed. During this time consultants were generally defined by the consultation model they followed (Kurpius & Robinson, 1978). The 1980s and 1990s saw expanded versions of the models from the 1970s. Today, these models are used to outline the general ways in which the consultant might bring him- or herself into the system; they will be discussed later in this chapter.

The latter part of the 20th century also brought us the proliferation of theories of consultation. Many of these theories are similar to the counseling theories examined in Chapter 4 but applied within a consulting framework. Unlike the models of consultation that speak to the consultant's general style, his or her theoretical perspective represents the prism through which the consultant will come to understand the system and affects how he or she will devise strategies for change. Some of these theories will be discussed later in the chapter.

Recent Trends

A SYSTEMIC PERSPECTIVE

> *Whether implicitly or explicitly, current models of organizational consultation are based upon systems theory.* (Brown, Pryzwansky, & Schulte, 1987, p. 89)

Today, a systems perspective has become an essential component to the consultation process (see General Systems Theory, Chapter 6). Consulting with one person regarding another not only involves the three primary individuals (the consultant, consultee, and "other"), but also involves the complexity of the interrelationships of all the systems in which the other individuals work, live, and play (Campbell, Coldicott, & Kinsella, 1995; Klein, Gabelnick, & Herr, 2000). Figure 8.1 shows a sample of some of the various subsystems that consultants need to consider when doing consultation. A systems perspective assumes that the consultant must examine the complex interrelationships among all components of the system (Fuqua & Kurpius, 1993; Kurpius, 1985), make suggestions for change based on this kind of thinking, and assist the consultee in viewing the system contextually if change is to maintain itself:

> *Perhaps one of the most significant changes in the practice of consultation is in helping the consultee become more conceptual in understanding the multiple ways of viewing a problem. . . . Peter Senge (1990) referred to this intervention as a learning organization and systems-thinking process and stressed that this cognitive activity is essential to any helping relationship.* (Kurpius & Fuqua, 1993d, p. 596)

A DEVELOPMENTAL AND PREVENTIVE PERSPECTIVE Traditionally, consultation had a disease model orientation, whereby the consultant would be called in to remediate or solve the problem (Kurpius & Fuqua, 1993c). More recently, however, consultants have begun to see their role as assisting people and organizations through a process that will prevent future problems while developing the individual's or system's fullest potential (Albee & Ryan-Finn, 1993; Peters, 1999). This developmental and preventive process assumes that individuals and organizations will pass through a series of predictable stages as they work toward positive change. Although there is little doubt that many consultants today are still called in to an organization to deal with existing problems, the modern-day consultant will both assist in remediation of the problem and help the organization move toward the future (Zins, 1993).

FIGURE 8.1
A Sample of the Many Subsystems in Consultation

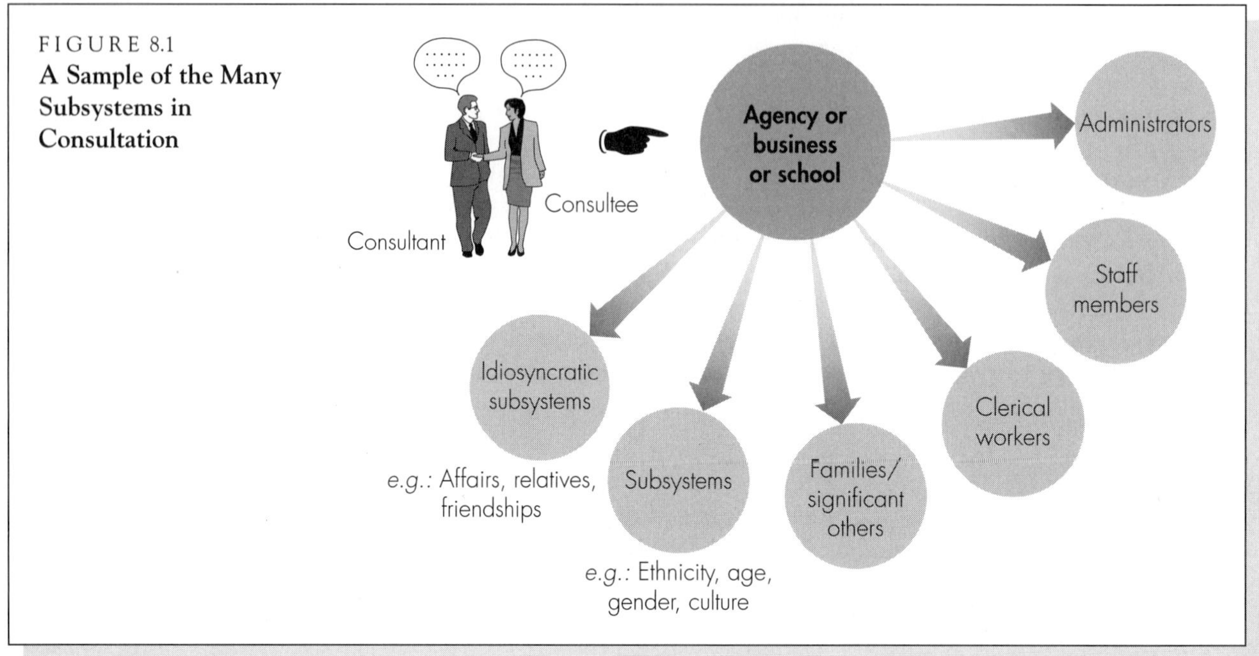

Models (Styles) of Consultation

Models of consultation speak to how a consultant brings him- or herself into the consulting relationship. Reminiscent of the models of consultation during the 1940s and 1950s, current models fall into one of two general orientations: consultant-centered, where the emphasis is on the consultant offering suggestions and advice for system change; or system-centered, where the consultant assists others to use their resources for system change. Because consulting today is more complex than it was during the 1950s, consultants will generally integrate their model with their theoretical perspective.

Consultant-Centered Consultation

1. *Expert consultant*. Here the consultant is seen as responsible for coming into the system and finding a "cure" (see Schein, 1969).
2. *Prescriptive consultant (prescription mode)*. Here the consultant collects information, diagnoses the problem, and makes the recommendations to the consultee on how to solve the problem (see Kurpius, 1978; Kurpius & Brubaker, 1976).
3. *Trainer and/or educator*. In this mode, the consultant is hired to come into a system and teach or train the staff (see Becker & Harris, 1973; Chandler, 1973).

System-Centered Consultation

1. *Consultant negotiator and/or facilitator*. Here the consultant helps individuals within the system communicate with one another, understand each other, and resolve conflicts among themselves (see Harrison, 1972; Rubenstein, 1973).

2. *Consultant as collaborator.* The consultant in this case acts as a facilitator of the change process by working jointly with the individuals involved. This partnership uses the consultant's expertise and relies on the individuals in the system to offer input into the problems and solutions (see Blake & Mouton, 1976, 1982; Kurpius, 1978).
3. *Process-oriented consultant.* This consultant either believes that he or she does not have the answer or withholds expertise with the belief that the most effective resolution, resulting in the highest self-esteem and sense of ownership of the problem, would be for the system members to find their own solution. Using this approach, the consultant has faith that system members can change if the consultant is able to offer a conducive environment for such change to occur (Kurpius & Fuqua, 1993c; Schein, 1969).

In choosing a model, the consultant needs to know his or her personality style, with whom he or she is working, and the problem to be addressed. For instance, a consultant who is consulting with master therapists would be likely to choose a different model than one who is working with beginning counseling students. A consultant whose natural style is directive would have a more difficult time taking on a system-centered style. And a consultant working with counselors who are providing less-than-adequate care on a suicide hotline would be likely to take on a different style than a consultant working with counselors providing quality care in a mental health center.

Theories of Consultation

While models of consultation speak to how the consultant brings him- or herself into the consulting relationship, theories of consultation provide a conceptual framework from which the consultant practices. Sometimes there is overlap between models and theories. For instance, a person-centered consultant would find it difficult to take on a consultant-centered style.

Practically any theory of consulting could be applied to consultation. What appears most important in choosing a theory is how it: (1) defines itself relative to consultation, (2) is used to conceptualize the consultee's problem, (3) uses intervention strategies to solve problems, (4) deals with problems unique to that theory, and (5) handles termination and follow-up (Brack, Jones, Smith, White, & Brack, 1993). Keep in mind that almost all consultants today integrate their model of consultation with their theoretical orientation while maintaining a systemic and developmental approach.

The following are a few brief examples of theories that have been applied to consultation, but be reminded that other approaches also exist (Brack et al., 1993). Within this section, I took the liberty of matching what I consider to be the best style (system-centered or consultant-centered) with each theory noted. As you read the theories, consider the approach with which you most identify.

Person-Centered Consultation

By its very nature, person-centered consultation is system-centered, because it is the purpose of this consultant to facilitate the change process in a nondirective fashion. This consultant would enter a system and attempt to understand each person's perspective on the nature of the system. The use of the basic core conditions of empathy, genuineness, and positive regard are therefore crucial for this consultant. Sometimes the person-centered consultant might run groups within the organization in an attempt to have individuals more effectively hear one another's points of view and with the belief that the natural process of the group will assist the system in healing itself. With the permission of the people in the organization, this consultant might share his or her findings with the whole organization.

Learning Theory

From a learning-theory perspective, it is crucial that the problem be clearly defined. This requires a careful initial analysis of the system, especially in light of the problem as presented by the consultee. Basic counseling skills are crucial to the beginning of this process. Later, as the problem increasingly becomes defined, the learning-theory consultant can use behavioral principles, cognitive principles, and social learning theory (modeling) to address identified problem areas and to set identifiable goals. A consultant from this perspective might do well by starting out system-centered and ending by being consultant-centered as he or she designs strategies for change.

Gestalt Consultation

As in Gestalt therapy, the Gestalt-oriented consultant's main goal is to increase the experience of the consultee and others involved in the consultation in an effort to decrease defenses and reduce neurotic behaviors. Gestalt consultants believe that by merely bringing the consultant into the system, change will occur. Therefore, this consultant enters the system with a particular way of being that encourages the expression of feeling and the letting down of boundaries in an effort to promote increased awareness and true encounters with self and with one another. This generally takes a combination of a system-centered and consultant-centered style, as the consultant on one hand wants to hear the experience of others while suggesting that others allow themselves to experience and express their feelings and thoughts more fully.

Psychoanalytic Approaches to Consultation

Relative newcomers to consultation, psychoanalytic approaches are particularly interested in looking at how unconscious behavior might be affecting the consultee's environment. The main goal of the consultant, therefore, is to make sense of the unconscious forces that are the route of problems (Brack et al., 1993). Problems are seen as projections of the individuals' unconscious processes. Resistance is seen as an important defense that protects the individual from examining his or her unconscious processes while at the same time protecting the system from undue stress (e.g., "If I really expressed my anger, things would truly get out of hand"). The consultant works cautiously with members in the system, being careful not to abruptly remove members' resistances and cause chaos and mental decompensation. Eventually, consultants will attempt to explain resistances and assist the members in attempting to understand their part in maintaining systemic problems.

The psychoanalytic-oriented consultant would do well starting out system-centered, as the consultant attempts to understand unconscious processes and move toward a consultant-centered approach as he or she explains the resistances in the organization.

Chaos Theory

As opposed to traditional counseling theories, which attempt to describe cause-and-effect in a linear fashion, chaos theory assumes that the world is largely unpredictable because of the vast number of inputs that can affect the functioning of a system (Peters, 1999). For instance, chaos theory, which has been applied to scientific and social systems, would assume that the dropping of leaves in China would affect, in some unknown ways, the weather across the globe. Therefore, it would be crucial to attempt to discover as many inputs as possible that might be affecting the system in an effort to reduce, as much as possible, the unpredictability of the system while keeping in mind that we all must live with a certain amount of chaos.

For consultants, it is important that they attempt to understand, as fully as possible, the chaos in the system. After an initial understanding of the chaos is achieved, the consultant takes a proactive role in which he or she makes suggestions for change in ways that may be experimental and creative in an attempt to alter the dynamics that have been creating the problematic situation. Although currently a long way from an exact science, chaos theory offers a new and interesting perspective to consultation. Chaos theory consultants would probably work best starting from a systems-centered perspective and later move to a consultant-centered approach as they become more proactive and engage individuals in the change process.

The Consulting Process: Stages of Consultation

A number of authors have defined the process of consultation in an effort to explain how a consultant enters a system, facilitates change, and leaves (Beer & Spector, 1993; Fuqua & Kurpius, 1993; Hall & Lin, 1994; Ross, 1993). One such model, by Kurpius, Fuqua & Rozecki (1993), describes six stages, not all that different from the stages of counseling noted in Chapter 5.

Stage 1: Preentry

In the initial stage of consultation, the consultant conceptualizes and articulates to self and to others what he or she has been asked to do. The consultant therefore must have a clear approach to consultation and how that may be implemented in the particular situation. This preentry stage involves an initial contact with the consulting system, in which the consultant explains the purpose of consultation and his or her approach. Some ways to do this are through letters to employees, preentry meetings, or by having the consultee (e.g., an administrator who initially contacted the consultant) or a designated employee explain the purpose.

Stage 2: Entry, Problem Exploration, and Contracting

The second stage of consultation is actually a three-pronged process that includes making contact with the consulting system, exploring the problem, and defining the contract between the consultant and the consulting system. Consultants make contact with the consulting system in many ways. For instance, one consultant might call a series of meetings with all the different work groups, while another consultant might decide to meet individually with each employee. A third consultant might do both. These stylistic differences are based largely on the consultant's conceptual model of consultation.

After contacting the members of the system, the consultant needs to probe the system in such a way that he or she will obtain an initial understanding of the problem. This enables the consultant to discuss the contract with the organization. Such issues as confirming fees; setting up meetings; defining materials needed; deciding purpose, objectives, and ground rules; and setting an approximate termination date are just a few of the items to be determined in the contracting phase of the second stage.

Stage 3: Information Gathering, Problem Confirmation, and Goal Setting

The first phase of the third stage, information gathering, is essentially a data-retrieval process. Based on the initial assessment of the problem and the contract decided in stage 2, the consultant is well situated to obtain reliable and valid data. This data-collection process ranges from obtaining specific hard numerical data, to sending out questionnaires to employees, to generating data (information) from small group sharing and individual meetings with employees. The data is then analyzed, synthesized, and interpreted. This process allows the consultant to confirm, deny, or revise the initial identification of the problem obtained in stage 2. The final identification of the problem allows the consultant to set achievable goals for the organization and to begin to examine methods for change.

Stage 4: Solution Searching and Intervention Selection

During the fourth stage the consultant begins to determine strategies for change. Although interventions can vary widely as a function of the consultant's style and theoretical orientation, regardless of style or orientation, the problem addressed should more or less be the same. So despite the fact that one consultant may be behaviorally oriented and prescriptive while another is psychodynamically and process oriented, in their unique ways, each will be working on the same identified problem. In addition, each consultant will define the problem contextually and push the system to make deep changes that will prevent future problems (systemic and developmental).

Stage 5: Evaluation

A good consultant wants feedback. He or she wants to know what worked, what didn't work, and what were his or her strengths and weaknesses. Evaluation includes asking participants for their judgments regarding the interventions that were made and whether or not the stated goals (change processes) were accomplished. Evaluation can be accomplished through a statistical analysis of the behaviors that were to be changed (summative evaluation), and/or completing ongoing evaluations by the members involved in the consultation process as it is happening (formative evaluation). Formative evaluation can be done verbally or in writing. At times, the consultant who learns through continual feedback that he or she is off track may need to reevaluate what he or she is doing.

Stage 6: Termination

The final stage of the consultation relationship is termination, which signifies the end of the consulting relationship either because success is pending or because the goals were not met. Termination occurs at a preset time determined during the contract phase of stage 2, although at times the predetermined termination date will be revised based on new information gathered during the consulting process. Whether the consultation is successful or not, it is important that the consultant reviews, with all parties involved, the results of the consulting relationship. If not successful, consultant and individuals involved should try to process what occurred so future plans can be made to rectify the situation. In either case, the ending of any relationship involves loss, and individuals involved should be given the opportunity to share feelings about ending the consulting relationship .

The Counselor as Consultant

Counselors have long been consultants. In fact, for some, this is their major role. The list of the consultees with whom the counselor may consult is long and includes: other counselors and helping professionals, school administrators, parents, teachers, college student services staff and administrators, college professors, administrators of social service agencies, clinical directors, clerical staff, managers in business and industry, and so forth. Let's take a brief look at some of the consultation activities of counselors who work at college counseling centers, schools, and community agencies.

Consultation and the College Counselor

Consultation has been a part of college counseling centers almost since their inception, and in many ways the process is not different from consultation in other settings (Stone & Archer, 1990; Westbrook et al., 1993). Although the college counselor has a wide range of activities to perform and spends just 10% of his or her time on consultation activities, consultation is the one activity that makes the center most visible (Gilbert, 1989; Stone & Archer, 1990).

Consultation by college counselors may be defined as any activity where advice and assistance based on psychological activities are provided to a group, office, department, club, and others (Stone & Archer, 1990). This should be distinguished from a closely related activity called outreach, which includes "an organized program, workshop, media effort, class, or systematic attempts to provide psychological education" (Stone & Archer, 1990, p. 357).

The kinds of consultation services offered by college counselors are so diverse that their extent could not be covered here. However, some of the major areas where college counseling centers have used consultation include consultation of the staff with the following (Jordan & Denson, 1990; Pinkerton & Rockwell, 1994; Stone & Archer, 1990; Westbrook et al., 1993):

1. Faculty, concerning the emotional distress of college students.
2. Administration, over diversity issues on campus.
3. Directors of residence life, over potential psychological stressors that students might face.
4. Students, about their concerns regarding other students.
5. Academic advisors, over high-risk students.
6. Disability services, in an effort to increase opportunities for the physically challenged.
7. Many aspects of the university community, in an effort to increase communication between employees and supervisors.
8. Parents, over concerns about their child (e.g., the child is a victim of date rape).

Consultation at college counseling centers may be consultant-centered or system-centered, depending on the group to which services will be provided. It is therefore crucial that the college counselor knows his or her audience and considers the topic to be discussed. For instance, where it may be important to come from an expert mode if discussing chemical dependence with students, the same group of students discussing issues of diversity might very well do better with a process orientation. In the same vein, faculty and administrators can be very turned off by consultants who take on a prescriptive role. Consultants who work with this population may want to be collaborative, which can be a little less threatening to administrators.

Consultation at college counseling centers is a wide-ranging service that is becoming increasingly popular. It offers the college counselor one more activity in which he or she can positively affect the lives of others.

Consultation and the Community Agency Counselor

During the 1950s there were relatively few community mental health agencies in this country. Then, in 1963, Congress passed the Community Mental Health Centers Act, and a new era in the delivery of mental health services was upon us. Providing federal funds for the creation of comprehensive mental health centers across the country, the act provided grants for short-term inpatient care, outpatient care, partial hospitalization, emergency services, and consultation and education services. For the first time there was an acknowledgment that consultation was an important factor in the prevention of mental health problems. The problem was that consultation in reference to community agencies was not yet firmly defined. However, this was soon to change. Consultation in community agencies went in two directions, outward and inward.

CONSULTING OUTWARD The focus of outward consultation is assisting individuals who have mental health concerns but are not clients directly involved with the agency. For instance, the agency counselor often consults with the parents and teachers of a client (e.g., helping them to cope with a child who has behavioral problems), as well as with other mental health professionals the client might be seeing (e.g., setting up meeting to assure that future treatment strategies aren't at cross purposes). The community agency counselor may also consult with schools, hospitals, businesses, and other social service agencies in any number of ways. For example, one consultant might assist teachers and administrators from a school system in understanding the meaning of students' national test scores and help them devise productive ways of using the scores. Another consultant might be asked by a local business to help reduce the general stress level of its employees, and a third consultant might help a social service agency understand some of its employees internal conflicts.

CONSULTING INWARD In 1970, Gerald Caplan published his *Theory and Practice of Mental Health Consultation*, which became one of the most well-known consultation delivery models. Similar to some of the models of consultation we looked at earlier, Caplan's theory defined the role of the consultant in agencies and made suggestions on ways to intervene in organizations. His theory, which is still very much in use today, looks inward at an agency, with the major focus being concern for the clients the agency serves. He described four types of consultation in agencies that are focused on the consultant: (1) offering specific suggestions to a counselor who has asked for help in working with a client, (2) assisting a counselor in identifying problems the counselor has in working with a cli-

BOX 8.1

An Example of Program-Centered Consultation at a Mental Health Center

A consultant is called in by the administrative director of a local mental health center. The director is concerned about morale at the center, saying that he has heard that people are unhappy and that there is a depressed mood throughout. Not only is he concerned about morale, but he is worried that the number of billing hours has dropped in the past six months as a result of the mood in the agency. He asks the consultant to evaluate the situation and to make recommendations.

The consultant first writes a letter to all staff and assistants explaining who he is, his consulting style, when he will be coming to the agency, what he will be doing, and approximately how long he will be there. In addition, he discusses the limits of confidentiality, noting that after meeting with everyone at the agency, he will be sharing general feelings, dynamics, and systemic problems that seem to be occurring. He notes that he will keep individual issues confidential, but that his experience as a consultant has shown him that when people begin to discuss personal concerns, things sometimes leak out into the agency. He encourages all agency personnel to avoid this if possible.

Before actually coming to the agency, the consultant develops a hierarchical plan to visit each workgroup. He starts with the administration, meeting separately with the clinical, medical, and administrative directors; next he meets with the heads of each unit in the center (e.g., outpatient direct, day treatment director, and so forth); he then meets with therapists and mental health assistants from each unit, followed by a meeting with the secretarial and clerical staff. He finishes by meeting with the janitorial staff. Using empathy and basic listening skills, he meets first with each group and then individually with each member. While meeting with the staff, the consultant is also gathering data from the agency on changes in client flow, the economic status of the agency, salaries, types of degrees necessary for varying jobs, information flow (e.g., paperwork trails), and so forth.

Following the consultant's initial contact with each unit and member of the agency, he gathers all his information and spends two or three weeks determining what he considers to be the major problems in the agency. A report is written with the issues defined, and strategies for change are suggested. This report is sent to the agency director and distributed to the agency personnel. Two weeks later he meets with the whole agency for a feedback session from agency personnel. Based on the feedback, a revision to the report is written and distributed.

After approval from the agency, the consultant begins to implement the strategies for change. Throughout this process, he is receiving process feedback concerning what is working and what is not. He adjusts his strategies based on this feedback. Finally, after a certain amount of change is completed and directions for continuing the change process in the future are determined, the consultant begins his termination from the agency. Closure is made through a series of agency group sessions where all who want can come and give feedback in person. An anonymous written evaluation is also made available to all personnel. A follow-up evaluation is completed six months later to see if change was indeed maintained.

ent or a number of clients, (3) facilitating communication in the agency and educating agency staff and administrators on identified problems so that the agency runs more smoothly and clients get better service (see Box 8.1), and (4) working solely with administrators to facilitate communication and educating them on identified problems so that the agency runs more smoothly and the clients get better service.

Inward consultation and outward consultation activities are extremely important components of the community agency counselor's job. Such consultation activities clearly assist in providing better services for clients.

The School Counselor as Consultant

Consultation has long been an important aspect of the school counselor's role and, since the late 1960s, has consistently been listed, along with counseling and guidance functions, as one of the major responsibilities of the school counselor (Fall, 1995; Muro &

Dinkmeyer, 1977). With schools becoming increasingly more complex, collaborating with other essential staff in the school is one way that school counselors can help meet the needs of students (Shoffner & Briggs, 2001). If a school counselor can assist teachers in helping students or students in helping other students, then that counselor is expanding the helping relationship from one level to many levels. A few of the many ways that school counselors act as consultants include (Baker, 2000; Dougherty, 1992a; Muro & Dinkmeyer, 1977; Schmidt, 1991):

1. Assisting teachers in understanding the psychological, sociological, and learning needs of students.
2. Assisting teachers in classroom management techniques.
3. Assisting teachers, administrators, and parents in understanding the developmental needs of children and how they might affect learning.
4. Meeting with students concerning issues they have with other students (e.g., how to handle name-calling).
5. Meeting with other professionals in the community concerning the needs of a particular student with whom the counselor is working.
6. Meeting with parents, teachers, and specialists regarding the individual education plan of a special needs student.
7. Assisting students in becoming peer counselors and conflict mediators.
8. Assisting in setting up a school environment that is conducive to learning for individuals from all cultures.
9. Offering organizational consulting skills to assist administrators and others in the efficient running of the schools.
10. Offering administrators, parents, teachers, and students assistance in understanding the purpose of assessment instruments and how to interpret their results.

The school counselor is in much more of a precarious position in his or her role as a consultant than is the community agency counselor or college counselor. A school is a very tightly knit organization with clear boundaries between the various professionals. Teachers, administrators, and counselors have very different roles, and they all have responsibilities to the students and their parents. Teachers sometimes don't want to be bothered by counselors or administrators. Counselors sometimes don't want to be bothered by teachers. Parents often have views on their children that differ dramatically from the teacher, counselor, and administrator. The school counselor needs to learn how to balance his or her role as consultant so that each component of the school feels heard and responded to. Ultimately, this balancing act is the most challenging part of a school counselor's job. It is therefore essential that the school counselor understand the unique systemic qualities of the school where he or she works if change is to take place (Forman, 1995). The school counselor's training in interpersonal communication skills, consultation skills, and contextual thinking makes him or her particularly able to do this task. When a school counselor is seen siding with the administration, teachers, students, or parents, his or her consultative techniques have gone awry.

Although schools have their own unique systemic qualities, consultation in the schools can follow many of the same models that have been discussed. Therefore, a school counselor as consultant may be found to be consultant-centered at times (e.g., prescribing a communication skill to a parent or a new behavioral management skill to a teacher), or system-centered (e.g., collaborating with the school psychologist, teacher, specialist, and parent on the individualized plan for a student).

Consultation in the schools is one of the main functions of the school counselor and may be the most challenging, invigorating, and creative aspect of the job, as the counselor attempts to find strategies for change that will lead to an increase in self-esteem and learning for all students while satisfying the needs of parents, teachers, and administrators.

Supervision

Whether one is a counselor in a community agency or at a school or college, supervision has become an expected and crucial part of a counselor's professional responsibility (Borders & Cashwell, 1992; Borders & Usher, 1992; Usher & Borders, 1993). This is evidenced by (1) licensing boards requiring increasing numbers of hours of clinical supervision, (2) licensing boards setting more rigid standards for clinical supervisors, (3) agency and school administrators increasingly supporting the need for supervision, (4) the development of Ethical Guidelines for Counseling Supervisors (ACES, 1993, 1995), and (5) the adoption by ACA of The Standards of Counseling Supervisors, which sets standards of preparation and practice of supervisors (ACES, 1990; Dye & Borders, 1990). But, what exactly is supervision, and how is it related to consultation?

Supervision Defined

Supervision: A Special Kind of Consultation

> *Me and you talking about him or her with the purpose of some change.*
> (Fall, 1995, p. 151)

Remember this simple quote from earlier in the chapter? Although written to define consultation, it aptly speaks to supervision, which also focuses on change in others. Supervision has been defined as an intensive, interpersonally focused relationship in which one person is designated to facilitate the development of therapeutic competence in one or more other persons (Loganbill et al., 1982).

Supervision is a type of consultation in which the counselor consults with the supervisor in order to enhance his or her ability to work with clients. Although a type of consultation, supervision differs from most other forms of consultation. For instance, whereas most forms of consultation are time limited, supervision often involves an ongoing relationship between the supervisor and supervisee. Whereas most forms of consultation do not involve an intense interpersonal relationship that focuses on the consultee, supervision generally does, with the consultee being the supervisee. And, whereas in most forms of consultation the consultant generally does not have a direct evaluative responsibility for the consultee, in supervision the supervisor, in one fashion or another, is evaluating the supervisee (Benshoff, 1944; Bernard & Goodyear, 1998).

Supervision: A Systemic Perspective

Like consultation, supervision by its very nature involves a number of systems. The most basic system is that of the supervisor ↔ (supervisee/counselor) ↔ client. As in all homeostatic mechanisms, if you change one component, the whole system changes. That is the wonderful part of being a supervisor. Impart knowledge to and facilitate growth in your supervisee, and soon you will see his or her clients change. The system is responding. Take this one step further, and we see other systems change. A rebounding effect occurs where the client now affects the systems in which he or she is involved—perhaps his or her family. Didn't someone once say, "Throw a rock in a pond and the ripples expand indefinitely"?

The manner in which systems are affected in supervision is complex. First and foremost, the simple act of supervision fine-tunes the counselor's skills and ultimately can have a positive effect on the client and the systems in which he or she is involved. However, another process may be occurring. Called *parallel process* (Sumerel, 1994), it has long been known that the client–counselor relationship is often mimicked in the supervisor–supervisee relationship. It is believed that this occurs because the counselor unconsciously takes on the traits of the client, which are repeated in the supervisory relationship. Parallel process is generally viewed as something to be avoided (e.g., taking on the client's anxiety and repeating it in supervision). However, if discussed in supervision, parallel process can be worked through and ultimately be helpful to the client–counselor relationship (Pearson, 2001).

Sometimes it is argued that a reverse parallel process occurs, such as when positive qualities in a supervisor (e.g., good empathic responding) are taken on by the counselor and subsequently passed on to the client. It is hoped that these qualities will ultimately be passed on by the client to others in his or her life.

Whether it is a simple improvement in the knowledge base of the supervisee or the complexity of parallel process, it is clear that supervision involves a system that can have far-reaching effects (Lonergan, 1994).

Who Is the Supervisor?

The Association for Counselor Education and Supervision (ACES) defines supervisors as:

> *[c]ounselors who have been designated within the university or agency [or school] to directly oversee the professional clinical work of counselors. Supervisors also may be persons who offer supervision to counselors seeking state licensing and so provide supervision outside the administrative aegis of an applied counseling setting.*
> (ACES, 1995, p. 271)

The supervisor has a number of roles and responsibilities, including assuring the welfare of the client; making sure that ethical, legal, and professional standards are being upheld; overseeing the clinical and professional development of the supervisee; and evaluating the supervisee (ACES, 1993, 1995). Like the effective therapist, the good supervisor is empathic, flexible, genuine, and open (Borders, 1994b). In addition, the good supervisor is able to be an evaluator of the supervisee and is comfortable with being an authority figure (Bradley & Gould, 1994). Good supervisors know counseling, have good client conceptualization skills, and are good problem solvers.

Who Is the Supervisee?

ACES (1995) defines the supervisee as:

> *Counselors-in-training in university programs at any level working with clients in applied settings as part of their university training program, and counselors who have completed their formal education and are employed in an applied counseling setting.* (p. 217)

One role of the supervisor is to evaluate the supervisee. The supervisee, in contrast, is learning from the evaluative process and building a professional identity (Bradley &

Gould, 1994). The supervisee thus is in a vulnerable position, subject to the evaluation of the supervisor. It is inevitable, therefore, that at some point in the supervisory relationship supervisee resistance will occur. Of course the amount and kind of resistance will depend on a number of factors, including: (1) supervisor characteristics, such as style of supervision, age, race, gender and sex role attitudes, power issues, and other relationship dynamics; (2) the personality style of the supervisee; (3) the match between supervisor and counselor styles; and (4) the amount of defensiveness the supervisee brings to the relationship (Bernard & Goodyear, 1998; Dye, 1994).

Individual or Group Supervision

Supervision usually occurs one-on-one or in small groups, with there being a number of advantages and disadvantages to both of these types of supervision. For instance, group supervision allows for collaborative learning, as supervisees have the opportunity to be exposed to many different perspectives (Prieto, 1996). Also, group supervision offers clinicians the opportunity to experience a group and thus enhance their group facilitation skills through modeling (Newman & Lovell, 1993). In addition, some research has shown that group supervision may be as effective as individual supervision and affords the supervisee the opportunity to gain support, learn new techniques and case conceptualization skills, work on interpersonal issues, and increase insight and self-awareness (McAuliffe, 1992a; Ray & Altekruse, 2000; Werstlein, 1994).

From a practical standpoint, group supervision allows a number of supervisees to receive supervision at one time. Therefore, whether taking place in graduate school or at an agency or school, group supervision allows an often limited number of supervisors to supervise a number of supervisees, usually three to seven. For those who may be paying for supervision, group supervision is generally much less expensive than the $50 to $100 an hour a counselor might pay for individual supervision.

Although there are many benefits to group supervision, it may not offer the intimacy and intensity found in individual supervision, and research on its effectiveness has been mixed (Prieto, 1996). Some would argue that supervision, which at moments can be like therapy, can only work if the supervisee is able to disclose at deeply intimate levels, which may not be attainable in group supervision. Finally, individual supervision can result in the development of a mentoring process in which the supervisee becomes the student of a master counselor. This is less likely to occur in group supervision.

Models of Supervision

Today, most supervisory styles can fall into three categories: (1) developmental models, (2) orientation-specific models, and (3) integrated models (Leddick, 1994).

Developmental Models

Developmental models have as their core the belief that there are stages, like patterns of development, through which the supervisee will pass as he or she obtains supervision. Therefore, the supervisor can rely on a certain amount of predictable growth as well as resistance, depending on the stage of the supervisee. Of course, individual supervisees may move faster or slower through these stages based on their personality style, their ability, and their fit with their supervisor. Awareness of developmental stages can assist

TABLE 8.1

Counselor Trainee Characteristics as a Function of Level of Development

	SELF- AND OTHER-AWARENESS	MOTIVATION	AUTONOMY
LEVEL 1	Trainee's focus is primarily on self as he or she attempts to deal with anxiety related to fears of evaluation. Insight and empathy may be difficult due to this anxiety and self-doubt.	High degree of motivation based on keen desire to be a counselor. Wants to help people and learn the correct techniques and strategies to use.	Characterized by dependence on supervisor. Wants to be advised by supervisor and has strong desire to leave major decision making to supervisor.
LEVEL 2	Trainee is better able to focus on the affect and cognitions of client. Trainee might become greatly involved with client's pain and have difficulty detaching. Counselor begins to see the impact he or she has upon client.	Doubt about skills proficiency arises as counselor begins to understand the complexity of the counseling relationship. Trainee may seesaw between these self-doubts and confidence as he or she becomes increasingly more proficient with interventions and receives positive feedback from the client and supervisor.	Characterized by dependency/autonomy conflict as trainee becomes more confident in skills and wants independence but at the same time fears it.
LEVEL 3	Counselor is able to move into the client's world and out of own world and process client's situation. Allows counselor to understand which techniques have the most impact on client change.	Counselor begins to integrate own style of therapy and work on strengths and weaknesses. Seesawing slows, and counselor feels more consistent about skills. Is freely able to receive feedback from supervisor.	Here the trainee feels comfortable about functioning in an independent fashion. When doubts arise, trainee feels as if he or she can consult with others without losing his or her sense of professional identity.

SOURCE: Stoltenberg and Delworth, 1987.

the supervisor in developing strategies for growth based on the supervisee's particular stage (Nixon & Claiborn, 1987).

Although there have been a number of developmental models over the years, probably the best known is that of Stoltenberg and Delworth (1987), who focus primarily on counselors-in-training. Stoltenberg and Delworth believe that trainees will pass through three levels of development as they grow and change in three areas: self- and other-awareness, motivation, and autonomy (see Table 8.1). In brief, they believe that during the course of supervision, counselors-in-training (1) become increasingly aware of client needs and the interventions that might suit them, (2) become increasingly less dependent on the supervisor as faith is gained in their own ability, and (3) go through a roller-coaster ride in motivation, at first feeling very enthusiastic, later feeling less so as trainees doubt their skills, and later again feeling motivated (see Figure 8.2). Although Stoltenberg and Delworth's model is still being researched (Lovell, 1999b), there is some beginning evidence that graduate trainees do undergo positive changes in the three areas they identified (McNeill, Stoltenberg, & Romans, 1992; Tryon, 1996).

Orientation-Specific Models

Many counselors who have adopted a particular type of therapy (e.g., Gestalt, person-centered, behavioral, and so forth) believe that the best kind of supervision for them is to have a master therapist/supervisor who practices a similar approach and can therefore give

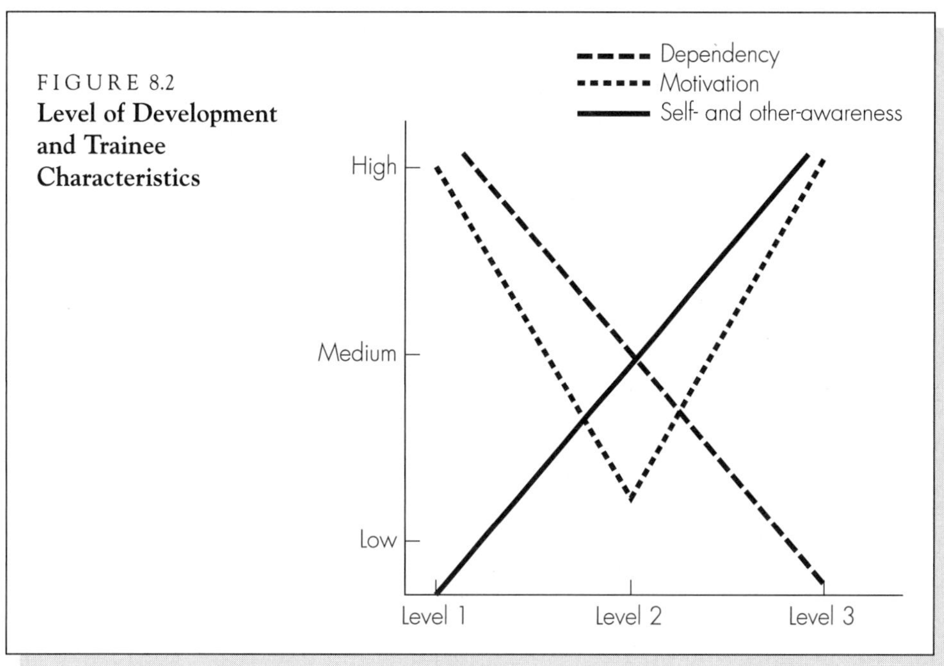

FIGURE 8.2
Level of Development and Trainee Characteristics

them training in that approach. There are two ways this can occur. The first is when the supervisor structures the supervision so that it models the particular approach that the supervisee is using in counseling (Bernard, 1992, 1997; Cashwell, 1994; Freeman, 1992). Therefore, a behavioral supervisor would model a behavioral approach by identifying problems in supervision, collaboratively set goals to work on, and then use techniques to reach those goals. The psychoanalytic supervisor would do analysis with the supervisee, while the person-centered supervisor would use empathy, show unconditional regard, and be genuine with his or her trainee.

In the second orientation-specific model, the supervisor uses his or her knowledge base to gently guide and teach the supervisee (Freeman, 1992). For instance, if a trainee were working with a client behaviorally and not making progress, the supervisor might offer advice on some new behavioral techniques. A psychoanalytic supervisor might suggest a specific psychoanalytic technique and show the counselor how to use it (e.g., dream analysis), and a person-centered supervisor might suggest the trainee work on his or her empathic responses and show the trainee how he or she could make better responses.

Integrated Models

Perhaps more appropriately called meta-theories, integrated models are not theory specific and can be used regardless of the theoretical approach of the supervisee. One such model is Bernard's discrimination model (Bernard, 1992, 1997; Bernard & Goodyear, 1998). Dependent on the needs of the supervisee, this model examines three roles that supervisors might take on at differing times during the supervisory relationship. These include (1) a didactic role in which the supervisor is a teacher, (2) an experiential role in which the supervisor is a limited counselor assisting the supervisee in working through issues that are affecting his or her ability as a therapist, and (3) a consultant role, in which the supervisor is an objective colleague assisting the supervisee. A major focus of this model is how the trainee uses his or her skills to conceptualize and process client issues.

Interpersonal process recall (IPR), another integrated model that was developed by Norm Kagan (1980), has been particularly popular over the years (Cashwell, 1994). In many ways this model relies on the trainee to uncover his or her own strengths and weaknesses. In this type of supervision, the supervisor and the trainee meet together with an audio- or videotape of the trainee with a client. The trainee, supervisor, or both can control the tape, starting and stopping it when it is believed that there is an important moment in therapy. The supervisor's role is to attend accurately to the feelings and thoughts of the supervisee and, when appropriate, ask leading questions to deepen the session. The following questions have been used in this inquiry session:

1. What do you wish you had said to him or her?
2. How do you think he or she would have reacted if you had said that?
3. What would have been the risk in saying what you wanted to say?
4. If you had the chance now, how might you tell him or her what you are thinking and feeling?
5. Were there any other thoughts going through your mind?
6. How did you want the other person to perceive you?
7. Were those feelings located physically in some part of your body?
8. Were you aware of any feelings? Does that feeling have any special meaning for you?
9. What did you want him or her to tell you?
10. What did you think he or she wanted from you?
11. Did he or she remind you of anyone in your life?

In the tradition of some of the humanistic therapies, IPR is a model of supervision that gives the trainee the ability to explore feelings and thoughts about a therapeutic relationship within a trusting and safe environment. The trainee can therefore get in touch with those aspects of him- or herself that are preventing the client from moving forward in counseling.

All of the above models offer a slightly different take on the supervisory process and are not necessarily exclusive of one another. For instance, one can adopt a developmental model and either be orientation-specific or use an integrated approach. In choosing a supervisor, if given the choice, a supervisee should of course pick the supervisor who offers the approach that will best facilitate his or her learning process as well as the therapeutic experience of the supervisee's clients.

Finally, as with the counseling relationship, there is some evidence that the strength of the alliance or bond between the supervisor and supervisee, regardless of model, may be the most crucial factor for effective supervision (Ladany & Friedlander, 1995). Thus, the supervisor who has exceptional knowledge in supervision may be ineffective if he or she cannot build a relationship with the supervisee.

Supervision of Graduate Students

Graduate students in CACREP-approved counseling programs—and, we hope, all counseling programs—will have a number of opportunities to receive supervision. Although the manner in which this occurs will vary from program to program, counseling programs generally offer a course early on that provides supervision of basic counseling skills. Within this course students usually have the opportunity to audio- and/or videotape a session with a client or with a fellow student. Supervision of the graduate student is generally given by the professor, an advanced graduate student, and/or by peers. Usually, students will also have the opportunity to obtain supervision in a practicum and in the culminating graduate school experience, the internship. Supervision in these courses is almost always given by an advanced graduate student, a professor, and/or a field supervisor.

CACREP requires, and most graduate programs offer, supervision of taped or live sessions. There are a number of ways this can be accomplished. First, there is the tried-and-true fashion of tape recording a counseling session. Although videotaping certainly offers broader feedback to the trainee than audiotaping, either can be an invaluable tool for supervisor feedback. Although anxiety-provoking for many, most counseling programs today require some kind of live supervision that offers opportunities for immediate feedback that other kinds of supervision cannot (Costa, 1994). Counseling programs generally have rooms equipped with one-way windows that allow the student to be viewed by supervisors or peers as the student is involved in a live counseling session or role-play. Students can receive immediate feedback through a number of methods such as a telephone or a "bug-in-the-ear." Although effective at offering immediate feedback, these methods can be somewhat intrusive. The use of a computer monitor facing the counselor and next to the client, with the keyboard located on the opposite side of the one-way mirror, is considerably less intrusive (Neukrug, 1991). Using this method, supervisors and/or fellow students can type in feedback via the keyboard to the monitor, which is seen by the counselor in the adjoining room. Finally, the use of e-mail, real-time video linkups, and other promising electronic communication advances offers trainees the opportunity of speaking with supervisors immediately even though they may be hundreds of miles away (Casey, Bloom, & Moan, 1994; Myrick & Sabella, 1995).

There is one more way of obtaining feedback about your client – writing case notes. Well-thought-out and well-written case notes can be invaluable to the counselor-in-training and are one more way in which counselors can obtain feedback from their supervisors (Tallent, 1993).

Supervision of Practicing Counselors

> *Increasingly, clinical supervision is being viewed as a critical component in counselor development across the life span. . . .* (Usher & Borders, 1993)

Although ongoing supervision has become more popular in recent years, the frequency and kind of supervision varies depending on setting. Today, many counselors receive individual supervision, while a substantial number receive group supervision or peer supervision (Benshoff, 1994). School counselors have significantly less supervision than agency or private practice counselors, with up to 45% of them receiving no supervision at all (Borders & Usher, 1992). Counselors tend to prefer a supervisor who is relationship oriented and collegial over someone who is task oriented and a supervisor who focuses on conceptual and counseling skills as opposed to professional issues (Usher & Borders, 1993).

Unlike other counselors, school counselors are in the unique position to be supervised by more than one person (Agnew, Vaught, Getz, & Fortune, 2000). Clinically, school counselors will often be supervised by one or more of the following: the director of guidance for the school system, the head guidance counselor in a school, colleagues via peer supervision, or a private supervisor whom they may hire on their own. Administratively, school counselors are often supervised by building administrators (e.g., assistant principals) to assure that they work effectively within the system; that they are in compliance with local, state, and federal laws; and that they have good working relationships with school staff and parents (Henderson, 1994).

Although any style of supervision can be applied to any counseling setting, a number of authors have suggested altering supervisory techniques to fit a particular counseling specialty. Marriage and family therapists, addictions counselors, school counselors, agency counselors, college counselors, and so forth all have unique job functions that might call for changes in the supervisory process (Coll, 1995; Juhnke & Culbreth, 1994; McAuliffe, 1992a; Usher & Borders, 1993; West et al., 1993). Counselors are urged to read the literature on supervision in their respective specialty area.

Multicultural Issues

Multicultural Consultation within a System

The consultant is in a unique position relative to multicultural issues. Being brought into a system means that one will be dealing with dynamics within the organization, and cultural differences will undoubtedly be affecting such dynamics. Thus, when entering a system, the consultant must do his or her best to understand the culture of the system, the culture of subsystems, and the unique background of each individual within the system (Homan,1994; Jackson & Hayes, 1993).

Because issues of race and ethnicity are often difficult to broach, there is generally tension related to cross-cultural issues among individuals within the system. Sometimes this tension may simply be a function of ignorance of differing cultural backgrounds. In other cases deep feelings of hatred and racist attitudes may prevail. The consultant must assess the degree to which cross-cultural issues play a role in the daily functioning of the system and, based on this assessment, include methods of dealing with these issues in his or her strategies for change. To be successful at this, the consultant must have an understanding of his or her biases, knowledge of other cultures, and knowledge of the kinds of intervention strategies that can effect positive change in the system.

Multicultural Consultation and Supervision with an Individual

When conducting individual consultation or supervision, such as a brief consult with a colleague or long-term supervision of a counselor, the effective consultant or supervisor should consider the possibility that cross-cultural differences are a major source of tension between the consultee or supervisee and the client (Daniels, D'Andrea, & Kim, 1999). Thus, the consultant/supervisor needs to have knowledge of multicultural issues and be able to suggest strategies for helping the consultee or supervisee work with his or her clients.

In long-term consulting relationships, such as supervision, Fong (1994) suggests a number of techniques that can be used to explore cross-cultural issues. They include: (1) planned discussions concerning culture and its relationship to counseling, (2) exploration of the cultural backgrounds of the supervisor and supervisee, (3) reviews of videotape sessions with clients to examine nonverbal behavior and how that might reflect cultural differences, (4) modeling of cross-culturally appropriate behavior by the supervisor, (5) consideration of cultural issues during the intake and in all written reports, and (6) experiential exercises in supervision to highlight cross-cultural issues.

Ethical, Professional, and Legal Issues

Ethical Issues

Ethical Issues in the Consulting Relationship

A number of authors have illuminated ethical issues specific to the consulting process (ACA, 1995a; Dougherty, 1992b; Newman, 1993). Some of them include:

1. *Confidentiality in consultation:* the right to privacy and confidentiality within the consulting relationship.
2. *Consultation as an option:* the right to seek consultation from other competent professionals.
3. *Consultant competency:* the importance of having the necessary qualifications to offer the kind of consulting necessary.
4. *Understanding with clients:* the importance of developing a clear understanding of the problem and devising reasonable goals for change.
5. *Consultant goals:* the importance of having as a major consultant goal the encouragement of client growth toward self-direction.
6. *Informed consent:* informing clients about the procedures to be used and probable course of treatment for the consulting relationship and having clients consent to participate in it.
7. *Dual relationships:* avoiding any dual relationships that may cause harm to the consulting process.

Ethical Issues in the Supervisory Relationship

Because supervision is technically a kind of consultation, when supervising one should be aware of the issues listed above. However, because additional concerns arise in supervision (see Bernard, 1994), ACES (1993, 1995) has developed Ethical Guidelines for Counseling Supervisors. Thus, in addition to the above, ACES suggests supervisors be knowledgeable about ethical concerns related to:

1. *Relationship boundaries*: Supervisors are aware of the differential in power between themselves and their supervisees and are thus respectful of appropriate boundaries professionally and socially.
2. *Sexual relationships*: Supervisors do not engage in sexual relationships with supervisees.
3. *Preparation in supervision*: Supervisors have the necessary training to offer supervision.
4. *Responsibility to clients*: Supervisors have a responsibility to assure that adequate counseling is taking place between the supervisee (counselor) and the client.
5. *Endorsement*: Supervisors do not endorse unqualified supervisees for credentialing but rather attempt to take steps to help them become qualified.

Professional Issues

Standards in Counseling Supervision

As noted earlier in this chapter, in an effort to assure that supervisors are properly trained, The Standards of Counseling Supervisors was developed by ACES and approved by ACA (ACES, 1990). These standards delineate 11 core areas in which supervisors should have expertise: (1) effectiveness as a counselor; (2) healthy personal traits and characteristics; (3) knowledge of ethical, legal, and regulatory issues; (4) knowledge of the nature of the supervisory relationship; (5) knowledge of supervisory methods and techniques; (6) knowledge of counselor development; (7) competency in case conceptualization; (8) competency in the assessment and evaluation of clients; (9) competency in oral and written report writing; (10) ability to evaluate counselors; and (11) knowledge of research in counseling and counseling supervision.

Values in Consultation and Supervision

Whether one is supervising a counselor or consulting with an agency, the consultant/supervisor is in a position of power that affords him or her the opportunity to influence clients. One way we can influence clients is through the expression of our values. The expert consultant/supervisor must accept the fact that he or she has the ability to influence others through the expression of his or her values and examine how he or she can do so in a nonmanipulative and positive manner (Newman, 1993).

Legal Issue: Liability in Consultation and Supervision

Because consultants and supervisors are directly or indirectly in a position to effect change in clients, they can be held responsible for any potential negative results of their consultation or supervision (Guest & Dooley, 1999). This particularly came to light during the Tarasoff decision (see Chapter 4). After learning that a client was threatening to harm his ex-girlfriend, the client's therapist, a psychologist at a campus counseling center, broke confidentiality and told campus police, who subsequently picked up the client for questioning. The psychologist's supervisor reprimanded the psychologist for breaking confidentiality. The ex-girlfriend was subsequently killed by the client, and her parents sued everyone involved in the case, including the supervisor. The supervisor, among others, was found liable for not assuring the safety of the client's ex-girlfriend. Thus we see how consultants/supervisors can be held responsible for the work they perform.

The Counselor in Process: Committed to Ongoing Consultation and Supervision

Consultation is not something you read about in a book. It is your professional responsibility. You are responsible for consulting when you are working with a difficult client, responsible for consulting when you are not sure of the best direction in which to move with a client, responsible for consulting when you think you may be working outside your area of competence. Consultation and supervision are living processes. Those who do not seek consultation are dead to the profession and are likely harmful to their clients. If we are to be the best at what we do and are committed to the growth of our clients, we must assure that throughout our professional lives we are forever seeking out consultation and supervision.

Summary

This chapter examined two important types of helping relationships: consultation and supervision. We noted that although there is no universally accepted definition of consultation, there is some general agreement on what it is. We thus defined consultation as a triadic relationship where the consultant has been contracted by the consultee to deliver direct service to a person, group, organization, or community in an effort to assist the individual or system in working through difficulties.

In this chapter, we gave a brief history of consultation, noting that it first became popular during the 1940s and 1950s and was more systematically developed during the 1960s and 1970s. As we moved into the 1980s and 1990s, we identified a number of models or styles of consultation, noting that they tended to fall in one of two categories: consultant-centered, where the consultant uses his or her body of knowledge to offer suggestions and advice for system change; or system-centered, where the consultant assists people in the system to use their own resources in the change process. This same time period saw the rise of a number of theoretical approaches to consultation. Sampling some of these theories, we briefly discussed the following approaches as applied to consultation: person-centered, learning (cognitive and behavioral), Gestalt, psychoanalytic, and chaos theory. We noted that consultants generally have a style or model of working related to the theoretical approach to which they adhere.

Regardless of the approach of the consultant, we noted that there is a trend today to view consultation from a systemic and developmental perspective; that is, the consultant wants to understand problems from a contextual perspective and hopes not only to alleviate the presenting problem but also to work toward bringing positive and predictable change in the future. Regardless of the approach a consultant uses, we noted that there are a number of predictable stages to the consulting process. We explored one model that included the following six stages: preentry; entry, problem exploration, and contracting; information gathering, problem confirmation, and goal setting; solution searching and intervention selection; evaluation; and termination. Finally, we examined some of the consultation activities of school counselors, agency counselors, and college counselors.

This chapter also examined the process of supervision. Supervision was defined as an intense interpersonally focused relationship that involves a number of systems, the most basic being that of the supervisor ↔ (supervisee/counselor) ↔ client. We described supervision as a special type of consultation and noted similarities and differences between the two. Both consultation and supervision focus on the change process, are systemic, are therapeutic but are not therapy, and involve talking with a third person(s) about another party. Noting differences, we stated that consultation, unlike supervision, is time limited and does not have a direct evaluative responsibility to the consultee.

This chapter examined three models of supervision that have evolved over the years. The developmental model speaks to predictable stages a supervisee will go through while in supervision. The orientation-specific approach uses a specific counseling theory as its basis for the supervisory process, while integrated models are not theory specific and can be integrated within one's theoretical orientation. It was noted that any of these models can be practiced in individual or group supervision.

Highlighted as a crucial component to graduate school training, we observed that supervision is generally provided during skills classes and field work experiences. We noted that a large percentage of practicing counselors continue to obtain supervision after graduate school and that the majority of practicing counselors receive individual supervision, while a lesser but substantial number receive group or peer supervision. It was found that counselors of all kinds tend to prefer a supervisor who is relationship oriented and collegial over someone who is task oriented and a supervisor who focuses on conceptual and counseling skills as opposed to professional issues.

We examined the importance of multicultural issues when consulting with agencies or organizations. We noted that whenever entering a system a consultant must do his or her best to understand the culture of the system, the culture of subsystems, and the unique background of each individual within the system. Knowledge of the various cultures within the system is the first step toward helping individuals understand how cross-cultural issues affect their interpersonal relationships. We also highlighted that cross-cultural issues are particularly important when practicing consultation or supervision with an individual. We offered a number of techniques that could assist the consultant or supervisor in examining how multicultural issues affect his or her relationships with clients or supervisees.

We noted in this chapter that a number of ethical issues are particularly important to the consultation and supervision process and include: confidentiality, consultation as an option, consultant competency, understanding the problem clearly with clients, helping clients work toward self-direction, informed consent, and not having dual relationships. Additional ethical issues particularly important to the supervisory relationship include knowing relationship boundaries, not engaging in sexual relationships with supervisees, being adequately prepared as a supervisor, having responsibility to the supervisee's clients, and not endorsing unqualified supervisees for credentialing. We stated the importance of knowing The Ethical Guidelines for Counseling Supervisors and of being competent in all of the areas delineated in the Standards of Counseling Supervisors. We discussed the importance of understanding that consultants and supervisors wield much power and that they must effect change without abusing this power. We noted that this power does not come without cost; because we affect the lives of others, we can be held liable if we do not act competently as consultants and supervisors.

Finally, we concluded this chapter by stressing that consultation and supervision should be an ongoing component of the counselor's job. Without consultation and supervision, we are an island unto ourselves, left only to our own resources.

INFOTRAC and Other Information Resources (e.g., ERIC and PsycINFO)

Note: When relevant, key words are in quotation marks.

1. Research more fully a "consultation model" or "consultation theory" of your choice.
2. Research the ethical and legal responsibilities of supervisors ("ethical clinical superv," "legal clinical superv").
3. Delve more deeply into a "model of supervision" of your choice.

SECTION **IV**

The Development of the Person

Overview

The common theme running through the three chapters in this section is the focus on human development. Although each chapter focuses on a specific area in the development of the person, they all offer us a manner of conceptualizing ourselves and our clients as a function of a developmental process. Chapter 9 does this by offering a lifespan approach to understanding normal development in a number of important domains, including physical, cognitive and moral development, and the development of faith. Chapter 10 identifies theories that hypothesize about the development of abnormal behavior and presents a way of classifying behavior, and Chapter 11 offers a view of how personality is reflected through one's career development process.

As you read through this section, you might want to consider the developmental aspects of your life. Reflect back on your childhood and the kinds of transitions through which you passed. Then consider the transitions you've experienced in your adult life. Think about the impact they had upon you and your family. As you continue through this section, reflect on how you developed your sense of self and your state of mental health. Think about how you became you! Finally, think about why you are considering a career in counseling. What kinds of developmental issues have affected this important choice in your life? Clearly, this section offers a framework for working with clients, but it also presents a number of models to help you understand who you are today.

CHAPTER 9

Development Across the Lifespan

With each passage from one stage of human growth to the next we, too, must shed a protective structure. We are left exposed and vulnerable but also yeast and embryonic again, capable of stretching in ways we hadn't known before. These sheddings may take several years or more. Coming out of each passage, though, we enter a longer and more stable period in which we can expect relative tranquillity and a sense of equilibrium regained. (Sheehy, 1976, p. 29)

I remember going on a trip out west with my parents and my brother. I was 13, and my brother was 8. I was miserable. I sat in the back seat of the car going through the pains of having just reached puberty. My parents, I think, just thought I was going through a miserable stage. No matter where we went or what we did, I only thought about being in love. Oh yeah, and sex of course. Somewhere in the middle of this trip, we stopped at a small gift shop. There was a girl who worked there with whom I fell in love. I was shy but managed to have some small talk with her. No one knew my passion for her; it was my secret. My parents took us to national parks, visited incredible sites where they "oohed" and "ahed," and I just thought about her. I even sent her a postcard with a short note and my return address. I hoped so much that I would hear from her. I did not. Even today when thinking back on that trip, in my mind I have a hazy picture of the Grand Canyon, Mesa Verde, and Old Faithful, but I have an indelible picture of her. Puberty is a very powerful experience, and it's a part of our normal developmental patterns.

I struggled through puberty. There was no one to talk with. My parents grew up in a time when sex was not talked about; well, there could be a few dirty jokes, but no real conversations about sex. There was no school counselor to go to. And my friends, well, those conversations were certainly limited. I was left to my own devices, struggling with my own needs, desires, and wondering if this was all normal. Like most people, I struggled through this normal phase of development.

This chapter is about normal development across the lifespan. The chapter's goal is to provide you with an understanding of the counselor's role in helping to ease clients through what can sometimes be painful transitions through normal developmental stages. As with my struggle through puberty, we all manage to get through a series of normal and predictable developmental stages in our journey through life. No doubt I would have struggled through puberty even if I had had Carl Rogers to talk with. However, with Carl by my side, I probably would have felt that what I was going through was normal.

We will start this chapter by briefly reviewing some of the physical and psychological developmental milestones that children, adolescents, and adults face. Next, we will explore the cognitive and moral development of childhood, or how children develop their ways of knowing the world. This will be followed by an examination of constructive development in adults, or how adults develop their ways of understanding and constructing reality. Next we will examine lifespan development, or the kinds of tasks and challenges that individuals face as they pass through life stages. Then we will examine a model of faith development. Defining faith in a very broad manner, the theory we will examine reflects concepts from all the theories in this chapter. We will conclude the chapter by examining multicultural, ethical, professional, and legal issues related to normal development.

A Little Background

The counseling profession has long prided itself on having a developmental focus. However, the actual practice of counseling from a developmental perspective was, until recently, greatly lacking (Blocher, 1988). In fact, what in the past was called a "developmental perspective" tended to be more of a humanistic approach that included some vague notion that the individual can develop over time. Despite the fact that the 1960s saw some attempts at applying developmental models in the schools and in college settings, generally, the concept of ". . . development seemed little more than a catchword" (Blocher, 1988, p. 14). It was not until the 1980s that the application of theory to practice became a reality.

The early 1980s heralded in the true era of developmental counseling. The establishment of the CACREP standards in 1981, which included human development as one of its core curriculum content areas, highlighted development as a crucial element in the counseling profession. Then, in 1983, the American Personnel and Guidance Association changed its name to the American Association for Counseling and *Development* (now ACA). It was becoming increasingly clear that the profession wanted a name that mirrored a developmental perspective in practice.

We have come a long way in the past 20 years. Today, we find developmental models being applied to school counseling (Muro & Dinkmeyer, 1977; Muro & Kottman, 1995; Neukrug, Barr, Hoffman, & Kaplan, 1993), in clinical settings (Ivey, 1990, 1993; Ivey & Goncalves, 1988), with college students (Evans, Forney, & Guido-Dibrito, 1998; King, 1994), in the training of counseling students (McAuliffe et al., 2000), with the supervision of counselors (Stoltenberg & Delworth, 1987), and in everyday life (Sheehy, 1976, 1995). But what do we really mean by development?

Understanding Human Development

The development of a person is complex and occurs on many levels. Over the years a number of models of human development have been described that can assist the counselor when working with clients. Although these models differ tremendously in how they apply developmental theory, they tend to share common elements. For instance, most hold the belief that development is continual, is orderly, implies change, is by its nature painful and growth-producing, can be applied with many differing counseling approaches, and is preventive, optimistic, and wellness-oriented. Let's explore some of these concepts.

Development Is Continual

Development refers to change over the lifespan and comes in many different forms. After birth, and until we die, we start a journey in many different domains, including: cognitive, physical, interpersonal, intrapsychic, moral, and spiritual. Our journey along these domains is nonstop and continuous. Once we step on the ride, we can't get off (DiLeo, 1996).

Development Is Orderly and Sequential and Builds Upon Itself

Models that describe human growth have a predictable pattern of development from earlier to later stages, in which the latter stages build on what has already been experienced and integrated into our lives:

> *Development proceeds stage by stage in orderly sequence, and although there are individual variations, these do not basically alter the ground plan that is typical of our species. . . .* (DiLeo, 1996, p. 3)

This predictable pattern of growth allows the counselor to assess the developmental level of the client and predict the next developmental hurdle the client will face. If an individual does not successfully accomplish a developmental task when it is prime for its ascendancy, then there is greater likelihood of pathological development occurring, or at the very least, it is more likely that the individual will struggle as a result of not completing a stage (Langer, 1969).

Development Implies Change, but Our Core Remains More or Less the Same

As we walk down our developmental path, we encounter much that is new to our current understanding of the world. Generally, we *assimilate* this new information, which means that we take it into our existing understanding of the world. Periodically, however, we move into a state of readiness for a dramatic shift in the way we live in the world, and with support we *accommodate* or dramatically change the way we understand the world. Our core remains the same; but, as we assimilate and accommodate to the world, we appropriately adapt. Like a piece of clay we can be molded, sometimes torn apart and then put back together, but we are always clay. Each piece has a different shape, and it can come in different colors, different weights, and different consistencies, but it is all clay.

Development Is Painful, Yet Growth-Producing

Developmental theory suggests that there are transition points from one developmental level to another. Such points are generally earmarked by disequilibrium as the individual accommodates to a new way of living in the world. Transitions will often be experienced as a state of confusion, anxiety, depression, fear, and/or exhilaration, and they can occur quickly or can last for years.

Transition will be less disequilibrating if the individual has had success in passing through previous developmental milestones and if there is support in the individual's environment to ease him or her through the transition. Support for change comes in many forms; it can be the nurturing needed for the infant to grow physically, the reinforcement given to an adolescent as he or she begins to think in increasingly complex ways, or the psychological support needed by the adult going through a career change. The support can be given by a parent, a friend, or a counselor. However you go through them, transitions ultimately mean that you are growing toward something greater than you were previously.

Developmental Models Are Transtheoretical

Developmental theories can be used in conjunction with most counseling approaches. Developmental theory acknowledges the importance of the interplay between the environment and the person and attempts to determine the effects of both on the development of the person. It therefore can be used with counseling approaches that stress environmental or intrapsychic approaches to the individual. A counselor who understands development and the milestones faced by individuals can choose counseling strategies from many theoretical approaches when working with specific developmental issues.

Development Is Preventive, Optimistic, and Wellness-Oriented

The nature of developmental theory lends itself toward prevention and a wellness model of mental health. For instance, by knowing the expected transitions an individual will be facing, the counselor can develop workshops and educational seminars that can assist individuals in understanding their natural progression from one developmental level to another. A developmental perspective offers the counselor a model from which he or she can understand the client's predicament as well as a framework from which to develop strategies to assist the client, who may want to revisit past developmental tasks that remain unfinished. Whereas pathological models assume that the person has an inborn deficit that probably cannot be fixed, developmental models view pathology as either a normal response to a developmental transition point or an important signal that we need to complete a past developmental task that has remained unfinished:

> *. . . most modern developmental theories are optimistic. They see growth and development as the natural tendency of the organism. Even when environmental circumstances are less than optimal, individuals do their best to learn and grow, often showing considerable resourcefulness. Often adult behaviors that seem "symptomatic" are in fact coping strategies that enabled the individual to survive hardship in childhood.* (Wallen, 1993, p. 1)

In summary, human development is continuous, orderly, sequential, painful yet growth-producing, and a natural and potentially positive part of our existence. Developmental counseling offers the counselor a unique perspective when working with clients. The developmentally astute counselor knows (1) a variety of developmental theories, (2) the types of social issues and personal problems often experienced by clients as they pass through specific developmental stages, and (3) the kinds of counseling techniques that might work with clients as they past through the stages (Thomas, 1990). Clearly, knowledge of human development can go far in assisting the counselor in his or her work with clients.

A Brief Overview of Physical and Psychosocial Development

Development in Childhood

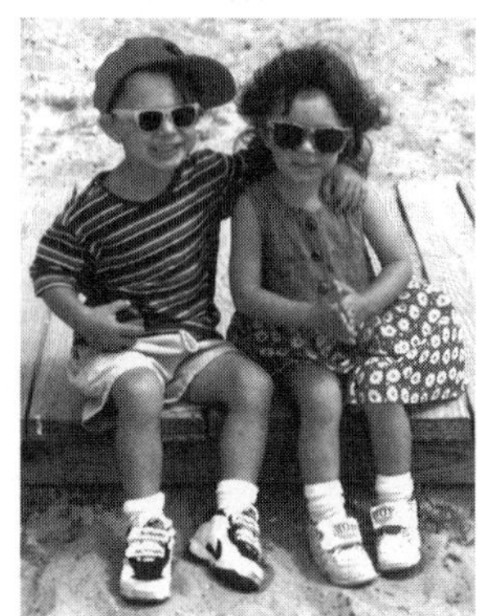

The developing child undergoes major physiological, social, and cognitive changes in the first few years of life (Rice, 2001). Of course, until puberty and usually sometime afterward, there are great gains in height and weight. Gross and fine motor skills change quickly in the first few years of life, and the nervous system, which seems structurally complete, is actually functionally incomplete and will not finish growing until early adolescence. For instance, the myelin sheath that covers the nerve continues to develop until the child is 2, which accounts for the jerky movements of infants, and the cerebral cortex will not be complete until approximately age 12. As the nervous system continues to develop, there are rapid increases in the child's sensory development, speech and language ability, and cognitive and intellectual functioning. Increased physical abilities are soon to affect the child's psychosocial development. For instance, increased mobility allows the toddler to explore more of his or her environment, and toddlers who are reinforced for their exploratory behavior will develop higher self-esteem than those who are reprimanded.

Because the vast majority of children will develop at fairly predictable rates, a counselor or child specialist who is aware of physiological timetables normed for children can assess whether or not a child is on target for his or her physiological development. Normative physical and social development have been described by Arnold Gesell, as well as others, and have been used to determine a child's developmental maturation in such things as readiness for kindergarten (Gesell & Ilg, 1943; Rice, 2001).

Although the rate of children's physical development is fairly consistent, the scope of a specific child's development is based on the genetic predisposition of the child in interaction with the environment. For instance, although most children will be able to do multiplication by the fourth grade, their rate of learning and range of ability will vary based on genetics and environment. Along these lines, a brilliant child is at a major disadvantage if he or she is brought up in a home that has lead paint and lead in the water or neglectful parents, while a child who is less able can shine if placed in a stimulating and nurturing environment (see Figure 9.1).

Evidence of the importance of a nurturing environment in a child's development can be seen through the success of the Head Start Program. Since the 1970s, Head Start has provided disadvantaged preschool children intellectually stimulating and nurturing environments. On average, these children have done noticeably better academically and socially than children of a similar background who have not received such an opportunity (Lee, Brooks-Gunn, Schnur, & Liaw, 1990; Lee & Loeb, 1995; Pelligrini, Perlmutter, Galda, & Brody, 1990).

FIGURE 9.1
The Bender Visual Motor Gestalt

The Bender Visual Motor Gestalt is an assessment instrument that is used to determine possible psychological, physiological, and developmental problems in children and adults. In giving the instrument, you ask the individual to reproduce nine figures which are presented to him or her in sequence (the figures are actually much larger than depicted below). For children, difficulties in reproducing some of the figures could be indications of a learning disability, developmental delay, or emotional problems. Below are reproductions of four of the figures of two children who are developmentally on target. When Hannah couldn't reproduce figure 6, she became very frustrated and drew the lines below. Look at how much easier it is for the older child to reproduce the figures.

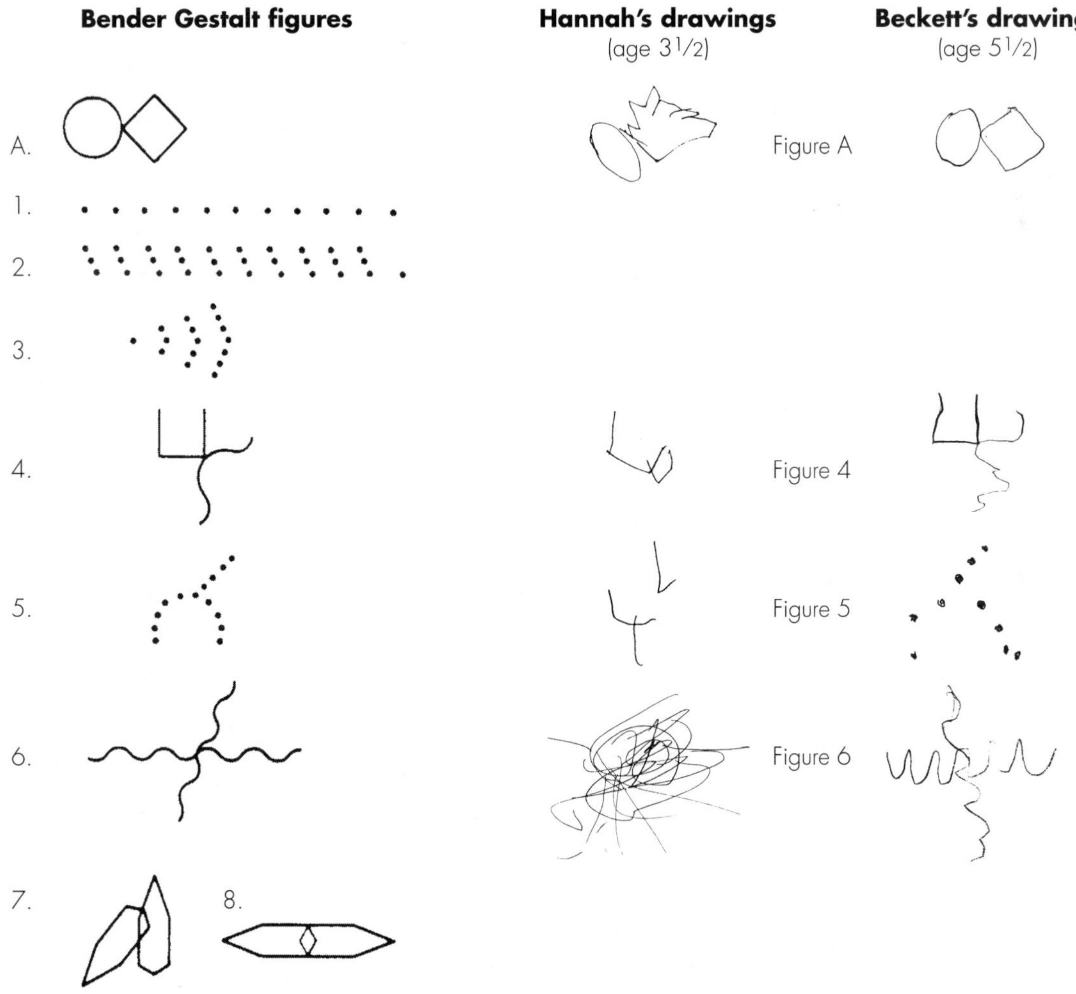

Development in Adolescence and Adulthood

As children grow into adolescence, they face the major task of dealing with the physical and psychological aspects of puberty. Of course, changes in their bodies can greatly affect how they feel about themselves. Adolescence is the time when teenagers will compare themselves to each other as they develop a sense of their identity. In adolescence, many teenagers face a myriad of social issues with which they will struggle, including drug use, crime and violence, dating, sexual identity, and sexually transmitted diseases. Late adolescence marks the time when teenagers will begin to consider their future plans. Older adolescents have to decide whether or not to go on to college or to work and consider a career and/or a college major.

Adolescence and young adulthood bring with them the blossoming of a person's sexuality. Of course, how this is dealt with can affect the individual for the rest of his or her life. Body image issues become particularly important now, especially for women who feel pressure to reflect the image of the beautiful and slender models portrayed in the media (Muth & Cash, 1997).

Young adulthood is highlighted by making career choices and, for some, making lifelong commitments. Thus, issues of intimacy and how the young adult fits into the world of work are prominent at this time. These issues become increasingly more important as the young adult moves into what is called by some *early adulthood*. Success at having a love relationship and committing to a career is often reflected in one's psychological adjustment to the world in this time of life.

As individuals move into middle adulthood, they begin to recognize the slow decline in their physical abilities. When men and women reach their forties most will see slow weight gains and changes in vision, reaction time, strength, and motor ability. The psychological associations to death and dying are likely to increase, especially as parents and grandparents become ill and die. Women will soon face menopause, and many men, an increasingly larger stomach. Adults will begin to assess their worth in the world of work and begin to think about their entrance into late adulthood. Those who have been raising families are likely to reflect on how the family has grown, and those who have not raised families are likely to ponder what it is like not to leave a legacy through their children.

As we move on in life, slow physical changes continue, and in later adulthood disease, ill health increase, and changes in physical abilities occur. These include changes in hearing, taste, smell, visual acuity, and memory, as well as an increasingly fragile skeletal system. As many are now living into their late eighties and nineties, additional health problems become increasingly prevalent. Psychologically, many older adults reflect on their lives and assess whether or not they are satisfied with what they have accomplished.

The Development of Knowing: Cognitive and Moral Changes in Childhood

This section of the chapter will examine cognitive and moral development of children. However, much of what you will read also applies to adults. This is because most individuals do not reach the higher stages until much later in life, and some never reach them. These theories present the earliest ages at which all people could achieve these stages if given the appropriate environmental stimulus.

Jean Piaget and Cognitive Development

How does a child come to understand the world? This is the question that Jean Piaget asked when he first began exploring the cognitive development of children (Flavell, 1963). Piaget found that children learn through a process of assimilation and accommodation. Assimilation occurs when the child uses his or her existing way of understanding the world to make sense out of new knowledge. Accommodation, on the other hand, occurs when the child changes his or her previous ways of knowing to make sense out of this new knowledge (Piaget, 1954).

Piaget stated that, in accommodating to the world, *schemata* (new cognitive structures; e.g., new ways of thinking) are formed that allow an individual to adapt and change his or her ways of thinking and understanding the world. This process of assimilation, forming new schemata, and accommodation can occur throughout the lifespan but is most obvious during childhood. Piaget showed that there were a number of concepts that a child can understand only at the age-appropriate level (Box 9.1).

Through his research on child cognitive development, Piaget determined that children pass through predictable stages of development, each highlighted by a particular way of understanding the world (Inhelder & Piaget, 1958; Piaget, 1954). In the *sensorimotor stage* (birth through 2), the infant responds almost exclusively to his or her physical and sensory experience. In this stage the child hasn't acquired full language ability, is not able to maintain mental images, and responds only to the here-and-now of experience. A parent attempting to have a rational conversation with a 1-year-old is pretty much wasting his or her time, as this child is almost exclusively responding to the here-and-now of sensory experiences. However, it may be good practice for the child to periodically hear the tone of rational talk as the child readies him- or herself for the next stage of development.

The *preoperational stage* (2 through 7) is marked by the development of language ability, the ability to maintain mental images and to manipulate the meaning of objects (e.g., a doll is a baby, a block is a car) (Muro & Dinkmeyer, 1977). The child in this stage responds intuitively to the world. Not yet able to think in logical sequences or in complex ways, the child responds to what seems immediately obvious as opposed to what might be logical. Unless the child is on the verge of entering the next stage of development, trying to explain logical principles would be difficult and usually impossible. Imagine trying to explain to Hannah that the M&Ms had different amounts of mass. She just wouldn't get it!

BOX 9.1

Hannah's Developmental Readiness

When my daughter was two years old, she loved M&Ms, which we attempted to give to her sparingly. At one point we discovered small M&Ms, which were about half the size of the regular ones. Giving her a bunch of these small candies made Hannah ecstatic. After all, now she could have *more* than she had on previous occasions. Hannah has not yet learned the concept that more in number does not necessarily mean more in volume or mass. Although *we* understood that five large M&Ms are about the same as ten small ones, this was not yet logical to Hannah. She could not think differently at this young age. At some point, in the not-too distant future, she would understand the concept of differences in size, shape, and mass.

From ages 7 through 11 the child enters the *concrete-operational stage*, in which he or she can begin to figure things out through a series of logical tasks, can begin to classify things, and is able to understand a sequence of events. Children can now make mental comparisons in their minds and mentally manipulate images. For instance, a child in this stage could create a mental image of a map of how to get to a friend's house. Children in this stage are often adamant about their logical way of viewing the world. For instance, when I was helping a friend's son with a math problem, he became angry when I suggested another way at finding the solution. He did not yet have the cognitive flexibility to examine other ways of knowing.

Children in the concrete-operational stage will have difficulty with metaphors or proverbs, because they haven't developed the capacity to think abstractly. However, when children (or adults!) move into Piaget's final stage, *formal operational* (11 through 16), they are able to apply more complex levels of knowing to their understanding of the world. A child in this stage can understand that objects might have symbolic meaning (e.g., the Liberty Bell is more than just a bell), can test hypotheses, understand proverbs, and consider more than one aspect of a problem at a time.

Piaget's research on child development has greatly assisted us in understanding how children learn and gives us a healthy respect for age-appropriate developmental limitations. Such knowledge has greatly affected styles of teaching, ways to parent effectively, and methods of counseling children.

Kohlberg's Theory of Moral Development

Like Piaget, Kohlberg wondered how children come to understand the world. However, he was particularly interested in how they come to understand and justify their moral behavior. Although Piaget had written about the process of moral development, Kohlberg greatly extended Piaget's original thoughts (Muro & Dinkmeyer, 1977).

By having children respond to moral dilemmas (problem situations of a moral nature with no clear-cut answer), Lawrence Kohlberg (1969) discovered that moral reasoning developed in a predictable pattern that spanned three levels of development, each containing two stages. The first level, *preconventional* (roughly ages 2 through 7), is based on the notion that children make moral decisions out of concern of being punished by someone more powerful than themselves. In stage 1 of this level, moral decisions are made to avoid punishment from individuals in authority, while in stage 2, decisions are made with an egocentric/hedonistic desire to satisfy one's own needs and to gain personal rewards. Imagine two 6-year-old children vying for the same toy, both yelling, "I want it!" A parent comes over and asks the children to share, with which they comply (wanting to avoid punishment from authority). Suddenly, one of the 6-year-olds gives the other a piece of candy and says, "Here, you have this and give me the toy" ("You scratch my back and I'll scratch yours" as long as I leave with a little bit more).

In Kohlberg's *conventional* level, moral decisions are based initially on "social conformity and mutualism" and later on "rule-governed behavior." In stage 3 of this level, the individual responds in a manner to please others and in hopes of avoiding the disapproval of significant others. Most children will reach stage 3 by age 13 (Gerrig & Zimbardo, 2002). An example of a stage 3 behavior is a 10-year-old who justifies making fun of a child at school because his friends are encouraging him to, they all do it, and he does not want to displease them. Ask this child to defend his behavior, and he might say, "Well, everyone else was doing it, so I didn't think it was wrong." Ask this same child to state what would be the morally correct behavior if a bunch of kids were calling another kid names and he was asked to do the same, he might respond that it would not be right to call the kid names. This is because within this context, he would want to please you and therefore would respond with what he knows to be the socially correct response.

In stage 4 of the conventional level, adolescents and adults will emphasize a system of laws and rules as a means of maintaining a sense of order in their lives. Here, some 10-year-olds will reason that it is not right to make fun of other kids in school because it is against the rules at school. This stage represents an important shift from externality to internality from a need to receive approval from others to following a set of internalized rules.

Kohlberg believed that the final level of development, *postconventional* morality, requires formal-operational thinking and found that most individuals will never reach this level because of the cognitive complexity involved. The postconventional thinker believes in the process of democratically devised social contracts (e.g., laws) that can be analyzed, interpreted, and changed, but that ultimately take precedence over individual needs (stage 5). In this stage, an individual would be likely to follow the law because there are governing moral principles that have been used in their development. However, such a person is willing to examine inconsistencies in laws and work on changing laws not seen as good for society.

In stage 6 of the *postconventional* level, moral decisions are based on a sense of universal truths, personal conscience, individual decision-making, and respect for human rights and dignity (Rice, 2001). Here an individual would consider moral truths in his or her decision-making process and, after deep reflection, might choose to break a law, deciding that such an action is taken out of respect for the dignity of people and for the betterment of society (Sprinthall, Sprinthall, & Oja, 1998) (see Box 9.2). For instance, during the civil rights movement of the 1960s some individuals broke laws to advance the cause of civil rights for all people.

Although Kohlberg identified the lowest ages at which some individuals had reached conventional and postconventional thinking, he found that some young adults and adults have not mastered conventional thinking, while most have not reached postconventional thinking. He therefore advised that it would not be unusual to find same-aged adults at different levels of moral development.

Gilligan's Theory of Women's Moral Development

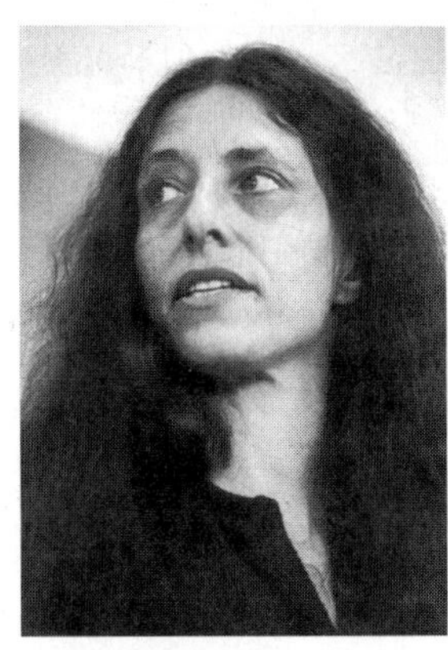
Carol Gilligan

In 1982, Carol Gilligan wrote a book called *In a Different Voice*, which questioned some of Kohlberg's assumptions. Gilligan, who had been a colleague of Kohlberg's, noted that most of his research had been done on a small group of boys, and she proposed that moral reasoning for females might be based on a different way of knowing or understanding the world. She noted that Kohlberg's theory stressed the notion that high-stage individuals make choices that stress autonomy and individuality, whereas her research seemed to indicate that women at high levels of development value connectedness and interdependence and view the relationship as primary when making moral decisions. In describing the differences between men and women, Gilligan notes the responses of one of Kohlberg's subjects and compares him to a woman she interviewed:

> *Thus while Kohlberg's subject worries about people interfering with each other's rights, this woman worries about "the possibility of omission, of your not helping others when you could help them."* (Gilligan, 1982, p. 21)

BOX 9.2

Going to Jail for Reasons of Personal Conscience

For fourteen months my brother-in-law Steve (lower left) was incarcerated because he and others broke into a naval shipyard, snuck onto an Aegis destroyer, poured their own blood onto the ship, and banged on the ship as protest against nuclear missiles. Some might say that Steve is in Kohlberg's Stage 6, that he has chosen to break the law for the betterment of society and out of his deeply held belief that nuclear arms can only harm people. If Steve has thoroughly reflected upon this, considered all points of view, and come to this decision in a deeply personal and thoughtful manner, he would be in Stage 6. If he did this act out of approval of his social group or a system of rules which he adhered to strongly, such as the rules of his group, he would be in Stage 3 or 4. Often people can do the same acts and be at different stages. You must know the person to determine the stage. I believe Steve is in Stage 6.

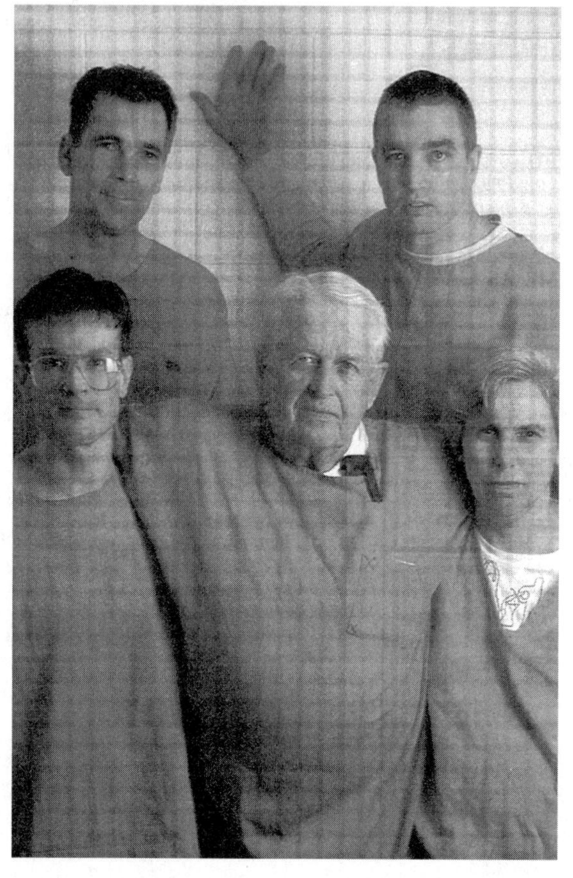

Jailed activists

(Republished with permission of Globe Newspaper Company, Inc., from the July 27, 1997, issue of *The Boston Globe*, © 1997.)

Gilligan stated that in the development of moral reasoning, especially in stages 3 and above, women will emphasize a "standard of caring" in moral decision making; that is, a concern for the other person will be a core ingredient when making moral decisions. She noted that women are more likely to be concerned about the impact their choices might have on others, whereas men are more concerned about a sense of justice being maintained (Zimbardo & Gerrig, 1996). Noting these male and female differences, Gilligan states:

> *Given the differences in women's conceptions of self and morality, women bring to the life cycle a different point of view and order human experience in terms of different priorities.* (Gilligan, 1982, p. 22)

More specifically, the level 1 preconventional girl is not dissimilar to Kohlberg's level 1 boy, in that her moral reasoning is narcissistic; she reasons from a survival, self-protective perspective. For Gilligan, the level 2 conventional woman shows a concern for others and feels responsible for others, as opposed to Kohlberg's level 2 person, who is concerned about pleasing others or following the rules. Gilligan's level 3 postconventional woman is a complex thinker who recognizes the interdependent nature of humans and that every action a person takes affects others in deeply personal ways.

Consider how an adolescent or adult woman might respond if her moral reasoning is grounded in a standard of care for others and a sense of responsibility to others as opposed to the individualistic and rule-following perspective of many men. Also, you might want to consider Steve's moral choices (Box 9.2). In determining Steve's moral decision-making process, one would have to determine if Steve was driven more out of a sense of personal conscience and what he thought would be best for the world or out of a sense of personal conscience and a standard of care—a concern for how his actions would affect others.

Gilligan has added a unique perspective to the concept of moral development and brings to the forefront major differences that men and women hold toward moral reasoning. Understanding such differences is crucial in helping us understand why men and women view moral reasoning in very different ways.

Comparison of Cognitive and Moral Development

There is a logical association between Piaget's stages of cognitive development and Kohlberg's and Gilligan's levels of moral development. The preoperational thinker responds intuitively and cannot think logically or in complex ways. From a perspective of moral development, this person can only be in the preconventional level, responding on a gut level to the rudimentary morality of punishment and reward and acting in a self-centered manner. Although Kohlberg and Gilligan offer different perspectives on their understanding of the conventional person, reflection on self or complex thinking concerning higher moral principles is not possible at this level. Therefore, it is likely that you would find the concrete-operational person exhibiting moral reasoning from this level. Finally, for both Kohlberg and Gilligan it is clear that the kind of introspection and consciousness necessary for the post-conventional thinker can only be found by the individual who has conquered formal-operational thought (see Table 9.1).

Adult Cognitive Development

For years, the development of knowing in the adult took a backseat to understanding the cognitive development of children. However, recently a number of theories have offered an explanation of how adults make sense of the world. Like their child-development counterparts, which reach upward and attempt to explain pieces of adult development, these theories extend downward and have something to say about child development. However, in practice, these theories tend to be applied to adults. Two of the theories that have gained some prominence in recent years are Kegan's constructive development theory and Perry's theory of epistemological reflection (Kegan, 1982; Perry, 1970).

Kegan's Constructive Developmental Model

Kegan believes that our understanding of the world is based on how we construct reality as we pass through the lifespan. His subject-object theory, which was discussed briefly in Chapter 1, states that there are specific developmental stages through which individuals

TABLE 9.1

A Comparison of Piaget to Kohlberg and Gilligan

PIAGET'S STAGES	PIAGET	KOHLBERG/GILLIGAN LEVELS	KOHLBERG	GILLIGAN
Sensorimotor	Responds to physical and sensory experience.			
Preoperational	Intuitive responding. Maintenance of mental images. No logical thinking.	Preconventional	1. Punishment/reward. 2. Satisfy needs to gain reward (you get from me, I get from you).	Concern for survival and self-interest.
Concrete-operational	No complex thinking. Uses logical thinking sequencing, categorizing, to figure things out. Rigid in ways of knowing.	Conventional	1. Social conformity/ approval of others. 2. Rules and laws to maintain order.	Caring for others. Sacrifice of self for others. Responsible to others.
Formal-operational	Abstract thinking. Complex ways of knowing.	Postconventional	1. Social contract/ democratically arrived at. Rules that can be changed through a logical process. 2. Individual conscience.	Decision making from an interdependent perspective. All that we choose affects everyone else.

NOTE: Kohlberg's levels are each divided into two stages, as shown.

pass that reflect their meaning-making system. Movement from a lower to higher stage necessitates a letting go of the earlier stage. This is not done easily, and Kegan suggests that movement occurs most successfully if there is challenge to one's existing view of the world within a supportive environment (Kegan, 1982).

Kegan (1982) suggests there are six stages of cognitive development (stages 0 to 5), with stages 3, 4, and 5 representing ways in which the adult views the world. Kegan states that the self-absorbed infant, being born into the *incorporative* stage, is all reflexive and has no sense of self as separate from the outside world. However, as the very young child begins to experience the world, reflexes are no longer the primary focus; instead the young child attempts to have his or her needs met through attainment of objects outside of self. In this *impulsive* stage the child has limited control over his or her actions and acts spontaneously to have needs met. No wonder the second year of life is often called the "terrible twos":

> *In disembedding herself from her reflexes the two-year-old comes to have reflexes rather than be them, and the new self is embedded in that which coordinates the reflexes, namely, the "perceptions" and the "impulses."* (Kegan, 1982, p. 85)

As children gain control over their impulses, they move into the *imperial* stage, where needs, interests, and wishes become primary and impulses can now be controlled (see Box 9.3). For instance, here the child begins to recognize what he or she wants, can recognize the desire for it, and can now have some control over how to try to obtain the toy.

BOX 9.3

Garrett: Responding from the Imperial Stage

Garrett is the 12-year-old son of a friend of mine. Recently, when wanting to spend time with a friend of his, he was told that this friend had already made plans to spend time with another boy. Garrett felt rejected and left out. If Garrett had still been in the impulsive stage, he might have thrown a temper tantrum. Instead, having passed into the imperial stage, he had control over his impulses and devised a way to get his needs met. He manipulated a way to spend time with both of them, disregarding their need to be with one another. You see, in the imperial stage one can control impulses and therefore develop plans to have one's needs met, and in this stage there is little empathy for other people's desires. Therefore, Garrett did not yet have the ability to talk over his feelings with his friends. Hopefully, when he's a little older, he'll be able to share his feelings of being left out and understand (have empathy for) his friends' desire to be with one another.

When his father was explaining this situation to me he said that at first he was going to try to talk with his son about the other kids' feelings but then he realized that Garrett just couldn't hear that yet. If you're in the imperial stage and not yet ready to give it up, there's little you can do to "make" a person be in the interpersonal stage.

Although some adults are in the imperial stage of development, most are in the last three stages. During the *interpersonal* stage, the individual is embedded in relationships; that is, relationships are primary, and needs and wishes are met through the relationship. Symbolically, the interpersonal person lives by the following statements, "I am you, you are me. I do not have an existence without the other. You make me who I am." As opposed to the narcissistic orientation of the imperial person, the interpersonal person begins to show glimpses of empathy. After all, if your existence is contingent on your relationship with others, you had better periodically show them understanding. However, mostly this stage is symbolized by its dependency on others. The interpersonal person's need for relationship can be seen in many of the popular songs of our era, which are often highlighted by dependency needs such as "I will die without you" or "I am no one if you are not in my life."

The individual who moves out of embeddedness in another moves into the *institutional* stage, where a sense of autonomy and self-authorship of life is acquired. Relationships in this stage are still important but no longer seem like the essential ingredient for living. In this stage the individual's understanding of his or her values and interests become important. Here the individual may choose a partner because the other person shares similar values; however, the person in this stage does not need the partner as he or she does in the interpersonal stage. The institutional person can sometimes become quite arrogant about his or her point of view. Feeling independent and strong, this person can sometimes angrily stake out his or her position. Some of my colleagues joke that all New Yorkers are in this stage of development.

Kegan's final stage, the *interindividual* stage, highlights mutuality in relationships; that is, the individual can share with others and learn from others in a nondependent way. Here there is a sharing of selves, without a giving up of self, and difference is tolerated and even encouraged at times. In an effort to be continually self-reflective, this individual encourages feedback about self. Finally, the interindividual person has respect for self and for all others, regardless of their stage. One might say that this person is the epitome of the self-actualized human.

BOX 9.4

The Life of Malcom X

The life of Malcolm X is a good example of movement through Kegan's stages (see Haley, 2001). As a young adult, Malcolm X found himself involved in a life of crime and drug addiction as he narcissistically tried to have his needs met (imperial stage). Given a ten-year jail sentence for robbery, in prison he was introduced to the Nation of Islam, a Black Muslim religion headed by Elijah Mohammad. Malcolm readily gave up his former lifestyle and became embedded in the values of the Nation of Islam. He lived, slept, and breathed *their* values, and his identity became the values held by the Nation of Islam (interpersonal stage). However, as he grew as a person, he realized that he did not agree with some of their ideas, and he moved from embeddedness in their values to a strong sense of his own religious, cultural, and moral values. Although still an activist, and still somewhat closed to other points of view, he had matured to the point in which he was now embracing his own set of values (institutional stage).

Following a pilgrimage to Mecca, he changed his name to Al Hajj Malik al-Shabazz and again modified his views "to encompass the possibility that all white people were not evil and that progress in the black struggle could be made with the help of world organizations, other black groups, and even progressive white groups" (*Encyclopedia of Black America,* 1981, p. 544). Clearly, Al Hajj Malik al-Shabazz had evolved to Kegan's interindividual stage. He could now hear other points of view, be open to feedback, and yet have a clear sense of his own uniqueness in the world.

Kegan's developmental model stresses the interpersonal nature of development. Growth is based on our ability to interact with others and to let go of past, less effective types of relating. Although Kegan gives some general time lines for when movement into higher levels could occur, it is usual to find older adults who have not moved out of the interpersonal and sometimes even the imperial stages. The life of Malcolm X is an extraordinary example of a person's movement through the stages (see Box 9.4).

Perry's Theory of Intellectual and Ethical Development

William Perry's theory of epistemological reflection (Perry, 1970), discussed briefly in Chapter 1, was developed to examine the cognitive development of adults, particularly college students. The Perry scheme, as it is known, describes movement through four stages (King, 1978). In the first stage, *dualism*, students view truth categorically, as right or wrong, and they have little tolerance for ambiguity. Dualists take on all-or-nothing thinking and believe that experts have answers to almost all questions. Therefore, they believe that they can get the "truth" from their professor. As individuals develop, they begin to doubt some of their absolutist-type thinking and move into multiplicity, or, as reported by some, transition (Magolda & Porterfield, 1988), in which a beginning recognition of the limits of authorities occurs.

In the next stage, *relativism*, students are able to think more abstractly and become interested in knowing about differing opinions. In relativism, a student comes to understand that there may be many ways of constructing reality and of defining truth; that the professor has a body of knowledge, but others have knowledge as well; and that learning can be a joint sharing process between the professor and students. Individuals in this stage are often ambivalent about what values and relative truths to call their own.

Perry's last stage is called *commitment to relativism*. In this final stage, individuals have the capacity to maintain their relativistic outlook while also committing themselves to specific behaviors and values that guide them. Such individuals make a commitment to a specific way of viewing the world (e.g., pro-life, pro-choice), are open to changing their commitments if given new facts, and can hear different points of view. For example, the committed relativist may make a specific religious or job commitment while at the same time recognizing the possibility that new information may modify that choice (Widick, 1977).

Perry's theory has been actively used in college settings to understand how college students think and the cognitive changes they go through while attending college (Magolda & Porterfield, 1988). However, the theory may have broader implications, because it may be able to describe a general orientation as to how individuals interact in the world, with some people reflecting the rigid, inflexible themes found by the dualists, while other people are capable of the multiple-perspectives-taking of the relativist. At the very least, some research has indicated that the Perry scheme is related to a counselor's ability at being empathic, being nondogmatic, and having an internal locus of control (Neukrug & McAuliffe, 1993).

Although Perry did not set age limits for individuals who are dualistic, relativistic, or committed in relativism, it would not be too difficult to approximate the lowest ages in which you might find each. The dualist could be as young as the individual in the concrete-operational stage (around 12), while the relativist would need minimally to be in Piaget's formal-operational stage and Kegan's institutional stage to take on multiple perspectives (ages 16 to 18). The individual who is committed in relativism would also have to be in formal operations and seems to hold many of the same qualities as Kegan's interindividual person (minimal age of 40).

Comparison of Adult Cognitive Development Theories

Although Kegan's theory is much more broadly based than Perry's, there are many similarities between the two. For instance, both examine how the individual constructs reality and makes meaning in his or her life. Both suggest that as individuals develop, their view of reality is one that becomes increasingly more complex, more open, and seems to embody many of the characteristics of what we might call the self-actualized person. Finally, both theories state that adult development is likely to occur if the individual is afforded an environment that is supportive yet challenging to one's current way of making meaning.

Lifespan Development

Some models of understanding the development of the person have taken a lifespan perspective; that is, the individual is seen as continuing to grow over the lifespan with development not being viewed as suddenly ending in childhood or starting in adulthood. In addition, the previous models we have examined offered stages through which all people could pass, although many will not reach the highest stages of development. Lifespan models offer stages through which every person will pass.

One of the more prevalent models of lifespan development has been Erikson's stages of psychosocial development, which examine how psychosocial forces affect the development of the person. Another model offered by Levinson examines stages of development experienced by men over the lifespan.

Erikson's Stages of Psychosocial Development

Although Erik Erikson started out studying Freud's psychoanalytic approach, he later developed a model that rejected many of Freud's original tenets. Contrary to Freud, he felt that the individual was not determined by instincts, early childhood development, and the unconscious. Instead he posited that psychosocial forces, in combination with biological and psychological factors, were major motivators in the development of a healthy personality. As opposed to Freud's deterministic philosophy, Erikson had faith in the ability of the individual to overcome many of his or her problems. Erikson felt that as the individual passes through life, he or she has age-related developmental life tasks to overcome. A healthy ego is contingent on the individual's ability to master these critical periods of development, said Erikson. If a positive identity is created, the individual can successfully move on to the next critical period. On the other hand, the individual who is not able to cope with age-specific developmental tasks will develop a low self-image and a bruised ego and will carry these dysfunctions into the next levels of development, therefore making it difficult to successfully complete later developmental tasks. Erikson's eight lifespan stages are often referenced as a means of assisting the helper in understanding typical developmental tasks of the individual (Erikson, 1963,1968, 1980, 1982).

Trust versus mistrust (birth to 1 year). During this first stage the infant develops a sense of trust or mistrust based on the ability of his or her parents to nurture and provide a sense of psychological safety.

Autonomy versus shame and doubt (1 to 2 years). During these years the toddler is beginning to explore the environment and gain control over his or her body. Promoting a child's newfound abilities leads to a sense of autonomy; inhibiting the child leads to a sense of shame and doubt.

Initiative versus guilt (3 to 5 years). As the child continues to grow physically and intellectually, he or she increases exploration of the environment. Parents can either reinforce the child taking initiatives or make the child feel guilty by thwarting such initiatives.

Industry versus inferiority (6 to 11 years). In this stage, the child is beginning to understand the world and obtain a basic sense of what he or she does well, especially in relationship to peers. The child begins to set goals based on his or her self-assessment of strengths. The ability of the child to feel a sense of accomplishment in achieving goals can lead him or her toward a sense of self-worth. Not achieving goals can lead to feelings of inferiority.

Identity versus role confusion (adolescence). As adolescents begin to identify their temperament, values, interests, and abilities, they begin to recognize the specific attributes that define their personality. Lack of role models or experiences that discourage such self-understanding can lead to identity confusion.

Intimacy versus isolation (early adulthood). Once the young adult has achieved a sense of self, he or she is ready to develop intimate relationships. On the other hand, lack of self-understanding leads to isolation from others and/or an inability to have mutually supporting relationships that encourage individuality with interdependency.

Generativity versus stagnation (middle adulthood). The healthy adult in this stage is concerned about others and about future generations. This individual is able to maintain a productive and responsible lifestyle and can find meaning through work, volunteerism, parenting, and/or community activities.

Integrity versus despair (later life). In this last stage of development, the older person examines his or her life and can feel a sense of fulfillment or despair. Successfully mastering the developmental tasks from the preceding stages will lead to a sense of integrity for the individual.

Erikson's lifespan model is often used as a cornerstone for helping individuals understand expected crises through which they may be passing. Such understanding can sometimes help normalize problems that may feel quite unbearable in the moment.

Levinson's The Seasons of a Man's Life

Daniel Levinson's book *The Seasons of a Man's Life* (1985) examined developmental changes of men through the lifespan. His research, which was the basis for the well-known book *Passages* (Sheehy, 1976), examined men in a number of occupational groups, and although he wrote a book on the lifespan development of women (Levinson, 1996), it never gained the popularity of his original work.

Through an intensive biographical interview with each man, Levinson identified four eras in men's lives, including: *childhood and adolescence*, *early adulthood*, *middle adulthood*, and *late adulthood*. In addition, he later suggested that because men are living longer, there is most likely another era called late, late adulthood. Eras are preceded by transitional periods in which the individual adapts for the upcoming life stage. Eras are subdivided into periods, each of which has its own unique issues that will be faced by men (see Figure 9.2). Levinson believed that the eras are universal, cross-cultural, and

FIGURE 9.2
Developmental Periods in Early and Middle Adulthood
SOURCE: Levinson, 1978, p. 57.

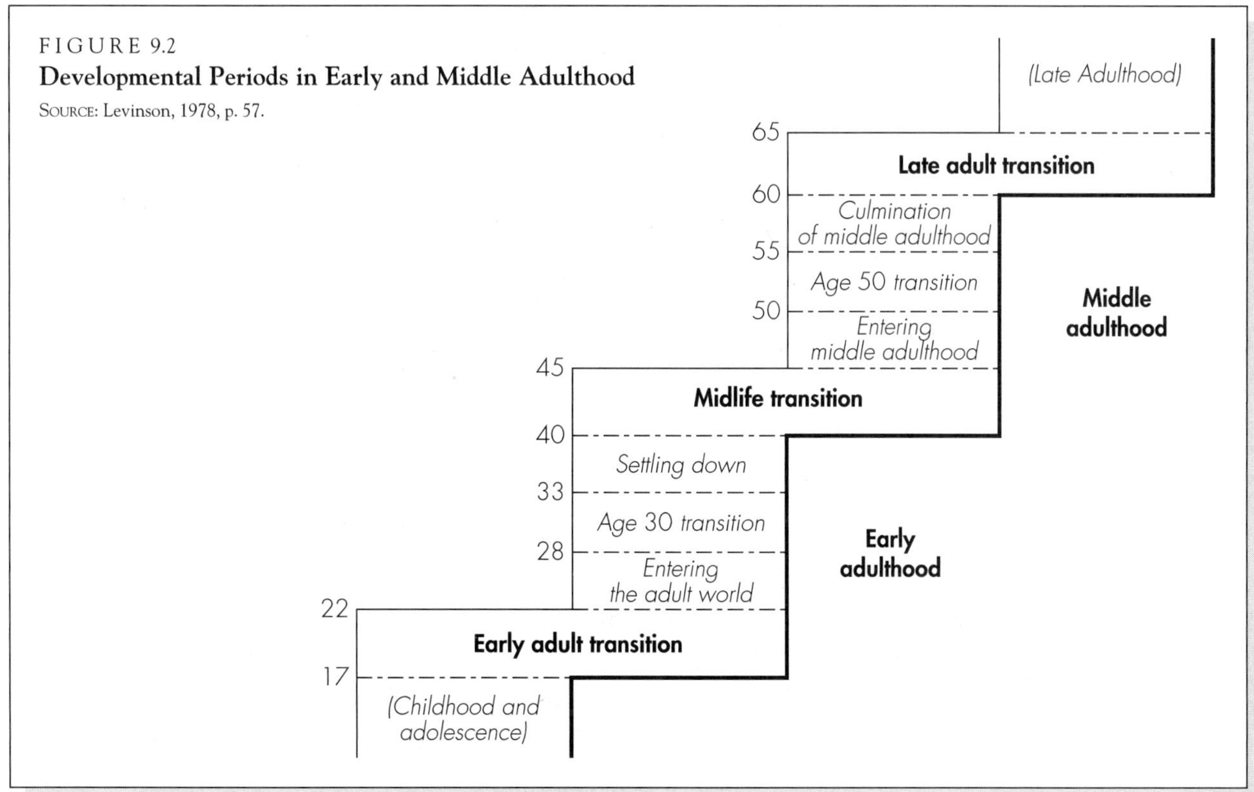

TABLE 9.2

Developmental Periods of Levinson

Early adult transition (17–20): Leaving the family and adolescent groups, going to college, military service, marrying.

Entering the adult world (22–28): Time of choices, defining goals, establishing occupation and marriage; conflict between desire to explore and desire to commit.

Age 30 transition (28–33): Period of reworking, modifying life structure; smooth transition for some, disruptive crisis for others; growing sense of need for change before becoming locked in because of commitments.

Settling down (33–40): Accepting a few major goals, building the structure around central choices; establishing one's niche, working at advancement.

Midlife transition: (40–45): Midlife crisis, link between early and middle adulthood; review and reappraise early adult period; modify unsatisfying aspects of life structure; adjust psychologically to the final half of life; intense reexamination causes emotional upset, tumultuous struggles with self, questioning every aspect of life.

Entering middle adulthood (45–50): End of reappraisal, time of choices, forming a new life structure in relation to occupation, marriage, locale; wide variations in satisfactions and extent of fulfillment.

Age 50 transition (50–55): Work further on the tasks of midlife transition and modification of structure formed in the mid-40s; crisis if there was not enough change during midlife transition.

Culmination of middle adulthood (55–60): Building a second middle adult structure; time of fulfillment for those who can rejuvenate themselves and enrich their lives.

Late adult transition (60–65): Conclude efforts of middle adulthood, prepare for era to come; major turning point in life cycle.

Late adulthood (65+): Confrontation with self, life: need to make peace with the world.

Late, late adulthood (80+): Further psychosocial development or senescence.

SOURCE: Rice, 1983.

predetermined by a complex interaction of social forces, our biology, and psychological factors. Within each period are what Levinson called life structures, which are tasks or challenges that are faced by each man in the following areas: career, love relationships, marriage and family, relationships with self, uses of solitude, roles in social contexts, and relationships with individuals, groups, and institutions.

Levinson identifies the ebbs and flows of the developmental process for men. Noting that within each era there are periods of great stability and of great fluctuation, he offers us an understanding of the normal life tasks that will be faced by most men (see Table 9.2).

Comparison of Lifespan Development Theories

A number of similarities exist between the lifespan theories of Erikson and Levinson. For instance, both state that there are specific developmental stages through which all individuals must pass. Both suggest that these stages are age specific; that is, you can assume that each individual will be dealing with specific developmental tasks within a specified age span. Both theories are sequential but not hierarchical; that is, although stages follow one another in an orderly manner, and difficulty in one stage can affect later stages, no stage is considered better than another. Finally, Erikson and Levinson suggest that their developmental tasks are a function of biological, psychological, and sociological factors and are probably universal across cultures.

> *If this developmental sequence does hold to some degree for the species, its origins must be found in the interaction of all these influences as they operate during a particular phase. . . .* (Levinson, 1978, p. 322)

Fowler's Theory of Faith Development

Drawing on the work of Erikson, Piaget, and Kohlberg, James Fowler developed a theory of faith development (Fowler, 1976, 1984, 1991, 1995). Fowler believes that faith is universal and inherent in our nature and relates to how we make meaning. Faith, as defined by Fowler, is much broader than a singular examination of one's religious orientation. It has to do with a person's core values, the images of power that drive the person, and the stories that motivate the individual consciously and unconsciously throughout life (e.g., the stories of Jesus, Martin Luther King, Jr., Muhammad, the unique stories that drive our families, and so forth):

> . . . *We shape commitments to causes and centers of value. We form allegiances and alliances with images and realities of power. And we form and shape our lives in relation to master stories. In these ways we join with others in the finding and making of meaning.* (Fowler, 1991, p. 22)

This broad definition of faith means that the atheist, agnostic, fundamentalist, and communist all have some faith experience, for faith is not dependent on a belief in God (Fowler, 1991). In fact, faith is deeper than one's belief system because it includes unconscious motivations.

Based on his research, Fowler (1976, 1991) identified six stages of faith development with minimal ages at which Fowler believes a person can enter a specific stage. Within Fowler's model one can see pieces of each of the theories we examined in this chapter. Thus, as we read through Fowler's theory, consider how all of the developmental models examined might explain different aspects of his theory. This can act as a mini review for this chapter.

STAGE 0, PRIMARY FAITH (INFANCY) Based on Erikson's first psychosocial stage of trust versus mistrust, Fowler believes that infants have a predisposition toward a trusting relationship, which, if developed, will be the basis for the development of faith later in life.

STAGE 1, INTUITIVE-PROJECTIVE FAITH (MINIMAL AGE: 4) Based on Piaget's preoperational stage, children in this stage respond mostly to stories, feelings, and imagery. Their world is not logical; it is a symbolic mystery and can be greatly affected by adult views of faith. Symbols and stories are swallowed whole and can be used to expand a child's vision of the world; however, they can also be used to instill fear:

> *My friend told me that the devil will come up out of a hole in the ground and get me if I'm not careful, so now I won't play in the backyard by myself.*
> (Fowler, 1984, pp. 54–55)

In this stage, children are quite malleable and will mimic those around them. This stage offers opportunity for faith development, yet it can also restrict a person's ability to develop faith (see Box 9.5) if he or she is placed in a fearful environment.

STAGE 2, MYTHIC-LITERAL FAITH (AGE 6½ TO 8) Having entered Piaget's concrete-operational stage, children in this stage are particularly susceptible to literal interpretations of faith. Symbols, stories, and beliefs from one's traditions are taken one-dimensionally and literally. They are what they are. Children are logical, believe in causation, and

BOX 9.5

A Child with Intuitive-Projective Faith

A friend of mine had twin 5-year-old boys whom she placed in a fundamentalist Christian day-care center. She was of a different faith but found this center to be the most convenient for her. One evening, about two weeks after the boys had started at that day-care center, I was having dinner at their house when one of the boys asked me, "Do you believe in God?" I began to respond by saying, "That's a difficult question," and before I could say any more he yelled out, "You're going to hell!" It was clear that the day-care had been promoting a view of the world that he unquestioningly took as his own. These new authorities in his life held a lot of power, and he imitated what he was hearing. My friend soon took her sons out of this day-care center.

My friend's son, in just a few short weeks, had taken in a fearful belief from a newfound social force in the environment—the day-care center. He projected his newfound fear onto me, telling me I would go to hell (he had learned that he would go to hell if he did not believe).

rely on the truth held by authorities, such as one's parents. Therefore, others play a particularly powerful role in developing the child's meaning-making system. These ways of making sense out of the world are strikingly similar to what Perry calls dualistic thinking.

STAGE 3, SYNTHETIC-CONVENTIONAL FAITH (12 TO 13) As the child moves into adolescence, he or she enters Piaget's formal-operational stage and takes on an increasingly complex and abstract view of the world. The individual is now able to reflect on his or her interactions with others and consider what is important for the development of a value system. Ultimately, the individual in this stage synthesizes all viewpoints from his or her social sphere into a unique meaning-making system. However, because the individual remains embedded within his or her social sphere, this meaning-making system is still naive because it reflects only those values within that sphere. One's faith is therefore unique to one's self, yet based on those close to him or her. This may be compared to Kegan's interpersonal stage of development, where the person is embedded in others for definition of self.

STAGE 4, INDIVIDUATIVE-REFLEXIVE FAITH (18 TO 19) Like the individual in Kegan's institutional stage, the individual in this stage has the ability to take responsibility for his or her own faith development. This is epitomized by being able to let go of values that are based solely on one's immediate social sphere and being able to develop a new meaning-making system through reflection and introspection. This relativistic individual now recognizes different types of faith experiences and may forcefully move toward a new ideology (e.g., the college student who grew up Baptist and becomes a Buddhist). Certainly, the beginning ability to reflect on self and see different points of view are indicative of postoperational and postconventional thinking. In addition, we can see remnants of Levinson's early adult transition stage as the individual is symbolically leaving his or her family.

STAGE 5, PARADOXICAL-CONJUNCTIVE FAITH (30 TO 32) This relativistic experience of faith happens when the individual is able to honor and affirm others who have different faith commitments while not denying his or her own faith. There is a newfound understanding of symbols and metaphors related to one's own faith tradition, as well as the faith traditions of others. There is an openness to other points of view, a commitment to one's own point of view, and a sense of humility regarding all that is known (or not known). This stage has strong leanings toward what Perry called "commitment in relativism."

STAGE 6, UNIVERSALIZING FAITH (38 TO 40) Few individuals reach this stage of faith, which involves a true acceptance of all others, regardless of stage or faith tradition. Fowler calls this "decentration from self," or the ability to fully understand the views of others, to be able to see the world through their eyes, a true knowing of others. The individual in this stage experiences faith as universal, beyond particular ideological beliefs, and this person is therefore able to embrace all others. This individual is able to integrate beliefs from many disparate viewpoints and synthesize them into a faith experience that is unique to him- or herself. This stage shares many similarities with Kegan's interindividual stage where the person may be described as self-actualized:

> *Stage Six bears the burden and challenge of relating to persons and issues concerned at . . . other stages and levels of development. It must do so with patience, compassion and helpfulness.* (Fowler, 1976, p. 202)

Other Developmental Theories

Many other developmental theories exist. For instance, Loevinger (1976) developed a theory of ego development that examined how individuals develop interpersonally, cognitively, and morally over the lifespan. In studying college students, Chickering developed a theory of college student development that elaborates on Erikson's stages of identity and intimacy (Chickering & Reisser, 1993) and assists counselors and others to understand college student development (see Chapter 18). Similarly, Gould (1972, 1978) and Vaillant (1977) have both examined adult development over the lifespan and offer stages similar to those of Erikson and Levinson. Other models include Belenky's developmental model of women's ways of understanding the world (Belenky et al., 1997); Stoltenberg and Delworth's supervision model, which was discussed in Chapter 8; Donald Super's (1984) model of career development, which will be examined in Chapter 11; and Michael D'Andrea's stages of racism, which will be explored in Chapter 14 (D'Andrea & Daniels, 1992). The theories mentioned in this chapter offer us a beginning look at some of the more popular developmental theories.

Applying Knowledge of Development

Counselors can assist people of all ages in making smooth psychological transitions as they develop. For instance, a counselor who has knowledge of normative growth in children will be alerted to developmental lags, which can be caused by such things as abuse, poverty, lack of parenting skills, and biology. In the areas of cognitive and moral development of children, knowledge of the developmental stages can give the counselor insight into the child's way of understanding the world and help identify stage-appropriate ways to work with children (McAuliffe, 2001). Similarly, knowing the predictable psychological pitfalls of adolescence can help counselors develop appropriate counseling skills, groups, and workshops to help youth through this often difficult time and make appropriate referrals when necessary.

Adult cognitive development models can offer counselors great insight into understanding how their clients construct reality and thus help them develop treatment plans that are appropriate to the client's developmental level. Also, such models can be used by school counselors and college student development specialists when trying to help teachers understanding their students. These models can then be used to develop new ways of teaching students that are developmentally appropriate. Finally, adult cognitive development models can be used by mental health professionals as a possible alternative to some of the pathological models of development.

Cognitive development models have direct application to counselor training. Beginning research reveals a strong positive relationship between level of adult cognitive development and the helper's ability to be empathic, nondirective, flexible, and nondogmatic and to have an internal locus of control (Basseches, 1984; Benack, 1984, 1988; Lovell, 1999a; Neukrug & McAuliffe, 1993). By assessing their developmental levels, graduate students can examine potential weaknesses and strengths that they may bring with them to the counseling relationship. In addition, counselor educators can adapt their training practices to the developmental level of the student (McAuliffe & Eriksen, 2000).

Through a knowledge of lifespan models and the stage-specific developmental issues that clients face, counselors can better comprehend the problems of clients and be less likely to pathologize normal developmental crises. When an issue of adjustment is found to be directly related to a current developmental crisis or unresolved issues from past developmental stages, counselors can devise appropriate strategies that can assist the client in the resolution of the crisis.

Finally, knowledge of faith development can help counselors understand the values, images, and stories of our clients and help us fully appreciate their uniqueness. The felon and the model citizen, the child and the older person, the individual from diverse cultures and the individual from mainstream culture, all have been driven by values, images, and stories. Know these and you know your client. Know your client, and you are much more likely to develop effective treatment strategies.

Comparison of Developmental Models

The varying models of development we have looked at in this chapter offer differing dimensions in our understanding of the person. Some of these models looked at cognitive functioning, others at lifespan development, and still others at moral reasoning and the development of faith. A model's seeming focus on one dimension (e.g., lifespan development) does not mean it may not hold some of the qualities of other models (e.g., cognitive development). With some of the models, the individual will pass through each of the stages; in others, he or she may only pass through some of the early stages. Although all of the models are sequential (stages build upon stages), only some of the models are hierarchical, which implies that each stage is considered better than the previous stage. Figure 9.3 offers a visual comparison of the varying models we looked at in this chapter.

Multicultural Issue: The Development of Cultural Identity

Like many characteristics, how we identify with our culture/ethnic group can be explained as a developmental process. Thus, we can examine how we have grown and changed as men, as women, as gay or heterosexual men and women, as blacks, as whites,

FIGURE 9.3 **A Comparison of Developmental Models**

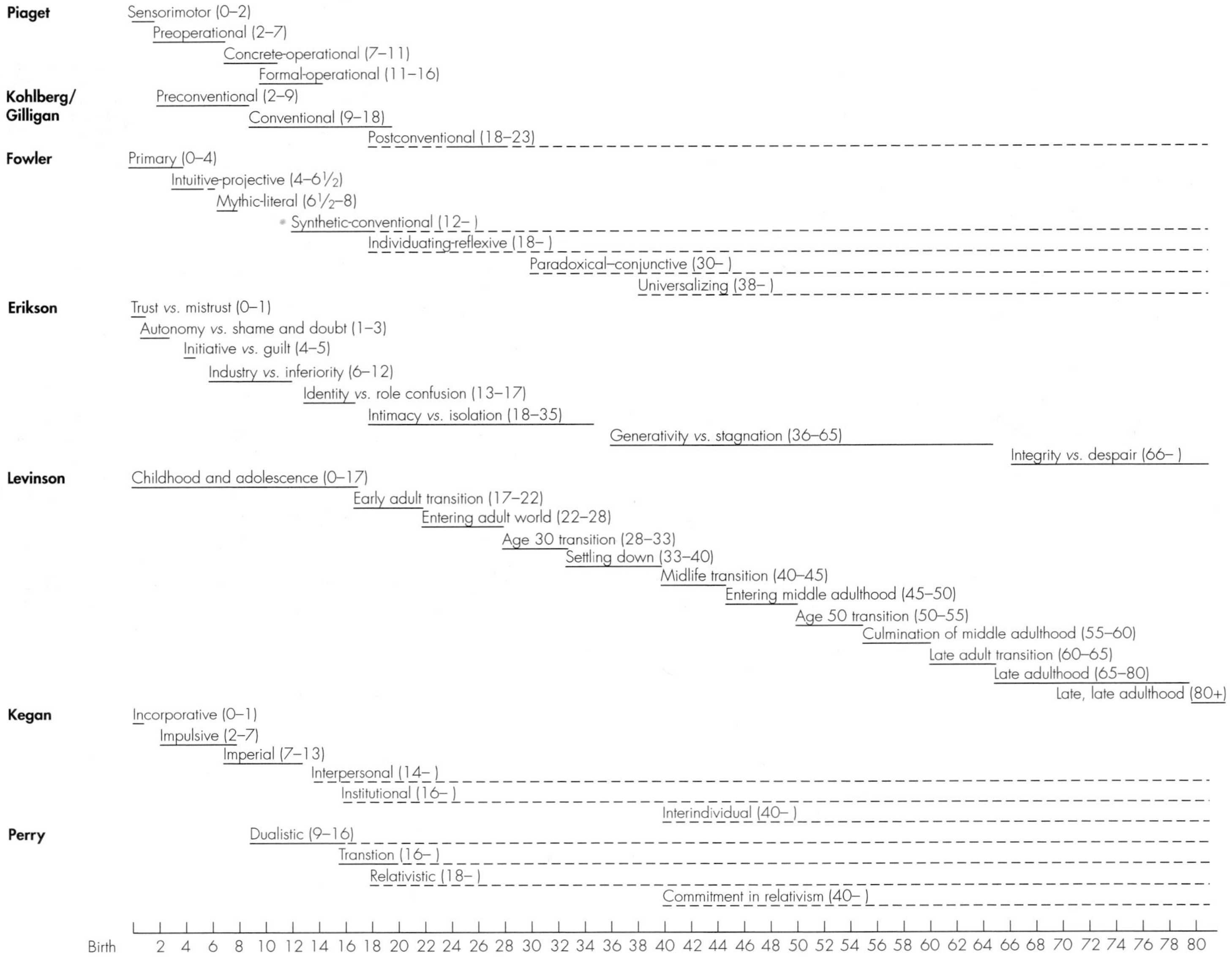

Note: The onset of certain stages can vary by several months in childhood and several years in adulthood, In fact, in many of the above developmental schemes, an individual may never reach the later stages of possible development. A dashed line represents the age range in which an individual could potentially attain a particular stage. A solid line represents the age range in which an individual is more likely to attain a particular stage.

as Asians, and so forth (Atkinson et al., 1998; Sabnani, Ponterotto, & Borodovsky; 1991). These models assume there is a predictable progression through stages of development of cultural/ethnic consciousness. In Chapter 14 we will have the opportunity to explore some of these models in detail.

With some research tentatively showing that racial identity might be related to one's ability as a counselor, particularly when counseling culturally different clients (Ottavi, Pope-Davis, & Dings, 1994), it is imperative that as students of counseling you assess where you are in the development of your cultural/ethnic identity. Counseling programs can assist students in examining themselves; but, ultimately, if we are to move toward an identity that embraces and effectively works with all cultures, each of us must be willing to actively and purposefully look inward (D'Andrea & Daniels, 1992).

Ethical, Professional, and Legal Issues

The ACA Code of Ethics: A Developmental Emphasis

The counseling profession today prides itself on having a positive, growth-oriented, developmental focus. This emphasis is reflected in the preamble of the ACA code of ethics (1995):

> *The American Counseling Association is an educational, scientific and professional organization whose members are dedicated to the enhancement of human development throughout the life span.*

As a counselor there is no doubt that you will come across and work with some clients whom you might consider to be abnormal, mentally ill, or, at the very least, a little out of the mainstream. We may even diagnose and label them, but we must always have respect for our clients' dignity and honor their unique developmental journey. Through our caring, our knowledge of development, and our effective use of skills, we can help lift some of the burdens clients feel and assist them in their journey through life.

Professional Associations

Although the entire counseling profession has a developmental foundation, two divisions of ACA particularly focus on development across the lifespan: the Association for Adult Development and Aging (AADA), which publishes the journal *Adultspan*; and the Counseling Association for Humanistic Education and Development (C-AHEAD), which publishes the *Journal of Humanistic Education and Development*. If you have a particular interest in the knowledge of developmental theory, you might consider joining one or both of these divisions.

Legal Issue: Missing Problems Because We're Too Positive

Psychiatrists, and some clinical psychologists, often get a bad rap for being too oriented toward psychopathology. They tend to diagnose and label, and this tunnel vision can sometimes prevent client growth. Counselors sometimes have the opposite problem. By seeing only the positive side of human nature, they may sometimes miss serious pathology, suicidal or homicidal thoughts, and deeply troubling feelings. A counselor who misses a serious problem can damage the counseling process and may even have some responsibility for a client's suicide or homicide. Clearly, this opens the counselor up to lawsuits.

Counselors must not be fearful of seeing the dark side of people. One can help a person look at his or her shadow and yet still have an optimistic view of the person. In fact, some would say that only through looking at one's darkest side can healing and growth occur.

The Counselor in Process: Understanding Your Own Development

Recently, a friend of mine was telling me about a theory of development that, unlike Levinson, suggests that we are always in transition, we never have periods of rest. Um, I thought to myself, that certainly feels like my life,—it's kind of a roller coaster that sometimes moves fast and smoothly, while other times it feels like an uphill climb and chugging along. Maybe there are short periods of rest, but they sure do seem to last only a moment or two. I guess I can either go along for the ride or get off. I think I'll keep moving. But maybe while on this roller coaster of life, I can do my best to make sure the ride is as smooth as possible—kind of oil the wheels, make sure I'm in the seat snugly, and get to know the person sitting next to me.

Our lives can be unexplored and bumpy, or, as we move along our unique paths, we can check ourselves out, look at the path ahead of us, and make sure that things are as smooth as possible. This, I believe, means exploring our own development. It means examining the physical, social, and psychological forces that have impinged upon us and continue to affect us. It means looking at the developmental crises in our past that may still be impinging upon us, exploring the developmental phases we are currently experiencing, and thinking about where our future development might take us.

Knowledge of our own development increases our self-knowledge and helps us understand the ways in which we interact with others. But perhaps what is most important, understanding our own development helps us understand the relationships we form with our clients.

Summary

This chapter looked at development: child development, adult development, cognitive development, moral development, lifespan development, and the development of faith. We started by noting that, by their nature, developmental theories are continual; are orderly and sequential; build upon themselves; are painful yet growth-producing; are transtheoretical; are preventive, optimistic, and wellness oriented. A developmental framework allows us to understand the common characteristics of people at different ages and stages, the typical problems experienced by people as they pass through the lifespan, the causes of some problems, and therapeutic strategies for change.

The chapter began by presenting an overview of development through the lifespan and particularly focused on some of the physical and associated psychosocial changes that occur in childhood, adolescence, and adulthood. It was noted that development occurs at fairly predictable rates, and a counselor or developmental specialist who is aware of physiological and psychological timetables can assess whether or not a person is on target for his or her development.

Within the chapter we examined a number of developmental models. We started by looking at cognitive and moral development. We noted that Piaget examined how cognitive development unravels and identified a number of stages that he called sensorimotor, preoperational, concrete-operational, and formal-operational. He found that as children move through these stages there is an orderly progression that begins with the child's ability to maintain mental images and language skills, leads to the child's ability to think logically and orderly, and culminates in adolescence with the child's ability to think abstractly and in complex ways.

We next examined Kohlberg's theory of moral development, in which he identifies three levels of development called preconventional, conventional, and postconventional thinking. These stages reflect Kohlberg's belief that moral reasoning goes through a series of stages that move from extreme narcissism toward concern for democratic principles and one's personal conscience. We also noted that Gilligan argued that unlike men's moral development, which tends to be individualistically oriented, women's development includes a standard of care whereby women are concerned with how their choices affect others.

Looking at adult cognitive development, we examined two theories: Kegan's theory of constructive development and Perry's theory of epistemological reflection. Both Kegan and Perry believe that we continually construct reality and that this occurs in stages, with many individuals never having the opportunity to reach the higher stages of development. Although Kegan's stages span the life cycle, his theory is mostly applied to adult development. His stages are called incorporative, impulsive, imperial, interpersonal, institutional, and interindividual. Kegan believes that in adulthood individuals move from a narcissistic position, to a position of mutuality, to a place where the individual develops a strong sense of self, to the final position where the person is a complex thinker who can perceive situations from many perspectives, have a strong sense of self, and be able to hear feedback.

Perry's theory, which focuses mostly on college students, mapped the potential changes of young adults as they move from being dualistic, black-and-white thinkers toward becoming relativistic people who can see differing perspectives. The highest stage for Perry is the person who is committed in relativism, epitomized by the person who can see varying perspectives yet have a strong commitment to specific values.

Lifespan development was another frame from which we examined the development of the person. Reviewing the theories of Erikson and Levinson, we noted that both present age-specific stages through which all people must pass (Levinson only focuses on men). Erikson's stages include: trust versus mistrust, autonomy versus shame and doubt, initiative versus guilt, industry versus inferiority, identity versus role confusion, intimacy versus isolation, generativity versus stagnation, and integrity versus despair. Levinson's theory identified four periods in a man's life: childhood and adolescence, early adulthood, middle adulthood, and late adulthood. Levinson believed that each era is marked by transition and periods of stability and has its own unique tasks to master.

The final theory we examined was Fowler's model of faith development. Defining faith as a person's core values, the images of power that drive that person, and the stories that motivate the individual consciously and unconsciously, we stressed that Fowler's model is much broader than a religious focus on faith. Presenting six stages of faith development, Fowler suggests that the development of faith parallels many other developmental theories and moves from a rigid adherence to a point of view, toward a relativistic understanding of varying points of view, to an acceptance of and love for many different perspectives while simultaneously having one's own faith experience.

In this chapter we also noted that like many characteristics we examined, our identity with our culture/ethnic group can be explained as a developmental process. We stressed the fact that if we are to work effectively with all clients, we must risk looking inward and gain an understanding of our own cultural/ethnic identity.

As we neared the end of the chapter we highlighted the notion that the foundation of our profession is developmental and noted that ACA has two divisions that focus on development. This developmental focus stresses the dignity of the client and client growth and change while discouraging labeling and diagnosing. While on the one hand this is our strength, we warned that at times this positive, future-oriented focus may make some counselors become too lax and miss a serious client problem. This could have devastating effects and lead to ethical complaints and lawsuits against the counselor.

Finally, we stressed that knowledge of our own development can greatly assist us in understanding ourselves, the ways in which we interact with others, and the ways in which we form relationships with our clients.

INFOTRAC and Other Information Resources (e.g., ERIC and PsycINFO)

Note: When relevant, key words are in quotation marks.

1. Research any of the "developmental theories" in more depth.
2. Compare and contrast "developmental issues" related to "counseling children" and "counseling adolescents."
3. What unique "developmental issues" are related to "counseling adults."

CHAPTER **10**

Abnormal Development, Diagnosis, and Psychopharmacology

My second job after my master's degree was as an outpatient therapist at a community mental health center. Suddenly, I was working closely with clinical psychologists and psychiatrists. I had a caseload that included a number of clients with serious emotional disorders. Every time I conducted an intake interview, I was required to follow it up with a consultation with the psychiatrist. Invariably, he wanted me to talk diagnosis and clinical terms I had never considered or learned about at school or in past jobs. I had to catch up quickly. However, part of me didn't want to because I really didn't believe in this diagnosis stuff anyway. I had to use this book called the *Diagnostic and Statistical Manual-II (DSM-II)*. It had descriptions for the various emotional disorders. It soon became my bible.

Well, I rather quickly learned about making diagnoses, and I didn't find it half bad. It helped me categorize clients, which seemed to help organize my thinking about them. It helped me understand which medications might be appropriate for specific diagnoses. And it sometimes helped me in treatment planning. However, I was still doubtful–a part of me thought, "Is this real, or are we making up these categories? I've experienced moments of all these diagnoses at different times in my life. And maybe diagnosing these people increases the likelihood that they'll remain ill, like a self-fulfilling prophecy. We see them that way, we label them that way, and they become that way." Most of all it bothered me when some of the other clinicians would smugly say things like, "Oh, he's borderline, he can't act any other way."

It's more than 25 years later now, and I hope I've learned and have become a little more sophisticated about abnormal behavior and diagnosis. However, whenever I listen to someone diagnosing another, there's still a part of me that asks, "Is this real?" I believe this is a healthy part of me and is reflective of the history of our profession–a profession that has, in the past, balked at the use of diagnosis and the concept of "abnormal behavior." On the other hand, maybe there is something to categorizing behavior and using diagnosis. I would hope that I could understand abnormal behavior, reap the possible benefits of using diagnosis, and continue to have a healthy questioning attitude.

This chapter will examine the concepts of abnormal behavior, diagnosis, and psychopharmacology, concepts that some of us may continue to question. We will start by examining reasons why these concepts may be important and examine the close relationships among them. We will then describe psychopathology from genetic, biological, psychodynamic, learning theory, and humanistic perspectives and present a brief description of how a large number of counselors today integrate these perspectives. This will be followed by an overview of the *Diagnostic and Statistical Manual-IV-TR (DSM-IV-TR)*, the current diagnostic system used in the United States and through much of the world. We will also offer a brief overview of many of the psychotropic medications currently used in the treatment of various disorders. As usual, we will conclude the chapter with an examination of multicultural, ethical, professional, and legal issues related to the concepts we are studying.

Why Study Abnormal Behavior, Diagnosis, and Medication?

- John is in fifth grade and has been assessed as having a conduct disorder and attention deficit disorder with hyperactivity (ADHD). John's mother has a panic disorder and is taking antianxiety medication. His father is bipolar and taking lithium. Jill is John's school counselor. It is written into John's individualized educational plan (IEP) that he should see Jill for individual counseling and for group counseling. Jill must also periodically consult with John's mother and father.
- Tenesha is a sophomore in college. She has just broken up with her boyfriend, is severely depressed, and cannot concentrate on her school work; her grades have dropped from A's to C's. She comes to the counseling center and sobs during most of her first session with her counselor. She admits having always struggled with depression but states that, "This is worse than ever; I need to get better if I am going to stay in school. Can you give me any medication to help me so I won't have to drop out?"
- Eduard goes daily to the day treatment center at the local mental health center. He seems fairly coherent and generally in good spirits. He has been hospitalized for schizophrenia on numerous occasions and now takes Haldol and Cogentin to relieve his symptoms. He admits to Jordana, one of his counselors, that when he doesn't take his medication he believes that computers have consciousness and are conspiring through the World Wide Web to take over the world. His insurance company pays for his treatment. He will not receive reimbursement from his insurance company unless Jordana specifies a diagnosis on the insurance form.

With evidence that a large percentage of Americans have or will experience an emotional disorder (Hersen & Van Hasselt, 2001), it is clear that regardless of where you are employed, you will be working with clients who (1) have serious emotional problems that are sometimes labeled as abnormal behavior or as an emotional disorder, (2) have been given or are in need of a diagnosis for treatment purposes and/or for legal reasons, and (3) are taking or in need of medication. Although controversy exists about defining "abnormality," diagnosing, and using psychotropic medications, these topics must be addressed by counselors today (Fong, 1995; Hinkle, 1994a, b; Hohenshil, 1994). This has not always been the case.

Counselor educators and counselors have historically had a disdain for diagnosing and labeling and have at times opposed the use of psychotropic medication. In fact, within counseling programs, training in abnormal development was practically unheard of until recently. The reasons for this were many. First, the early history of the counseling profession was largely influenced by the humanistic approaches to counseling, which downplayed the notion of abnormal behavior, the role of diagnosis, and the use of medication. This influence also led counseling professionals to believe that training in psychopathology and diagnosis would unduly stigmatize individuals. In addition, many counselors and counselor educators believed that counselors should be working with "normal" individuals and in a preventive and wellness role. Seeing no practical purpose for having training in psychopathology, they felt that the role of the counselor should be to focus on developmental issues and the positive side of human nature. Recently, however, many counseling programs have begun to include in their curriculum a focus on psychopathology, diagnosis, and psychopharmacology (Hinkle, 1994a; Hohenshil, 1993a, 1994). There are many reasons for this change:

1. Counselors in all specialty areas are increasingly working with clients who are severely disturbed.
2. In contrast to past years, when most graduates from counseling programs obtained jobs in schools where they infrequently encountered serious emotional disorders, a large portion of graduates now work in community agencies, often with individuals with mental illness.
3. Federal and state laws (e.g., PL94-142) now require that students with severe emotional disorders be serviced in the schools. Thus, today's school counselor is more likely to be dealing with students with severe emotional problems.
4. Many counselors accept that they need to know diagnostic procedures if they are to receive reimbursement from insurance companies.
5. Society has increased tolerance for individuals with emotional problems and mental disorders, and there is less stigmatizing of individuals with diagnosis.
6. A diagnostic system offers clinicians a common language with which to discuss client issues.
7. There has been a retreat by some from the rigid adherence to a philosophy that all mental illness is a social construction.
8. Diagnosis can sometimes be helpful in the development of treatment plans, and treatment plans sometimes may include the use of medication.
9. There is a growing body of evidence that our biology contributes to, and in some cases may even determine, some forms of mental illness.
10. Some people get better with medications, and we now understand that we had best not throw out the baby with the bathwater (the concepts of abnormal behavior and of diagnosis are inextricably tied to the use of medications).

You Can't Have One without the Other: Abnormal Behavior, Diagnosis, and Medication

Webster defines *abnormality* as "not conformed or conforming to rule; deviating from a type or standard; irregular; unnatural; contrary to system or law." This is not too different from Davison's and Neale's (2001) more clinical definition:

> *Patterns of emotion, thought, and action deemed pathological for one or more of the following reasons: infrequent occurrence, violation of norms, personal distress, disability or dysfunction, and unexpectedness.* (glossary, p. 1)

If you believe that there are deviations from the norm, sometimes dramatic ones, you're probably going to want to classify and understand them. This is what diagnosis does. Therefore, such classification systems as the *Diagnostic and Statistical Manual-IV-TR (DSM-IV-TR)* (APA, 2000) offer clinicians a mechanism for understanding how some individuals deviate from more typical behavior. In addition, if you can classify individuals into different categories, you can research which treatment strategies, including the use of medications, will best apply to each diagnostic category. For instance, it is now clear that psychoanalytic therapy does little for a person who has an obsessive–compulsive disorder, and today one would be hard-pressed to find someone recommending using a stimulant for depression. Well, this used to be the treatment of choice!

Today, there is less controversy about the concept of abnormality, with most clinicians believing that psychopathology is a function of genetic, biological, sociological, and psychological factors. We may and probably should argue about the term *abnormal,* but no matter what you call it, there are individuals who exhibit some rather unusual or deviant behaviors from the norm. We may and probably should argue that diagnosis is stigmatizing, but there are individuals who are helped because there was an adequate diagnosis and a subsequent treatment plan. And we probably should argue about the overuse of medication, but it is clear today that some people are helped, and even miraculously changed, due to medication.

Personality Development and Abnormal Behavior

Genetic and Biological Explanations

Genetics, which is the science of hereditary characteristics, is a subset of biology, which is the science of life. Biology therefore includes genetic factors, but genetics does not include all biological factors. For instance, if we say that biological factors can affect the development of intelligence in children, we are referring to such things as prenatal care, nutrition, exposure to toxins, hormonal changes, genetics, and so forth. However, when we assert that genetics can affect the development of intelligence in children, we are referring to how the expression of genes, not other factors, can affect cognitive ability.

The nature versus nurture debate as it relates to personality formation has a long and turbulent history and continues today. However, the schisms among genetic determinists, environmental advocates, and intrapsychic zealots are clearly much less than ever before. This may be partially because the concept of heritability has changed, with genes no longer being seen as deterministically causing behavior. Today's views of genetics assume that in most cases there are complex environmental influences on the action of genes (Nigg & Goldsmith, 1994). In addition, the belief that genes determine one's personality at birth has been dismissed, with the current thinking being that genetic influences "are dynamic over the life span" (Nigg & Goldsmith, 1994, p. 349):

> *The general misconception that genetic models are uniquely deterministic is an obstacle to the necessary integration of research across diverse levels of analysis, including genetic and psychosocial models of behavior. . . . Psychotherapy may*

> *remain the most accessible avenue of intervention for many personality problems, even if genetic influences are discovered. . . .* (p. 372)

Clinicians today realize that research on the effects of genetics and other biological factors generally supports the view that there is a genetic predisposition to many forms of mental illness and even to many less severe emotional problems. It is assumed, for instance, that temperament, or that part of our personality that is biologically based and stable across time, is probably developed "through [a] bidirectional interplay between inborn, temperamental attributes [e.g., genetics] and external demands, supports, and circumstances" (Teglasi, 1995, p. 4). Therefore, one's temperament can act as a buffer against or be predisposed toward the expression of certain personality characteristics (e.g., emotional disorders) (Teglasi, 1995). For instance, when two individuals are placed in a nurturing environment, symptomatic behavior may not be observed in either. However, place these same two individuals in a stressful environment, and one may develop an anxiety disorder while the other's temperament may act as a buffer against the development of a disorder. In examining child development, Niehoff (1994) pulls together some of the most recent findings on the interaction between biology, environment, and personality formation:

> *. . . the denial of basic needs, antecedent stresses of mistreatment and abuse, and extremes of parental behavior . . . are cited as "toxic" factors that in conjunction with biological causes, supersede other environment enhancing forces and cause more children to grow into adulthood with dysfunctional behaviors.* (pp. 3–4)

The linking of biology, including genetics, with environmental factors in the development of personality moves the counseling profession toward an approach that is truly holistic. Understanding the intricate interaction among these variables can be very powerful in the effective use of counseling. Clinicians in today's world should no longer be shy about consulting experts familiar with genetics and biology as these efforts can help to provide the most broadly based treatment for their clients.

Which emotional disorders are most likely to be biologically based? In an exhaustive review of the literature, Nigg and Goldsmith (1994) found that most personality disorders found on Axis II (see p. 268) have a basis in genetics. Other disorders have also been suspected to be genetically linked. In fact, it may be that most emotional problems have some genetic component, including something as basic as being prone to anxiety and pessimism (grumpy, fearful neurotics . . . , 1996; Lesch et al., 1996).

It would seem to make intuitive sense that if a disorder is at least partly biologically based, one might consider using biological interventions in addition to psychotherapy. Biological interventions can be defined broadly and can include such things as stress reduction, exercise, how we eat, how we sleep, the amount of light we receive, and of course psychopharmacology. All of these, in some manner or another, affect one or more major biological systems and can positively or negatively affect our mood (Norden, 1996). In addition, it should also be of no surprise that research on some forms of mental health problems shows that the combination of counseling and the use of psychotropic medications is more effective than either counseling or medication alone (Conte, Plutchik, Wild, & Karasu, 1986; Norden, 1996).

Freud's Model of Psychosexual Development

As we remember from Chapter 4, Freud believed that we are born with sexual and aggressive instincts that unconsciously affect our behaviors throughout life. He identified a structure of personality that includes the id, the depository of all of our instincts; the ego, the development of the rational part of our mind; and the superego, which constitutes the moral part of our mind. Freud believed that infantile sexuality is an expression of instinctual body urges associated with different bodily functions. Based on these pleasure zones, Freud identified stages of development through which each individual will pass. The satisfaction of these erogenous zones, or lack thereof, is crucial to the establishment of our ego and superego and ultimately to the healthy functioning of the individual or to abnormal behavior (Appignanesi, 1990; Corey, 2000a).

Born all id, the infant is immediately thrust into the first stage of psychosexual development, the oral stage, in which pleasure is received through feeding. The hungry infant wants to be fed, and his or her main goals are to obtain pleasure through feeding and to reduce stress caused by hunger and lack of tactile stimulation received through the mouth. The major developmental task of this stage, which occurs between birth and age 1½, is how the child becomes attached to the mother (or the major caretaker) as a function of feeding. Therefore, this relationship becomes the prototype or model for a number of personality characteristics, including the ability to be trusting, tenacity, the ability to refuse, aggression, greediness, acquisitiveness, and sarcasm. Corey (2000a) notes that personality problems from this stage can include "the development of a view of the world based on mistrust, fear of reaching out to others, rejection of affection, fear of loving and trusting, low self-esteem, isolation and withdrawal, and inability to form or maintain intense relationships" (p. 76). From this perspective, one can see how abusive or neglectful parenting can lead to pathological behavior.

During the anal stage, the child receives pleasure from bowel movements, and the child's instinctual urges become focused on the anal erogenous zone. This stage, which occurs between ages 1½ and 3, is distinguished by a child's physiological readiness to be toilet trained. The main function of this stage is for the child to develop his or her capacity to retain or evacuate, which becomes a metaphor for the child's ability to master his or her impulses. The parents' attempt to introduce the idea that there are socially appropriate behaviors (the prototype being using the potty) is significant in the development of the child's ego and superego. However, defecating is pleasurable, and the child resists interference with this pleasurable experience. Consequently, the child becomes embroiled in a battle of control, independence, power, and doing the socially correct thing (Hall, 1954). Ultimately, the child has to learn how to control his or her feelings of aggression, housed in the id, and does so by the development of the ego, which learns to deal rationally with the world, and through the use of defense mechanisms, which are now being spawned in an effort to have the child restrain murderous impulses.

Parental attitudes about defecation, cleanliness, control, and responsibility have a major effect on personality development. For instance, parents who are particularly strict may have children who retaliate and aggress against them and who ultimately grow into adults with little respect for authority, who are irresponsible, messy, disorderly, extreme, and controlling of others. On the other hand, some children with punitive and strict parents may assume their parents were right and become extremely neat, fastidious, compulsive about orderliness, and disgusted by and fearful of dirt, and generally exhibit other over-controlled behavior (Hall, 1954). You might say that these individuals are constipated in their relationship to the world.

Other parents, who extensively praise children on their ability to go to the potty, can lead them to have an exaggerated sense of self. As adults, these individuals may make things to please others or may be generous, philanthropic, and charitable. On the other hand, too much emphasis on toilet training may leave the child with the feeling he or she has lost something when defecating, ultimately leading toward a sense of depression and anxiety of future losses. These individuals may hoard things and be thrifty in an attempt not to feel loss. Finally, becoming fixated upon the erotic pleasure of defecating can lead to an adult need to collect and possess things, or, in a defensive posture, these individuals may respond in the opposite way by becoming reckless, gambling, and giving away possessions.

In the third stage of development, the phallic stage, which occurs from ages 3 to 5, the erogenous zone again shifts, this time to the child's genitals. The child becomes aware not only of his or her genitals but also of the genitals of the opposite sex. The child in this stage receives pleasure from self-stimulation. The types of permission parents give the child in this stage can greatly affect the child's attitudes and values and are crucial in the development of the individual's superego.

During this stage an Oedipus or an Electra complex is awakened in which the child identifies with the same-sex parent. As a result of this identification, instinctual urges take over, and the child wishes to possess the opposite-sex parent and eliminate the same-sex parent. However, the child soon realizes this is not achievable. The subsequent guilt felt as a result of the child's attempts to possess the opposite-sex parent is eventually resolved by the child developing a sense of moral responsibility toward the world—there are things that we cannot have, and we must live in this world responsibly. These values are stored in the superego. Thus, this stage is crucial for the development of the nature of attachments to significant men and women in one's life, the identification with masculinity or femininity, and the development of the superego. The superego is crucial for later development as its internalized version becomes our parents within us and the morality of our social system.

The latency stage, ages 5 through puberty, is a period of relative relaxation for the child where he or she replaces earlier sexual feelings with a focus on socialization. Here the child becomes more aware of peers, and there is increased attention placed on peer-related activities. Freud's final stage of development, the genital stage, begins at puberty and continues through the lifespan. Sexual energy, in this stage, is focused on social activities with peers and on love relationships. During this stage we discover whether earlier stages of development were resolved adequately, as the adult's behavior will reflect unresolved issues from the earlier stages. These issues will often be cloaked by defense mechanisms but can generally be deduced through analysis.

As reflected in the above, parenting behaviors through the developmental stages affect the formation of the ego and superego and establish the precarious balance among the id, ego, and superego:

> *Thus the superego takes up a kind of intermediate position between the id and the external world [the ego]; it unites in itself the influences of the present and the past. In the establishment of the super-ego we have before us, as it were, an example of the way in which the present is changed into the past. . . .* (Freud, 1969, p. 64)

Ultimately, how the id, ego, and superego impinge on our lives, unconsciously and to a lesser degree consciously, determines the individual's level of health or dysfunction. Our defense mechanisms, created to ward off anxiety resulting from tension among the id, ego, and superego, give us a peek into our early development and the kinds of parenting that we received.

Conclusion

Freud was quite specific in his description of disorders and their roots, with the oral, anal, and phallic psychosexual stages holding the potential for the later development of dysfunctional behavior. However, some of these assertions have not held up under research. Despite this fact, the basic core of his theory remains tenable. For instance, the concept that development occurs as we pass through a series of erogenous zones and that early parenting can affect personality formation is considered, at the very least, to be an important factor in understanding emotional disorders. Also, the concept that there is an unconscious that affects our behaviors has remained an important factor for most therapists in their understanding of behavior. Finally, the idea that we can explore our early development and examine how it has affected our personality style is important in almost all counseling approaches. Whether or not one agrees with most of what Freud conceptualized, it is clear that the lens through which counselors and others view the developing person has been greatly affected by the psychoanalytic view of development.

Learning Theory and the Development of the Person

> *The child is born empty of psychological content into a world of coherently organized content. Like a mirror, however, the child comes to reflect his environment; like an empty slate he is written upon by external stimuli; like a wax table he stores the impressions left by these stimuli; and like a machine he may be made to react in response to stimulating agents.* (Langer, 1969, p. 51)

This radical quote, reflecting early behavioral thought, shows the rigid views that many learning theorists held about the development of the person. Drastically differing with Freud's notion on instincts, Skinner and other early learning theorists believed that "the most important causes of behavior are environmental and [that] it only confuses the matter to talk about inner drives" (Nye, 2000, p. 80). However, the vast majority of learning theorists today have a much broader view of development, with many now believing that genetic factors, cognitive structures, and even intrapsychic forces play a role in personality development. However, the basic core of this nonstage theory is still learning theory.

As we learned in Chapter 4, learning theorists believe that individuals learn behaviors through operant conditioning, classical conditioning, or modeling (social learning) and therefore place emphasis on how positive or negative reinforcement, models, and the pairing of an unconditioned stimulus with a conditioned stimulus affects our personality development (Bandura et al., 1963; Skinner, 1971; Wolpe, 1969). Operant conditioning is generally considered to be the most common type of conditioning and occurs when behavior is reinforced, thus increasing the probability of that response occurring again. Over the years, through rigorous research, Skinner and others delineated many principles of operant conditioning, each of which is crucial to the shaping of behaviors and the development of personality. A small portion of these include:

1. *Positive reinforcement:* Any stimulus that, when presented, increases the likelihood of a response.
2. *Negative reinforcement:* Any stimulus that, when removed, increases the likelihood of a response.
3. *Punishment:* Following a response with an aversive stimulus to a decrease a specific behavior. Punishment is often an ineffective method of changing behavior as it may lead to undesirable side effects (e.g., counteraggression).
4. *Schedules of reinforcement:* The numerous ways in which a stimulus can be arranged to reinforce behavior; based on elapsed time and frequency of responses.
5. *Discrimination:* The ability of a person to respond selectively to one stimulus but not respond to a similar stimulus.

6. *Generalization:* The tendency for stimuli that are similar to a conditioned stimulus to take on the power of the conditioned stimulus.
7. *Extinction:* The ceasing of a behavior because it is not reinforced.
8. *Spontaneous recovery:* The tendency for responses to recur after a brief period of time after they have been extinguished.

Skinner and other learning theorists maintain that reinforcements often occur very subtly and in ways that we may not immediately recognize (Nye, 2000; Skinner, 1971; Wolpe, 1969). Therefore, things like changes in voice intonation, subtle glances, TV shows that appeal to us, or body language could subliminally affect our personality development. They note that by examining a situation closely enough, one could attain an understanding of the types of reinforcement contingencies that were instrumental in shaping an individual's behavior.

Recently, many learning theorists have included a cognitive framework within their conceptualization of development. Such cognitive therapists as Ellis (1962), Meichenbaum (1977), and Beck (1976) believe that not only does the behavior of the individual become reinforced, but also the ways in which the individual thinks. Therefore, thinking can dramatically affect behavior, and behavior can dramatically affect thinking in a complex interaction. Cognitive-behaviorists have challenged the beliefs of the original behavioral purists and have changed the manner in which most learning theorists conceptualize the development of the individual.

Because abnormal development is seen as a result of reinforcement contingencies, learning theorists believe that change can occur at any point in the life cycle. Therefore, one can identify dysfunctional behaviors and irrational thinking, determine the reinforcers that continue the dysfunctional ways of living in the world, and devise methods of reinforcing new behaviors and different cognitions.

Summarizing some of the major factors that can lead to healthy or abnormal development, modern-day learning theorists believe:

1. The individual is born capable of developing a multitude of personality characteristics.
2. Behaviors and cognitions are continually reinforced by significant others and by cultural influences in our environment.
3. Reinforcement of behaviors and cognitions is generally very complex and can occur in very subtle ways.
4. Abnormal development is largely the result of the kinds of behaviors and cognitions that have been reinforced (other factors such as genetics may also affect development).
5. By carefully analyzing how behaviors and cognitions are reinforced, we can understand why an individual exhibits his or her current behavioral and cognitive repertoire.
6. Through the application of principles of learning, old dysfunctional behaviors can be extinguished and new healthy behaviors can be learned.

Conclusion

Learning theory offers a unique, objective, straightforward method of understanding personality development (Myers, 2001). Maladaptive behavior is believed to be the result of dysfunctional behaviors and faulty cognitions that are reinforced, sometimes in very subtle ways. Because maladaptive behavior is believed to be at least partly learned, it can be unlearned and new functional behaviors can be adopted. Thus, modern-day learning theorists generally have an optimistic view of the person in that they believe the person can change his or her way of living in the world. Today's behaviorists, therefore, have an antideterministic view of human nature in that they believe people can use reinforcement contingencies and biological interventions (e.g., medication) to become better human beings.

The Humanistic Understanding of Personality Development

The humanistic approaches that have probably had the most impact on our understanding of the development of the individual have been the person-centered approach of Carl Rogers (1951) and the hierarchical approach of Abraham Maslow (1968, 1970). Rogers's and Maslow's ideas are in stark contrast to the views of psychoanalysts and the learning theorists:

> *I think it is now possible to be able to delineate this view of human nature as a total, single, comprehensive system of psychology even though much of it has arisen as a reaction against the limitations (as philosophies of human nature) of the two most comprehensive psychologies now available behaviorism (or associationism) and classical, Freudian psychoanalysis. . . . In the past I have called it the "holistic-dynamic." . . .* (Maslow, 1968, p. 189)

Maslow stated that people have what he called a hierarchy of needs, with lower-order needs having to be satisfied before the next need on the hierarchy can be assimilated (see Figure 10.1). This has great implications for understanding the motivations of individuals. For instance, by examining Figure 10.1 we can see that an individual who is hungry or in need of shelter probably has little ability to focus on the needs of love and belonging; the individual who feels unloved and does not have some sense of a social support will necessarily have lowered self-esteem; and so forth. The highest need to be satisfied, stated Maslow, was self-actualization, in which one is in touch with one's feelings, has high self-worth, is alive and spontaneous, and has developed a sense of one's own spirituality.

Although Rogers's theory is not a hierarchical theory of development, on many occasions he stated his support for the ideas of Maslow and implied that an individual who is given a nurturing environment would develop according to Maslow's hierarchy. He believed there was a natural fit between his and Maslow's ideas.

Rogers believed that individuals are born good and have a natural tendency to actualize and obtain fulfillment if placed in a nurturing environment that includes empathy, congruence, and positive regard. As opposed to Freud, Rogers did not emphasize the importance of instincts, the unconscious, or developmental stages in the formation of personality development. As opposed to Skinner, Rogers did not place much value on reinforcement contingencies in creating the personality of the individual. In fact, in the 1960s, Rogers and Skinner did a series of debates that highlighted their differences. One such difference was Rogers's strong belief that the quality of the relationship between the child and his or her major caretakers is one of the most significant factors in personality development (Rogers, 1951, 1957, 1980a).

Rogers believed that we all have a need to be loved. He stated that significant people in our lives often place upon us conditions of worth or ways we should act in order to

FIGURE 10.1
Maslow's Hierarchy

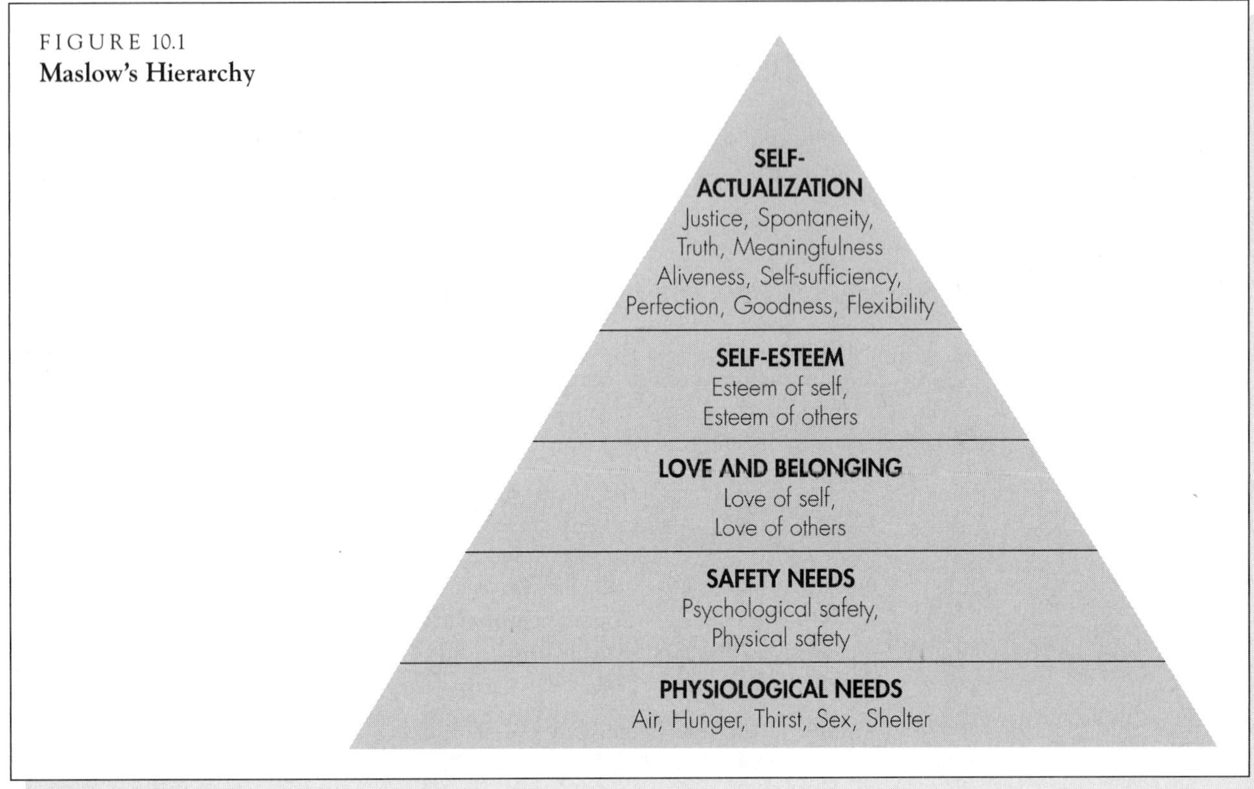

receive their love. Therefore, as children we will sometimes act in ways to please others in an effort to obtain a sense of acceptance even if the pleasing self is not our real self. In essence, the child has learned that by acting in an incongruent or nongenuine fashion, he or she will receive acceptance. This nongenuine way of living then becomes the way of relating to the world and prevents the person from becoming self-actualized, becoming one's true self. This is when our self-actualizing tendency is thwarted.

Rogers would not have used the term *abnormal*. He felt strongly that this term and terms like it are stigmatizing and are not accurate. He believed that all dysfunctional behaviors were the result of individuals having conditions of worth placed upon them that would eventually result in disengagement from self. In fact, he believed this response to conditions of worth was a natural reaction to an unhealthy environment. The story of Ellen West epitomizes this kind of response to an untenable situation, with unfortunate results (see Box 10.1).

Conclusion

The humanistic approach downplays, and in many cases challenges, the concept of abnormality. Instead, so-called abnormal behavior is seen as an attempt by reductionistic and dispassionate clinicians to objectify and isolate the client. If we call the individual abnormal, we take away his or her humanness and no longer need to deal with this person as a

BOX 10.1

The Story of Ellen West

As described by Rogers (1961), Ellen West, was a client who underwent psychotherapy by a number of well-known nonhumanistically oriented therapists (a client Rogers knew about but never saw himself). Rogers noted that Ellen felt that she had to follow her father's wishes (conditions of worth) and not marry the man whom she loved. Consequently, she disengaged herself from her feelings by overeating and becoming quite obese. A few years later, she again fell in love but instead married a distant cousin due to pressure from her parents. Following this marriage she became anorectic, taking 60 laxative pills a day, again as an apparent attempt to divorce herself from her feelings. She saw numerous doctors, who gave her differing diagnoses, treated her dispassionately, and generally denied her humanness. Eventually, disenchanted with her life, Ellen West committed suicide.

This story, Rogers noted, gives a poignant view of what it's like to lose touch with self—to be incongruent. As Ellen West felt she needed to gain the conditional love of her parents, she gave up the most valuable part of self—her "real" self. Losing touch with self led to a life filled with self-hate and a sense of being "out of touch." Eventually, she was viewed by therapists as mentally ill, which Rogers implied might have added to her feelings of estrangement and her eventual suicide.

human being. In fact, humanists would say that abnormal behavior is a healthy response to an unhealthy situation. In other words, abnormal behavior is the individual's attempt to survive in a world that places conditions of worth on the person. What is abnormal, say the humanists, is the attempt to call something abnormal that is actually natural.

Comparison of Models

Table 10.1 shows a comparison of the four models we examined. Each approach offers a unique perspective on the development of the person, and, until recently, they were viewed as fairly exclusive of one another. Today, attempts have been made to integrate these approaches. Table 10.1 has included treatment approaches that, with the exception of the biological model, were described in Chapter 4.

Integrating Theories

Although the biological, psychoanalytic, learning, and humanistic approaches to abnormal development seem in stark contrast to one another, most individuals today find a way of merging these four approaches (see Box 10.2). Today, it is common for counselors to believe that the individual is affected by a myriad of forces including experiences in early childhood, the kinds of reinforcements received throughout the person's life, the kinds of supportive or nonsupportive relationships experienced, and biological and genetic factors. The battles of the 1960s over the correctness of one theory over another have subsided as individuals now move toward merging these approaches. In fact, ignoring an approach because it does not fit your view of human nature in some cases could be seen as incompetent and unethical if it might work faster or be more effective in treatment of clients with specific disorders.

TABLE 10.1

Comparison of Models of Personality Development

	BIOLOGICAL	PSYCHOANALYTIC	LEARNING THEORY	HUMANISTIC
DEVELOPMENTAL STAGES	Some traits exhibit at varying times based on our biological timetable; other traits we're born with.	Psychosexual stages of development are oral, anal, phallic, latency, and genital.	There are no developmental stages; learning occurs from birth, and people can continue to learn throughout the lifespan.	Maslow's hierarchy may loosely be considered developmental with no age parameters. People are capable of moving toward self-actualization.
MAJOR THEMES	Some traits are inherited. Some inherited traits are expressed only with certain conditions present. Some personality traits are developed through exposure to environment, regardless of genetics (e.g., alcohol-related delirium).	Psychosexual stages. Structure of personality: id, ego, superego. Unconscious. Instincts. Defenses.	Reinforcement contingencies. Schedules of reinforcement. Learning/relearning. Generalization. Discrimination. Recently: Intervening cognitions.	People are born good. Qualities for growth include empathy, UPR, and genuineness. Conditions of worth. Regard for others versus regard for self. Tendency toward self-actualization.
DEVELOPMENT OF HEALTHY SELF	Traits may be a function of the draw of the cards (genes). Environment can affect biology and ultimately development of healthy self (e.g., prenatal care).	Early healthy parenting is crucial, as is ability to master psychosexual stages and suitable development of id, ego, and superego.	Reinforcement of specific behaviors and/or thoughts will lead to a healthy sense of self.	Conditions in environment need to be conducive for the individual to expose his or her true self. Conditions include empathy, UPR, genuineness. The true self is always healthy.
TREATMENT	Genetic engineering, healthy environment, care of body, and medication.	Psychodynamic therapy, long-term treatment, and resolution of unresolved conflicts.	Identifying problem behaviors, setting goals, and using behavioral and cognitive change strategies.	Exposure to environment that will be conducive to development of one's true self (can be through therapy).

Diagnosis and Abnormal Behavior: What Is DSM-IV-TR?[1]

Derived from the Greek words *dia* (apart) and *gnosis* (to perceive or to know), the term *diagnosis* refers to the process of making an assessment of an individual from an outside, or objective, viewpoint (Segal & Coolidge, 2001). Although attempts have been made to classify mental disorders since the turn of the last century, it was not until 1952 that the American Psychiatric Association published the first comprehensive diagnosis system, called the *Diagnostic and Statistical Manual (DSM-I)*. Although *DSM-I* had many critics and was indeed a crude effort at a diagnostic system, it did represent the first modern-day attempt at the classification of mental disorders. *DSM-I* was revised numerous times over the years to its current edition, the *DSM-IV-TR*. This version, which is a distant cousin

[1] Parts of this section are paraphrased from *DSM-IV-TR* (APA, 2000).

BOX 10.2

Causing Dysfunctional Behavior In Children

In examining the varying models of psychopathology, Niehoff (1994) has found that in addition to biological and genetic factors, the following 16 behaviors can cause dysfunctional behavior in children if done habitually. Consider how each of these may be described from a psychoanalytic, learning, or humanistic perspective.

1. Making the child (beyond infancy) helpless and dependent on you and what you think.
2. Restricting, interfering, or controlling.
3. Ignoring a problem when you know there is one.
4. Failing to supervise the child's activity.
5. Engaging in emotional abuse, such as harsh verbal punishment, threatening, aggression, judging, terrorizing, or any form of rejecting or putting down of the child's feelings or needs, in order to control.
6. Reacting in a state of frantic anxiety to the child, living in chaos, engaging in emotional explosions, or communicating in a habitually critical or negative tone.
7. Using physical punishment or pain as a way of control; in other words, physical abuse.
8. Using a child as a target or object in any way that has to do with sex, having any activity you consider sexual with children, making jokes about their sexuality; in other words, sexual abuse.
9. Acting untruthfully to yourself or to the child, treating the child inconsistently, doing things that you insist the child not do.
10. Shunning, avoiding physical contact, isolating the child, or not communicating with the child.
11. Being absent from the child and not having the child with people he or she feels safely and warmly adjusted to.
12. Avoiding taking care of something for the child considered important for children, neglecting a child, or depriving the child of basic needs (food, clothing, shelter, medical care, and the like) as practice in parenting.
13. Coercing the child to take care of what you want or need for you own pleasure and convenience, having children perform in roles for which they are not developmentally prepared where it might not seem good for them or where the child feels, or is, unsafe.
14. Holding the child responsible for the way the family life is going or for the needs of the family.
15. Shaming the child, "making the child feel bad," to get your way.
16. Doing anything compulsive with or around the child. (Niehoff, 1994, pp. 20–22).

of the original *DSM-I*, offers explicit ways of determining a diagnosis and presents a five-part multiaxial diagnostic system (APA, 2000; Hinkle, 1994b). It should also be stressed that *DSM-IV-TR* does not favor one theory of etiology over another and does not offer treatment plans, although the diagnostic categories are often used by clinicians in the treatment planning process (Jongsma & Peterson, 1999; Seligman, 1996).

Although the *DSM-IV-TR* has its critics, it has become the most widespread and accepted diagnostic classification system of emotional disorders (Seligman, 1999; Wakefield, 1992). Although many clinicians do not use all five axes, a good number will find two or more of the axes useful. Axis I describes "Clinical Disorders and Other Conditions That May Be a Focus of Clinical Attention." Axis II delineates "Personality Disorders and Mental Retardation." Axis III explains "General Medical Conditions." Axis IV describes "Psychosocial and Environmental Problems," while Axis V offers a "Global Assessment of Functioning." The following are very brief descriptions of the five axes.

Types of Disorders (Based on DSM-IV-TR)

DSM-IV-TR offers a wealth of information on disorders that are used by clinicians in making sound diagnostic judgments. The following very brief overview summarizes hundreds of pages of information from Axis I and Axis II of *DSM-IV-TR*. For an in-depth review of the disorders, please see *DSM-IV-TR* (APA, 2000).

Brief Overview of Axis I Disorders

This axis includes all disorders except for those classified as personality disorders or as mental retardation (Axis II disorders). Generally, these disorders are considered treatable in some fashion and are often reimbursable by insurance companies as a function of mental health or related services. The following lists and very briefly defines the disorders.

DISORDERS USUALLY FIRST DIAGNOSED IN INFANCY, CHILDHOOD, OR ADOLESCENCE The disorders in this section are generally found in childhood; however, at times individuals are not diagnosed with the disorder until they are adults. Particularly important for school counselors, the disorders include: learning disorders, motor skills disorders, communication disorders, pervasive developmental disorders, attention-deficit and disruptive behavior disorders, feeding and eating disorders of infancy or early childhood, tic disorders, elimination disorders, and other disorders of infancy, childhood, or adolescence.

DELIRIUM, DEMENTIA, AMNESTIC, AND OTHER COGNITIVE DISORDERS Delirium, dementia, and amnestic disorders are all cognitive disorders that represent a significant change from past cognitive functioning of the client. All of these disorders are caused by a medical condition or a substance (e.g., drug abuse, medication, allergic reaction).

MENTAL DISORDERS DUE TO A GENERAL MEDICAL CONDITION This diagnosis is made when a mental disorder is found to be the result of a medical condition and include catatonic disorder, personality change, and mental disorder not otherwise specified. Other disorders that may at times be the result of a medical condition are listed under the following specific diagnostic categories: deliruim, dementia, amnestic disorder, psychotic disorder, mood disorder, anxiety disorder, sexual dysfunction, and sleep disorder.

SUBSTANCE-RELATED DISORDERS A substance-related disorder is a direct result of the use of a drug or alcohol, the effects of medication, or exposure to a toxin. They include alcohol, amphetamine, caffeine, cannabis, cocaine, hallucinogens, inhalants, nicotine, opioids, phencyclidine (PCP), sedatives, and hypnotics.

SCHIZOPHRENIA AND OTHER PSYCHOTIC DISORDERS All disorders classified in this section share one thing in common: psychotic symptomology as the most distinguishing feature. The disorders include schizophrenia, shizophreniform disorder, schizoaffective disorder, delusional disorder, brief psychotic disorder, shared psychotic disorder, psychotic disorder due to a general medical condition, substance-induced psychotic disorder, and psychotic disorder not otherwise specified.

MOOD DISORDERS The disorders in this category share a common feature, mood disturbances of the depressive, manic, or hypomanic type. The mood disorders are divided into four broad categories: depressive disorders, bipolar disorders, mood disorder due to a general medical condition, and substance-induced mood disorder.

ANXIETY DISORDERS There are many types of anxiety disorders, each with its own discrete characteristics. They include panic attack, agoraphobia, panic disorder with or without agoraphobia, agoraphobia without history of panic disorder, specific phobia, obsessive–compulsive disorder, posttraumatic stress disorder, acute stress disorder, generalized anxiety disorder, anxiety disorder due to a general medical condition, substance-induced anxiety disorder, and anxiety disorder not otherwise specified.

SOMATOFORM DISORDERS Somatoform disorders are characterized by symptoms that would suggest a physical cause. However, no such cause can be found, and there is strong evidence that links the symptoms to psychological causes. Seven somatoform disorders include: somatization disorder, undifferentiated somatoform disorder, conversion disorder, pain disorder, hypochondriases body dysmorphic disorder, and somatoform disorder not otherwise specified.

FACTITIOUS DISORDERS As opposed to somatoform disorders, which describe individuals who believe that their physical symptoms have a physiological etiology, factitious disorders are found in individuals who intentionally feign physical or psychological symptoms in order to assume the sick role. Two subtypes include factitious disorder with predominantly psychological signs and symptoms and factitious disorder with predominantly physical signs and symptoms.

DISSOCIATIVE DISORDERS Dissociative disorders occur when there is a disruption of consciousness, memory, identity, or perception of the environment. Five dissociative disorders include dissociative amnesia, dissociative fugue, dissociative identity disorder (formerly called multiple personality disorder), depersonalization disorder, and dissociative disorder not otherwise specified.

SEXUAL AND GENDER IDENTITY DISORDERS This section includes disorders that focus on sexual problems or identity issues related to sexual issues. They include sexual dysfunctions, paraphilias, gender identity disorders, and sexual disorder not otherwise specified.

EATING DISORDERS These disorders focus on severe problems with the amount of food intake by the individual that can potentially cause serious health problems or death. They include anorexia nervosa, bulimia nervosa, and eating disorders not otherwise specified.

SLEEP DISORDERS These disorders have to do with severe sleep-related problems and are broken down into four subcategories: primary sleep disorders, sleep disorder related to another mental condition, sleep disorder due to a general medical condition, and substance-induced sleep disorder.

IMPULSE CONTROL DISORDERS NOT ELSEWHERE CLASSIFIED Impulse control disorders are highlighted by the individual's inability to stop him- or herself from exhibiting certain behaviors. They include intermittent explosive disorder, kleptomania, pyromania, pathological gambling, trichotillomania, and impulse-control disorder not otherwise specified.

ADJUSTMENT DISORDERS Probably the most common disorders clinicians see in private practice, adjustment disorders are highlighted by emotional or behavioral symptoms that arise in response to psychosocial stressors. The subtypes of this diagnosis include adjustment disorders with depressed mood, with anxiety, with mixed anxiety and depressed mood, with disturbance of conduct, with mixed disturbance of emotions and conduct, and unspecified.

Brief Overview of Axis II Disorders

Axis II diagnoses tend to be long-term disorders in which treatment almost always has little or no affect on changing the presenting symptoms of the individual. The two kinds of Axis II disorders are mental retardation and personality disorders.

MENTAL RETARDATION Characterized by intellectual functioning significantly below average (below the second percentile) as well as problems with adaptive skills, mental retardation can have many different etiologies. There are four categories of mental retardation: mild mental retardation (IQ from 50–55 to approximately 70), moderate mental retardation (IQ from 35–40 to 50–55), severe mental retardation (IQ from 20–25 to 35–40), and profound mental retardation (IQ below 20–25).

PERSONALITY DISORDERS Individuals with a personality disorder show deeply ingrained, inflexible, and enduring patterns of relating to the world that lead to distress and impairment in a person's life. Such an individual may have difficulty understanding him- or herself and others and may be labile, have difficulty in relationships, and have problems with impulse control. Personality disorders are generally first recognized in adolescence or early adulthood and often remain throughout one's lifetime. There are three clusters of personality disorders, with each cluster representing a general way of relating to the world.

Cluster A includes paranoid, schizoid, and schizotypal personality disorder. Individuals with these disorders all experience characteristics that may be considered odd or eccentric by others.

Cluster B disorders include the antisocial, borderline, histrionic, and narcissistic personality disorders. Individuals suffering from these disorders are generally dramatic, emotional, overly sensitive, and erratic.

Cluster C includes the avoidant, dependent, and obsessive–compulsive personality disorders. Common characteristics found within this cluster are anxious and fearful traits.

Axis III: General Medical Conditions

Axis III provides the clinician the opportunity to report relevant medical conditions of the client. If the medical condition is clearly related to the cause or worsening of a mental disorder, then the medical condition is listed on both Axis I and Axis III. If the medical condition is not a cause of the mental disorder but will affect overall treatment of the individual, then it is listed only on Axis III. An example of an Axis III medical condition that could be a cause of an Axis I diagnosis would be the development of heart disease that caused an adjustment disorder. In this case the heart disease would be noted along with the adjustment disorder on Axis I, as well as separately on Axis III. *The International Classification of Diseases*, 9th revision *(ICD-9-CM)*, an abbreviated form of which is found in the *DSM-IV-TR*, is used to code the Axis III medical condition. Axis I uses the *DSM-IV-TR* classification and includes a reference to the medical condition:

> Axis I: Adjustment Disorder with Depressed Mood as a response to congestive heart failure (309.0)
>
> Axis III: Failure, Congestive Heart (428.0)

On the other hand, if an individual has a sleep disorder and subsequently develops acute prostatitis (infection of the prostate) that worsens, but did not cause, the sleep disorder, it would be written as:

Axis I: Narcolepsy (347)

Axis III: Prostatitis (618.9)

If there is no Axis III diagnosis, then a notation of "Axis III: None" is listed.

Axis IV: Psychosocial and Environmental Problems

Psychosocial or environmental problems that affect the diagnosis, treatment, and prognosis of mental disorders as listed on Axes I and II are noted on Axis IV. Generally, such problems will only be listed on Axis IV, but in those cases where it is believed that such stressors may be a prime cause of the mental disorder, a reference should be made to them on Axis I or II. General categories of psychosocial and environmental problems include the following: problems with one's primary support group, problems related to the social environment, educational problems, occupational problems, housing problems, economic problems, problems with access to health care services, and problems related to interaction with the legal system/crime. An example of an Axis IV diagnosis might include:

Axis IV: Job Loss

Axis V: Global Assessment of Functioning (GAF)

Axis V is a scale used by the clinician to assess the overall functioning of the client and is based on the psychological, social, and occupational functioning of the client. The GAF scale ranges from very severe dysfunction to superior functioning, and a score of 0 means there is inadequate information to make a judgment (see Table 10.2). In giving a GAF rating, the clinician can report current functioning, the highest functioning within the past year, or any other relevant GAF ratings based on the uniqueness of the situation.

Making a Diagnosis

The *DSM-IV-TR* offers decision trees to assist the clinician in differential diagnosis. Thus, if one is considering two or more diagnoses that share similar symptoms, the decision tree walks the clinician through a series of steps designed to assist in choosing the most appropriate diagnosis. This is particularly important as the eventual diagnosis chosen affects treatment planning and choices of psychotropic medication. It is possible to have more than one Axis I and Axis II diagnosis, and in those cases the additional diagnoses should be reported. A typical multiaxial assessment may look something like the following:

Axis I 309.0 Adjustment Disorder with Depressed Mood

Axis II 301.82 Avoidant Personality Disorder

Axis III No Diagnosis

Axis IV Divorce

Axis V GAF = 60 (current); 75 (highest in past year)

Sometimes part of treatment can be the use of psychotropic medications as an adjunct to counseling. The next section will give a brief overview of some of the more common medications used in the treatment of emotional disorders.

TABLE 10.2

Global Assessment of Functioning Scale (GAF)	
Code*	(*Note:* Use intermediate codes when appropriate, e.g., 45, 68, 72)
100 | 91	**Superior functioning in a wide range of activities; life's problems never seem to get out of hand, is sought out by others because of his or her many positive qualities. No symptoms.**
90 | | 81	**Absent or minimal symptoms** (e.g., mild anxiety before an exam), **good functioning in all areas, interested and involved in a wide range of activities, socially effective, generally satisfied with life, no more than everyday problems or concerns** (e.g., an occasional argument with family members).
80 | | 71	**If symptoms are present, they are transient and expectable reactions to psychosocial stressors** (e.g., difficulty concentrating after family argument); **no more than slight impairment in social, occupational, or school functioning** (e.g., temporarily falling behind in schoolwork).
70 | | 61	**Some mild symptoms** (e.g., depressed mood and mild insomnia) **OR some difficulty in social, occupational or school functioning** (e.g., occasional truancy, or theft within the household), **but generally functioning pretty well, has some meaningful interpersonal relationships.**
60 | 51	**Moderate symptoms** (e.g., flat affect and circumstantial speech, occasional panic attacks) **OR some difficulty in social, occupational, or school functioning** (e.g., few friends, conflicts with peers or coworkers).
50 | 41	**Serious symptoms** (e.g., suicidal ideation, severe obsessional rituals, frequent shoplifting) **OR any serious impairment in social, occupational, or school functioning** (e.g., no friends, unable to keep a job).
40 | | | 31	**Some impairment in reality testing or communication** (e.g., speech is at times illogical, obscure, or irrelevant) **OR major impairment in several areas, such as work or school family relations, judgment, thinking, or mood** (e.g., depressed man avoids friends, neglects family, and is unable to work; child frequently beats up younger children, is defiant at home, and is failing at school).
30 | | 21	**Behavior is considerably influenced by delusions or hallucinations OR serious impairment in communication or judgment** (e.g., sometimes incoherent, acts grossly inappropriately, suicidal preoccupation) **OR inability to function in almost all areas** (e.g., stays in bed all day; no job, home, or friends).
20 | | 11	**Some danger of hurting self or others** (e.g., suicide attempts without clear expectation of death; frequently violent; manic excitement) **OR occasionally fails to maintain minimal personal hygiene** (e.g., smears feces) **OR gross impairment in communication** (e.g., largely incoherent or mute).
10 | 1	**Persistent danger of severely hurting self or others** (e.g., recurrent violence) **OR persistent inability to maintain minimal personal hygiene OR serious suicidal act with clear expectation of death.**
0	Inadequate information

SOURCE: American Psychiatric Association, 2000, p. 34.

Psychopharmacology

Today, there are a host of medications that can be used as an adjunct to counseling in the treatment of many disorders (Kalat, 2001; Schatzberg & Nemeroff, 1998). For instance, research on the effectiveness of psychotropic medication on depression has shown that the combined use of medication with therapy has a better outcome than either treatment on its own (Conte et al., 1986; Norden, 1996).

Whether or not medication should be used as an adjunct to counseling and how one broaches this possibly delicate topic with clients are ever-increasing issues for the counselor and other mental health professionals (Ingersoll, 2000; Sarwer-Foner, 1993). In fact, it is now common for counselors to consult or refer to a physician, generally a psychiatrist, who can assess the client and prescribe appropriate psychotropic medications. Therefore, it is important for counselors to have a basic working knowledge of psychopharmacology, more than could be offered in this brief overview.

For the treatment of a wide array of emotional disorders, we will classify medications into five groups: antipsychotics, antimanics, antidepressants, antianxiety agents, and stimulants (Donlon, Schaffer, Ericksen, Pepitone-Arreola-Rockwell, & Schaffer, 1983; National Institute of Mental Health, 1995).

Antipsychotics

During the early 1950s the first wave of antipsychotic drugs was discovered. These were soon to dramatically change the field of mental health. For the first time, individuals with severe psychotic symptoms could be treated with some success. This would subsequently be one of the major impetuses for the release of hundreds of thousands of individuals from mental institutions around the country (see Chapter 2). Antipsychotic drugs are used to treat all types of psychoses and are also occasionally used in the treatment of bipolar disorder, depression with psychotic features, paranoid disorders, and delirium and dementia (Donlon et al., 1983; Marder, 1998; Raskind & Peskind, 1998).

There are seven groups of antipsychotic drugs, which include the phenothiazines, thioxanthenes, butyrophenones, dihydroindolones, dibenzoxazepines, diphenylbutylpiperidine, and dibenzodiazepine (Marder, 1998; National Institute of Mental Health, 1995; Owens & Risch, 1998; Pirodsky & Cohn, 1992). Some of the earlier antipsychotic drugs that became very popular and are still in use today are known by their trade names: Thorazine, Haldol, Mellaril, Stelazine, and Prolixin. More recently Clozaril and Risperdal have been two of the more popular antipsychotic drugs in use.

Antipsychotics can dramatically alter the course of an individual who is having an acute psychotic episode. This is important, because the quicker an individual can recover from a psychotic episode, the greater the likelihood of eliminating or at least decreasing the intensity of future psychotic episodes.

Although antipsychotic medications can help an individual who has a long history of psychotic behavior live a more normal life, they are often not a cure. For these individuals, normal cognitive functioning is often not returned, and they are frequently left seeming somewhat stilted in their thinking and ability to respond. Depending on the type and dosage of medication, a number of side effects may occur. For instance, some individuals may have autonomic side effects that include dry mouth, blurred vision, constipation, urinary retention, and a decreased libido. Extrapyramidal side effects, which can include muscle spasms, Parkinson-type symptoms, and motor restlessness, can be found in many individuals who take antipsychotic medications. Tardive dyskinesia, which includes involuntary movements of the tongue, lips, and facial muscles, can occur in some individuals who have taken high dosages of antipsychotic medications over a long period of time, although it has occasionally been seen when the medications are taken for short periods in lower doses. Serious blood disorders have been found with some of the newer antipsychotic medications. A few of the other possible side effects include a fast heartbeat, sedation, weight gain, and skin pigmentation.

Antimanic Drugs

Around 150 years ago an element called lithium was discovered that was found to have positive affects for the treatment of a number of bodily afflictions (Lenox & Manji, 1998). In the early 1950s, lithium was rediscovered as an effective treatment for bipolar disorder (then called manic-depression). Lithium seems to act particularly well in lessening the effects of manic symptoms in an individual with bipolar disorder. Because it does not have the same dramatic effects with the depressive end of the illness, antidepressants are often also prescribed. For individuals who take lithium, the level of drug in the system has to be assessed through a blood test, because too much lithium can cause severe side effects and too little will be ineffective in treatment. Like the antipsychotics, lithium can produce a number of side effects including gastrointestinal problems, neurological problems, hypothyroidism, edema, weight gain, and others, although they are generally viewed as less serious than those of the antipsychotic medications. Although lithium has been used in the treatment of other disorders (Lenox & Manji, 1998), generally it is often an early treatment of choice for bipolar disorder.

Lithium has been shown to be a very effective drug for the treatment of bipolar disorder, oftentimes restoring an individual to a normal lifestyle. However, some individuals do not respond to treatment with lithium. For those individuals, a number of anticonvulsant medications, such as Depakote, have been shown to be somewhat effective. In addition, some benzodiazepines (antianxiety drugs) may also be helpful in treating manic episodes (Keck & McElroy, 1998).

Antidepressants

The use of amphetamines during the 1930s was one of the first attempts to treat depression psychopharmacologically (Pirodsky & Cohn, 1992). Known as "speed," this medication did little except to temporarily stimulate a person's central nervous system, which often would eventually lead to a crash and more serious depression. In addition, consistent use of amphetamines can lead to paranoia and health problems.

The 1950s saw a dramatic shift in the treatment of depression with the identification of two classes of antidepressants called monoamine oxidase inhibitors (MAOIs) and tricyclics (Krishnan, 1998; Potter, Manji, & Rudorfer, 1998). Until recently, these classes of drugs were the medications of choice in the treatment of depression, with the tricyclics being used more frequently because they tended to have fewer side effects. However, the last few years have seen the widespread use of a new class of antidepressants called selective serotonin reuptake inhibitors (SSRIs) (Norden, 1996; Tollefson & Rosenbaum, 1998). The SSRIs have been called miracle drugs by some due to their limited side effects and often dramatic results. In fact, these drugs have been so effective that there is some evidence that they can help make an individual who already feels relatively well feel even better. For these reasons, such drugs as Prozac, Luvox, Paxil, and Zoloft have very quickly become commonplace in American society. In addition to the treatment of depression,

SSRIs also show promise in treating other disorders, including obsessive–compulsive disorder, panic disorder, some forms of schizophrenia, eating disorders, alcoholism, obesity, and some sleep disorders.

Besides the SSRIs, there are a number of what have been called "atypical" antidepressants that also have fewer side effects than the tricyclics or the MAOIs and seem to be promising in the treatment of depression. Some of these include Serzone, Effexor, Wellbutrin, and Remeron.

Antianxiety Medications

The use of modern-day antianxiety agents started with the discovery of Librium, which came on the market in 1960 and was soon followed by Valium. These medications and other benzodiazepines were better tolerated and less addictive than barbiturates, the previous drug of choice (Ballenger, 1998). However, tolerance of and dependence on benzodiazepines can be developed, and there is a potential for overdose on these medications.

Today, benzodiazepines, such as Valium, Librium, Tranxene, and Xanax, are frequently used for generalized anxiety disorders as they have a calming effect on the individual. In conjunction with psychotherapy, these medications can be an effective agent in treating such disorders. Benzodiazepines have also been shown to be helpful in reducing stress, for insomnia, and in management of alcohol withdrawal (Nishino, Mignot, & Dement, 1998). In addition, they have been used in conjunction with some antidepressants for the treatment of obsessive–compulsive disorder (OCD) and in treating social phobias and posttraumatic stress disorder (Ballenger, 1998). One other drug, a nonbenzodiazepine called Buspar, has been found to be effective for use in generalized anxiety disorders and can be an alternative to the use of the more popular benzodiazepines (Ninan, Cole & Yonkers, 1998; Taylor, 1998).

Stimulants

Probably the first modern-day stimulant used to treat emotional disorders was cocaine, which was first discovered in the mid-1800s. However, due to its addictive qualities, cocaine has never become a treatment of choice in this country. In 1887 amphetamines, which had many of the same stimulant qualities of cocaine but were less addictive, were synthesized (Fawcett & Busch, 1998). Over the years amphetamines were used, mostly unsuccessfully, as diet aids, as antidepressants, and to relieve the symptoms of sleepiness. However, during the 1950s amphetamines were found to have a paradoxical effect in many children diagnosed with attention deficit disorder (ADHD), in that amphetamines seemed to calm them down and help them focus. Today, the use of stimulants in the treatment of attention deficit disorder is widespread, with the three most common drugs being Ritalin, Cylert, and Dexedrine. In addition to treating attention deficit disorder, stimulants have also been found to be successful in the treatment of narcolepsy and are somewhat successful in treating residual attention deficit disorder in adults.

Psychopharmacology has come a long way since the 1950s when the first modern-day psychotropic medications were introduced. Increasingly, the medications used for a wide array of disorders are more effective and have fewer side effects than in the past. As the mechanism for psychological disorders becomes understood, new and even more effective medications can be developed to specifically target the underlying physiological mechanism causing the disorder.

Multicultural Issue: The Misdiagnosis of Minority Clients

People from different cultures may express feelings in different ways, and symptomology may differ as a function of culture (Hinkle, 1994b; Solomon, 1992). Thus, some have argued that although the use of diagnosis and *DSM-IV-TR* can be helpful in treatment planning, it can lead to the misdiagnosis of culturally different clients because of ignorance, bias, and stereotypes held by clinicians.

An even more radical view held by some is that a diagnosis is a way of legitimizing socially unacceptable behavior, thus giving those in positions of power the ability to legally oppress the culturally different (Eysenck, Wakefield, & Friedman, 1983; Horwitz, 1982, cited in Hinkle, 1994b). In fact, Szasz (1970) years ago warned that the "aim of psychiatric classification [diagnosis] is to degrade and socially segregate the individual as a mental patient . . . and the creation of a class of justifiably persecuted scapegoats" (p. 239).

The issue of misdiagnosis is particularly true for African Americans, as nonblack clinicians do not have a clear sense of the cultural context from which some symptoms arise (Garretson, 1993). An obvious example of this is the diagnosis of paranoia, when in fact African Americans have lived in an oppressive society and have a real cultural context within which to feel paranoid (sometimes when you think people are out to get you, they are!). In contrast, sometimes clinicians miss a diagnosis because of cultural stereotypes, such as the clinician who views a withdrawn Asian American as exhibiting culturally typical behavior when in actuality he or she is depressed.

In an effort to alleviate some of the potential problems with the misdiagnosis of minority clients, the writers of *DSM-IV-TR* have included a section called the "Glossary of Culture-Bound Syndromes." This glossary lists 25 syndromes that are afflictions or illnesses specific to some cultures that could be falsely mistaken for any of a number of diagnoses found in *DSM-IV-TR*. For instance, read the explanation of the affliction known as koro, which is mostly found in south and east Asia:

> *A term, probably of Malaysian origin, that refers to an episode of sudden and intense anxiety that the penis (or in females, the vulva and nipples) will recede into the body and possibly cause death. . . .* (APA, 2000, p. 900)

Although *DSM-IV-TR* gives us some culture-bound syndromes of which we all should be aware, it does little to rid clinicians of their biases and stereotypes, which can continue to lead to the misdiagnosis of culturally different clients.

Ethical, Professional, and Legal Issues

The Proper Diagnosis of Mental Disorders

Noting the potential misuse and abuse of diagnosis, the ACA code of ethics addresses two important issues when making a diagnosis (ACA, 1995a, Standard E.5):

a. *Proper diagnosis*. Counselors take special care to provide proper diagnosis of mental disorders. Assessment techniques (including personal interview) used to determine client care (e.g., locus of treatment, type of treatment, or recommended follow-up) are carefully selected and appropriately used.

b. *Cultural sensitivity*. Counselors recognize that culture affects the manner in which clients' problems are defined. Clients' socioeconomic and cultural experience is considered when diagnosing mental disorders.

Challenging Abnormality and Diagnosing

Terms like *abnormal behavior*, *mental illness*, and *diagnosis* have firmly planted themselves in the field of mental health and perhaps into the fabric of society. For this reason, counselors are called upon to examine the meanings of these terms and to understand the basics of diagnostic categories. However, Corey and associates (1998) summarize some of the reasons that clinicians might want to be tentative when making a diagnosis. They state that:

- Diagnosis is an objective process in which the person making the diagnosis is really not in the shoes of the person being diagnosed.
- Diagnosis tends to rob people of their uniqueness.
- Diagnosis can lead to a self-fulfilling prophecy for both the client and clinician (I think, therefore I am).
- Diagnosis leads to tunnel vision where the clinician attempts to fit all problems into the specific diagnostic category.

Some authors have argued that important distinctions can be made about the causes of emotional problems and the efficacy of using a diagnostic classification system (Glasser, 1961; Ivey & Ivey, 1998; Laing, 1967; Rogers, 1961; Szasz, 1961, 1970, 1990). These authors disagreed with some of the more common ways in which emotional problems are conceptualized, the use of diagnosis and terms like *mental illness*, *abnormal*, and *psychopathology*. For instance, both Laing and Szasz viewed mental illness as a normal response to a stressful situation. In fact, Laing even encouraged people to get in touch with their own psychosis as a means of letting go of their stressors and would periodically allow himself to "go insane" in his own hospitals. Szasz believed psychopathology is the client's way of communicating about social and cultural forces that impinge on him or her (Davison & Neale, 2001). In a similar vein, Glasser believes that psychopathology is irresponsible behavior and is the individual's attempt to control his or her world. If you can identify and change such behaviors, the person can then show responsible or normal behaviors.

Finally, Ivey and Ivey suggest that psychopathology can be viewed from a developmental and contextual perspective. Rather than assuming that there is something inherently wrong with a person, they suggest that an individual's diagnosis is the result of problems in development and responses to the issues of family, community, and cultural stressors. This positivistic approach does not suggest discontinuing the use of diagnosis but offers a humanistic and antideterministic way of approaching diagnoses.

This controversy is hardly over, and regardless of what side of the fence you find yourself on, it is suggested that you keep an open mind to the arguments on the other side.

The Over-Diagnosis of Mental Illness

Swenson (1997) notes that clinicians who are trained in diagnostic procedures will tend to over-diagnose. This is probably because the medical model suggests that it is better to judge a well person sick than a sick person well. Clearly, what is best is to diagnose a person accurately or, if in doubt, to consult and discuss your doubts. A dramatic case of

BOX 10.3

On Being Sane in Insane Places (Rosenhan, 1973)

A group of eight pseudopatients presented themselves to mental hospitals. One was a psychology graduate student, three were psychologists, one a pediatrician, one a psychiatrist, one a painter, and one a housewife. These subjects presented themselves to 12 mental hospitals in five states. The only symptoms they displayed in the admissions offices were saying that they felt their lives were empty and hollow and that they heard voices saying "empty, hollow, thud." The researchers chose these symptoms because they could not find one case of "existential psychosis" in the literature. Once admitted, the pseudopatients ceased showing any symptoms at all. Mental health professionals diagnosed all but one of these people as schizophrenic, and the length of hospitalizations ranged from 7 to 52 days. The professional staffs of the hospitals never detected the fraud, although many actual patients were suspicious and questioned the fake patients (Swenson, 1997, p. 449).

over-diagnosis was shown in a study conducted by Rosenhan, *On Being Sane in Insane Places* (1973; cited in Swenson, 1997), in which eight healthy people were inaccurately diagnosed and placed in mental hospitals for a range of 7 to 52 days (see Box 10.3).

Because Rosenhan's study was conducted in the early 1970s, we can hope that times have changed and we would not see a repeat of the above. However, the tendency to over-diagnose by clinicians trained in *DSM-IV-TR* is probably still here.

Confinement against One's Will

As a result of the Donaldson *v.* O'Connor (1975) decision (see Chapter 2), individuals in mental hospitals cannot be held against their will for extended periods of time if they are not in danger of harming themselves or others. However, a person can still be involuntarily hospitalized if it can be shown that he or she is in danger of harming him- or herself or others or if he or she is gravely ill. This initial hospitalization is usually for a short period of time, perhaps two to three days. At that point a certification by two or more experts or a court hearing is generally needed to continue short-term hospitalization of two or three weeks. Any long-term confinement against the patient's will would necessitate a court hearing and is very unusual in today's world.

The Counselor in Process: Dismissing Impaired Graduate Students

I have at times sat in a faculty meeting when a faculty member brought up the name of a student and suggested that the student be approached because it seemed apparent that he or she had severe emotional problems. Sometimes I have agreed with the faculty member's assessment; other times I have not. For me, this issue is similar to the old debate concerning the use of the term *abnormal behavior.* In terms of students, it first challenges me to define "severe emotional problem," and secondarily asks me to ponder whether or not I believe such students can be assisted to the point that they can be effective counselors (see Bradey & Post, 1991). The ACA ethical guidelines suggest the following:

> *Professional counselors, through continual evaluation and appraisal, are aware of the academic and personal limitations of students and supervisees that might impede future performance. Professional counselors assist limited students and supervisees in securing remedial assistance and dismiss from a training program students and supervisees who are unable to provide competent service.* (ACA, 1995a, Section F.3)

If conceptualizing a "problem student" from a developmental and wellness perspective as presented in Chapter 9, I would assume that he or she could change. However, if I were to look at this student from an abnormal development perspective, I might think that there is something inherently wrong with him or her, and that change would be particularly difficult if possible at all. I might ask the student to drop out of the program. Perhaps there is a middle point between these two extremes; however, the issue remains: Do we believe that any student can eventually overcome his or her personal limitations and be effective as a counselor, or do we think that some individuals are simply too impaired? What do you think?

Summary

This chapter examined the concepts of abnormal behavior, diagnosis, and psychopharmacology, noting that the three are inextricably connected. Whereas it used to be unusual for counseling programs to examine these concepts, because of changes in the field, it is becoming increasingly common and important.

The chapter examined four models of abnormal development. The genetic and biological model assumes that there are inherited factors that, when expressed, will show certain personality traits. It also asserts that some genes only get expressed when exposed to certain environmental factors. In addition, the biological model states that environmental factors can greatly affect the development of certain traits regardless of one's genetics. The psychoanalytic model, on the other hand, assumes that abnormal development is a function of the ability to master the psychosexual stages. Individuals who are parented poorly as they pass through the first five years of life will develop a precarious balance among their id, ego, and superego, which ultimately will lead to dysfunctional ways of being. This model is particularly deterministic, stating that personality development occurs very early in life and is difficult to change. In contrast, the learning perspective assumes that what was learned can be unlearned, and new behaviors and ways of thinking can be learned. Learning theorists believe that we are born as blank slates and, through operant conditioning, classical conditioning, and modeling, we learn either healthy or dysfunctional ways of living. In recent times, most learning theorists have included a cognitive perspective stating that our cognitions are also reinforced and can lead to healthy functioning or to irrational ways of thinking. Finally, the humanistic perspective believes that there is a natural growth force in people, and, if placed in a nurturing environment, the individual will develop a healthy personality and high self-esteem. However, if conditions of worth are continually placed upon the person, growth will be thwarted and there will be a tendency toward dysfunctional ways of living in the world. Humanists believe that the individual can change at any point in his or her life if placed in a supportive environment.

If one believes that there are deviant behaviors, then it is natural to want to classify them. This is what diagnosis achieves. The chapter therefore offered an overview of the *DSM-IV-TR*, the major diagnostic classification system for emotional disorders. We noted that the *DSM-IV-TR* is a multiaxial system. Axis I describes "Clinical Disorders and Other Conditions That May Be a Focus of Clinical Attention." Axis II explains "Personality Disorders and Mental Retardation." Axis III describes "General Medical Conditions." Axis IV describes "Psychosocial and Environmental Problems," while Axis V offers a "Global Assessment of Functioning." The *DSM-IV-TR* offers a system of differential diagnosis to assist the clinician in distinguishing among similar diagnoses. This ultimately can greatly assist in treatment planning.

If an accurate diagnosis is made, then treatment planning becomes easier, one aspect of which may be the use of psychotropic medication. Therefore, we examined five classes of drugs often used in the treatment of a wide range of emotional disorders. They included the antipsychotics, antimanics, antidepressants, antianxiety agents, and stimulants. A brief history of the use of various psychopharmacological agents was described along with descriptions of some of the major psychotropic medications currently in use.

In this chapter we explored problems inherent in the use of diagnosis for some minority clients. It was noted that bias, prejudice, and ignorance can lead to a misdiagnosis because culturally different clients may express symptomatology in different ways from majority clients. In its ethical guidelines, ACA highlights the importance of proper diagnosis, especially when working with the culturally different client.

One professional issue we discussed in this chapter was how diagnosis is viewed by some as the way that society legitimatizes the oppression of minorities. We reviewed the ideas of Szasz, Glasser, Rogers, and Laing and noted that they all refused to use the term *mental illness*, stating that it tends to depersonalize and oppress the individual. Regardless of one's belief in mental illness, we discussed the fact that research seems to indicate that clinicians who are trained in the use of diagnosis will tend to overuse it.

In this chapter we also discussed that it is no longer easy to confine a person in a mental institution against his or her will. Today, evidence that a person is in danger of harming self or others or is gravely ill must be presented if a person is to be committed for a short period of time, and a court hearing is needed for long-term confinement.

Finally, we ended the chapter with a brief consideration of the impaired graduate student and whether counseling programs should view these students as incapable of change and therefore problematic for continuation in a program.

INFOTRAC and Other Information Resources (e.g., ERIC and PsycINFO)

Note: When relevant, key words are in quotation marks.

1. Pick a diagnosis from the "DSM-IV-TR" (you may need to use the keyword "DSM-IV") categories and research it in more detail.
2. Review any of the "theories of psychopathology" in more detail.
3. Examine how "psychopharmacology" is used within a treatment category of your choice.

CHAPTER **11**

Career Development: The Counselor and the World of Work

My father was a building contractor; when I was young he used to take me to various construction sites, and I would watch buildings slowly getting built. As a teenager, during the summers, I assisted a carpenter or laborer at the sites. I remember getting picked up at five-thirty in the morning, cramped half-asleep in the cab of a well-seasoned truck, to be taken on a bumpy ride to work. I would think to myself, "Is this what I want to do for the rest of my life?" Luckily, because I did well in school, I knew I'd be going on to college; but to do what?

Majoring in biology and thinking I would not be accepted to medical school, I chose dentistry as my eventual occupational choice. My mind was made up, I thought. But something did not feel right. Although a part of me said, "Go to dental school," another distant voice said, "This is not for you, you have other things to do in your life, other things that involve helping people in other ways." These divergent feelings and thoughts were certainly an outgrowth of many things, including my family values, placement in my family, my interests, my own emerging values, and my abilities.

Although it was a tough decision, I eventually chose to listen to my inner voice, and I switched my major to psychology. Eventually, through selected trial and occasional error, I ended up in the field of counseling. No doubt my life would have been made somewhat easier if I had had the benefit of a career counselor who could assess my likes and dislikes, my values, and my abilities; help me understand my personality; facilitate self-knowledge and self-reflection; and assist me in applying all of this knowledge to my career development journey.

As I proceeded in my career, I continued to be faced with a number of choices. Should I go on for a doctoral degree? Should I go toward clinical work or academia? Should I change career paths totally? Again, my choices often seemed to be a product of trial and error. I would try something out to see if I liked it, if I was good at it, and would then make a decision about my future career direction. However, as I gained more awareness and began to more fully understand the career development process, I saw that I could choose my own direction in life if I had adequate knowledge of myself and knowledge of the world of work. No longer would my career decision making be an accident. I began to choose my future!

Despite the fact that I have been pretty satisfied with my chosen occupation, there were times when my life did not feel complete. Therefore, other activities began to fill in some of the empty spaces. In my mid-twenties I began to jog. As the years continued, running and aerobics became a focal point in my life. They offered an outlet for my stress, a place for me to meet other people, and an activity that took me away from my work. In my early forties I married, and soon after, I was a father. As new life roles emerged, I found that I had to balance my roles of professor, clinician, exerciser, and writer with those of husband and father.

My story, with its twists and turns, is fairly common. People tend to haphazardly go through life without the benefit of guidance. Sometimes people intuitively move in the direction that serves them best, but many people are unhappy with their jobs and other life roles.

If afforded the opportunity for career counseling, many would have an easier time in their journey through life. They would be able to make smart occupational and life choices. That is why this chapter is so important. It explains the career development process, its importance to life satisfaction, and the role of the counselor in facilitating career development.

This chapter will survey the career development process and specifically examine how individuals make career choices, the meaning of work in people's lives, the major theories of career development, and some of the career information systems available. In addition, we will conclude the chapter by examining multicultural issues related to career development, and ethical, professional, and legal issues in the realm of career development.

Some Definitions

The career development process is perhaps the most misunderstood counseling-related subject. Therefore, it is particularly important to start out with some basic definitions. The following definitions, synthesized by some prominent authors, are terms related to the career development process (Herr & Cramer, 1996; Isaacson & Brown, 2000; Sears, 1982; Super, 1976; Wise, Charner, & Randour, 1978). Keep in mind that some of these definitions may not be the same as our common, lay definitions.

Avocation. A chosen activity, not necessarily pursued for money, that gives satisfaction to the individual and fulfills an important aspect of the person's life.

Career. The totality of work and life roles through which an individual expresses him- or herself. A career represents not only one's efforts at occupations, but how all life roles are an expression of self.

Career awareness. One's consciousness about career-related decisions, which can be facilitated through a self-examination of one's values, abilities, preferences, knowledge of occupations and life roles, and interests.

Career development. All of the psychological, sociological, educational, physical, economic, and other factors that are at play in shaping one's career over the life span.

Career counseling. Individual or group counseling with a focus to increase career awareness and to foster decision making relative to career goals.

Career guidance. A program, designed by counselors, that offers information concerning career development and facilitates career awareness for individuals.

Career path. The sequence of positions and/or jobs, which typically signifies potential advancement, available to persons within an organization or business.

Jobs. Positions within a specific work environment (e.g., school, agency, business) that are similar in nature.

Leisure. Time taken from required effort (e.g., job or occupation) in order to pursue self-chosen activities that express one's abilities and/or interests.

Occupation. Jobs of a similar nature that can be found within several work environments and connote the kinds of work a person is pursuing. Occupations are definable outside of the person; careers are defined by the person's total work and life roles.

Work. Effort expended at a job, occupation, or avocation in order to produce or accomplish something.

Is Career Development Developmental?

You might be wondering why a chapter on career development is included in a section on human development. In fact, career development is human development because it examines the development of the person, and it is developmental because it occurs in distinct stages over one's lifetime. Unfortunately, I find that when most people think about career development, they think that it is a process of finding a job. In actuality, it is much more than that. In fact, career development includes all of the following:

- The 3-year-old who plays house or hammers a peg into a hole.
- The 5-year-old who joins a T-ball league.
- The 10-year-old inner city youth who has few role models.
- The 12-year-old who begins to examine his or her abilities and likes and dislikes.
- The 14-year-old who suddenly discovers that her parents are getting divorce.
- The 17-year-old who considers what college to go to and the 17-year-old who ponders what job to take after high school.
- The 25-year-old who takes a new job and also leads an aerobics class.
- The 30-year-old who gives up a full-time job to do child care.
- The 37-year-old who is promoted and is vice-president of the local PTA.
- The 45-year-old who hates her job but continues to work at it to make money while maintaining an exciting hobby on the side.
- The 50-year-old who wonders, "Is this all there is?"

- The 60-year-old who ponders whether or not he should retire in a couple of years.
- The 70-year-old who never worked, has raised a family, and has become a fairly good tournament bridge player.
- The 85-year-old who reflects back on his or her various life roles.

Career development is lifespan development (Super & Hall, 1978). It is expressed through the job, occupations, leisure activities, and avocations we have chosen. Most important, it is how we experience ourselves in all of our life roles. It is affected by the kinds of messages we received from our parents, from our community, from our religious affiliation, and from society. It is ongoing, ever transforming, and doesn't end until we die.

Why Career Development and Career Counseling?

I hope by now you see that career development is not just the process of finding a job, but the development of all of our various life roles and the factors that go into shaping them. It is reflected in how each of us expresses our identity through the roles we choose. Career counseling is helping the 3-year-old develop a sense of self, assisting the 12-year-old in understanding what she is good at and what she likes, helping the 17-year-old choose a college or a job, helping a client weigh the relative importance of being a parent and working at a job, helping a person work through midlife issues, assisting an individual as she readies for retirement, and reminiscing with an older person about his life. Career counseling helps to raise a person's awareness about the choices he or she is making in life.

Adequate career counseling can assist us in making smart choices around our work and other life roles. The work we choose is a large part of our career development process and serves a number of important economic, social, and psychological needs for the individual (see Table 11.1). Numerous studies show that career planning and career counseling are related to job satisfaction and positive mental health (Assouline & Meir, 1987;

TABLE 11.1

Different Purposes Work Can Serve

ECONOMIC	SOCIAL	PSYCHOLOGICAL
Gratification of wants or needs	A place to meet people	Self-esteem
Acquisition of physical assets	Potential friendships	Identity
Security against future contingencies	Human relationships	A sense of order
Liquid assets to be used for investment or deferred gratifications	Social status for the worker and his or her family	Dependability, reliability
Purchase of goods and services	A feeling of being valued by others for what one can produce	A feeling of mastery or competence
Evidence of success	A sense of being needed by others to get the job done or to achieve mutual goals	Self-efficacy
Assets to purchase leisure or free time	Responsibility	Commitment, personal evaluation

SOURCE: *Career guidance and counseling through the lifespan* (5th ed.), by E. L. Herr and S. H. Cramer, p. 70.

Spokane, 1985). It is not a big leap to realize that adequate career planning and career counseling can help us feel better about our lives. This is why career counseling is so vital to facilitating a client's career development.

A Little Bit of History

The counseling profession owes its existence to vocational guidance. At the turn of the 20th century, on the heels of the industrial revolution, there came many demographic changes throughout the United States. Almost overnight, there was a large influx of people who moved from rural areas to the cities, an increased number of immigrants who settled mostly in urban areas, and, with this, a large increase in the number of children in city schools. Shifts in the types of available jobs were evident as was the need to assist these new city dwellers and students in their vocational development.

One of the first persons credited with developing a systematic approach to vocational guidance was Frank Parsons (McDaniels & Watts, 1994). As noted in Chapter 2, Parsons was a man who envisioned systematic vocational guidance in the schools, a national vocational guidance movement, and the importance of counseling to assist individuals in their vocational development (Jones, 1994). Parsons, known to be a humanitarian, later became known as the founder of vocational guidance and suggested that vocational guidance involved a three-step process that included knowing oneself, knowing job characteristics, and making a match between the two through "true reasoning" (Parsons, 1909, 1989). Realizing the importance of vocational guidance, others joined the bandwagon. Individuals like Jesse Davis in Grand Rapids, Michigan; Eli Weaver in New York City; and Anna Reed in Seattle established guidance services in their respective school systems (Aubrey, 1977).

In 1932, during the midst of the Depression, the Wagner O'Day Act was passed establishing the U.S. Employment Services, which provided vocational guidance for the unemployed. Also around this time, the testing movement began to spread. The merging of vocational guidance with testing was a natural partnership because assessment offered a relatively quick and reliable means of determining individual traits. It was also during this time frame that the U.S. Department of Labor published the *Dictionary of Occupational Titles*, which represented one of the first attempts at organizing career information. Now, individuals could assess their traits and match them to existing jobs.

During the 1950s there was a shift from vocational guidance to career development. Instead of focusing only on making a job choice, the emphasis was now placed on one's lifelong career patterns, with the concept of career being defined very broadly. Now, leisure activities, avocations, occupations, and post-vocational patterns related to retiring would all be considered important components of one's "career development." One theory, proposed by a team composed of an economist, a sociologist, a psychiatrist, and a psychologist (Ginzberg, Ginsburg, Axelrad, & Herma, 1951; Ginzberg, 1972) and a second theory, developed by Donald Super (Super, 1957, 1990), were instrumental in transforming vocational guidance to developmental career guidance and counseling (Walsh & Ossipow, 1988).

With the emergence of humanistic approaches to counseling, as well as government initiatives such as the National Defense Education Act, which stressed career guidance in the schools, new comprehensive models of career guidance were developed in the 1960s and 1970s. These models viewed career guidance broadly and included:

(1) focusing on lifelong patterns of career development; (2) assisting individuals in making choices that reflected their sense of self; (3) the examination of leisure and avocational activities when working with clients; (4) viewing career development as a flexible and changeable process as compared to the rigid, irreversible process of earlier times; and (5) an emphasis on the individual, not the counselor, as the career decision-maker (Herr & Cramer, 1996).

The 1980s and 1990s expanded the notion that career development was a lifespan process to which counselors could assist individuals in their life roles. In addition, the computer age brought about a wealth of accessible information that allowed for quick exploration of the world of work. The evolution of career development models in conjunction with this new technology made career exploration an exciting and in-depth process.

Today, career guidance and career counseling are important components of what all counselors do. This is one of the reasons career and lifespan development has been selected by CACREP as an important content area for graduate programs in counseling.

Theories of Career Development

Since the beginning of the vocational guidance movement, and particularly in the past 20 years, a number of career development models have focused on assisting the individual in understanding his or her career choices. Although their goals are similar, these models approach the career counseling process in distinct ways. For instance, self-efficacy theory states that the types of choices we make are based on our beliefs about whether or not we can do certain behaviors (Albert & Luzzo, 1999; Bandura, 1997; McAuliffe, 1992b). Social learning theory, on the other hand, asserts that career decision making is a function of learned experiences and that clients can be taught new ways of enhancing the quality of their lives (Krumboltz, 1994; Krumboltz, Mitchell, & Jones, 1976; Mitchell, Levin, & Krumboltz, 1999). Decision-making theory contends that how a client understands him- or herself is crucial to the manner in which he or she makes career decisions (Tiedeman & Miller-Tiedeman, 1984; Tiedeman & O'Hara, 1963). Situational theories (Warnath, 1975), on the other hand, state that the choices we make are often out of our control (e.g., unavailability of jobs due to a recession).

Although all of the above theories offer interesting ways of approaching the career development process, the theories that we will examine in some detail include modern-day trait-and-factor theory, John Holland's personality theory of occupational choice, Ann Roe's psychodynamic theory, Super's lifespan development theory, and cognitive development approaches. These theories are broad in nature and seem to have gained the most attention these days. We will conclude this section by examining how an effective career counselor can draw from many different theories when working with clients.

Trait-and-Factor Approach

The trait-and-factor approach, initially proposed in the early work of Frank Parsons, was the major career development theory for many years, maintaining its popularity until the 1950s. This approach originally was a straightforward process that involved the counselor assisting the client in assessing his or her strengths, examining the availability of jobs, and using a rational process to make career decisions. The approach, which focused largely on assessment of ability and interests, was largely didactic and directive.

Although trait-and-factor theory has maintained its emphasis on the importance of a fit between the individual and the environment, current-day trait-and-factor counselors have expanded their role greatly. The following summarizes some of the important features of current-day trait-and-factor theorists (Brown, 1984; Herr & Cramer, 1996; Miller, 1974, Swanson, 1994):

1. Individuals have unique traits that can be measured, discussed, and examined. Some of these include: aptitudes, needs and interests, values, stereotypes and expectations, psychological adjustment, the propensity to take risks, and aspirations.
2. Occupations necessitate that individuals have certain traits if they are to be successful in that occupation.
3. The better the ability of the individual to match his or her traits to occupations, the more likelihood the individual will have success and feel satisfied.
4. The interaction between client and therapist is a dynamic process that includes both affective and cognitive components.
5. The ability of an individual to match his or her traits with occupations is a conscious process that can occur in a deliberate fashion. However, such matching can only be effective if a person has insight into self and knowledge of his or her unique traits and the situational factors that may affect potential decisions.

Today's trait-and-factor counselor does not simply match abilities and interests with jobs but uses a variety of techniques to examine how the vast array of the client's skills, interests, and personality variables might affect eventual career choices. This is done in a dynamic manner in which the counselor, through the use of modern-day counseling techniques, facilitates client understanding of self and assists the client in making decisive career choices.

John Holland's Personality Theory of Occupational Choice

John Holland developed a theory of occupational choice that states that people express their personality through the career choices they make (Holland, 1973; Holland & Gottfredson, 1976). Holland believed that genetic and environmental influences lead people to develop "a hierarchy of habitual or preferred methods for dealing with social and environmental tasks" (Herr & Cramer, 1996, p. 220). Holland identified six personality types that he believed represented the major ways in which individuals differ and gave them names that reflected their orientation: realistic, investigative, artistic, social, enterprising, and conventional (see Box 11.1). Holland asserted that there are numerous occupations that can fit one's personality type. Thus, individuals with similar personality types yet differing abilities could find a number of jobs in which they could express their personality type.

Although one can be a pure type, it is more usual for an individual to have two or more types that predominate. By listing in order of preference an individual's top three types, we can find what is called one's occupational code. Holland conducted research that supported the notion that the six personality types could be viewed on a hexagon, with adjacent types sharing more common elements than nonadjacent ones (see Figure 11.1). Generally, an individual's predominant type and secondary types are close to one another on the hexagon. For instance, if an individual was highest in the social type, than it would not be surprising if the artistic and enterprising types were also high because they are next to the social type on the hexagon.

BOX 11.1

Holland's Personality and Work Types

Realistic: Realistic persons like to work with equipment, machines, or tools, often prefer to work outdoors, and are good with manipulating concrete physical objects. These individuals prefer to avoid social situations, artistic endeavors, or intellectual tasks. Some settings in which you might find realistic individuals include filling stations, farms, machine shops, construction sites, and power plants.

Investigative: Investigative persons like to think abstractly, problem solve, and investigate. These individuals feel comfortable with the pursuit of knowledge and with dealing with the manipulation of ideas and symbols. Investigative individuals prefer to avoid social situations and see themselves as introverted. Some settings in which you might find investigative individuals include research laboratories, hospitals, universities, and government-sponsored research agencies.

Artistic: Artistic individuals like to express themselves creatively, usually through artistic forms such as drama, art, music, and writing. They prefer unstructured activities in which they can use their imagination and creative side. Some settings in which you might find artistic individuals include the theater, concert halls, libraries, art or music studios, dance studios, orchestras, photography studios, newspapers, and restaurants.

Social: Social people are nurturers, helpers, and caregivers and have high concern for others. They are introspective and insightful and prefer work environments in which they can use their intuitive and caregiving skills. Some settings in which you might find social people are government social service agencies, counseling offices, churches, schools, mental hospitals, recreation centers, personnel offices, and hospitals.

Enterprising: Enterprising individuals are self-confident, adventurous, bold, and sociable. They have good persuasive skills and prefer positions of leadership. They tend to dominate conversations and enjoy work environments in which they can satisfy their need for recognition, power, and expression. Some settings in which you might find enterprising individuals include life insurance agencies, advertising agencies, political offices, real estate offices, new and used car lots, sales offices, and in management settings.

Conventional: Individuals of the conventional orientation are stable, controlled, conservative, and sociable. They prefer working on concrete tasks and like to follow instructions. They value the business world and clerical tasks and tend to be good at computational skills. Some settings in which you might find conventional people include banks, business offices, accounting firms, and medical records offices.

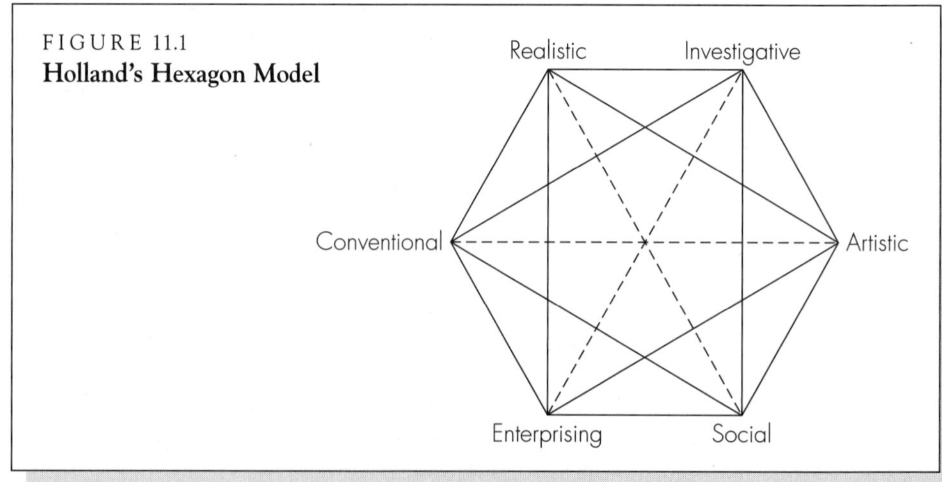

FIGURE 11.1
Holland's Hexagon Model

Holland also asserted that jobs could be classified by type. Thus, he hypothesized that if you accurately matched an individual's code to a job that has the same code, you increase your chances of having a person who is satisfied at the job and ultimately in his or her career. Thus, the individual with the SAE code could be matched with occupation "counselor," which has the same corresponding code. Research on the Holland codes has been plentiful and has shown that accurate matches do indeed increase the chances for job satisfaction (Assouline & Meir, 1987; Jagger, Neukrug, & McAuliffe, 1992). Keep in mind, however, that there are many other SAE choices besides counselor.

Holland and others have worked hard to identify the codes that would best fit in various jobs. For instance, Gottfredson, Holland, and Ogawa (1996) identified the occupational codes for more than 12,000 jobs and published these codes in the book *The Dictionary of Holland Occupational Codes*. By taking one or more of a number assessment instruments (e.g., *Strong Interest Inventory*, Consulting Psychologists Press, 1994; *Self-Directed Search*, Holland, 1994), an individual can determine his or her Holland code and then match it with occupational codes. You might want to take the exercise in Figure 11.2 if you would like a crude yet quick way of obtaining your Holland code.

FIGURE 11.2
Finding Your Holland Code

Realistic: People who are practical, robust, have good physical skills, like the outdoors, and who avoid social situations, intellectual pursuits, and artistic endeavors.

Investigative: People who like to investigate, think abstractly, and do problem solving, but avoid social situations and tend to be introverted.

Conventional: People who are concrete, like to work with data, and prefer routine problem solving. They prefer clerical tasks and tend to be neat, follow instructions, and look for social approval.

Artistic: People who express themselves through art, are creative and imaginative, like unstructured activities, and tend to be sensitive, introspective, and independent.

Enterprising: People who are persuasive, self-confident, like to lead, and see themselves as stable, sociable, adventurous, bold, and self-confident.

Social: People who are concerned for others, nurturers, introspective, and responsible; who like social situations and are verbally skilled.

Take the first letter of the group for each of the first three groups that you picked, in the order that you picked them; this is your code. For instance, I picked the social group first, the artistic group second, and the enterprising group third. Therefore, my Holland code would be SAE.

Holland's theory has been used extensively by career counselors, and it is to his credit that numerous assessment instruments to determine one's code have been developed. In addition, research has consistently shown the importance of the Holland theory when working with clients. John Holland has certainly added much to career counseling.

Ann Roe's Psychodynamic Theory

In 1956 Ann Roe developed a rather elaborate theory that based career choice to a large degree on the kinds of early parenting received. Roe hypothesized that parents can be classified as either warm or cold and that these two styles result in one of three types of emotional climates: emotional concentration on the child, acceptance of the child, or avoidance of the child (see Figure 11.3). The type of emotional climate in the home will result in one of six types of parent–child relationships, which influences the kinds of occupational choices the child will eventually make (Roe & Siegelman, 1964). Parenting style, said Roe, ultimately results in the individual having one of the following eight orientations toward the world of work: service (I), business (II), organization (III), technology (IV), outdoor (V), science (VI), general culture (VII), and arts and entertainment (VIII).

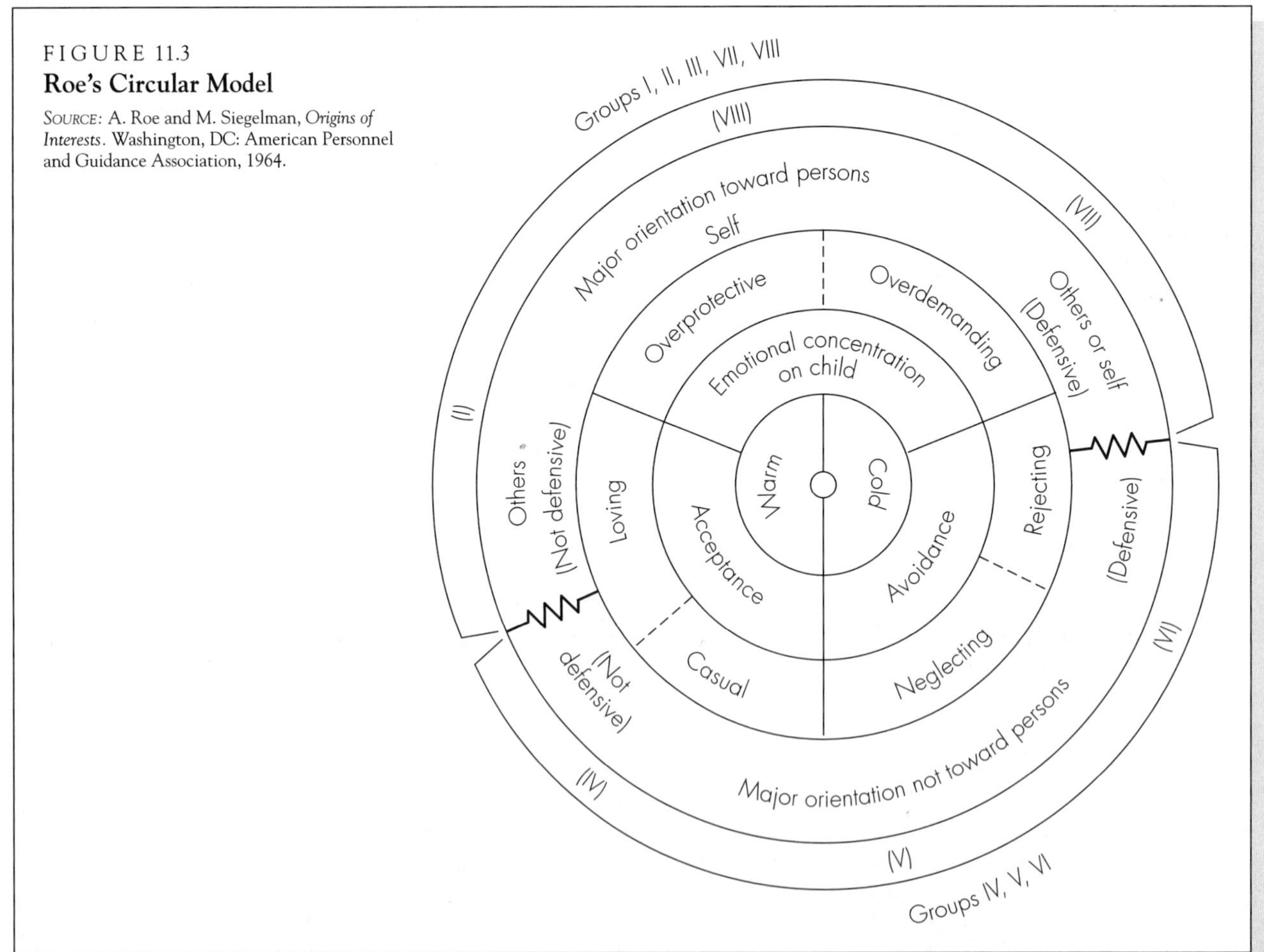

FIGURE 11.3
Roe's Circular Model

SOURCE: A. Roe and M. Siegelman, *Origins of Interests*. Washington, DC: American Personnel and Guidance Association, 1964.

Peterson, Sampson, and Reardon (1991) describe Roe's different parenting styles and the possible influences they have on occupational choice:

1. *Protective*. The parents are indulgent and demonstratively affectionate and give the child special privileges. The home may be described as child-centered. Children from such homes tend to gravitate to the service, arts, or entertainment fields.
2. *Demanding*. The parents set forth high expectations for accomplishment and impose strict regulation and obedience. Children growing up in this type of environment may be oriented to general culture (lawyers, teachers, scholars, librarians) or to the arts and entertainment fields.
3. *Rejecting*. The parents do not accept the child as a child, perhaps not even as an individual. They are often cold, hostile, and derogatory, making the child feel inferior and unaccepted. Rejected children tend to pursue science occupations.
4. *Neglecting*. The parents simply ignore the child; they give little attention, either positive or negative. They provide minimum physical care and less emotional sustenance. Neglected children tend to develop science and outdoor interests.
5. *Casual*. The parents give emotional and physical attention to the child, but only after higher-priority issues in their own lives have been attended to. Children treated casually tend to gravitate to technological occupations (engineers, aviators, applied scientists) or organizational occupations (bankers, accountants, clerks).
6. *Loving*. The parents are warm, helpful, and affectionate. They set limits and guide behavior through rational problem solving. They help the child with activities but are not intrusive. Children whose parents are loving tend to gravitate to service or business-contact occupations (promoters, salespersons). (pp. 55-56)

Although Roe believed that early parenting styles were instrumental in shaping occupational choice, she also believed that such factors as gender, the economy, physical appearance, chance factors, family background, temperament, and one's genetic makeup and how it impacts on interests and abilities could affect career choice. She believed that these factors interacted with one another in complex ways. Although research on Roe's model has been mixed (Herr & Cramer, 1996; Isaacson, 1985), she has contributed much by being one of the first theorists to relate occupational choice to personality style. Such a focus has dramatically changed the way that counselors work with clients as it suggests the importance of looking at early family dynamics when practicing career counseling.

Super's Lifespan Development Approaches to Career Counseling

Like the lifespan approaches studied in Chapter 9, lifespan developmental approaches to career counseling involve a series of sequential and predictable stages through which individuals pass. During the 1950s Donald Super developed a theory that drew from a number of developmental models (Super, 1957, 1990). His theory, which became known as a developmental self-concept theory, soon became prominent in the field (Ossipow, 1996). Super's theory contended that:

1. Career development is an ongoing, continuous, and orderly process starting in early childhood and ending with death.
2. People's abilities, personality traits, and self-concepts differ, and individuals are qualified for a number of different types of occupations based on their characteristics.

3. Occupations tend to be specifically appropriate for people with certain kinds of qualities, although there is enough variability in occupations to allow for some differences in the kinds of people who will be drawn to them.
4. Self-concept is both a function and result of one's career development process and can change as one passes through developmental stages.
5. Movement from one occupational level to another is influenced by a number of factors, including parental socioeconomic level, status needs, values, interests, skill in interpersonal relationships, economic conditions, and intelligence.
6. Starting in early childhood and continuing into late adulthood, career development can be assisted by helping individuals understand and develop their abilities and interests and by assisting them in understanding their strengths and weaknesses.
7. By understanding the developmental level of the individual, counselors can make appropriate interventions that can assist individuals in learning about themselves and their career development process, thus making occupational choices more likely to lead to satisfaction at work and a high self-concept.
8. Career development is generally irreversible, although some people who face important development crises may recycle through the stages at any point in their career.

Super saw career development as a five-stage process, with each stage having substages distinguished by unique developmental tasks (see Figure 11.4). During the growth stage (ages birth through 14), children identify with others, gain an awareness of interests

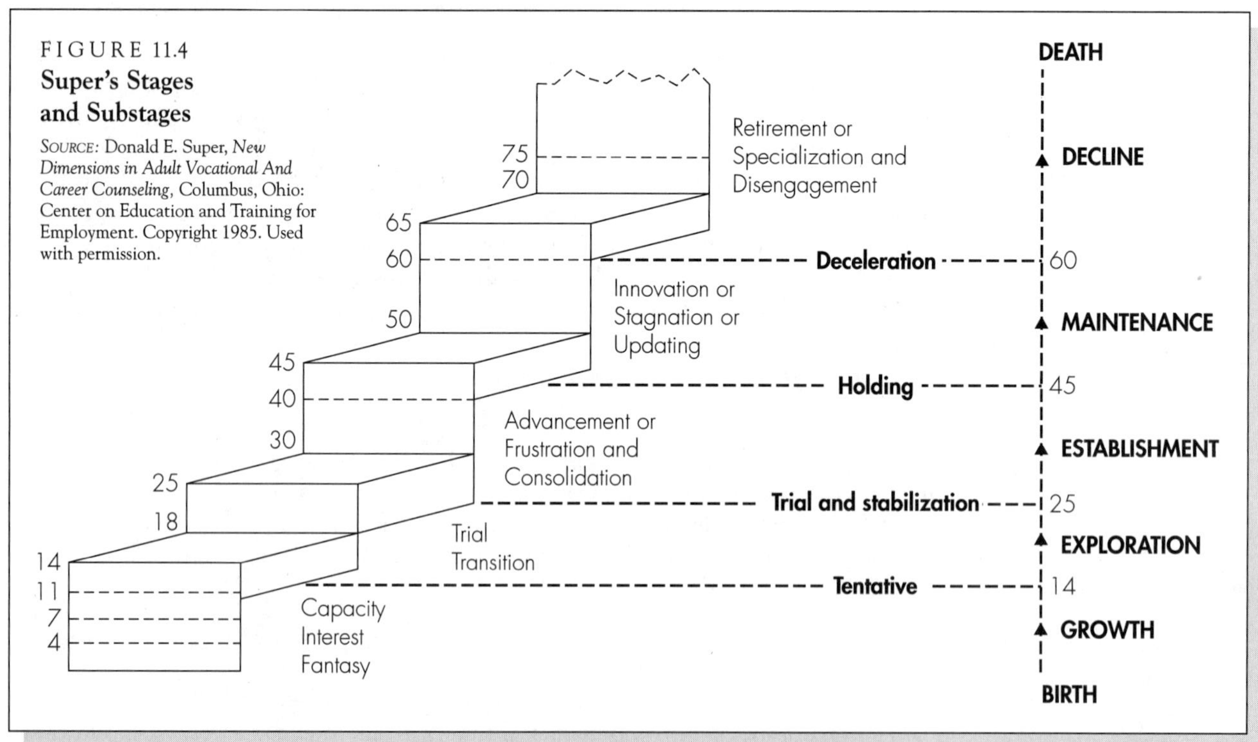

FIGURE 11.4
Super's Stages and Substages

SOURCE: Donald E. Super, *New Dimensions in Adult Vocational And Career Counseling*, Columbus, Ohio: Center on Education and Training for Employment. Copyright 1985. Used with permission.

and abilities, and begin to develop a career self-concept. Included in this stage is the very young child's beginning awareness of the world of work and the middle school youth who compares his or her abilities and interests to peers. In the exploration stage (ages 14 through 24), adolescents and young adults begin to tentatively test out their occupational fantasies through work, school, and leisure activities. Later in this stage individuals begin to crystallize their vocational preferences by choosing an occupation or further professional training. The establishment stage (ages 24 through 44) involves stabilizing career choices and advancing in chosen fields, while the maintenance stage (ages 44 through 64) encompasses the preservation of one's current status in the choices made and avoidance of stagnation. During the decline stage (ages 64 through death), people begin to disengage from their chosen fields and increasingly focus on retirement, leisure, and/or avocational activities.

If counselors are going to design effective strategies that will work with clients, they should be familiar with each stage and substage so they can tailor their techniques to the particular tasks unique to that developmental milestone. For instance, an elementary school counselor would be foolish to assist a child in making specific career choices, and a college counselor would be amiss to encourage a college student to quickly become established in a career.

Super's developmental approach has added an important dimension to the understanding of the career development process by making us aware of the universal developmental tasks that people face throughout their lifetimes.

Cognitive Development Approaches to Career Counseling

The most recent addition to career development theory has been promulgated by cognitive development theorists who believe that career decision making is related to how individuals make meaning out of the world of work (McAuliffe, 1993; Peavy, 1994). Cognitive developmentalists argue that most career development theories do not explain changes in cognitive functioning over the lifespan. They suggest that cognitive changes take place developmentally, and we could assist clients by initially determining their cognitive developmental stage and subsequently devising strategies to help them move to a higher stage (Knefelkamp & Slepitza, 1976; McAuliffe & Eriksen, 1999). Movement to higher-stage thinking would mean that clients would have changed their ways of understanding the world. Such movement occurs by supporting the client's current way of understanding the world and then gently challenging him or her to understand the world differently.

In describing the basic tenets of cognitive development theories, Peterson, Sampson, and Reardon (1991) highlight the following points:

- Cognitive development occurs in a series of predictable stages, which are the same for all people.
- People will differ in their rate of progression through the stages, and some may become arrested in a stage.
- Each stage is qualitatively different from the next, but they do overlap with one another.
- Higher stages are distinguished by more complex and more sophisticated ways of understanding the world.
- Sometimes, when faced with stressful situations, people may respond at lower stages.

In applying the above tenets, counselors have relied on different cognitive development theories. For instance, whereas McAuliffe explains meaning making through Kegan's constructive development theory, others use Perry's theory (see Chapter 9). Let's explore how a cognitive developmental theorist would work with a client using Perry's theory.

If you remember from Chapters 3 and 9, Perry talked about two kinds of people, the dualist and the relativist. Briefly, the dualist sees the world as black or white and believes that authorities have answers. Relativists, on the other hand, see the world as having relative truths with many ways of explaining a phenomenon or of understanding the world. Now, consider the dualistic college student who seeks career counseling. This student sees the career counselor as having knowledge to help him or her find the correct occupation, thus closing off other potential occupational choices. An effective cognitive developmental career counselor wants to support the student's current way of thinking and then gently challenge him or her to understand the world, and in this case, the career counseling process, in different ways. Therefore, this counselor would want to devise strategies to help the student move toward a relativistic outlook, one in which the student saw many possible occupational choices instead of seeing just one right occupation. In addition, this changed student would see the career counseling process as collaborative as opposed to a one-way directive counselor-to-client process.

Cognitive developmental theory is an exciting new approach in which client growth is possible if the counselor is able to identify the cognitive developmental stage of the client, understand the unique ways that individuals in that stage view the world, and support and challenge the client to new ways of understanding the world. This approach challenges counselors to understand the world of the client in an effort to free the client from the constraints of his or her meaning making system:

> *Seemingly simple [cognitive development] transitions can be opportunities for deep structural transformation. The counselor's tasks are to assess clients' implicit meaning-making stances and challenge and support clients to face dilemmas and become open to new possibilities.* (McAuliffe, 1993, p. 1)

Integrating Models of Career Development

When some of the major theories of career development are examined, it is clear that they approach working with the individual in very different ways. This is why most counselors doing career counseling integrate the various theories. Look at Angela (Box 11.2), and then let's examine how each theory discussed could offer a different and important perspective to her situation.

Trait-and-Factor Theory and Holland's Personality Theory

The modern day trait-and-factor counselor can help Angela explore her traits, such as her interests, aptitudes, values, and personality qualities, by taking some interest inventories, personality measures, and/or ability tests. In addition, the trait-and-factor counselor might help Angela explore the stereotypes she holds about specific occupations, as well as her beliefs about the kinds of occupations she thinks she can do (e.g., self-efficacy). This counselor would help Angela examine the world of work and assist her in understanding all of the occupations that might fit her personality type (e.g., Holland) as well as the situational factors that could affect her choices.

BOX 11.2

Integrating Career Development Theories: Angela

Angela is a 24-year-old first-year graduate student in counseling. Her mother, who is a school counselor, and her father, who is a head nurse, have both encouraged her to go into the counseling profession. Angela has a brother, John, who is two years older and going to medical school. She describes her relationship with her parents as loving but sometimes a little overwhelming and claustrophobic. Angela lives at home and is beginning to feel frustrated because her parents continue to want to know where she is most of the time. Angela has done particularly well in school, especially in the sciences and math. In fact, she switched majors her junior year from psychology to chemistry. Although Angela is doing well in her courses, she continues to have a "funny feeling" about being a counselor. Deep inside, she thinks that maybe she should be doing something else.

Developmental Theory

Angela is in the exploration stage of her career development process. A person in this stage usually wonders about the choices he or she has made and considers other options. Knowing this, the counselor might want to assure Angela that it is usual for young adults to be questioning their decisions. At the same time, it would be important for the counselor to understand the kinds of doubts Angela has about her decision to be a counselor. Ultimately, the goal of the counselor would be to help Angela move toward a more stable position relative to whatever career-related decisions she makes.

Psychodynamic Theory

The psychodynamic career counselor would assume that, in unconscious ways, Angela's parents have strongly influenced the kinds of career choices she has made. Having had loving parents who were a little overprotective and who are both in service occupations could lean Angela toward a service occupation such as counseling (see Ann Roe). However, one would not want to rule out many other service occupations. In addition, examining the kinds of early modeling and messages she received from her parents, as well as general parenting style and how that may have affected her personality development (e.g., dependency needs), can offer the counselor a wealth of information about Angela. Also, the counselor would want to examine Angela's position in her family and understand what it was like being the youngest in the family, the only daughter in the family, and the younger sister of a successful older brother.

Cognitive Development Theory

From this perspective the counselor would want to understand how Angela makes meaning out of her career decisions. Ultimately, the counselor wants to determine Angela's cognitive developmental level then help her move toward higher-stage thinking and a more stable position relative to career-related decision making. Using Perry, for example, the counselor might hypothesize, based on her age and her situation, that Angela is in transition from dualism to relativism. The counselor may want to find answers to the following questions in an attempt to understand Angela and affirm or revise this hypothesis:

- What is it about counseling that attracts Angela, and how does it fit her view of self?
- What is important in Angela's life?
- How does Angela make sense of the choices she has made?
- How has Angela's family influenced her?
- How does Angela make decisions?

If the counselor's hypothesis is affirmed, he or she would recognize that, having been a dualist, Angela had rigidly believed she should be a counselor and was not open to hearing other options. However, now that she appears to be in transition to relativistic thinking, she is beginning to question her past views and may be open to hearing about other choices. Supporting Angela while challenging her to find her own voice can help her in this difficult career decision making process.

Bringing It All Together

As you can see, each theory offers us a unique perspective on Angela; when used together, they can provide Angela the best opportunity to understand herself and make choices that would work best for her. As you can imagine, to fully assist Angela would take some time. It would include exploring her past and the influences it has had on her, assessing her lifespan developmental level, taking time to understand her present ways of making sense out of the world, assessing her traits, helping her examine opportunities that are available to her, and assisting her in making a transition to a new way of perceiving the world. Indeed, we are not simply talking about finding Angela a job or changing her major but helping Angela to gain deep knowledge about herself so she can make the wisest decisions for her life.

The Use of Career-Related Information

An extensive amount of occupational information is available in the field of career development. In the career counseling process, career information assures that all people have access to knowledge about careers, assists clients in understanding the nature of work, helps the counselor understand the client, and increases client self-understanding (Fredrickson, 1982). This section will examine some of the more prevalent informational resources available. Keep in mind that these represent just a few of the many ways of obtaining information about the world of work.

Occupational Classification Systems

The Dictionary of Occupational Titles (DOT)

The *DOT*, which is published by the U.S. Department of Labor (1999), is a comprehensive classification system of occupations. The *DOT* provides a short description for close to 30,000 occupations and offers a nine-code classification system for each job. The first series of three numbers of the classification system places jobs in general occupational groups; the second series of three numbers presents the complexity of worker traits related to the use of data on the job, the type of interactions with people at work, and the use of

BOX 11.3

An Example from the *DOT*: Counselor, Marriage and Family (*DOT* Number: 045.107.954)

Provides individual, marital, and family counseling services to adults and children, to assist clients to identify personal and interactive problems, and to achieve effective personal, marital, and family development and adjustment: Collects information about clients (individuals, married couples, or families), using interview, case history, and observation techniques, funnel approach, and appraisal and assessment methods. Analyzes information collected to determine advisability of counseling or referral to other specialists or institutions. Reviews notes and information collected to identify problems and concerns. Consults references material, such as textbooks, manuals, and journals, to identify symptoms, make diagnoses, and develop therapeutic or treatment plan. Counsels clients, using counseling methods and procedures, such as psychotherapy and hypnosis, to assist clients in gaining insight into personal and interactive problems, to define goals, and to plan action reflecting interests, abilities, and needs. Evaluates results of counseling methods to determine reliability and validity of treatment used. Interacts with other professionals to discuss therapy or treatment, new resources or techniques, and to share information. (Department of Labor, 1991, p. 52)

different types of things on the job (e.g., equipment, food) (see Box 11.3). Each of the three numbers range from 0 to 9 with the level of complexity increasing as you approach 0. The last three digits distinguish jobs that have the same first six digits. For instance, school counselor and mental health counselor have the same first six digits but are distinguished by the last three digits.

The Guide for Occupational Exploration (GOE)

The GOE was originally published in 1979 as a companion volume to the *DOT*. The *GOE* uses occupational categories that are based on well-known interest inventories and is considered to be simpler to use than the *DOT* (Sharf, 1993). The *GOE* is designed around 12 interest factors that include artistic, scientific, plants and animals, protective, mechanical, industrial, business detail, selling, accommodating, humanitarian, leading-influencing, and physical performing. These 12 groups are further divided into numerous subgroups. The *GOE* can be used by simply examining the various jobs in an interest factor and selecting those jobs that have some appeal. The GOE also offers detailed descriptions on approximately 2500 jobs.

The Occupational Outlook Handbook (OOH)

The *Occupational Outlook Handbook (OOH)* (2000-2001a) includes information on the nature of work of an occupation; working conditions; employment statistics; training, other qualifications, and advancement; job outlook; earnings; related occupations; and sources of additional information. Although the handbook only examines approximately 250 jobs and is not always perfect in its predictions, it accounts for approximately seven out of eight jobs in the economy and is a good source of information concerning general categories of work. The *OOH* can now be accessed on the Internet (see Box 11.4).

BOX 11.4

Selected Excerpts from the *OOH:* Counselors

Job Outlook

Overall employment of counselors is expected to grow *faster than the average* for all occupations through the year 2008. In addition, replacement needs should increase significantly as a large number of counselors reach retirement age.

Employment of school counselors is expected to grow as a result of increasing enrollments, particularly in secondary and postsecondary schools. . . .

Demand is expected to be strong for rehabilitation and mental health counselors. . . .

Similar to other government jobs, the number of employment counselors, who work primarily for State and local government, could be limited by budgetary constraints. . . .

Earnings

Median earnings for full-time educational and vocational counselors were about $38,650 a year in 1998. The middle 50 percent earned between $28,400 and $49,960 a year. The lowest 10 percent earned less than $21,230 a year, while the top 10 percent earned over $73,920 a year.

Following are median annual earnings for 1997 in the industries employing the largest numbers of vocational and educational counselors:

Elementary and secondary schools	$42,100
State government, except education and hospitals	35,800
Colleges and universities	34,700
Job training and related services	24,100
Individual and family services	22,300

Self-employed counselors who have well-established practices, as well as counselors employed in group practices, generally have the highest earnings, as do some counselors working for private firms, such as insurance companies and private rehabilitation companies. . . .

(Occupational Outlook Handbook, 2000–2001b)

Assessment Instruments

Interest Inventories

Over the years a number of assessment instruments have been developed to assist individuals in their career exploration process. Probably the most important of these have been the interest inventories, such as the *Strong Interest Inventory* (Consulting Psychologists Press, 1994), the *Career Decision-Making System (CDM)* (Harrington & O'Shea, 2000), and the *Career Assessment Inventory (CAI)* (Johansson, 1996). Interest inventories examine a client's interests in such areas as school subjects, types of people, types of occupations, amusements, and/or personal characteristics. Some interest inventories, like *The Self-Directed Search* (Holland, 1994), and the Strong (again) examine an individual's personality orientation toward the world of work and usually provide occupations in which the client might find a good fit.

Assessment of Aptitude

Aptitude testing allows an individual to examine whether or not occupational preferences match his or her ability. For instance, an individual who has interest in becoming a researcher but has little math ability may have a difficult time achieving his or her occupational goals, and a person who is found to have high mechanical ability might consider various jobs that relate to this aptitude. Some of the popular aptitude tests include the Differential Aptitude Test (DAT), published by the Psychological Corporation; the General Aptitude Test Battery (GATB), published by the U.S. Department of Labor, Employ-

BOX 11.5

Shayna's Personality Profile

Shayna had definitely decided that she was interested in an occupation that would provide her with an opportunity to help people. A personality inventory indicated that she was very reserved and nonassertive and deferred to others. She agreed with the results of the personality inventory and further agreed that these characteristics would make it difficult for her to accomplish her occupational goal. Shayna became convinced that she would have to modify these personality characteristics through a variety of programs, including self-discovery groups and assertiveness training. (Zunker, 2001, pp. 222–223)

ment and Training Administration; and the Armed Services Vocational Aptitude Battery (ASVAB), which was developed for the military and is sometimes given in high schools for free.

Personality Assessment

Numerous personality tests have been used in conjunction with career counseling. Tests such as *The Myers-Briggs Type Indicator* (Consulting Psychologists Press, 1985), and *The California Psychological Inventory* (Consulting Psychologists Press, 1996) can help a client focus on basic personality dimensions and examine whether or not his or her personality profile might fit with certain jobs (see Box 11.5).

Computer-Assisted Career Guidance

The expansion in the use of personal computers has made career information systems available to a vast array of individuals. Computers offer an easy and quick method of accessing large amounts of career information. Today, there are numerous computer programs that allow us to assess abilities, interests, values, and skills and also let us obtain all kinds of occupational information. Below are some of the ways that the computer is used today in career guidance.

Comprehensive Computer-Based Programs

Increasingly, computer-based programs are being developed that allow the individual to examine his or her values, interests, and skills and contain information on such things as occupations, college and trade schools, college majors, job availability, and financial aid. Many of these computer programs can be found in schools, colleges, business and industry, public employment and labor-related agencies, and private career counseling agencies. Some of the more popular programs include *Guidance Information System (GIS)* (Riverside Publishing Company, 1992), *Discover* (ACT Discover Center, 1998), and *System of Interactive Guidance and Information-Plus (SIGI-Plus)* (Educational Testing Services, 1993).

Testing

It is now possible to offer many interest and ability tests on computer; and, increasingly, counselors will no longer have to send tests out to be scored or spend a lengthy amount of time hand-scoring an instrument. Many of the traditional assessment instruments are rapidly being developed for computer usage.

The Internet

The amount of occupational information that can be found on the Internet is astronomical and will continue to increase. For example, the *Dictionary of Occupational Titles* can be downloaded, for a fee, from the Internet, and the *Occupational Outlook Handbook* can be accessed for free. Also, most publishing companies have now begun to sell software on the Internet; and, in many cases one can, for a fee, download the software directly. Finally, there is an ever-increasing number of sites, some well done, some that are rather unprofessional, that offer career guidance, usually for a fee.

Other Sources of Occupational Information

The amount of occupational information available is enormous, and much of it is free! For instance, printed materials can be obtained from a number of government agencies, commercial publishers, professional associations, educational institutions, and periodicals. In addition, many colleges and trade schools have career centers available for use by their students and even sometimes for the general public. In addition to free materials, numerous books offer career information materials. Today, there are even best-selling paperbacks that assist us in our career development (e.g., *What Color is Your Parachute?* Bolles, 2001). Finding information about occupations is relatively easy if one spends just a little bit of time.

The Clinical Interview: The Lost Child in Career Development

The field of career counseling is so replete with theories, career information, and career assessment instruments that sometimes it seems like our most precious counseling tool, the clinical interview, is forgotten. A good clinical interview can help the counselor gain an enormous amount of information about a client, information that can be effectively used in helping the client make career choices. The clinical interview is our way of operationalizing our career development theories. It can be used to assess family-of-origin issues that have had an impact on the client's career development, the meaning-making system of the client, client desires and wants, how the client tends to present him- or herself, and emotional problems that might interfere with an individual seeking out or maintaining certain jobs.

The clinical interview is a major part of the total assessment process for the client, and the counseling skills learned in a graduate program are the vehicle for that assessment. If career counseling meant only assessing traits and matching those traits with jobs, we would be operating out of a turn-of-the-last-century paradigm and would hardly need an advanced degree to work with clients.

Integrating Theory, Career Information, and Career Assessment

Between the numerous theories of career counseling and the enormous amount of occupational information available to counselors, you may be asking, "Where do I start when doing career counseling?" McAuliffe's (1998) Context Phase Stage and Style (CPSS) model suggests that when working with adults, one should begin by examining the context in which the client lives (culture, community, family), the developmental phase or stage in which the client finds himself or herself (e.g., Erikson, Kegan, Super), and the client's personality style toward the world of work (e.g., Holland code, early childhood patterns). This model offers a lot of promise in integrating the various elements talked about in this chapter.

Based on many of the same elements offered by McAuliffe, let me suggest some specific strategies when doing career counseling with adults:

1. Conduct a thorough clinical interview. Assess factors crucial to the client's career development process, including:
   - How early childhood issues have affected the client's propensity toward certain careers.
   - How socioeconomic status of the family of origin has had an impact on the client's aspirations.
   - How the parents' career development has had an impact on the client's aspirations.
   - How emotional problems may interfere with career decision making.
   - How situational issues may interfere with career decision making.
   - The determination of developmental level (e.g., Super) of the client.
   - The determination of cognitive development level (e.g., Kegan).
2. Assess the client's abilities, interests, and personality characteristics through the use of appropriate assessment instruments (e.g., Holland code, the CPI, the Strong).
3. Based on your clinical interview, the client's developmental level, and your assessment of your client thus far, devise treatment strategies in collaboration with your client that are congruent with his or her developmental readiness.
4. Make available appropriate informational resources that can be used in conjunction with your treatment plan.
5. Assist the client in understanding the world of work and factors that may potentially affect career choice (such as economic conditions or market saturation).
6. Have the client make tentative career decisions.
7. Explore the practicality of the career decisions chosen and begin to crystallize a choice.
8. Have the client take preliminary steps toward choosing a career path by doing such things as informational interviews with individuals who have taken a similar path, shadowing people at a job, and reading literature about the career path.
9. Follow up with the client to assure satisfaction and closure of the career development process.
10. Recycle if necessary. If the client is unsatisfied with his or her progress, start the process over, and reexamine all the issues.

As you can imagine from the above, a thorough career assessment can be a rather lengthy process. However, the use of such a process creates career choice and not career happenstance.

Multicultural Issues

Multicultural Career Counseling: Coming of Age

> *. . . more and more career counselors and vocational psychologists are also considering the manner in which they need to prepare themselves to meet the upcoming challenges of increasing cultural diversity. . . .* (Leong, 1995a, p. 2)

For years, career development was approached from a particularly white male middle-class perspective. Much of the research that was produced was based on white male clients. Assessment instruments were developed that were predictive only for white male clients, and little attention was paid to the unique issues of people of color, women, individuals with disabilities, and other diverse groups. More recently, there has been a groundswell of literature written to address these concerns, and we are just now seeing major career development texts devoting multiple chapters to diversity (e.g., Herr & Cramer, 1996; Zunker, 2001), entire books on diversity in career development being written (Leong, 1995b), and entire journals being devoted to this important issue (Leong, 1991). Multicultural career counseling is coming of age, but there is still a long road ahead.

Multicultural Theory of Career Development

Although the unique ways of working with culturally diverse groups have, in recent years, been discussed and analyzed (Leong, 1995b), no general theory of multicultural career development has been devised (Ossipow & Littlejohn, 1995). However, there are some issues that should be considered when working with culturally diverse clients. They include the following (Betz & Fitzgerald, 1995; Ossipow & Littlejohn, 1995; Subich, 1996):

1. Cultural values and practices may make full access to the workplace more difficult for some people (e.g., certain religious practices, such as praying every day and taking time off for certain holidays may be frowned upon at the workplace).
2. Whereas mainstream America has lived a life of upward mobility, some cultures and classes have not lived this dream and approach career development with different goals and aspirations.
3. The expression of self and the development of self-concept is central to the career development process, regardless of cultural background.
4. The person environment (personality workplace) fit, regardless of cultural background, is crucial for satisfaction at work.
5. The better the client understands his or her cultural identity development (see Chapter 14), the easier it will be for the client to find a fit between self and environment.
6. Discrimination in attaining jobs and at the workplace is a reality and needs to be addressed and acknowledged by career counselors.
7. Discrimination and racism have resulted in some people having serious doubts about their ability to obtain jobs and be upwardly mobile.
8. Knowledge about the career development issues of specific cultural groups is crucial to being an effective multicultural career counselor.
9. There are probably more differences within a cultural group than between cultural groups. Avoid uniformity of assumptions or thinking that all clients from one culture are the same.

10. Know that assessment procedures, so prevalent in career counseling, may have inherent biases and may not have addressed how well they predict for culturally diverse groups and women.

Career Counseling in a Diverse Culture: Specific Steps

Although no specific theory of multicultural career development may be on the horizon, a model for working with minority clients has been developed which can greatly assist the counselor (Bingham & Ward, 1996; Fouad & Bingham, 1995). In brief, the seven steps include the following:

Step 1. Establish rapport/culturally appropriate relationship.

Step 2. Identify career issues.

Step 3. Assess impact of cultural variables.

Step 4. Set counseling goals.

Step 5. Make culturally appropriate counseling interventions.

Step 6. Make decision.

Step 7. Implement and follow up.

Ethical, Professional, and Legal Issues

Ethical Standards for Career Counseling and Consultation

In 1982 the National Board for Certified Counselors (NBCC) developed its own set of ethical standards, which was adopted by the National Career Development Association (NCDA) in 1987. Because NCDA is a division of ACA, these ethical guidelines should be read in conjunction with the overarching ethical guidelines of ACA. The guidelines contain six sections including: general ethical concerns, the counseling relationship, measurement and evaluation, research and publication, consulting, and private practice. In addition, the guidelines contain a statement on how to make an ethical complaint against a career counselor.

Competency Guidelines for Career Development

The National Career Development Association (NCDA) offers a broad-based description of competencies needed for all counselors who practice vocational and career counseling. These competencies include general counseling skills, information, individual/group assessment, management/administration, implementation, and consultation. Recognizing the complexity of career development over the lifespan, the NCDA has also developed specific competencies for those who work with elementary, middle/junior, or high school students, and/or with adults. These competencies address the skills, knowledge, behaviors, and attitudes necessary to be an effective career counselor at the various levels of development.

Professional Associations

The NCDA, and the National Employment Counselors Association (NECA), both divisions of ACA, are two associations oriented toward career development (reach these divisions through the ACA Web site: www.counseling.org). *The Career Development Quarterly*, published by NCDA, and the *Journal of Employment Counseling*, published by NECA, are circulated quarterly and are membership benefits to those who join the associations.

Optimizing Career Development

Recently, when teaching an undergraduate class in human services, I asked my students to share why they had decided to enter the helping professions. An African American student told me about her school counselor who she believed had treated most black students in her high school in a manner that would discourage them from pursuing jobs in professional fields. She said, "This is why I have decided to become a school counselor, so I could assist African Americans in reaching their potential." Unfortunately, this is not the first time I have heard a story such as this.

Career counselors should be optimizing choices for clients, whether they are school counselors working with marginal students, college counselors assisting college students in job choices, agency counselors working with middle-aged adults who are seeking a job change, vocational rehabilitation counselors working with individuals who recently became paraplegic, or graduate students considering their options concerning doctoral work. Counselors should never say, "I don't think you can make it, you don't have the ability, you don't have the skills, you won't be able to take the pressure." Instead, they should be encouraging people, increasing options, and helping people seek their potential. Be realistic, but don't be discouraging. At best, discouraging clients in the pursuit of career dreams is incompetent; at worst, it is racist, sexist, ageist, and discriminatory toward individuals with disabilities.

Important Laws

Carl Perkins Act. Passed in 1984, this act authorized grants for the expansion of career guidance programs for students who had vocational education needs, as well as adults, single parents, displaced homemakers, ex-offenders, incarcerated persons, and individuals with disabilities who have needs for vocational education (Herr & Cramer, 1996).

Americans with Disabilities Act. This law, passed in 1992, assures that qualified individuals with disabilities cannot be discriminated against in job application procedures, hiring, firing, advancement, compensation, fringe benefits, job training, and other terms, conditions, and privileges ("Americans with," 1992).

PL94-142 (The Education of All Handicapped Children Act). Concerning career guidance, this law, along with the Carl Perkins Act, requires that students in occupational education programs must be given vocational assessment to assist them in their career development.

PL93-112. This law requires colleges to provide career services to persons with disabilities. For instance, students who are visually impaired might be given materials in braille to assist them in career guidance activities.

Rehabilitation Act of 1973. The Rehabilitation Act of 1973 assured access to vocational rehabilitation services for adults if they meet three conditions: being severely physically or mentally disabled, having a disability that interferes with their ability to obtain or maintain a job, and assessing that employment with their disability is feasible.

School-to-Work Opportunities Act. Passed in 1994 by Congress, this act provides incentives to help schools and community colleges develop programs that integrate academic learning with on-the-job experiences.

Title VII and Title IX. Title VII of the 1964 Civil Rights Act and Title IX of the Education Amendments of 1972 prohibit discrimination against women and minorities in all aspects of employment. In addition, Title VII and subsequent amendments set standards for the use of tests to assure they do not discriminate against culturally diverse populations.

The Counselor in Process: Career Development as a Lifespan Process

Career counseling is a lifelong process. It starts at birth and continues until we die. It is not just the process of finding a job, but how we actualize all our life roles. An astute counselor understands this process. He or she views it much like navigating a flowing river–a river that has twists and turns; parts that seem shallow, dangerous, and scary; and parts that are deep, still, and stable. This counselor understands that the river starts to flow in infancy when the child first begins to imitate adult behaviors and continues into young childhood when the youngster wonders about the world of work. Such a counselor sees this river pick up speed in adolescence with the teenager who begins to explore his or her interests, values, and abilities, and watches it move more rapidly and dangerously in young adulthood when the individual tentatively chooses a career. This river soon deepens and slows in mid-adulthood with the middle-aged person who feels established, or suddenly takes sharp twists and turns with the middle-aged person who decides to take a fresh look at his or her career choices. The river begins to slow in later life with the individual who moves out of work and into leisure activities, or the person who decreases the amount of work he or she is doing. The committed and wise career counselor is willing to flow, for a short while, along this river with his or her client; and, perhaps, if the helper is a good navigator, he or she can assist in guiding the client down the river along the most direct and stable route.

Summary

This chapter examined the counselor and the world of work. We began by defining a number of terms relevant to understanding career development. We then examined some sociological, psychological, and economic reasons why work and adequate career planning are so crucial for job satisfaction and positive mental health.

We noted that career development, formerly called vocational guidance, is the origin of the counseling profession and can be traced back to the early 1900s with the work of Frank Parsons. We noted that vocational guidance started out as a concrete and somewhat directive trait-and-factor approach. However, with the advent of new theories by Donald Super and others, it became a more humanistically oriented, developmental approach and has since been called career development.

In this chapter we described a number of career development theories that have emerged over the years. We noted that the trait-and-factor theory expanded and began to assess how a wide range of client skills, interests, and personality variables might affect eventual career choices. We examined the psychodynamic theory of Ann Roe, who advanced the idea that early parenting styles were instrumental in shaping occupational choice. We looked at John Holland's theory, which states that people express their personality through the types of career choices they make. We examined Donald Super's developmental theory, which suggests a person's self-concept is both a function and result of one's career development process. Lastly, we reviewed cognitive developmental theory that stresses the importance of understanding how the client makes meaning of his or her career development process. We concluded by noting that most career counselors today attempt to integrate many of these approaches when doing career counseling.

The next part of this chapter examined some of the prevalent kinds of career-related information that is available. We presented an overview of occupational classification systems including the *Dictionary of Occupational Titles*, the *Guide for Occupational Exploration*, and the *Occupational Outlook Handbook*. We talked about how the assessment of interest inventories, aptitudes, and personality is important in career counseling. Finally, we discussed the growing use of computers in career guidance and noted that comprehensive computer-based programs, computer-assisted assessment, and career resources over the Internet are becoming increasingly popular.

Having discussed theories, occupational information, and assessment techniques, we highlighted the point that the clinical interview is one of the most important tools the counselor has when working with clients. We then presented an outline for the integration of career development theories, occupational information, assessment techniques, and the clinical interview when doing career counseling.

Although we noted that there was no theory of multicultural career development, we stated that some general guidelines should be considered when working with diverse clients. In addition, we elucidated a number of steps to use when counseling minority clients on career issues.

Near the end of the chapter, we reminded you of the two major associations in the field of career development, the NCDA and the NECA. We also noted that the NCDA offers ethical guidelines and suggests competencies in the training of career counselors. We discussed the fact that counselors should be optimizing choices for clients, not limiting them, and we noted some important laws related to career counseling and career guidance.

Lastly, we emphasized that career counseling is a lifelong process that has twists and turns and that an effective career counselor helps to guide the client toward making this ride a little more satisfying.

INFOTRAC and Other Information Resources (e.g., ERIC and PsycINFO)

Note: When relevant, key words are in quotation marks.

1. Research any "career development theory" of your choice in more detail.
2. Explore the expanding role of "computers and career assessment."
3. Examine the effect of the "Americans with Disabilities Act" or other relevant laws on career choice and career development.

SECTION V

Research, Program Evaluation, and Appraisal

Overview

Research, program evaluation, and appraisal have much in common, and it is therefore natural to find them together in Section V of this text. For instance, some form of quantification is involved with the application of research, program evaluation, and appraisal. Program evaluation can be loosely seen as a kind of research, in that you are researching the value and worth of a program. Research often will use appraisal techniques to examine the research question at hand. Finally, research, program evaluation, and appraisal all involve close scrutiny of people. In research you are examining people in reference to a hypothesis or research question. In program evaluation you are examining how people respond to a program being offered, and in appraisal you are trying to determine a person's typical or habitual ways of responding. As you read through these chapters, consider the commonality of these important content areas and think about ways that you might apply research, program evaluation, and appraisal in your role as a counselor.

CHAPTER **12**

Testing and Assessment

There is much ignorance about very basic measurement, evaluation, and research topics among the practitioners . . . and among those who are ignorant, there is, on occasion, a fair amount of hostility toward some useful data. (Mehrens, 1992, p. 439)

One day while living in Cincinnati and working on my doctorate, I was walking down the street when a person came up to me and said, "Do you want to take a personality test?" I said, "Sure!" I was led into a storefront and proceeded to spend about 30 minutes completing an inventory. When I finished, I was asked to wait a few minutes while they scored it. Then, a person came into the room and said, "Well, you have a pretty good personality, and you're fairly bright, but if you complete Ron Hubbard's book on dianetics, you will have a better personality and be even brighter."

Ten years later, I was walking down a street in Minneapolis when I passed a store that was again selling books by Ron Hubbard. I walked in. Someone approached me and said, "Would you like to take a test?" I responded by noting that a number of years back I had taken such a test and was not convinced it was well made. We bantered back and forth, and finally the dianetics devotee and I came to an agreement. The deal was that I would purchase the book *Dianetics*, and at a later date read it, if and when the employee sent me information on the reliability and validity of the instrument, thus showing me that it is a well-made test. I gave him my home address. I never heard from him again.

You will be tested on this chapter! Just kidding; well, at least *I* won't be testing you on it. Tests create anxiety! Tests. Some of the most interesting, feared, misused, disliked, and potentially valuable tools we have as counselors are tests. What are they all about? This chapter will examine testing and assessment.

We will begin this chapter by asking why testing is important. Then we will give a brief overview of the history of tests and assessment. We will survey some of the many different kinds of tests and review the use of basic test statistics in the development and the interpretation of assessment instruments. We will discuss the concepts of reliability, validity, and practicality and offer ways of finding good tests. We will discuss the importance of writing test reports and review how the use of computers has affected the administration, scoring, and interpretation of tests. Finally, we will discuss multicultural, ethical, legal, and professional issues related to testing.

Why Testing?

The case for increased attention to appraisal based on the reality of counselor practice is strong and needs to be addressed through the combined efforts of CACREP, legislation, counselor education programs, and certifying bodies.
(Bubenzer, Zimpfer, & Mahrle, 1990, p. 51)

As a counselor you will be involved with testing (Anastasi, 1992). You may be administering tests. You are likely to interpret tests. You may be a consultant to others on the proper use of tests or supervise others who interpret tests. You may use tests in research and evaluation, and you will read about tests in the professional literature. Tests have permeated many aspects of our society, but there are only a handful of professionals who have sufficient knowledge about them to properly use them. As a counselor, you will be one of those few.

In most schools, counselors are the only individuals who have expertise in testing. The school psychologist, who is specifically trained in assessment, generally floats from school to school. The school administrators and teachers may have never taken a course in testing (Elmore, Ekstrom, Diamond, & Whittaker, 1993). And special education teachers and learning disability specialists, who generally have a strong background in diagnostic testing, have a limited focus.

Today, elementary, middle, and secondary school counselors all report that approximately 7% of their job function is testing (Partin, 1993; Wilgus & Shelley, 1988), and high school counselors report that they provide testing services to 20% to 37% of all students (Hutchinson & Bottorff, 1986). This includes all types of assessment, such as achievement testing, assessment of aptitude, assessment of interests, and personality assessment (Zytowski, 1982). The role of school counselors in relation to assessment varies and includes administering and interpreting tests, being a consultant to others about tests, using tests in program evaluation and research, and running schoolwide testing programs (Schafer & Mufson, cited in Schafer, 1995). In addition, school counselors sometimes provide workshops and individual consultation for teachers on test use and test interpretation (Elmore et al., 1993; Ginter, Scalise, & Presse, 1990; Schafer, 1995). Finally, school counselors will periodically receive and need to understand test reports from agency counselors who are working with students.

The likelihood that there are other professionals who have expertise in testing is greater in agencies and higher education settings than in the schools. However, there is still the possibility that in some settings, the counselor will be the only individual with such expertise. In either case, the probability is great that counselors will be asked to periodically administer and interpret educational and psychological tests for their clients (Bubenzer et al., 1990). In addition, counselors in these settings are often asked to understand test reports completed by other clinicians, and many counselors in these settings will be reviewing the test records of the children with whom they work. Finally, in these days of accountability, counselors are often asked to evaluate the efficacy of clinical programs, and assessment instruments are crucial for this process. It is clear that in agency and higher education settings testing has become a core component of the counselor's work.

Although tests have been criticized over the years for being poorly made and/or having bias, with advances in statistical analysis and improvement of test quality, tests today can offer us one additional way of exploring the inner world of our clients (Lewandowski & Saccuzo, 1976):

> *The effectively functioning counselor engages in a continuing cycle of hypothesis formulation and hypothesis testing about the particular individual. Each item of information whether it is an event recorded in a case history, a comment by the client, or a test score suggests a hypothesis about the person, which will be either confirmed or refuted as other facts are gathered.* (Anastasi, 1992, p. 611)

Why testing? Why not testing? Tests offer an additional venue in helping us understand the ability and personality of our clients. They can be useful in diagnosis. They can help in goal setting and treatment planning. And tests can be useful in research and evaluation. Based on our own past performance or our own personal biases, let us not assume that tests are of little value. Tests can be useful. Let's see how!

A Little Background

Broadly speaking, a test takes place whenever a person is asked to show the existence or amount of a particular trait or ability. In this sense, Abraham was given a test to show his faith when God asked him to kill his first-born son Isaac. And early Olympians were tested as they compared their performances to one another. One of the earliest tests, used for purposes with which we're more familiar, was developed in 2200 B.C.E. by the Chinese, who gave an essay-type test for the selection of what today would be called civil service employees. However, it was not until the 1800s that psychological and educational assessment turned into a more formal process.

The modern-day testing movement was formed out of two distinct processes occurring in the late 1800s. On the one hand, this period saw increased acceptance of Charles Darwin's theory that differences within a species and between species held the key to natural selection. Soon psychologists picked up the call to examine individual differences in people (Dawis, 1992). Individuals like Wundt and Fechner become particularly interested in experimental psychology and developed some of the first psychology labs. It was this impetus that led to an understanding that rigorous experimental control was crucial to scientific study of individual differences and that tests were often critical to this process (Kaplan & Saccuzzo, 1993).

One of the first assessment procedures was developed by Alfred Binet at the end of the 19th century. Hired by the Ministry of Public Education in Paris, Binet was asked to develop an instrument that could differentiate those who could function in a classroom from those who could not (Drummond, 2000). This scale, which was later revised by Terman at Stanford University, became known as the Stanford-Binet test of intelligence, a revised version of which is still in use today.

A number of developments at the beginning of the 20th century saw the spread of assessment instruments in a number of other realms. For instance, the popularity of psychoanalysis and its emphasis on personality development influenced the beginning of objective and projective personality assessment. In addition, on the heels of the Industrial Revolution there was an influx of people to large cities, and this resulted in a need for objective tests of achievement and of vocational assessment in the schools. Finally, World War I saw a sudden need for the widespread use of personality and ability tests to help in the placement of recruits in the military. The assessment movement had taken hold in the United States.

With advancements in statistical knowledge and its application to test construction, assessment instruments began to take on a modern look in the 1940s and 1950s. As we moved into the 1960s and the 1970s the advent of the computer made it easier to examine the statistical properties of tests and improve their quality. The 1980s saw the proliferation of personal computers, which increased the ability of researchers to examine the quality of tests (Sampson, 1995), and the 1990s saw a revolution in the ways that many tests are administered, scored, and interpreted. This revolution continued as we moved into 21st century.

Today, tests are pervasive throughout our society. There are long tests, short tests, extremely long tests, and very short tests; tests to measure knowledge and tests to measure passion; tests to see if you can be diagnosed and tests to see if you're self-actualized; tests for admission into graduate school and tests to finish graduate school. They are everywhere. Today, tests can be broadly categorized as formal or informal. Let's take a look at some of the different kinds of formal and informal tests in existence today.

Formal Assessment Tests

Although tests today are appreciably better than their distant relatives at the turn of the 20th century, the basic test categories have pretty much stayed the same. Formal tests are those tests that tend to be nationally made and given to large groups of individuals across the country. Formal tests can be *ability tests*, measurement in the cognitive domain; or *personality tests*, measurement in the affective domain. See Figure 12.1 for a visual outline of the different kinds of ability and personality assessment categories.

Assessment of Ability

Ability tests include *achievement tests*, or tests that measure all of what one has learned, and *aptitude tests*, or tests that measure all that one is capable of learning. Achievement tests include *survey battery*, *diagnostic*, and *readiness* tests. Aptitude tests include *individual intelligence tests*, *cognitive ability tests*, *special aptitude tests*, and *multiple aptitude tests*. Regardless of the type of ability test used, their purpose is to measure the cognitive development of the individual (Anastasi & Urbina, 1997).

Achievement Tests (Survey Battery, Diagnostic, and Readiness)

Survey battery tests are used to measure general achievement and are commonly administered in the schools, usually in large groups. Probably you are familiar with these types of tests through your own education. The *Iowa Test of Basic Skills* and the *Stanford Achievement Test* are two examples of survey battery achievement tests. The uses of survey battery achievement tests are many and include the assessment of a student's ability level, the determination of teaching effectiveness, and the examination of the general level of students' ability throughout a school or school system.

FIGURE 12.1
Typesof Assessment Instruments

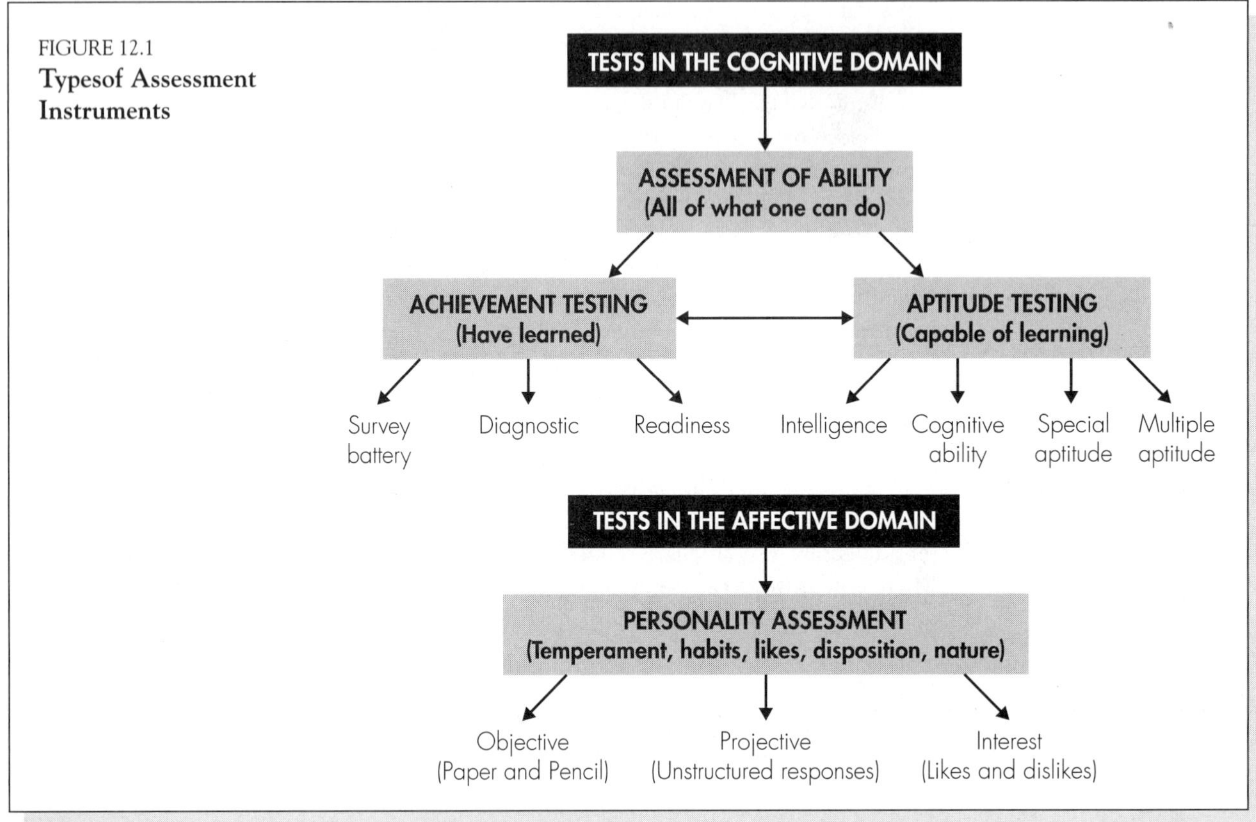

Diagnostic achievement tests, which are used to delve more deeply into areas of suspected learning problems, are often given one-to-one by an experienced examiner, usually a school psychologist or learning disabilities specialist. Oftentimes, these tests are recommended following the results of a survey battery achievement test and when, in consultation with parents and teachers, it seems probable that a student may have a learning disability. This means that it is suspected that the student's ability is much lower in one or more specified areas than his or her average ability in other areas. Today, if an individual is found to have a learning disability, laws protect the child's right to an education (see Box 12.1).

Readiness tests are used to assess an individual's ability to move on to the next educational level. These days, readiness tests are mostly used to determine if a child is developmentally ready to move on to first grade, since kindergarten-age children develop at different rates. It should be stressed that lack of readiness for kindergarten does not imply lack of innate ability but is likely to reflect developmental differences at an early age. For instance, a very bright child may be developmentally not ready to move into first grade. In fact, intellectual ability in young children varies so much from year to year that to make long-lasting decisions solely based on a child's intellectual ability at this young age would be unwise (Hutchens, Hamilton, Town, Gaddis, & Presley, 1991).

BOX 12.1

Public Law 94-142

In 1975, *Public Law 94-142* (PL94-142) was passed (Federal Register, 1977). This landmark legislation assured the right to an education, within the *least restrictive environment,* for any individual from age of 3 through age 21 who had a disability. The law asserted that any individual who was suspected of having a learning disability had the right to be tested, at the school system's expense, for the disability. Thus, diagnostic testing, usually administered by the school psychologist or learning disability specialist, has become one of the main ways of determining who might have a disability. Students who have been determined to be learning disabled must be given an *Individual Education Plan* that states the services that will be offered to assist the student with his or her learning problem. The law also proclaimed that whenever possible and reasonable, students must be placed with students in regular classrooms (mainstreamed).

Aptitude Tests

Four major kinds of aptitude tests include *individual intelligence tests, cognitive ability tests, special aptitude tests,* and *multiple aptitude tests.* Individual intelligence tests, which are tests that are given one-to-one to measure general intellectual ability, are administered by highly trained examiners, most often psychologists. These tests have a broad range of uses, such as helping to identify individuals who are learning disabled, developmentally delayed, or gifted, and can even be used as an indicator of personality characteristics. Usually, when a comprehensive assessment of an individual is requested, an individual intelligence test is included.

Cognitive ability tests are paper-and-pencil tests used to measure the cognitive skills necessary to be successful in school. These tests, which are often given in groups, are generally used to determine a student's capability in school or to predict how well an individual will do in school. Therefore, they are sometimes used for school placement and as predictors of ability in college (e.g., SATs), graduate school (e.g., GREs), and professional schools (see House & Johnson, 1993a,b; Stricker & Burton, 1996). Cognitive ability tests can also aid in identifying those who are gifted. Finally, these tests are often used as one method of determining which students may be learning disabled, as it is common for such students to score significantly higher on cognitive ability tests than achievement tests. This is because, due to their learning disability, these students are not achieving at their potential.

Special aptitude tests focus on measuring specific segments of ability (e.g., spatial ability, eye-hand coordination, mechanical ability) and are often used to predict the potential for success at specific jobs or training programs. For instance, one's aptitude on an eye-hand coordination test may be used to predict success at operating complex machinery in a factory. Or a drawing test may be used to predict success in art school. Multiple aptitude tests, which measure a number of specific segments of ability, are used to understand an individual's aptitude on a broad range of abilities which can subsequently be used in occupational decision making. Some examples of multiple aptitude tests include the *Differential Aptitude Test (DAT)*, which is frequently used by high school counselors; the *Armed Services Vocational Aptitude Battery (ASVAB)*, which is given by the military (often for free in the schools); and the *General Aptitude Test Battery (GATB)*, which is given by employment security offices.

Although achievement testing measures what a person has learned and aptitude testing measures one's potential for learning, in point of fact there is often much overlap between the two (see Figure 12.1). For instance, one would be naive to assume that the SATs or the GREs are not measuring what one has learned. However, because they are both used to predict future performance, they are considered aptitude tests.

Personality Assessment

The assessment of personality includes the measuring of one's temperament, attitudes, values, likes and dislikes, emotions, motivation, interpersonal skills, and/or level of adjustment (Anastasi & Urbina, 1997; Drummond, 2000; Gibson & Mitchell, 1999). Temperament, one of the most commonly measured attributes, is determined by biological and genetic factors and an array of environmental factors (e.g., parenting, reinforcement of learning, and so on). Because it is difficult to factor out temperament from environmental factors in the measurement of personality, with a few exceptions, resulting scores on personality tests represent a conglomerate of both factors (Teglasi, 1995). The three types of personality assessment that are most commonly used today are objective tests, projective tests, and interest inventories.

Objective Personality Tests

Objective personality tests are paper-and-pencil instruments used to measure some aspect of personality. Thus we might find tests measuring anxiety, depression, psychosis, suicidal tendencies, eating disorders, marital satisfaction, and on and on. Some of these tests, like the *Minnesota Multiphasic Personality Inventory-II (MMPI-II)*, measure psychopathology and probably measure at least some aspects of one's temperament, while others, like the *Myers-Briggs*, measure common qualities that are likely not to be related to temperament. A few of the many uses of objective personality tests are to deepen client insight, to help in the determination of clinical diagnosis, to make predictions about future behaviors, to determine personality characteristics for the court (e.g., child custody, child molestation accusations), and for hiring employees for sensitive jobs (e.g., working with children or nuclear arms).

Projective Tests

Projective tests attempt to assess personality characteristics by having an individual make responses to unstructured stimuli. Stimuli presented allow for a broad range of responses that are representative of conscious and unconscious needs, desires, likes, drives, and personal struggles. For instance, the *Rorschach*, one of the most widely used projective tests, uses inkblots as stimuli to which the individual responds. After all the responses are collected, the examiner interprets their meaning. Other types of projective tests include sentence completion, where the end of a sentence is left off and the client completes it with the first thing that comes to mind; drawings, where the client is asked to make a specific drawing, which is later interpreted (e.g., a drawing of the client's family all doing something together); and tests in which the individual is asked to develop stories from pictures that are presented.

Interest Inventories

Although they are, strictly speaking, a type of objective personality assessment, interest inventories are generally classified separately because of their popularity and very specific focus. Used to determine the likes and dislikes of a person, as well as an individual's personality orientation toward the world of work, interest inventories are almost exclusively used in the career counseling process. These instruments are to some degree able to predict job satisfaction based on occupational fit. For instance, if, based on the results of an interest inventory, a person chooses a job that seems to match his or her personality type, then that person is more likely to be satisfied in that occupation than a person who does not have an occupational fit (Jagger et al., 1992). With an estimated 3,000,000 interest inventories being given each year, these assessment instruments have been particularly successful as an adjunct to the career counseling process and have become big business in the world of assessment (Hansen, 1995; Zytowski, 1994). Although many interest inventories exist, two of the more popular include the *Strong Vocational Interest Inventory* (Consulting Psychologists Press, 1994) and the *Self-Directed Search (SDS)* (Holland, 1994).

Informal Assessment Procedures

Informal assessment instruments are generally developed by the individual giving the test (e.g., counselor, teacher), and although they may be less valid than other kinds of instruments, they offer us an important and relatively easy method of examining a slice of behavior of an individual. Although there are many kinds of informal assessment instruments, two of the most common are *rating scales* and *observation*.

Rating Scales

Rating scales allow an individual to give a subjective rating of a behavior on a scale. A few of the different kinds of rating scales include *Likert-type scales*, *semantic differential scales*, *rank order scales*, *numerical scales*, and *behavior checklists* (see Box 12.2).

BOX 12.2

Examples of Rating Scales

1. ***Numerical Scale:*** Pick the item that best describes you:
   (1) very outgoing and social
   (2) moderately outgoing and social
   (3) slightly outgoing
   (4) somewhat withdrawn
   (5) very much withdrawn

2. ***Likert-type Scale:*** Rate how much you liked this class.

   1_________2_________3_________4_________5
   not at all   a moderate amount   a lot

3. ***Behavior Checklist:*** Place an "X" next to the item that best describes you:

   ___extroverted ___shy ___anxious
   ___happy ___introverted ___nurturing

4. ***Rank Order:*** Place a 1 next the type of therapy you think is most effective, a 2 next to the one you think is second most effective, down to a 5 next to the one you think is least effective.

   ___psychoanalytic ___humanistic ___behavioral
   ___transpersonal ___cognitive

5. ***Semantic Differential:*** Place a mark on the lines that best represent the relative strengths of your attributes as listed below.

   introverted______________________extroverted
   happy______________________sad
   warm______________________cold
   anxious______________________calm

Observation

Observation, as the name implies, involves the viewing of an individual's behavior, either directly or indirectly. For instance, *time sampling* and *event sampling* are two kinds of observation in which a behavior is targeted for examination. In time sampling, a targeted behavior is identified for observation over a specified amount of time. For instance, if I wanted to evaluate the skills of a counselor trainee, I might listen to 5-minute segments from each of eight 30-minute audiotaped role-plays rather than listening to all 4 hours of the tapes. In event sampling, I target a specific behavior without concern for time. For example, in the case of the counselor trainee, I would listen to all of the eight tapes but only focus on one behavior, such as the empathic responses of the trainee. Often, time and event sampling are combined, such as in the case when I might listen to 5-minute segments of the eight tapes and listen only for empathic responses.

Besides event and time sampling, there are many other kinds of observational techniques. Some of the more common ones include *structured interviews*, in which designated questions are given orally to the person being evaluated and responses are noted; *journals*, such as dream journals or *diaries*; *cumulative records*, such as performance records and other personal information that may be noted in student or employee files; and *situational tests*, such as when an individual is placed in a "contrived naturalistic situation" and his or her responses are noted (e.g., role-playing with a client).

Norm-Referenced and Criterion-Referenced Testing

Generally, tests are either *norm-referenced* or *criterion-referenced*. In norm-referenced tests, the individual can compare his or her score to the conglomerate scores of a peer or *norm group*. Usually, norm groups consist of a national representative sample of individuals. Many tests that are sold by national publishing companies are norm-referenced.

In contrast, criterion-referenced tests are designed to assess specific learning goals of an individual. Achievement of these goals, as measured by a criterion-referenced test, shows mastery of the subject matter at hand. Oftentimes, criterion-referenced tests are used with individuals who are learning disabled, because goals can be individualized for the student based on his or her specific learning problem.

Standardized Testing and Nonstandardized Testing

Standardized tests are administered in the same manner and under the same conditions each time they are given. In contrast, *informal, nonstandardized* assessment procedures are not necessarily given under the same conditions and in the same manner at each administration. Often, formal tests are standardized and informal tests nonstandardized. However, this is not a hard-and-fast rule.

Examples of the Different Test Categories

An example of a formal, standardized, norm-referenced test is an individual intelligence test in which the test is given the exact same way across the country and an individual's score is then compared to national norm group scores. The NBCC exam, to become a Nationally Certified Counselor (NCC), is an example of a formal, standardized, norm-

TABLE 12.1

Comparison of Standardized, Nonstandardized, Norm-Referenced, and Criterion-Referenced Tests

	STANDARDIZED	NONSTANDARDIZED
NORM-REFERENCED	These assessment instruments must be given in the same manner and under the same conditions each time they're given. Often, they are highly researched objective instruments that are developed by publishing companies. Usually, large norm groups are available with which the individual can compare his or her results.	These assessment instruments may vary in how they are administered and generally are not as rigidly researched as the standardized tests. However, because of their informal nature, they may be more practical for the purpose in which they are being used. Scores that are later compared to a norm group should be viewed more tentatively than standardized tests.
CRITERION- REFERENCED	These instruments are given in a standard manner and have preset learning goals that are based on an individual's personal educational objectives. In these tests, often created by large publishing companies, individuals have the ability to tackle their individualized learning goals *and* have their results compared to national norm groups.	These instruments are informally made, often by teachers, and are based on the teacher's knowledge of his or her students and the content area being tested. The teacher can develop an individualized test that has preset learning goals for each student. The informal nature of these instruments means that norm groups are rarely available for comparisons.

referenced test. This objective paper-and-pencil test is given throughout the country at a specified date and time to all counselors who would like to obtain national certification.

Examples of a formal, standardized, criterion-referenced test are nationally made individual achievement tests, which are often given to learning disabled students. These tests are given the same way each time they are administered, but a student takes only those parts of the test relevant to his or her individual learning goals as defined by a special education teacher. This test could additionally be norm-referenced if a comparison to a national norm group is desired and available.

Using a checklist to measure self-concept while observing a child in a class and then comparing the child's scores to a local norm group (e.g., students in the school) might be an example of an informal, nonstandardized and norm-referenced test.

Finally, a teacher-made test that has targeted learning goals for students might be an example of an informal, nonstandardized, criterion-referenced test. Based on a teacher's knowledge of a student's ability and on the specific content under question, a test would be created to assess a student's ability. When a student has mastered his or her learning goals, he or she has passed the test.

Basic Test Statistics

Relativity and Meaningfulness of Test Scores

Jeremiah receives a score of 47 on a test, and Elise receives a score of 95 on a different test: How have they done? If Jeremiah's score was 47 out of 52, one might assume he has done fairly well. But, if 1000 people had taken this test and all others received a higher score than Jeremiah, we might view his score somewhat differently. And to make things even more complicated, what if a high score represents an undesirable trait (e.g., cynicism, depression, schizophrenia)? Then clearly, the lower he scores compared to his norm group, the comparatively better he has done, and vice versa.

What about Elise's score? Is a score of 95 good? What if it is out of a possible score of 200, or 550, or 992? If 1000 people take the test, Elise's score is the highest, and a higher score is desirable, we might say that she did well, at least compared with her norm group. But if her score is on the lower end of the group of scores, then comparatively she did not do well.

By comparing Jeremiah and Elise's scores to their peer or norm group, we put meaning to their scores. This is because norm group comparisons:

1. *Allow individuals to compare themselves to their peer group*. For instance, Jeremiah and Elise can examine how their scores are as compared to people who took the same test and are like them in some important way (e.g., similar age, same grade).
2. *Allow test takers who took the same test but are in different norm groups to compare their results*. For instance, a parent who has two children, two grades apart, could determine which one is doing better in reading (e.g., one might score at the 50th percentile, the other at the 76th relative to the peer groups). Or a school counselor might be interested in the self-esteem scores of all the fifth graders as compared to all the third graders.
3. *Allow an individual to compare his or her results on two different tests*. For instance, as noted earlier, it is sometimes valuable to know an individual's score on an achievement test as well as on a scholastic aptitude test, because a discrepancy between the two tests might be an indication of a learning disability. Or, when doing personality assessment, it is not unusual to give a number of different tests with an effort made to find similar themes running through the various tests (e.g., high indications of anxiety on a number of different tests).

It is important to remember that Jeremiah and Elise will have their own opinions about how they think they should do on the test. Thus, a high score to one person would be a low score to another. The individual who consistently scores at the highest percentiles on a math test may feel upset about a score that is in the average range, while an individual who consistently scores low may feel good about that same score. Similarly, an individual who has struggled with lifelong depression may feel good about a moderate depression score on the *Beck Depression Inventory*, while another person might be concerned about such a score.

Measures of Central Tendency and Variability

Measures of Central Tendency

Measures of central tendency tell us what is occurring in the midrange of a group of scores. Thus, if you know a person's score, you can compare that score to one of three scores that represent the midrange of the group. Three measures of central tendency include the *mode*, or the most frequent score; the *median*, or the middle score, the point at which 50% of the scores fall below and above; and the *mean*, or the average of all of the scores. Although measures of central tendency do not tell you a whole lot about the group of scores, they do at least give you a sense of whether a known score is higher or lower than the mean, median, or mode.

FIGURE 12.2
The Bell-Shaped Curve

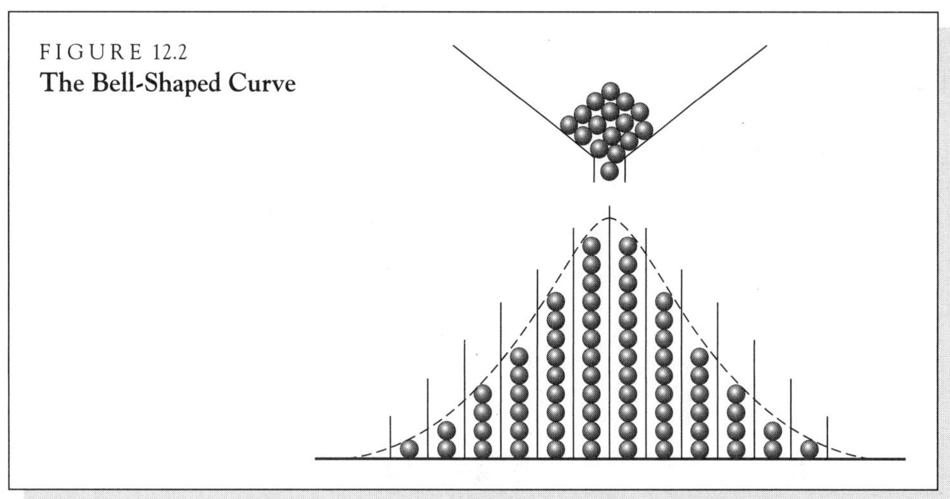

Measures of Variability

A number of years ago I was in the Boston Museum of Science, where I saw a device through which hundreds of balls were dropped at once (see Figure 12.2). Approximately every five minutes the balls would be dropped. After they were dropped, they would be automatically collected, readying for the next drop. All day long this machine would drop those balls over and over again. Now, this in and of itself was not so amazing. However, what did seem extraordinary was the fact that each and every time those balls were dropped they would distribute themselves in the shape of a *normal curve* (also called the *bell-shaped curve*). Now, mind you, they were not distributing themselves in that manner because they were being sent in that direction. No, they were distributing themselves like this by chance.

In point of fact, the resulting bell-shaped curve is a product of the natural laws of the universe and is explained through the laws of probability. However, no matter what label you use to describe it, it is amazing that such a predictable pattern occurs over and over again. What does this have to with testing? Like the balls dropping in this device, when we measure most traits and abilities of people, the scores result in a bell-shaped distribution. This is very convenient, for the symmetry of this curve allows us to understand measures of variability, particularly standard deviation, which is crucial to our understanding of norm-referenced tests.

Measures of variability tell us how much scores vary in a distribution. Three types of measures of variability include the *range*, or the number of scores between the highest and lowest scores on a distribution; the *interquartile range*, which measures the middle 50% of a group of scores; and the *standard deviation*, or the manner in which scores deviate around the mean in a standard fashion. Although all three measures of variability are important for the interpretation of test scores, in normally distributed curves the standard deviation takes on particular importance. For instance, examine the hypothetical curve in Figure 12.3 that might result from the distribution of scores of American adults on a test to measure depression. In this case, as in all normally distributed curves, the mean or average score always represents the 50th percentile and splits the distribution in half. In

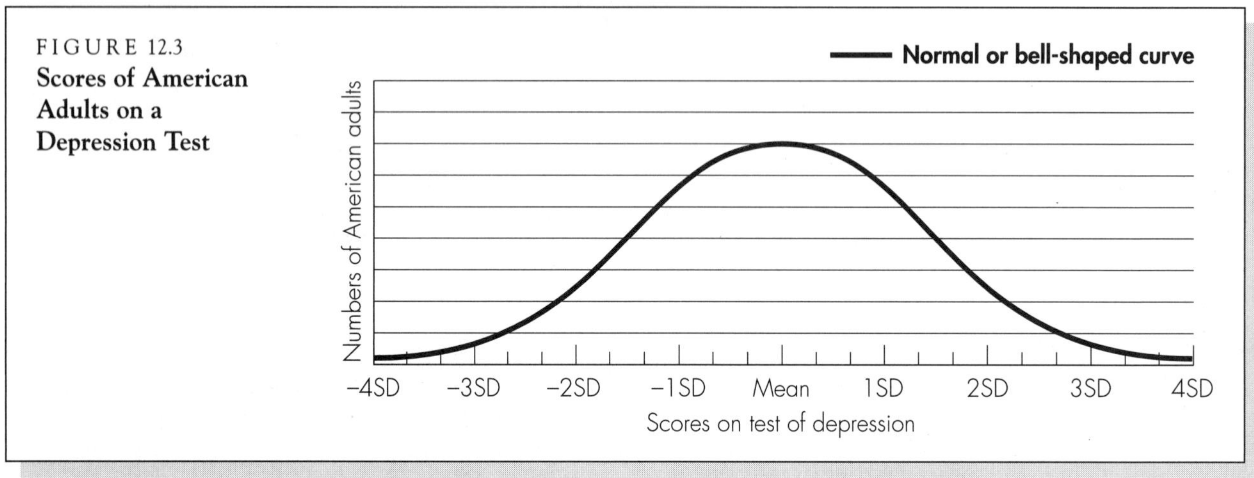

FIGURE 12.3
Scores of American Adults on a Depression Test

addition, the standard deviation distributes itself in a consistent manner. For instance, in all normally distributed curves, approximately 34% of the scores will fall between the mean and +1 standard deviation, and another 34% between the mean and –1 standard deviation. Similarly, 14% will fall between +1 and +2 standard deviations and 14% will fall between –1 and –2 standard deviations. Finally, 2% will fall between +2 and +3 standard deviations and another 2% between –2 and –3 standard deviations.

Furthermore, in the normally distributed curve in Figure 12.3, as in all tests that have a distribution that approximates a bell-shaped curve, certain assumptions can be made about how scores deviate around the mean. For instance, if an individual scores above the mean, we immediately know that he or she has scored better than 50% of the population who took the test. If the individual scores at about the point of one standard deviation, he or she has scored at approximately the 84th percentile, and so forth (see Figure 12.4).

Consider for a moment that a test has a mean of 52 and the standard deviation of 20. For this test, most of the scores (about 68%) would range between 32 and 72 (plus and minus one standard deviation; see Figure 12.4). On the other hand, a second test that had a mean of 52 and a standard deviation of 5 would include 68% of its scores between 47 and 57 (again, plus and minus one standard deviation). Clearly, even though the two tests have the same mean, the range of scores around the mean varies considerably. An individual's score of 40 would be in the average range on the first test but well below average on the second test. This example shows why measures of central tendency and measures of variability are so important in understanding test scores.

Derived Scores

Usually, when a large group of individuals takes an assessment instrument, each person's reported score is not the *actual* raw score obtained by that person. Similarly, the mean is generally not the actual mean of all the raw scores. Instead, to make scores easier to interpret, the raw scores are converted to what are called *derived* scores. You are probably already aware of a number of derived scores such as *percentiles*, *stanines*, or *SAT-type* scores. If scores were not converted in this fashion, every individual who wanted to interpret his or her score would have to have knowledge of standard deviation and how it varies from test to test. In addition, converting scores to derived scores makes it easier to compare

FIGURE 12.4
Comparison of the Variability of Two Different Normal Curve Distributions

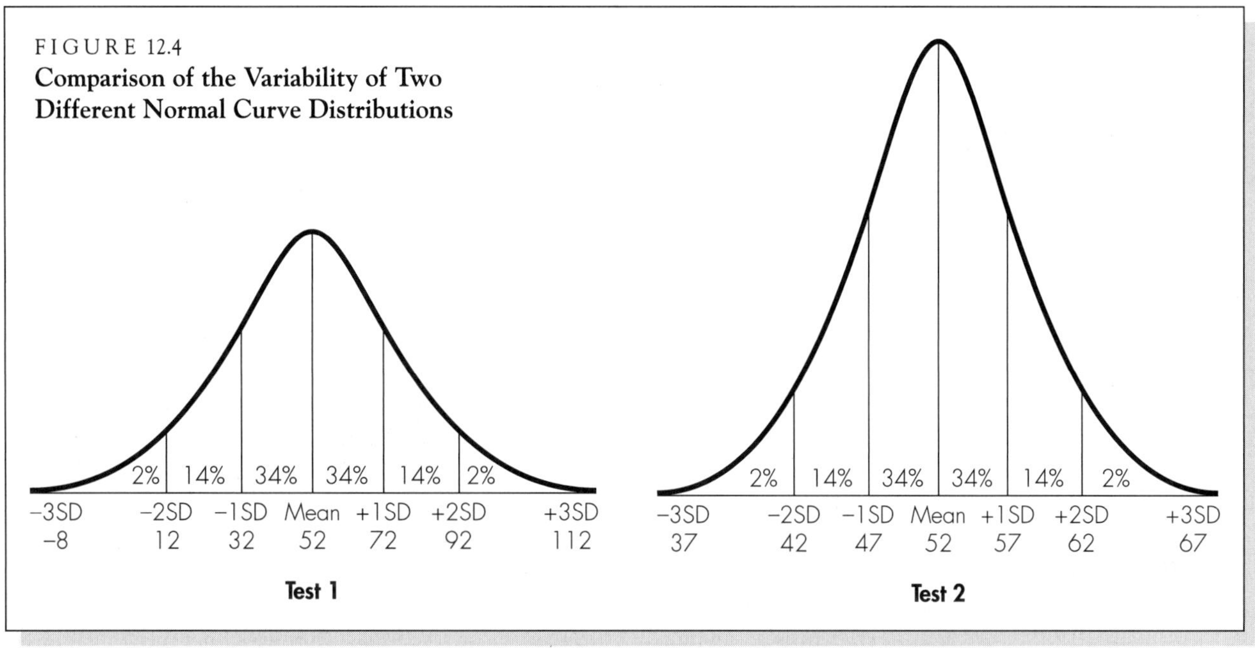

scores on different tests because their units of measurements are made comparable (e.g., percentiles on one test can be compared to percentiles on another).

Although the means and standard deviations of tests can vary dramatically, normally distributed curves will always have the same *percentage* of scores distributing between the mean and one standard deviation above the mean (approximately 34%) or below the mean (another 34%). Similarly, all normally distributed curves will have the same percentage of scores between the mean and two standard deviations above the mean (approximately 48%) or below the mean (another 48%) and, of course, between the mean and three standard deviations above the mean (approximately 50%) or below the mean (another 50%). This property allows us to convert scores from any test that is normally distributed to a derived score of our choice. For instance, imagine two persons taking the same test: One obtains a raw score of 32 and the other a raw score of 92. When we discover that the mean is 52 and the standard deviation is 20 points, we immediately know that the first person scored at the 16th percentile (one standard deviation below the mean, or 52 minus 20) while the second person scored at the 98th percentile (two standard deviations above the mean, or 52 plus 20, and plus 20 again) (see Figure 12.4, Test 1). Now we know that on this test one person scored at the 16th percentile while another scored at the 98th percentile; these are derived scores. They are derived from the original raw scores. However, there are also other types of derived scores. For instance, if this was a test to measure depression, we might use a derived score called a *T-score* (Transformed-score). Having a mean of 50 and standard deviation of 10, T-scores are often used with personality assessment. Therefore, for the two individuals noted above, the first would have obtained a T-score of 40 (one standard deviation below the mean), while the second would have obtained a T-score of 70 (two standard deviations above the mean).

In addition to comparing two individuals on the same test, derived scores allow us to compare the same individual on different tests or on different subtests of the same test. For instance, a person might receive a T-score of 56 on a test of depression and a T-score of 32 on a test that measures trait anxiety. Thus, on the first test that person scored above the mean (mean of T-scores is 50), and the same person obtained a score quite a bit below the mean (almost two standard deviations; e.g. 50 minus 10 and minus 10 again would be a derived score of 30). Below are some of the more typical derived scores that are used.

Percentile rank. A derived score that describes the percentage of scores that fall at or below a given score. Percentiles are used with many different types of tests.

T-scores. A derived score having a mean of 50 and a standard deviation of 10 and generally used with personality tests.

Deviation IQ. A derived score having a mean of 100 and a standard deviation of 15 and generally used with intelligence tests.

SAT/GRE-type scores. A derived score having a mean of 500 and a standard deviation of 100. Used mostly to report SAT and GRE scores.

Grade equivalent scores. A derived score generally used with achievement tests to determine an individual's position relative to his or her grade level. The grade level of the student represents the mean of the grade equivalent. Probably the most misunderstood of derived scores, grade equivalents above current grade level do not mean that the individual can thrive at that grade level. Instead, it means that the student is doing much better than those students within his or her own grade level.

Stanines. A derived score generally used with achievement tests. Stanines range from 1 to 9 with a score of 5 representing the mean and 2 stanines being equivalent to one standard deviation.

Idiosyncratic publisher-derived scores. On some tests, particularly survey battery achievement tests, publishers create a derived score unique for that test. Therefore, a specific achievement test might have a mean of 150 and a standard deviation of 20, or a mean of 200 and a standard deviation of 25, and so forth—whatever specific mean and standard deviation the publisher decides to use. Usually, test publishers pick numbers that allow test takers to interpret their scores relatively easily.

Correlation Coefficient

A basic statistic that is not directly related to the interpretation of tests but is crucial in test construction is *correlation coefficient*. Correlation coefficients show the relationship between two sets of scores, range from +1 to –1, and generally are reported in decimals of one-hundredths (see Figure 12.5). A positive correlation shows a tendency for two sets of scores to be related in the same direction. For instance, if a group of individuals took two tests, a positive correlation would show a tendency for those who obtained high scores on

FIGURE 12.5
The Range and Strength of Correlation Coefficients

−1, −.99,... −.80.......... −.51.... −.25... −.10... −.02, −.01,0, +.01, +.02... +.10... +.25.... +.51,.......... +.80... +.99, +1

strong **moderate** **low** **none** **low** **moderate** **strong**

the first test to obtain high scores on the second test and for those who obtained low scores on the first test to obtain low scores on the second test.

A negative correlation shows an inverse relationship between two sets of scores; for instance, individuals who obtain high scores on the first test would be likely to obtain low scores on the second test. A correlation that approaches +1 or –1 shows a particularly strong relationship, while a correlation that approaches 0 shows little or no relationship between two factors. For instance, if I wanted to show that the GREs predict college performance, I would have to show that the correlation coefficient does not approach zero and is significant enough to warrant its use (see House & Johnson, 1993a,b). Similarly, if I wanted to show that my newly made test of depression was worthwhile, I could correlate scores on my new test with an established test of depression. In this case I would expect to find a relatively high correlation coefficient as evidenced by the fact that individuals who scored high on my test would have a tendency to score high on the established test and individuals who scored low on my test would have a tendency to score low on the established test.

What Makes a Good Test Good?

Psychological tests and inventories, derived from and refined by scientific research, contribute to responsible practice by providing an empirical basis (sometimes the only empirical basis) for assessment and intervention. (Claiborn, 1991b, p. 456)

Four qualities that are particularly important in establishing the worthwhileness of a test are (1) *validity*, whether or not a test measures what it is supposed to measure; (2) *reliability*, the ability of a test to accurately measure a trait or ability; (3) *practicality*, the ease of administration and interpretation of the test; and (4) *cultural fairness*, whether or not the test measures what it is supposed to measure in a consistent manner for all subgroups to whom the test is given. Let's take a closer look at these qualities.

Validity

There are numerous ways that a test can be shown to be valid. Regardless of the method used, it is important to remember that validity is attempting to show that the test is indeed measuring the quality it purports to measure. Validity is a statement about the test, not about people taking the test. Generally, five kinds of validity are identified, with face validity being considered by most not to be a real type of validity. (After reading this section, see Table 12.2 for a summary of types of validity.)

Face Validity

Face validity examines the content of an assessment instrument to determine, in a cursory way, whether or not the items of the instrument seem related to the kind of instrument it purports to be. Face validity has much to do with how individuals who are being evaluated view the test and the relationship of their perception to the likelihood that they will give their maximum performance. For instance, an individual might be more motivated to take a career assessment instrument that asks questions about jobs, interests, and likes and dislikes as opposed to one that measures personality variables that may, on the surface, seem unrelated to careers, despite the fact that both can be used to predict satisfaction in a career. Or some people who are uneasy about feeling anxious may be less motivated and more defensive taking a test that obviously measures anxiety as compared to one that has the same validity but asks questions that on the surface do not seem to be measuring anxiety.

Content Validity

Content validity has to do with whether or not test items are constructed in a manner that shows they represent the defined body of knowledge being tested. Content validity is most important in ability testing, especially achievement testing, in which items picked to be included in the instrument need to be representative of the content area being tested. Content validity is generally achieved by surveying well-known texts, the professional literature, and experts in the test content area and then developing items based on the knowledge gained.

Criterion-Related Validity

Criterion-related validity exists when an assessment instrument is shown to be related, generally through the use of correlation coefficient, to some external criterion or reference. Two types of criterion-related validity are concurrent validity and predictive validity. Concurrent validity occurs when a test is shown to be related to a criterion in the present. For instance, using a correlation coefficient, a newly made test of depression can be correlated with an established test of depression or with experts' clinical judgments of clients' depression. A high correlation would show criterion-related validity. A low correlation would mean the test's validity is questionable. Predictive validity takes place when a test is shown to be predictive of a future criterion. For instance, again using a correlation coefficient, the SATs can be correlated with students' GPAs in college. A high correlation would show that the SATs can, to some degree, predict college grades. However, a low correlation would leave us questioning the ability of the test to predict college grades and the usefulness of the test for college admissions (see Stricker & Burton, 1996).

Construct Validity

Construct validity is used to show that a specific construct exists (e.g., depression), and to support a theoretical assumption associated with a construct being measured. If I wished to show that my construct existed and could be measured, I should be able to make some predictions based on scores from my instrument. For instance, a test to measure depression should be able to distinguish those who are depressed (e.g., psychiatric admissions for depression) from those who are not depressed (e.g., a group of identified nondepressed individuals), thereby showing that the construct depression is measurable. Some other examples of construct validity would be if the test could distinguish depressed individuals who were given an antidepressant from those who were not, or if the test could distinguish those who have typical symptoms of depression (e.g., lack of sleep, too much sleep, weight gain or loss, crying, and so forth) from those who do not have these symptoms.

Reliability

The second quality examined in determining the adequacy of an assessment instrument is reliability. Whereas validity is used to show that a test is measuring what it's supposed to measure, reliability examines the accuracy of test scores. As with validity, reliability is measuring the adequacy of the test and is not making a statement about the people taking the test. There are a number of ways of examining such accuracy. (After reading this section, see Table 12.2 for a summary of types of reliability.)

TABLE 12.2

Summary of Types of Validity and Reliability	
VALIDITY	RELIABILITY
Content: content analysis; experts contribute test questions and are consulted, and items are created from well-known sources.	*Test–retest:* the ability of a test to show consistency in scores from one testing to a second testing.
Concurrent: a kind of criterion-related validity. The relationship between the test and a criterion in the present (e.g., another test, expert judges' ratings).	*Parallel forms:* the correlation of one form of a test with a second equivalent form of the test.
Predictive: a kind of criterion-related validity. The relationship between the test and a future criterion.	*Split-half:* the relationship between items on one-half of a test with items on the second half of the test.
Construct: the ability of a test to show that a certain construct exists and can support a theoretical assumption of the test.	*Internal consistency:* the average of all possible split-half reliabilities.

Test–Retest Reliability

One of the most common types of reliability, test–retest reliability examines the relationship between scores on one administration of a test with scores on a second administration of the same test. For instance, if I wished to show that my test was accurate, I might administer the instrument to a large group of individuals and, a short time later, perhaps one week, administer it a second time. I would then correlate the scores from the first administration with the scores from the second administration of the test. A test that is poorly made (has a fair amount of error) will result in many individuals having large deviations between the first and second administrations of the test. One problem with this kind of reliability is in sorting out whether deviations between the first and second administration of a test are the result of changes in individuals or because of error in the test. For instance, if individuals are given a test to measure depression, then seek out therapy, and one month later are given the same test, it would be difficult to determine if changes in test scores are a result of therapy or reflective of a poorly made test. This is why other types of reliability that do not rely on a second administration of the test are often used in addition to or in lieu of test–retest reliability.

Alternative Forms Reliability

Sometimes called parallel forms or equivalent forms reliability, alternative forms reliability measures accuracy in a test by correlating one form of a test with a second form that is considered to be a close mirror to the first form. Because the two forms are generally given at the same time, the possibility that the correlation is a result of changes in the individual between the first and second administrations of the test is eliminated. One problem with this kind of reliability is the difficulty of making a second form that is a true mirror of the first. For many tests, it is not practical to devise a second, equivalent form of the test.

Split-Half Reliability

Split-half reliability eliminates the problem of having to create a second form of the test. In this kind of reliability, the instrument is split in half in some rational manner that assumes that scores on the first half of the test should be equivalent to scores on the second half of the instrument. The two halves of the test are then correlated to show the accuracy of the test. Errors of this kind of reliability revolve around the fact that one is correlating two halves of a test rather than two full-length tests.

Internal Consistency

Like split-half reliability, internal consistency reliability gives an estimate of consistency based on a single administration of a test. The reliability estimate found reflects the average of all split-half reliabilities. With the advent of computers, this kind of reliability has become quite popular.

Practicality

Suppose I have a test that can accurately assess mental health diagnosis, but each administration costs $1000. This test may be good at what it does, but the cost may be prohibitive for most people. Or, suppose we have an instrument than can accurately measure learning disabilities but takes a school psychologist two days to administer. These are some of the questions that we must struggle with when deciding whether or not a test is practical.

Practicality examines whether or not the test is realistic to give. It includes issues related to the cost of testing, the ease of administration, the length of the test, and the ease of interpretation. A test can have good validity and good reliability and be cross-culturally fair, and yet not be a practical test to give.

Cross-Cultural Fairness of Tests

> *. . . tests must be used in ways that, as far as possible, take advantage of the tremendous utility of test and other assessment data, while also facilitating optimal understanding and nurturance of a wide range of individual and cultural differences.* (Walsh & Betz, 2001, p. 424)

The last quality important in determining whether a test is worthwhile is whether it is cross-culturally fair. Although it is impossible to eliminate all bias from tests, one should expect that the bias is small enough to allow for justifiable interpretations of any individual's score. When examining cultural bias, test publishers should have exhaustively reviewed the extent to which the content of a test has cultural bias. For instruments used to predict future behavior, the test should be shown to be predictive for minority groups. This does not mean that it will predict in the same manner for all groups, but that the predictive validity of each subgroup was examined and the test was shown to predict accurately for each subgroup (Walsh & Betz, 2001). In fact, the U.S. Supreme Court case of *Griggs* v. *Duke Power Company* (1971) asserted that tests used for hiring and advancement at work must show that they can predict job performance for all groups.

Cross-cultural bias in testing is an important issue when assessment instruments are used with minorities. Examiners need to be aware of bias in testing, ethical issues related to assessment and multiculturalism, and state and national laws concerning the use of tests with minorities. (See Box 12.3.) Some related issues will be discussed later in this chapter.

Where to Find Tests

Today, there are well over 3000 tests available for sale (Thorndike, 1997). Because there are so many options, finding a test that meets one's specific needs is not always an easy

BOX 12.3

The Use of Intelligence Tests with Minorities: Confusion and Bedlam

The use of intelligence tests with culturally diverse populations has long been an area of controversy. Some states have found intelligence tests biased and have banned their use in certain circumstances with some groups (Swenson, 1997). Other states have not found widespread evidence of bias. If intelligence tests are used, the examiner needs to be astute to the proper way of administering and scoring the test with all clients.

The concern for bias in testing has gone so far in some circles that if the situation wasn't so serious, it would almost be comical. Take the case in California of Mary Amaya, who was concerned that her son was being recommended for remedial courses he did not need. Having had an older son who was found to *not* need such assistance only *after* he was tested, Ms. Amaya requested an intelligence test for her other son. However, since the incident with her first son, laws had been changed; California had decided that intelligence tests were culturally biased and thus banned their use for certain groups. Despite Ms. Amaya's request for an intelligence test, it was found that she had no legislative right to have it given to her son.

task. However, a number of sources are available to assist us in the proper selection of tests for use with a desired population. They include:

1. *Publisher resource catalogs*. Test publishing companies freely distribute catalogs that describe the tests they sell.
2. *Journals in the field*. Professional journals, especially those associated with measurement, will often describe tests they have used in research or give reviews of new tests in the field.
3. *Source books on testing*. There are a few comprehensive books that provide the names of the test author(s), the publication date, the purpose of the test, critical reviews, bibliographical information, information on test construction, the name and address of the test publishing company, the costs of the test, and other basic information about the test. Two of the most important source books are the *Buros Mental Measurement Yearbook* and its companion volume, *Tests in Print* (Claiborn, 1991b; Plake & Conoley, 1995; Plake, Conoley, Kramer, & Murphy, 1991).
4. *Books on testing*. Textbooks that present an overview of testing are usually fairly good at highlighting a number of the better-known tests that are in use today.
5. *Experts*. School psychologists, learning disability specialists, experts at a school system's central testing office, psychologists at agencies, and professors are some of the people who can be called upon for assistance with testing information.
6. *The Internet*. Today, publishing companies have home pages that offer information about tests they offer and from which you can purchase tests. In addition, the Internet has become an increasingly important place to search for information about testing. Of course, one needs to be careful to assure that any information from the Internet is accurate.

Writing Test Reports

In-depth information on the writing of test reports is not the purview of this text. However, because some counselors will write test reports and all counselors will read the test reports of others, it is crucial that they understand the basics of test report writing. Although the content of a report will vary based on the purpose of the testing, a test report will generally include the following categories: demographic information, reason for referral, relevant background information, behavioral observations of the client, test results, impressions, recommendations, and summary (Drummond, 2000; Goldman, 1971).

As with clinical case reports, test reports should not be longer than a few pages, and the examiner should use language that most professionals, even ones who have little or no background in testing, could understand. Some common problems that have been identified in the writing of tests reports include the overuse of jargon, focusing on the test(s) and downplaying the person, focusing on the person and de-emphasizing the test results, poor organization, poor writing skills, and failing to take a position about the person who was tested (e.g., not making specific recommendations) (Katz, 1985). Hopefully, as you proceed through your training program, you will obtain many opportunities to practice writing test and case reports.

Use of Computers in Testing

Computers have affected every area of testing (Sampson, 1990, 1995). Here are just a few of the ways that testing has changed as the result of computers:

1. *Test scoring and reporting*. Computers are now used to score tests in many different ways. Sometimes, such as at colleges or when publishing companies test thousands of individuals at once, mainframes are used to quickly scan and score the responses. Some testing companies offer an option in which the examiner can send them a computer-scanned answer sheet so they can score the test and promptly return it to the examiner. Finally, PCs are increasingly being used to administer and score tests. This allows for quick results that have been shown to improve client satisfaction (Flowers, Booraem, & Schwartz, 1993).
2. *Administration of tests*. PCs, as just noted, are increasingly used for the administration of a wide variety of ability and personality tests. Even the SATs and GREs are now be offered on a PC. It is easy to administer a test on a computer, and results can be obtained quickly.
3. *Interpretation of test material*. Today, computers can generate rather elaborate interpretations of test results. Such computer-generated reports can assist the counselor in explaining results to a client but will not replace the counselor, who is needed to explain what the test is about, to offer understanding about basic test statistics, and, most importantly, to listen keenly to the importance of the meaning test results have for the client.
4. *Access to tests on the Internet*. From the Internet we can now take tests, purchase tests, download tests, and find information about tests. There is little doubt that in a relatively short amount of time a large portion of the business of testing will be taking place on the Internet.
5. *Increased efficacy for the testing of individuals with disabilities*. Computer-adaptive test-taking devices now allow many individuals with disabilities to take tests with relative ease. Such devices reduce or eliminate the influence of those who inadvertently assisted individuals with disabilities while they were taking a test (Sampson, 1990).

Multicultural Issue: Caution in Using Tests

All testing should be considered within a framework of cultural diversity. (Anastasi, 1985, p. xxix)

In recent years there has been an increasing emphasis on test bias in the assessment of minorities (Watkins & Campbell, 1990). We have seen lawsuits filed that question the accuracy of some tests for culturally diverse individuals, laws passed preventing the use of other tests, and research conducted that considers the negative impact of tests. As a partial response to these problems, the Association for Assessment in Counseling (AAC), a division of ACA, has developed a set of multicultural assessment standards for the choosing, administration, and interpretation of tests (AAC, 1992; Prediger, 1994). These standards help counselors and others (1) understand the cultural bias inherent in tests, (2) know when a test should not be used because of bias, and (3) know what to do with test results when a test does *not* predict well for minorities. In addition to the standards, the ACA code of ethics speaks to the importance of the careful use of testing with minorities:

> *Counselors are cautious in using assessment techniques, making evaluations, and interpreting the performance of populations not represented in the norm group on which an instrument was standardized. They recognize the effects of age, color, culture, disability, ethnic group, gender, race, religion, sexual orientation, and socioeconomic status on test administration and interpretation and place test results in proper perspective with other relevant factors.* (ACA, 1995a, Standard E.8)

In the future, we are likely to see an increased emphasis on understanding the inherent bias in tests, the creation of new tests that are less biased, and new efforts to properly administer, score, and interpret tests given that they will, to some degree, have bias.

Ethical, Professional, and Legal Issues

Ethical Issues: Guidelines for the Use of Tests

To guide practitioners and the public, the ACA, APA, and AAC have developed a number of standards and guidelines specifically focusing on assessment. For instance, the ACA and APA have both targeted educational and psychological assessment as important components of their ethical guidelines. However, realizing that the ethical guidelines are not specific enough, both ACA and APA have formulated testing standards that include technical standards, professional standards, and standards for the administration and interpretation of tests (AAC, 1987; APA, 1999; Vacc, Juhnke, & Nilsen, 2001). In addition, the APA has also developed the Code of Fair Testing Practices in Education (APA, 1988). This code, which is written for the general public, explains the appropriate ways that test users (e.g., examiners) and test developers (e.g., publishers) should (1) develop and select appropriate tests, (2) interpret test scores, (3) strive for multicultural fairness in testing, and (4) inform test takers about their rights and test procedures. In a similar vein, AAC (2001) has developed the *Rights and Responsibilities of Test Takers: Guidelines and Expectations*. Finally, as previously noted, AAC has developed Multicultural Assessment Standards (AAC, 1992; Prediger, 1994).

Informed Consent

Informed consent implies that each person who is to be tested has been told the whys, whats, and hows of testing and has given permission for testing to take place (Thorndike, 1997). Generally, individuals have the right to refuse testing; however, in rare cases, such as court-ordered testing to assess fitness of a parent for a child custody case, a client may not have such a right.

Invasion of Privacy and Confidentiality

All tests invade one's privacy. However, concerns about invasion of privacy are lessened if the client has given informed consent, has some real choice in whether or not he or she can refuse testing, and knows the limits of confidentiality, such as when testing is court ordered.

Competence in the Use of Tests

To properly administer, score, and interpret test results, test givers must have adequate knowledge about testing and familiarity with any test they may use. In an effort to assist helpers in determining their level of competence, the American Psychological Association offers the following:

> *Level A tests are those that can be administered, scored, and interpreted by responsible nonpsychologists who have carefully read the test manual and are familiar with the overall purpose of testing. Educational achievement tests fall into this category . . .*
>
> *Level B tests require technical knowledge of test construction and use and appropriate advanced coursework in psychology and related courses (e.g., statistics, individual differences, and counseling) . . .*
>
> *Level C tests require an advanced degree in psychology or licensure as a psychologist and advanced training/supervised experience in the particular test. . . .*
> (APA, 1954, pp. 146–148)

More specifically, a bachelor's-level individual who has some knowledge of assessment and is thoroughly versed with the test manual can give a Level A test and, under some limited circumstances, a Level B test. For example, teachers can administer most survey battery achievement tests. The master's-level counselor or other helping professional who has taken a basic course in tests and measurement can administer Level B tests. For example, counselors can administer a wide range of personality tests, including most interest inventories and many objective personality tests. However, they cannot administer tests that require additional training, such as most individual tests of intelligence, most projective tests, and many diagnostic tests. These Level C tests are reserved for those who have a minimum of a master's degree, a basic testing course, and advanced training in the specialized test (e.g., school psychologists, learning disabilities specialists, clinical and counseling psychologists, master-level therapists who have gained additional training).

Other Ethical Issues

Many other ethical issues should be considered when giving and interpreting test results, and you are encouraged to carefully read the ACA ethical standards to familiarize yourself with them. Briefly, they include knowing how to (1) properly release test results; (2) select tests; (3) administer, score, and interpret tests; (4) keep tests secure; (5) pick tests that are current and up-to-date; and (6) assess that tests are properly constructed.

Professional Issues

Making Wise Decisions

Tests can help clients gain a greater understanding of themselves and assist them in making smart decisions. However, tests need to be used wisely, and, unfortunately, this has not always been the case. Problems with lack of competency in using tests have led to a difficult marriage between the counselor and testing (Bradley, 1994; Goldman, 1994). Counselors should know test manuals, know how to administer tests appropriately, and be able to properly interpret tests. Counselors should warn clients about the pitfalls of making decisions solely on the results of one test. If the results from one test can suggest a direction for a client, then two tests can do it better, and three tests can add more information, and three tests and a clinical interview can offer even more. Although a counselor can never assure that decisions that result from testing will benefit the client, he or she can make sure that the client has been given an appropriate test, has been administered the test properly, and has been afforded the best opportunity to understand the results.

Professional Association

Originally called the Association for Measurement and Evaluation in Guidance (AMEG), AMEG changed its name to the Association for Assessment in Counseling (AAC) in order to reflect a broader definition of assessment that includes the use of diagnosis, testing, interviewing, and other activities designed to understand the individual. Consider joining AAC if you are interested in testing, diagnosis, and the training and supervision of those who do assessment and/or if you are interested in developing and validating assessment products and procedures. AAC, a division of ACA, publishes *Measurement and Evaluation in Counseling and Development*. (You can reach AAC via www.counseling.org.)

Legal Issues: Laws That Have Had an Impact on Testing

A number of laws have been passed that impinge on the use of tests. Some of the more prevalent ones include:

The Buckley Amendment. Also known as the Family Rights and Privacy Act of 1974 (FERPA), this law affirms the right of all individuals to their school records, including test records.

The Freedom of Information Act. This law assures the right of individuals to access their federal records, including test records.

PL 94-142. As noted earlier, this legislative act assures the right of students to be tested, at a school system's expense, if they are suspected of having a disability that interferes with learning. The law, which applies to those from age of 3 through age 21, asserts that schools must make accommodations, within the least restrictive environment, for students with learning disabilities.

Carl Perkins Act (PL 98-524). This law assures that individuals with disabilities or who are disadvantaged have access to vocational assessment, counseling, and placement.

Americans with Disabilities Act. This law states that accommodations must be made for individuals who are taking tests for employment and that testing must be shown to be relevant to the job in question.

Civil Rights Acts (1964 and amendments). This series of laws asserts that any test used for employment or promotion must be shown to be suitable and valid for the job in question. If not, alternative means of assessment must be provided. Differential test cutoffs are not allowed.

The Counselor in Process: Assessment of Clients

Throughout this chapter, the term *testing* has been used interchangeably with the word *assessment*. However, within the counseling relationship, the assessment of clients is much broader than testing an individual. A holistic process, assessment includes a variety of activities to assist the client in his or her self-discovery process (Drum, 1992; Goldman, 1992; Hohenshil, 1993b). Assessment can certainly include the use of traditional tests; however, it may also include nontraditional techniques such as life lines, where a person reflects on the highs and lows of his or her life; self-assessment of abilities; diaries; the clinical interview; observation of the client, the review of past records (e.g., school, medical, etc.); and a variety of other techniques (Harrington, 1995; Juhnke, 1995).

Assessment is a continuous and ongoing process (Vacc, 1982). It begins the first moment the counselor and client meet. The counselor can then assist the client in gaining a baseline from which to compare future behaviors. As the helping relationship continues and deepens, the assessment process tends to move from being counselor-centered, in the sense that the counselor provides the tools to assist the client in his or her own self-assessment process, to being client-centered, whereby the client has learned how to assess self. In a sense, one might say that the process has moved from counselor assessment to client self-assessment. Although the counseling relationship will eventually reach an end, we hope that seeds have been planted for the client to continue with an ongoing and deepening self-assessment process throughout his or her life.

Summary

This chapter examined testing. We first examined why testing was important and noted that testing is one additional way that counselors can assess the inner world of the client. Testing can aid counselors in understanding the client's abilities and personality and can be useful in diagnosis, goal setting, treatment planning, and evaluation. We also found that testing is an important function of counselors in all settings, noting that counselors give and interpret tests, consult with others about tests, supervise those who do testing, read in the professional literature about how tests can be useful to our work with clients, and use tests in evaluation and research.

Within this chapter we noted that throughout history people have always been tested. We stated that the modern-day origins of testing can be traced back to the mid-

1800s when tests grew out of the focus on individual differences and the rigors of scientific method. With changing demographics and the industrial revolution, the turn of the 20th century saw the first need for the widespread use of tests, particularly vocational tests. With the advent of WWI, this impetus increased as ability and personality tests were developed to help with the placement of recruits. Soon, tests of all kinds could be found in use at many different settings. We noted that tests have been refined over the years, and that new statistical models and computers have particularly improved the quality of tests.

Today, there are many different kinds of tests, including ability tests, which comprise achievement and aptitude tests that measure ability in the cognitive realm; personality tests, which measure temperament, values, and interests in the affective realm; and informal forms of assessment, such as rating scales and observation. We noted that tests can be standardized and either norm-referenced or criterion-referenced; or nonstandardized and either criterion-referenced or norm-referenced.

In putting meaning to test scores, we noted that it is important to examine an individual's score relative to his or her norm group and to understand what the score means to the individual taking the test. We highlighted the fact that measures of central tendency and measures of variability can assist us in making comparisons between individuals who take the same test, or when comparing individuals who have taken different tests.

In examining basic test statistics, we explained how the standard deviation, one measure of variability, is particularly important in understanding norm-referenced tests. We also noted that the standard deviation helps us convert raw scores to derived scores. We discussed the fact that derived scores, such as percentiles, T-scores, deviation IQ scores, SAT/GRE-type scores, grade equivalents, stanines, and idiosyncratic publisher test scores, are used because they are easier to interpret than raw scores.

Within this chapter we discussed the importance of four qualities in making a test worthwhile. The first quality we highlighted was validity, or whether or not a test measures what it is supposed to measure. Then we defined reliability, or the ability of a test to accurately measure a trait or ability. The other two qualities we discussed were practicality, the ease of administration and interpretation of the test; and cultural fairness, whether or not the test measures what it's supposed to measure in a consistent manner for all groups.

We noted that today there are many sources that can help us find tests that have good reliability and validity, are practical, and have limited cultural bias. Some of these include publishers' resource manuals; professional journals; source books on testing, such as the *Buros Mental Measurement Yearbook;* textbooks on testing, experts in schools and agencies, and the Internet.

In this chapter we discussed the importance of writing good test reports and highlighted some potential problems in the writing of such reports. We also discussed how computers have changed the face of testing and the fact that they will continue to become increasingly more important.

Within this chapter we spoke of the inherent biases in tests when used with minority clients and that counselors should know the effects of bias on the administration and interpretation of test scores. We also raised other ethical and professional issues in testing, such as the importance of having the individual being evaluated give informed consent, the notion that all tests invade one's privacy, and that test takers should know the limits of confidentiality. We pointed out that three levels of test competency are associated with the proper administration, scoring, and interpretation of tests. Also, we noted that ACA, APA, and AAC offer ethical guidelines, standards of practices, and other important resources to help us in the administration, scoring, and interpretation of tests.

Noting some important legislative actions and their impact on testing, we briefly explained the Buckley Amendment, the Freedom of Information Act, PL94-142, the Carl Perkins Act, the Americans with Disabilities Act, and various civil rights acts and their amendments.

Finally, we concluded the chapter by contrasting the words test and assessment. We noted that within the counseling relationship assessment is an ongoing holistic process that can include testing as one of its components. We stressed that as the client continues in the counseling relationship, there tends to be movement from counselor assessment of the client to client self-assessment. We also noted that when a successful counseling relationship terminates, the client is able to continue the self-assessment process on his or her own.

INFOTRAC and Other Information Resources (e.g., ERIC and PsycINFO)

Note: When relevant, key words are in quotation marks.

1. Research, in more depth, any area of assessment highlighted in this chapter.
2. Examine the role "PL94-142" or other laws of your choice on assessment.
3. By examining the literature, conduct a critical review of a test of your choice.

CHAPTER 13

Research and Evaluation

Research has been maligned. Some criticize it, students fear it, and others approach it as if it were a virus, never coming too close to it. Unfortunately, many lose sight, or perhaps never gain the insight, that research "can be an exhilarating experience, analogous to adding pieces to a jigsaw puzzle." (Whitson, 1996, p. 622)

I remember a graduate student coming to me one day, bewildered after not finding significant results on a study she was conducting for her thesis. She had hypothesized that there would be a relationship between the number of years that one meditated and self-actualizing values; that is, the more you meditated, the more self-actualized you would be. She went to an ashram (a yoga retreat center) and had a number of meditators complete an instrument that measured how self-actualized they were, and then she collected information from these same individuals concerning how long they had been meditating. After collecting her data and performing a statistical analysis, she found no significant relationship. As she herself had meditated for years and was an ardent believer in meditation, she strongly felt that she would find such a relationship; she was clearly personally invested in the research. Upon finding no significant relationship, she said to me, "There must be something wrong with this research, because clearly people who have meditated for years are more self-actualized than those who have just started meditating." I suggested there was nothing wrong with the research, but that perhaps she had a bias because of her own experiences with meditation. I explained that this does not mean that meditation does not affect people, but that for this population, using this instrument, the evidence showed that no significant relationship existed. I went on to remind her that research is not how you feel something is, but what the results show. When she was able to see her own biases, she realized that perhaps I had a point.

A few years back I was conducting research on the relationship between dogmatism, internal locus of control, and attitudes toward learning in graduate students. I dutifully collected my data and was soon hoping to do my statistical analysis when a colleague of mine suggested it might also be interesting to look at how students make meaning in their lives. He suggested a process by which he would interview a number of students who had participated in my study and attempt to find patterns and themes in their responses. He eventually hoped to distinguish students from one another based on their ways of making meaning and suggested that we could relate meaning making to the other attributes I was examining. I suggested that his research seemed kind of soft. "How do you quantify interviews?" I asked. He was soon to teach me an important lesson about research: that research can be more than simply looking at numbers and that research comes in many different forms. He was suggesting integrating a qualitative approach with my quantitative analysis, two very different ways of doing research.

The federal government audited me once. A colleague and I had received a $70,000 grant to train helping professionals in the schools about substance abuse interventions. We ran a series of workshops and subsequently used a number of evaluation techniques to show the worthwhileness of the training program. These evaluation procedures served a number of purposes, including helping us examine what had been beneficial during the earlier workshops, assisting us in fine-tuning later workshops, helping us know the overall satisfaction of the participants with the total program, designing future training programs, and perhaps most significantly in this instance, having evidence to show the Feds that we were accomplishing our stated goals, that we were accountable.

Why do research and evaluation? Well, as you can see by the above examples, research and evaluation help us find answers to the questions we ponder, move us forward in our understanding of the world, help us show that what we are doing is worthwhile, are ways of expressing our creativity, and can even be interesting and fun!

This chapter will examine some of the more common research and evaluation techniques and, I hope, present them in a manner that is appealing and exciting. We will begin by defining the purpose of research and distinguish between two major forms of research, quantitative and qualitative. We will also compare the value of the different kinds of research. After surveying different research methods, we will offer an overview of evaluation methods and examine the relationship of evaluation to research. Finally, we will examine multicultural, ethical, professional, and legal issues related to research and evaluation.

Research

The Purpose of Research

The inquiry of truth, which is the love-making, or wooing of it, the knowledge of truth, which is the presence of it, and the belief of truth, which is the enjoying of it, is the sovereign good of human nature. (Sir Francis Bacon)

Best and Kahn (1997) describe research as "the systematic and objective analysis and recording of controlled observations that may lead to the development of generalizations, principles or theories, resulting in prediction and possibly ultimate control of events" (p. 18). In other words, research analyzes information in order to give us knowledge about the present, knowledge that may be helpful to us in making predictions about the future. Research comes in many forms and can be as varied as counting the number of times a child acts out during the day, surveying opinions of counselors, using intensive interviews to understand how moral development is established, or performing complex statistical analyses to determine which counseling skills are most effective.

Without research, knowledge remains stagnant, and new paradigms are unlikely to evolve (Kuhn, 1962). While our theories are interesting and are generally the basis for our research, theories hold little weight if they are not eventually grounded in research. Research validates what the counselor is doing and can suggest new avenues for approaching client change (Lambert, Ogles, & Masters, 1992). Research is the basis for evaluation that enables us to know if the programs and workshops we are conducting are effective. Without research, we are an ethereal profession with our heads in the air and little or no means of showing that what we do is meaningful.

Two Types of Research: Quantitative and Qualitative

Quantitative research assumes that there is an objective reality within which research questions can be formulated and scientific methods used to measure the probability that identified behaviors, values, or beliefs either cause or are related to other behaviors, values, or beliefs. Qualitative research, on the other hand, holds that there are multiple ways of viewing knowledge and that one can make sense of the world by immersing oneself in the research situation in an attempt to provide possible explanations for the problem being examined (Heppner, Kivlighan, & Wampold, 1992). In distinguishing qualitative and quantitative research, McMillan and Schumacher (2001) make several distinctions (see Table 13.1).

TABLE 13.1

Distinctions between Quantitative and Qualitative Research

	QUANTITATIVE	QUALITATIVE
Assumptions about the world	Objective reality that can be measured	Phenomenological: Reality is socially constructed
Research purpose	Explaining relationships between variables	Understanding phenomenon from participants' perspectives
Research methods and process	Preestablished design and statistical procedures	Emerging methods of examining the social phenomenon at hand
Prototypical studies	Studies designed to zero in on a problem and reduce error	Studies undertaken to broaden understanding of phenomenon being examined
Researcher role	Detached to avoid researcher bias	Immersed in study to gain an understanding of the phenomenon; "disciplined subjectivity" to understand data collected
Importance of the context in the study	To generalize results, studies developed to eliminate all influences except those being examined	Human behavior understood within its social context and therefore cannot be analyzed separately from it

Literature Reviews and the Statement of the Problem

Research offers us a mechanism to satisfy our innate curiosity about human nature. For instance, you have undoubtedly pondered the nature of emotional disorders and have wondered about effective ways to treat emotional problems. The only difference between you and a researcher is that the researcher uses specific procedures in an effort to seek out plausible answers to these questions. Where does the researcher start? At the beginning, of course with a hunch or an educated guess about a topic of interest that the researcher would like to explore. Then, the researcher must examine the prior research to see what has gone before.

The examination of prior research is called the *review of the literature* and is generally begun by conducting a computerized search of abstracts in the fields of education, psychology, and other disciplines that might be relevant to the research. Two particularly popular electronic searches are offered by Educational Resources Information Center (ERIC) and PsychINFO and can be completed at your library or via the Internet.

The *statement of the problem* places the research within its historical context, determines what research already exists on your topic, discusses why the issue at hand is important, limits the scope of what one is researching, distinguishes how your research departs from past research, and offers research questions, statements, and/or hypotheses that begin to delimit the type of research one will conduct (Charles & Mertler, 2002; McMillan & Schumacher, 2001). For instance, examine the statement of the problem on counselors' attendance in their own therapy presented in Box 13.1 and identify each of the above components.

Once the statement of the problem is developed, the research design can be formulated. Generally one's research design is based on a number of factors, including the researcher's bias toward quantitative or qualitative research and the kind of research that has previously been conducted, as evidenced in the literature review. Whether undertaking quantitative or qualitative research, a number of varying designs can be established. Let's take a look at some of the more prevalent research designs.

Research Designs

Qualitative and quantitative research approach the analysis of research problems differently. Thus, it is not surprising that their designs vary dramatically. Whereas quantitative research attempts to reduce the problem to a few very specific variables that can be experimentally manipulated, the aim of qualitative research is to make sense out of the problem by analyzing it broadly within its naturally occurring context. Therefore, we will separately examine the types of research designs offered by the quantitative and qualitative researcher, while keeping in mind that some researchers attempt to combine these two varying approaches (Schofield & Anderson, 1984).

Quantitative Research Designs

Quantitative research assumes that there is an objective reality that can be revealed through the use of research design and the statistical analysis of data. Quantitative research uses scientific method to show the plausibility that a hypothesis is valid or to find

BOX 13.1

Statement of the Problem

In order to enhance counselor self-understanding as well as client growth, many counselor educators have been proponents of personal therapy for counselor trainees and for practicing counselors (Corey et al., 1998; Guy & Liaboe, 1986). In summarizing the work of a number of other authors, Norcross, Strausser-Kirtland, and Missar (1988) noted that personal therapy is important because it will increase the emotional functioning of the therapist, assist the therapist in a deeper understanding of intra- and interpersonal functioning, ameliorate emotional burdens, add to the therapist's personal conviction about the ability of therapy to work, give the therapist an increased respect for the role of the client, and provide role models from which the therapist can learn.

More specifically, Watkins (1983) noted that personal therapy can diminish or eliminate "counselor acting out" behaviors including "attentional failures," "empathic failures," "aggressivity," "sexual and seductive behaviors," and "logistical failures" (mishandling of time issues, e.g., being late for appointments). Along the same lines, it has been suggested that psychotherapy can help the therapist look at his or her blind spots, widen the types of responses a therapist makes, and increase empathy and self-awareness (Ford, 1963; Pope, 1987; Strupp, 1955; Wampler & Strupp, 1976). So important is the belief that counselors should be in their own therapy that many graduate programs have required psychotherapy as part of counselor training (Garfield & Kurtz, 1976; Garfield, 1977; Greenberg & Staller, 1981; Wampler & Strupp, 1976).

The decision concerning which therapist to see is complex and related to the values held by the counselor who is considering seeking his or her own counseling. However, there are some qualities that seem to be more important for most counselors when choosing a therapist. For instance, when therapists from related helping professions rated a number of characteristics for choosing their therapist, competence, warmth and caring, and professional reputation were rated highly, while research productivity, cost per session, and flexibility were deemed less important (Grunebaum, 1983; Norcross et al., 1988).

Although attendance in therapy of psychiatrists, psychologists, and social workers has been explored, no research has examined the attendance in therapy of counselors. Thus, this study will examine the rates of attendance in therapy of ACA members and explore the reasons a counselor may choose a specific therapist when entering personal counseling.

possible answers to the research question being asked. Two main types of quantitative research are experimental and nonexperimental research.

Although both experimental and nonexperimental research use the scientific method and a reductionistic approach to understanding the research problem, there are some crucial differences between these two types of designs. In experimental research, the researcher is manipulating the experience of the participants (the treatment) in some manner to show a cause-and-effect relationship between it and specific outcome measures. Nonexperimental designs, on the other hand, tend to either look at relationships between variables or describe the attitudes, beliefs, and behaviors of a group being surveyed.

Experimental Research

TRUE EXPERIMENTAL RESEARCH In the realm of quantitative research, true experimental designs are considered *la crème de la crème* as they test, in a very controlled manner, for causal relationships between the variables being studied. In this type of research, the independent variable, or the variable being manipulated, is examined to determine if it has a direct effect on the dependent variable(s) or outcome measure(s).

In true experimental research, there is random assignment of subjects to treatment groups, which means that every subject has an equal chance of being in any of the treatment groups. There is a false belief by some that all true experimental research must have a control group. This is not the case; if the researcher is confident as a result of past research that any treatment is significantly different from no treatment, then he or she is not obligated to have a control group and may instead wish to compare different types of treatment.

One example of true experimental research would be a study of the effects of aerobics (the independent variable) on personality measures such as depression, anxiety, and internal locus of control (the dependent variables). Because aerobics is the variable being manipulated, various types of treatment (aerobics) must be offered; and, because this is true experimental research, I must have random assignment. Therefore, one design might be to randomly assign 100 individuals to four treatment groups: a control group that does no aerobic exercise, a group that participates in eight weeks of low-impact aerobics, a group that participates in eight weeks of a mixture of low- and high-impact aerobics, and a group that does eight weeks of high-impact aerobics. To assure that the personality of the aerobics leader is not a factor in the results, I could have multiple aerobics leaders, each of whom leads one class in each of the treatment groups.

Starting with the assumption that there would be no differences between these four groups, I would develop a null hypothesis that states, "There will be no difference on measures of anxiety, depression, and internal locus of control between individuals who participate in different types of aerobic exercise." When researchers use the null hypothesis, they hope to show that it is false; that is, the researcher wants to show that the treatment has caused difference between groups, thus demonstrating treatment effects. For instance, using the aerobics example, my assumption would be that if I randomly assigned 100 individuals to four groups, prior to aerobics (the treatment) these groups would look the same if I measured them on our personality measures. Therefore, following aerobic exercise (the treatment) any differences that are found between the groups would likely be due to the effect of the treatment and not due to other factors (see Figure 13.1).

Now, even if a treatment were totally ineffective, when measuring four groups of people on almost any characteristic you are likely to find some differences between groups just due to chance variables or fluctuations in scores. Therefore, in demonstrating that a treatment is effective, we are actually measuring the probability that these differences are due to the treatment and not due to chance of minor fluctuations. In fact, even in studies that showed that the probability was 999 out of 1000 that the results were due to the treatment, it could be that the results are spurious because you happened to hit that 1 in 1000 time that variations were due to chance alone. It's kind of like playing the lottery. You know that you're not going to win, but once in a while . . . In research, you can be pretty darn sure that if the probability is 1 in 100, your results are true–the treatment has shown effects. However, it could be that you hit the lottery, but in this case the lottery is not lucky, and you have found results that are not real. This is why researchers never speak of proving something but instead talk in terms of the probability that the treatment was effective (Leary, 2001).

In some ways the null hypothesis is used in our jurisprudence system. Criminal juries are operating from the null hypothesis, thus showing the probability that the criminal is guilty or not guilty. For instance, in a murder trial the defendant goes to court with the presumption of innocence, which is really the null hypothesis: "The defendant did not commit murder." The prosecution attempts to disprove the null hypothesis by show-

FIGURE 13.1
Comparison of Variability of Treatment Groups before and after Aerobics When Measuring Depression Scores

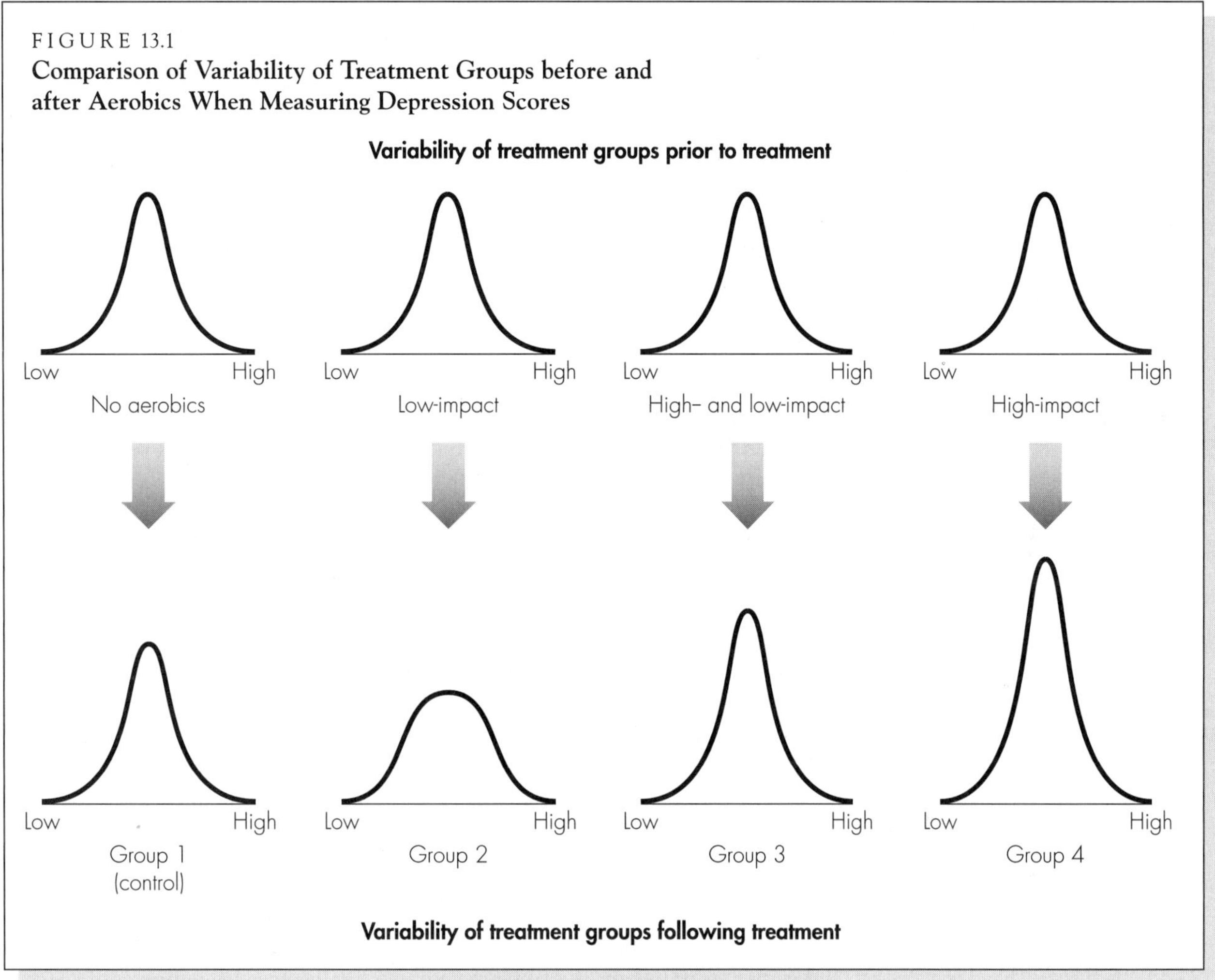

ing the probability that she committed the crime. If there is evidence beyond a reasonable doubt, you have disproved the null hypothesis, thus finding her guilty. On the other hand, if you have not convinced the jury of that probability, she is found not guilty, as opposed to innocent. We are not working with proof, but with probabilities. This is why a certain number of people who are innocent will always go to jail and a certain number of people will always be set free even though they are guilty. Science never gets to absolute truth, but perhaps close to it.

In doing true experimental research, there are a number of different kinds of design possibilities when deciding how to manipulate the independent variable and measure the dependent variable. Unfortunately (some of you may be saying fortunately!) this is not the purview of a text like this. However, regardless of the research design in use, in true experimental research we are examining whether or not the groups look the same after treatment as they did before treatment (see Figure 13.1).

BOX 13.2

A Failed Attempt at True Experimental Research

When I was living in New Hampshire, a colleague and I decided to do some research on the effects of aerobics on personality variables. After reviewing the literature, we found some possible links between aerobics and the personality variables of self-actualization, depression, and anxiety. We approached our local YMCA, which was running a rather extensive aerobics program. They agreed to let us talk with individuals who were about to start aerobics for the first time. They also agreed to let these people have eight free weeks of membership at the Y if half of them (randomly chosen) would not start aerobics for eight weeks. We found three instruments to measure anxiety, depression, and self-actualizing values with the intent of comparing, at the end of eight weeks, the group that started aerobics with the group that waited the eight weeks. We excitedly met with approximately 50 new "aerobians." We told them our plans—they looked at us and said, "Are you kidding? We want to start our aerobics classes now!"

Our good intentions obviously were not going to sway these individuals who were ready to get going with their exercise. Unfortunately for us, we were not able to implement our true experimental study. Instead, we had to consider using either a quasi-experimental or an ex post facto design, both of which would not be as powerful in showing treatment effects.

QUASI-EXPERIMENTAL RESEARCH As with true experimental research, in conducting quasi-experimental research one is attempting to determine cause and effect, and there is manipulation of the independent variable; however, there is no random assignment (Heppner et al., 1992). Instead of random assignment, this kind of research examines already existing intact groups and manipulates the treatment given to the groups (e.g., existing aerobics classes get different kinds of instructions, such as high- and low-impact aerobics).

Unlike true experimental research, the lack of random assignment in quasi-experimental research often results in less credibility in determining whether or not differences are due to the effects of the treatment. However, because the real world often does not provide us with opportunities to randomly assign individuals to treatment groups, true experimental research is frequently impractical to conduct, while quasi-experimental research and its use of intact groups can be more easily implemented (see Box 13.2). However, researchers are aware that intact groups, formed without random assignment, often carry with them a threat to internal validity (see Box 13.3).

SINGLE-SUBJECT DESIGNS Whenever a researcher has difficulty obtaining groups of individuals to examine, or when he or she is only interested in studying one or two subjects, such as in practice settings, single-subject designs may be implemented (Lundervold & Belwood, 2000). As in quasi-experimental research, there is no random assignment to treatment groups in single-subject designs, but there is manipulation of the independent variable, and such studies imply cause and effect. For instance, returning to our aerobics example, if I were working with a client who was struggling with anxiety and stress, I might design a study that examined the effects of aerobics, the treatment, on anxiety and stress as measured by a short anxiety scale and the client's resting heart rate. Using what is commonly called an ABA design, I would first obtain a baseline of my outcome measures (A), in this case anxiety and stress as measured on the anxiety scale and resting heart rate.

I would take a number of baseline measurements over a few weeks, then introduce the treatment, aerobics (B). I would continue to measure stress and resting heart rate over

BOX 13.3

Threats to Internal Validity

In all types of experimental research, there are many threats to internal validity that can result in researchers coming to false conclusions about their study if certain factors are not controlled. The following are very brief descriptions of 12 of these threats. A fuller understanding of them can be gained through a research course, a research text, and/or reading Campbell and Stanley (1963) and Cook and Campbell (1979), two classic books that describe these threats. The twelve threats include:

1. *History*, in which external events occur during the research which affects the treatment and results in invalid conclusions.
2. *Selection,* in which the ways that subjects are selected and assigned to treatment groups affect the results.
3. *Statistical regression,* where there is a statistical tendency for extreme scores to move closer to the mean if tested a second time. Therefore, regardless of the effect of the treatment, treatment groups with particularly high or low pretest scores may have scores move toward the mean during posttesting, thus leading to false readings concerning the effect of the treatment.
4. *Pretesting,* in which previously taking a test can affect the results, such as when a knowledge of the pretest affects the results of the posttesting.
5. *Instrumentation,* where changes in the instrument(s) can affect the results, such as when a more difficult pretest is used thus leading to the false conclusion that there were gains in posttesting.
6. *Subject attrition,* as when participants differentially drop out of treatment, thus leaving only the "better" or "worse" participants and results that are falsely attributed to the treatment.
7. *Maturation,* in which maturational changes in subjects, such as growing older or more tired or becoming hungry, affect the results.
8. *Diffusion of treatment,* in which subjects have knowledge of other treatment conditions, thus affecting their responses and leading to invalid results.
9. *Experimenter effects,* in which the researcher treats subjects differentially based on attributes not related to the treatment.
10. *Treatment replications,* in which the number of subjects does not accurately reflect the number of subjects undergoing treatment, such as when a group all receive a treatment *together*. Thus, only one replication of the treatment has been established as opposed to one replication for each member of the group.
11. *Subject effects,* when a participant exhibits positive or negative behaviors in response to the treatment because of the knowledge they are in a study.
12. *Statistical conclusion*, in which a violation of statistical inferences is made that results in invalid conclusions.

the next few weeks as the client participated in aerobics. Finally, I would remove the treatment and again take baseline measures over the next few weeks (A again). Evidence that the treatment is working should be indicated by a reduction in anxiety and stress levels during the treatment and a return to higher levels after the treatment. Often, to show additional efficacy of the treatment, the design is extended and made into an ABAB design, where the study finishes during a treatment phase with the expectation that the outcome measures should again produce change (Heppner et al., 1992). Figure 13.2 shows an example of an ABAB design for aerobics and its effect on anxiety and on stress.

Nonexperimental Research

CORRELATIONAL RESEARCH Correlational research includes research that attempts to understand the relationship between variables through the use of correlation coefficient. Generally, correlational research is of two kinds, simple correlational studies that explore the relationship between two variables or predictive correlational studies that are used to

FIGURE 13.2
Results from Hypothetical Study Examining the Effects of Aerobics on Anxiety Level and Heart Rate Using an ABAB Single-Subject Design

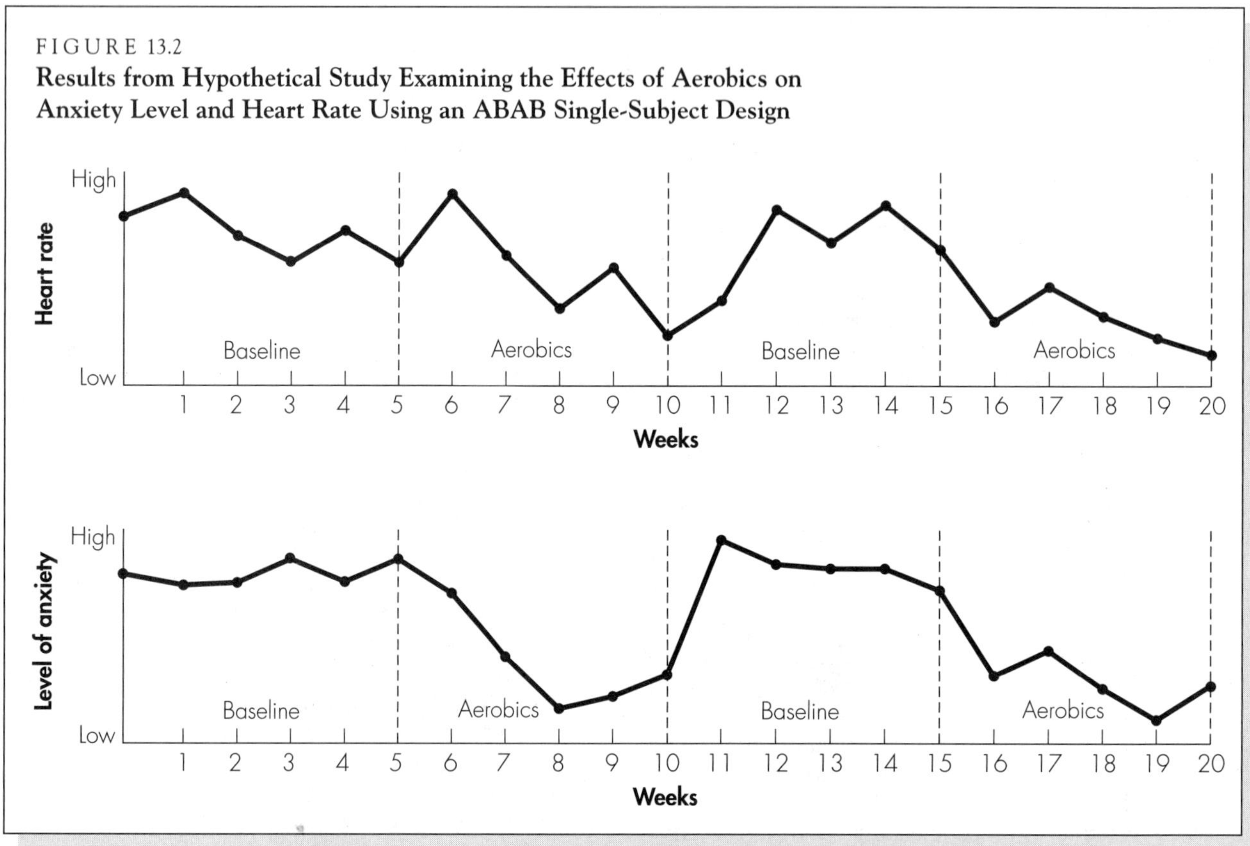

predict scores on a variable from scores obtained from other variables. If you remember from Chapter 12, correlation coefficients show the relationship between two sets of scores and range from –1 to +1. A positive correlation shows a tendency for one set of scores to be related to a second set of scores in the same direction. A negative correlation shows a relationship in opposite directions, and a correlation coefficient of 0 shows no relationship between variables. For instance, if I were interested in the relationship between the ability to be empathic and dogmatism, I could obtain scores from one group of individuals on these two variables and correlate them. In this case, you would expect to see a negative correlation that would indicate that individuals who were more empathic tended to be less dogmatic and vice versa. Generally, r is used in presenting the strength of the relationship. For instance, if I found a correlation coefficient of .89 between height and weight, I would say $r = .89$. Or, if I found that grades in graduate school had a mild negative correlation of –.24 with number of hours per week pursuing leisure activities, I would present the correlation as $r = -.24$.

SIMPLE CORRELATIONAL STUDIES In simple correlational studies, you examine selected variables that theory or past research suggests may be related to one another. Because correlational research does not show cause and effect and does not require random assignment, such research is generally easier to implement than experimental designs and is often used as preliminary research in an effort to check out a researcher's hunches.

TABLE 13.2

Intercorrelations between Cognitive Development, Age, GPA Internality, Dogmatism, and Empathy

VARIABLE	AGE	GPA	EXTERNALITY	DOGMATISM	EMPATHY
1. Cognitive development	$r = .26$*	$r = .21$	$r = -.24$*	$r = -.34$**	$r = .18$
2. Age	—	$r = .35$**	$r = -.15$	$r = -.13$	$r = .08$
3. GPA		—	$r = -.05$	$r = -.12$	$r = .28$*
4. Externality			—	$r = .65$**	$r = -.18$
5. Dogmatism				—	$r = -.18$
6. Empathy					—

*$p < .05$, **$p < .01$

One example of a simple correlational study is research I completed with a colleague where we examined the relationship among a number of factors that, based on the literature review, showed promise as being important in the development of helping skills for human service professionals (Neukrug & McAuliffe, 1993). Looking at the factors of cognitive development, age, GPA, internality/externality (internal locus of control), dogmatism, and empathic ability, we found the correlations noted in Table 13.2. Significant correlations are noted by placing one or two asterisks above the correlation coefficient. Based on the significance level noted, the probability is either 1 in 100 ($p = .01$), or 5 in 100 ($p = .05$) that such results would have been found by chance. Generally, research is considered not to be significant if the probability is greater than .05. In correlational research, significance is based on the size of the sample and the strength of the relationship, with larger sample sizes needing a smaller correlation to be significant. Based on your reading of Table 13.2, what variables are significant and what implications can you draw?

Correlational research is sometimes graphically represented in a scatterplot, as depicted in Figure 13.3. Look at how a correlation between externality and dogmatism differs as compared to the relationship between externality and cognitive development. Whereas there is a fairly strong relationship between the scores on externality and dogmatism, there is a mild to moderate relationship between cognitive development and dogmatism. What conclusions can you draw from this?

PREDICTIVE CORRELATIONAL STUDIES In contrast to simple correlational studies that examine the relationship between variables in the here and now, predictive correlational studies look at how one variable might be able to predict one or more other variables. The predictor variable is used to predict the criterion variable(s). It must be made clear, however, that although one variable can fairly accurately predict another, a cause-and-effect relationship has not been established. For instance, scores on the GREs should be predictive of GPA in graduate school, or they would not be useful for this purpose. Indeed, such scores have been shown to be moderately predictive of graduate school GPA in most subjects (*GRE Guide*, 1990). However, GRE scores certainly do not cause a certain GPA in graduate school.

Using a predictive correlational design, Jagger and colleagues (1992) measured the relationship between job fit and job satisfaction of over 100 successfully rehabilitated vocational rehabilitation clients. In this study, each former vocational rehabilitation client received a score based on the amount of congruence between (1) suggested occupational

FIGURE 13.3
Comparison of a Strong Positive Correlation with a Weak Negative Correlation on a Scatterplot

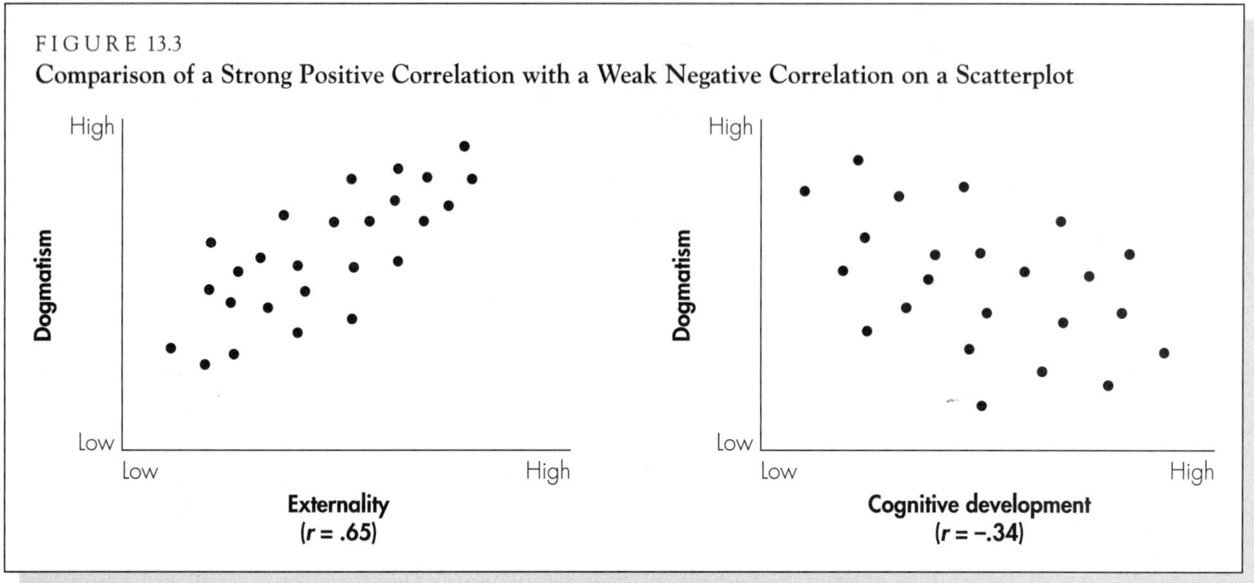

choice, as measured by a career inventory taken one year earlier; and (2) the eventual job attained. The more congruence, the higher the score; the less congruence, the lower the score. Thus, if my vocational testing a year ago suggested that I might fit well in the counseling field, and if I subsequently became a counselor, I would receive a high congruency score. If, on the other hand, my testing suggested I would find a better fit in jobs other than counseling, I would obtain a low congruency score if I ended up in the counseling profession. The congruency scores of all of the former clients were then correlated with current job satisfaction as measured by a job satisfaction scale administered to each former client. The eventual correlation between job fit and job satisfaction was shown to be +.39.

Although this study showed only a low-moderate correlation, the research suggests that the use of a personality instrument to assist individuals in eventual job placement could be helpful in predicting job satisfaction. However, a study such as this does not show causation between job fit and job satisfaction, as many alternative explanations for job satisfaction can be hypothesized. For instance, it could be that individuals who have higher congruency scores are more mentally stable, or brighter, or more skilled, thus leading to better job satisfaction. Unless further research in this area is explored, all or none of these possible explanations may be operating, because correlational research does not answer the question, "Why?" Although we cannot assume a causal relationship, we can assertively say that there are factors that lend themselves to satisfaction at work if one's personality fits the job obtained.

SURVEY RESEARCH In survey research, a questionnaire is developed or an interview designed with the purpose of gathering specific information from a target population. Surveys can gain interesting information about the values, behaviors, demographics, and opinions of a specific population and are used in a myriad of business, educational, and social science arenas. In describing the data obtained, survey research uses basic descriptive statistics such as frequency distributions, percentages, measures of central tendency, and measures of variability (see Chapter 12). Often, charts and graphs are used to illustrate some of the data obtained.

There are a number of steps that are usually followed when conducting survey research. For instance, McMillan and Schumacher (2001) suggest that researchers should (1) define their purpose and objectives, (2) determine the resources needed and the target population to be surveyed, (3) choose techniques for gathering data and give clear instructions to individuals completing the surveys, (4) decide on the sample of the target population, (5) develop a cover letter, (6) conduct a pilot test to uncover possible problems with the survey, (7) complete a follow-up of nonrespondents, and (8) account for reasons nonrespondents didn't reply to the survey and assess if they are different from those who did reply.

Although survey research can be quite interesting, it is not able to tell us the underlying reasons why we found what we found and often leaves gaps in our knowledge. For instance, in our research on counselors' attendance in their own therapy, we discovered that close to 80% of counselors had attended their own therapy. However, this information does not tell us the underlying reasons why they attended counseling. Do counselors attend therapy because they are more open to the experience, healthier, more dysfunctional? Therefore, survey research can be quite limiting although sometimes quite intriguing.

EX POST FACTO (CAUSAL-COMPARATIVE) RESEARCH Whereas experimental research involves random assignment and the manipulation of variables, *ex post facto* research, sometimes called causal-comparative research, examines the relationship of already existing intact groups. Ex post facto research is used when it is either impractical or impossible to manipulate the independent variable, such as when one might be examining the differential effects of gender, personality type, race, or when random assignment cannot be used (Heppner et al., 1992).

For instance, let's say we wanted to compare the scores on the National Counselor Certification (NCC) exam of students who graduated from CACREP-accredited counseling programs to those who graduated from non–CACREP-accredited programs. Obviously, we could not randomly assign students to graduate programs, and we cannot manipulate the independent variable, the type of graduate program attended. However, it would be a relatively easy process to obtain data from students who already had attended these schools and who subsequently took the NCC exam. It would then be a simple process to run a statistical analysis of which students scored higher on the exam.

Although ex post facto research is often more convenient than some experimental designs, there are inherent problems with this kind of research. For instance, because there is no manipulation of the independent variable and no random assignment, we cannot be sure if the independent variable is indeed responsible for the results. In our example above, if students from CACREP-accredited programs did do better, perhaps it's not the program that makes the difference on the NCC exam but the fact that CACREP-approved programs attract students who tend to do better in graduate programs. Or perhaps because students from CACREP-approved programs can take the exam sooner than those from non–CACREP-approved schools, the test material is fresher. Or perhaps faculty in CACREP-approved programs teach more to the test than do faculty in non-approved programs. And so forth.

In an effort to control for such rival hypotheses as those identified above, researchers will sometimes attempt to match treatment groups on variables that may be confounding the results. For instance, in our fictitious study above, students can be matched on

GRE scores and graduate GPA to assure that ability in both groups is similar. Also, students can be selected in a manner that assures that both groups of students have taken the exam within the same amount of time since graduation. On the other hand, it might be more difficult to control whether or not faculty are teaching to the test. Therefore, this rival hypothesis, along with any others that might be identified, should be noted as possible confounding variables in any discussion of results. In addition, other rival hypotheses, not identified by the researcher, could be affecting the results. Can you think of any other rival hypotheses in the study above? This is why researchers need to be very tentative when stating any conclusions in ex post facto research.

Qualitative Research Methods

Naturalistic-phenomenological philosophy is the basis of qualitative research (McMillan & Schumacher, 2001). This approach assumes that there are many ways in which reality can be interpreted and experienced by individuals. Rather than using the scientific method, as in quantitative research, qualitative research relies on the researcher to carefully observe and describe a phenomenon and to interpret the phenomenon within a social context. For these reasons, qualitative research allows one to examine phenomena that quantitative research cannot explore, like our understanding of abstract concepts such as empathy and the meaning we ascribe to God (Hanna & Shank, 1995). As a result, the findings of qualitative research offer us rich ways to apply research paradigms to specific clinical settings (see Collins, Collins, Botyrius-Maier, & MacIntosh-Daeschler, 1994; Froehle & Rominger, 1993; Segal-Andrews, 1994). Also, qualitative research can add important missing pieces of information that cannot be discovered through the reductionistic methods of quantitative research (Schofield & Anderson, 1984).

As opposed to the deductive, reductionistic methods of quantitative research, which identify variables, isolate them, and measure them, qualitative research relies on the case study method, a way of focusing and deeply probing and analyzing an event or phenomenon. This approach relies on a number of methods, often used simultaneously, in an effort to uncover themes and meaning about the phenomenon being studied.

Qualitative research generally uses research questions as opposed to hypotheses in providing direction for the research. Although qualitative research can take many forms, two types are ethnographic research and historical research.

Ethnographic Research

Ethnography refers to the description (*graphy*) of human cultures (*ethno*). Sometimes called cultural anthropology, ethnographic research was made popular by Margaret Mead, who studied aboriginal youth in Samoa by immersing herself with the people and their culture as she attempted to understand their lifestyle (Mead, 1961). Ethnographic research assumes that phenomena or events can best be understood within their cultural context. Take an event out of its context, and its meaning is likely to be interpreted from the context of the researcher as opposed to its original social context. Reality, therefore, is a social construction that, in order to be understood, needs to be examined within the phenomenological perspective from which it occurred. Thus ethnographers seek to understand events by understanding the meanings that people place on them from within their natural context.

The first step in conducting ethnographic research is to identify the group to be studied and to identify a general problem to be researched. Conducting a literature review can help the researcher gain a better understanding of the culture or group being studied

BOX 13.4

Disruptive Observation of a Third-Grade Class

While working in New Hampshire, I was once asked to "debrief" a third-grade class that had just finished a trial period in which a young boy, who was paraplegic and severely mentally retarded, was mainstreamed into their classroom. During this trial period, these third graders had a stream of observers from a local university come into their classroom to assess their progress. Because this was not participant observation, the observers would sit in the back of the classroom and take notes about the interactions between the students. This information was supposed to be used at a later date to decide whether it was beneficial to all involved to have the disabled student mainstreamed.

When I met with the students, they clearly had adapted well to this young boy who was disabled. Although the students seemed to have difficulty forming deep relationships with him, his presence seemed in no way to detract from their studies or from their other relationships in the classroom. However, almost without exception, the students noted that the constant stream of observers interfering with their daily schedule was quite annoying. Perhaps if participant observation was employed, where an observer interacted and was seen as part of the classroom, the students would have responded differently.

and assists the researcher in defining the purpose of the research and in developing hypotheses or research questions. Next, the researcher decides on what method he or she wishes to use to immerse him- or herself in the culture of the population. Prior to entering the culture, the researcher should develop a plan for implementing his or her data collection methods. Three common methods used in ethnographic research include observation, ethnographic interviews, and collection of documents and artifacts.

OBSERVATION Ethnographers will often observe a situation or phenomenon and describe, using extensive notes, what they view. Although sometimes qualitative researchers may take a nonengaged role when observing, more often they become participant observers. In this kind of observation the researcher immerses him- or herself with the group and may even live with the group (Burgess, 1995; Cole, 1975). However, it is important not interfere with the natural process of the group and to listen to and take scrupulous notes so that the observer understands the unique perspective of the group. It is only in this manner that the observer can obtain a rich appreciation for the ways in which the group constructs reality. It is particularly important that the observer record what role and what effect observing the group may have had on the group (see Box 13.4).

ETHNOGRAPHIC INTERVIEWS Ethnographic interviews are a second popular qualitative method of collecting data from a culture or group. Such interviews involve open-ended questions in an effort to understand how the interviewees construct meaning. Interviews may be informal; guided, in which questions are outlined in advance; or standardized, in which the exact questions are determined prior to the interview but the responses remain open-ended. Counselors are adept at doing ethnographic interviews because of their training in open-ended questioning. As with participant observation, it is important that the interviewer take scrupulous notes or record the interviews in order to obtain verbatim accounts of the conversation.

DOCUMENTS AND ARTIFACT COLLECTION Artifacts are the symbols of a culture or group and can help the ethnographer understand the beliefs, values, and behaviors of the group.

In this process it is helpful if the researcher knows how the artifact was produced, where the artifact came from, the age of the artifact, how the artifact was used, and who used it. Interpretation of the meaning of artifacts should be corroborated from observations and through interviews.

McMillan and Schumacher (2001) suggest the following major categories of artifacts: personal documents, such as diaries, personal letters, and anecdotal records; official documents, such as internal and external papers, records and personnel files, and statistical data; and objects that hold symbolic meaning of the culture (e.g., Native American headdresses).

Historical Research

The purpose of historical research is to describe and analyze conditions and events from the past in an effort to answer a research question. Historical research relies on the systematic collection of information in an effort to examine and understand past events from a contextual framework. When doing historical research, the researcher generally has a viewpoint in mind and needs to go to the literature to support this viewpoint. Then, the researcher will begin to collect data to show that his or her viewpoint has validity. At any point in this process, the researcher's point of view might change as he or she is influenced by the literature or by the sources of data obtained.

In collecting data for historical research, a number of sources can be used. Whenever possible, researchers attempt to use primary sources, or the original record, as opposed to secondary sources, which are documents or verbal information from sources that did not actually experience the event. Examples of primary sources include (Gay & Airasian, 2000; McMillan & Schumacher, 2001):

1. *Oral histories*. Oral histories are gathered when researchers directly interview an individual who had participated in or observed the event in question.
2. *Documents*. Documents are records of events that are generally housed in libraries or archival centers. Some examples include letters, diaries, autobiographies, journals and magazines, films, recordings, paintings, and institutional records.
3. *Relics*. Relics are any of a variety of objects that can provide evidence about the past event in question. Such things as books, maps, buildings, artifacts, and other objects are some examples of relics.

Statistics and Data Analysis in Quantitative and Qualitative Research

Although a text such as this cannot go into detail about the various kinds of statistical analyses that can be used, suffice it to say that the proper use of statistical procedures is critical to the eventual interpretation of research studies (Fong & Malone, 1994; Thompson, 1995a). Whereas quantitative research uses statistics to analyze results, qualitative research uses a process called inductive analysis.

Quantitative Research

Generally, the use of statistics in quantitative research can be separated into two broad categories: *descriptive statistics* which are used to summarize and describe results; and *inferential statistics* which are mathematical procedures used to make inferences about a larger population from the sample you are studying.

Largely discussed in Chapter 12, descriptive statistics includes: measures of central tendency, such as the mean, median, and mode; measures of variability, such as the range, variance, and standard deviation; derived scores, such as percentiles, stanines, T-scores, and DIQ scores; and measures of relationship, as in the correlation coefficient. Descriptive statistics are often used with survey research.

Inferential statistics are used to examine whether the differences or strengths of the relationships between treatment groups are likely to be found by chance alone. Some of the more common types of analyses include the *t test*, to measure differences between two means; the *analysis of variance(ANOVA)*, to measure differences between two means or among more than two means; *factorial analysis of variance*, used when there is more than one independent variable and the researcher is interested in examining each independent variable and how they might interact; *multivariate analysis of variance (MANOVA)*, used when two or more dependent variables are being examined; *significance of coefficient of correlation*, used when examining whether the relationship between two variables is statistically significant; and *chi square*, which is used to compare whether the observed frequency of scores differs from the expected frequency of scores. Generally, experimental research and ex post facto research use inferential statistics that measure differences between means, while correlational research examines the degree of relationship between variables.

Qualitative Research

Qualitative data collection relies on a process called inductive analysis, which means that themes and categories emerge from data (McMillan & Schumacher, 2001). Thus, the researcher who is examining the data collected through the various methods mentioned looks through the information for themes, ways of categorizing information, and ways of selecting important pieces of information. As this process continues, the researcher begins to see particular points emerge.

Generally, qualitative researchers classify their data by a process called coding. This process breaks down large amounts of data into smaller parts that seem to hold some meaning to the research question. For instance, if I were involved in a study to determine what problems at-risk high school students might have in a specific school, I might observe the youths; interview them; interview their teachers, school counselors, parents, and peers; and collect school records. I would then go through all of these pieces of information and identify and code themes that seem to emerge from the data. For instance, Box 13.5 shows pieces of interviews with (1) an at-risk student ("John"), (2) one of his teachers, and (3) his school counselor, as well as presents (4) a summary of his student records. Each of these four segments of information is broken down into themes. Similar themes are coded with the same superscript number.

My next step would be to place all similar themes (same coded numbers) together in a category that has a logical name (see Box 13.6). You can see in Box 13.6 that a number of categories have emerged from this process. Then I would continue this same process with all of the identified at-risk students. Finally, I would look at all the categories that emerged from all of the students and begin to look for similarities among students. It may be that some of the categories will merge with one another while other, new themes might emerge. For instance, if we consistently see youths-at-risk using humor to avoid issues (item 9 in Box 13.6), it may end up as a subtopic of defensiveness (item 13 in Box 13.6). Eventually, I would come up with a list of categories that represented the most relevant issues for at-risk students.

BOX 13.5

Emerging Themes through Data Analysis for an At-Risk Student

Segment of Verbatim Interview with John

I don't like school.[1] It's a waste of time.[1] The only thing it's good for is hanging out with my friends.[2] My dad never went to school, so why should I?[3] You don't learn nothing here anyway, nothing that's good for me. I don't care how I do on tests,[4] I just want to get some money[5] so I could buy some neat clothes. Then I could show off[6] to my friends and they would think I'm cool.[2] School sucks, I cut a lot[7]—I wish I could get out of here and get a job and make some money.[5] Can you get me a job?

Segment of Verbatim Interview with One of John's Teachers

John seems to be thinking of other things while in school and not interested in what's going on in class.[1] He is always talking to his friends in class, and seems to be in a clique,[2] that is, when he comes to school. He seems absent much.[7] He rarely does well on tests,[4] but I have noticed that he seems to do a little better if I let his mom know[8] that a test is coming up and when he's attending school consistently.[7] He always dresses very well and seems a little bit like a show-off.[6] He has a funny sense of humor,[9] although I would never laugh at his jokes in class because I don't want to reinforce his joking around. I think his scores in school are not reflective of how well he can do.[10] It's a shame. It's a wasted life.[11] I'm kind of sick of seeing this same pattern over and over again.

Documents and Records

a. Achievement test scores are low.[4]
b. Aptitude test scores are average.[10]
c. Records show that student seems to miss a lot of classes.[7]
d. An autobiography that he wrote for his counseling group seemed to show a number of painful events,[12] like his parents' divorce, that he may be covering up.[13]
e. He's gotten a number of detentions for "cutting up" in class.[9]
f. Poems he wrote in English were funny,[9], yet morbid about his future.[11]
g. A sentence-completion test he took with his counselor seemed to show an obsession with money.[5]

Segment of Verbatim Interview with John's School Counselor

John was in a group of students with high absenteeism, low grades, and an apathetic attitude toward school.[7,4,1] He was the jokester in the group.[9] He always had excuses for why he was absent.[6,13] On the one hand, he used his father as a role model for not having to finish school;[3] however, it seemed that his father is absent from his life and that he's hurt over this.[12] In general, I think his jokes are a way for him to gain attention[6,9] and cover up some inner hurts.[12] He's likable in many ways, but he's hard to reach.[13] He seems to have a wall around him.[13] His mother seems a source of comfort,[8] but his peer group is increasingly having more influence on him.[2] I'm concerned about his future.[11]

Although ethnographic research relies on coding and theme identification, as noted above, this can also be an important process in historical research when comparing different types of documents, relics, and possible interviews. In either case, this process is laborious, yet fruitful in finding out significant patterns and themes in qualitative research.

Issues of Quality in Research Studies

McMillan and Schumacher (2001) refer to validity as "the truth or falsity of propositions generated by research" (p. 167). Thus the degree to which our research design can come close to representing objective reality is a mark that a study has good validity. Two types of validity are *internal validity* and *external validity*.

BOX 13.6

Emerging Themes from Data Analysis

1. *Dislike of school:*	I don't like school. It's a waste of time. . . . Not interested in what's going on in class. . . . In a group of students with . . . an apathetic attitude toward school.
2. *Peer relationships:*	The only thing school is good for is hanging out with my friends . . . [If I wore neat clothes, my friends would think] I'm cool. . . . He is always talking to his friends in class . . . seems to be in a clique. . . . His peer group is increasingly having more influence on him.
3. *Dad as role model:*	My dad never went to school, so why should I? . . . Uses his father as a role model for not having to finish school. . . . Father is absent from his life.
4. *Test performance:*	I don't care how I do on tests. . . . He rarely does well on tests. . . . Achievement tests scores are low. . . . In a group of students with . . . low grades.
5. *Importance of money:*	I just want to get some money. . . . I wish I could get out of here and get a job and make some money. . . . An obsession with money.
6. *Narcissism:*	[If I had the neat clothes], I could show off. . . . He always dresses very well and seems a little bit like a show-off. . . . Jokes are a way for him to gain attention.
7. *Absenteeism:*	School sucks, I cut a lot. . . . He seems absent much. . . . [Does] better . . . when he's attending school consistently. . . . Records show that student seems to miss a lot of classes. . . . In a group of students with high absenteeism. . . . He always had excuses for why he was absent.
8. *Relationship with mom:*	. . . [Does] better [if his mom knows] a test is coming up. . . . His mother seems a source of comfort.
9. *Use of humor:*	He has a funny sense of humor. [He cuts up] in class. Poems he wrote in English were funny. . . . His jokes are a way for him to gain attention.
10. *Underachiever:*	His scores in school are not reflective of how well he can do. . . . Aptitude scores are average. [Achievement scores and grades are low.]
11. *Sense of future:*	It's a shame. It's a wasted life. . . . Poems . . . were funny yet morbid about his future. . . . I'm concerned about his future.
12. *Emotional pain:*	An autobiography . . . seemed to show a number of painful events. . . . His father is absent from his life and [he] hurts over this. . . . Jokes . . . cover up some inner hurts.
13. *Defensiveness:*	An autobiography . . . seemed to show a number of painful events. . . . He may be covering up. . . . He always had excuses for why he was absent. . . . He's hard to reach. He seems to have a wall around him.

Internal Validity

Internal validity represents the degree to which extraneous variables have been accounted for when drawing your conclusions and has already been briefly discussed (see Box 13.3). Studies that are more tightly controlled will have fewer threats to internal validity and therefore fewer rival hypotheses that may be an explanation for the data found. Clearly, quantitative studies are generally more tightly controlled than qualitative studies.

External Validity

External validity, on the other hand, refers to the generalizability of the results, or whether or not conclusions of the research can be applied to the larger population from the sample being investigated. The tight controls, small populations sometimes used, and reductionistic methods of quantitative research sometimes make it difficult to generalize to the larger population. In qualitative research, external validity has to do with the ability of the researcher to describe the research in ways that will be helpful to other researchers working with other populations. If reliable methods of obtaining information are used, and if the information is useful and based on sound theoretical underpinnings, then the implications of the research will be useful to other researchers. Put more simply, can we not learn something about our culture from studying the aborigines in Samoa?

Is Validity Valid in Qualitative Research?

Relative to qualitative research, some suggest that rather than using the term *validity*, qualitative research should be examining the credibility and trustworthiness of the research (see Lancy, 1993). The attempt to describe events in a reliable and valid (or credible and trustworthy) manner is difficult, as, by their very nature, events can hold multiple meanings depending on the frame of reference from which one is examining (see Box 13.7).

McMillan and Schumacher (1993) suggest that the ability to provide reliable and valid research in qualitative research is based on how well the researcher is able to record

BOX 13.7

Revisionist History and Multiple Perspective Taking

How is it that two intellectuals can have different takes on the same event? Lancy (1993) suggests that neither may be wrong, but that multiple perspectives on the same event may all be correct. For example, could it be that Thomas Jefferson could have owned slaves and have been both a racist *and* a champion for the rights of enslaved Africans?

Look at how Lancy (1993) suggests that different perspectives can both hold truth in justifying the different conclusions of two well-known historians concerning the motivations of turn-of-the-last-century reformers such as Jane Addams:

> *Who is right? That is a difficult question. Both accounts have elements of the "truth." Cremin is undoubtedly right in characterizing many progressive educators as human and compassionate reformers. On the other hand, Karier is probably correct in arguing that the effect of many policies they supported was to exacerbate existing inequalities, and preserve the advantages enjoyed by corporate elites then assuming control of American society. In other words, it is possible for both interpretations to be compatible, provided they do not directly contradict one another in interpreting a specific event or person's role in history. Remember, that historical explanations [and inferences from ethnography] need only be sufficient, not conclusive.* (p. 258)

information accurately and to use multiple methods in recording. For instance, they suggest taking verbatim accounts when interviewing people, using precise and concrete descriptions, using multiple researchers to get many perspectives and to look for similar themes among researchers, mechanically recording data, using primary data whenever possible, asking participants to make their own records and to match the researcher's understanding of events with participants' understanding of events, checking meanings with participants, and reviewing any data that seem atypical or discrepant.

After data have been obtained and authenticated, the researcher must go through a rigorous process of reviewing the data, synthesizing results, and drawing conclusions and generalizations. The researcher's original research question(s) may have been changed by this point as he or she has gone through the involved process of reviewing the literature and analyzing the sources. The final results of the research involve a logical analysis of the materials obtained as opposed to a statistical analysis as we find in quantitative research. Finally, the researcher needs to be careful not to get caught up in his or her point of view and should be open to offering opinions that both support and contradict the ultimate findings. The standards of excellence applied to qualitative research are an indication of the reliability and validity of the research (Best & Kahn, 1997; McMillan & Schumacher, 1993). See Box 13.8 to consider what methods a friend of mine used to establish standards of excellence in conducting historical research. Were his conclusions justified?

BOX 13.8

Historical Research: A New Temple for Corinth

My project began because I thought it might be interesting to take a new look at the letters of St. Paul. They have been extremely influential in the formation of Christianity, and yet they are rarely examined as artifacts of a world that existed 2000 years ago, a world very different from our own. Today, Christians look at them as theological treatises, but Paul wrote them as letters of guidance to specific Christian communities with specific challenges and problems.

I took one letter (1 Corinthians) and one image he uses (the community as a temple) in one passage (chapter 3, verses 16–17), and tried to see if traditional interpretations could be challenged by looking more closely at the actual historical and cultural context of the Corinthian people to whom Paul wrote. Traditionally, interpreters have assumed that Paul was spurning the Jewish temple in Jerusalem, the temple of his youth (since he was Jewish), and telling the Corinthian Christians that they were themselves *the* new temple of God. I knew this to be historically uncertain, since there was no external evidence that Paul ever turned his back on the Jerusalem temple. I wondered how else this text might be interpreted.

I began by studying the conventional ways that people interpret the target passage, and discovered some basic flaws in their views. To do this, I studied other primary texts to discover what functions temples played in cities like Corinth. Some of these texts were inscriptions found at archaeological sties, including Corinth. Others were literary texts by Roman authors. In addition, I studied the archaeological remains of the temples of Corinth, visiting the site three times, talking with archaeologists and biblical scholars who were also studying Corinth.

What I found was that it is likely Paul was *not* referring to the Jerusalem temple, since his audience was gentiles and there were plenty of other temples to which Paul could refer. And, I discovered that Paul was probably using the temple/community image to help the Corinthians understand who they were as a community, as opposed to attempting to get them to turn away from Jerusalem.

Past interpretations have unfortunately been used to support anti-Semitic attitudes, as it has been interpreted by some that Paul rejected his Jewish faith in favor of a new Christian one. This new, and I believe more historically accurate, interpretation supports the notion that Paul never stopped being a Jew; he just changed from being a traditional observer of Judaism to a Jew who believed that Jesus was the Messiah and was expressive of the fullness of Judaism. This sort of Jewishness was not rejected by other Jews until about 30 years after Paul died (see Lanci, 1997; 1999).

Reading and Writing Research

It is likely that some of you will be actively involved in doing research while all of you will be reading research. Certainly, if you are to remain professionally astute, it is your obligation to read the professional journals that offer the most current research in our field.

Reading quantitative and qualitative research follows a logical course that reflects what the researcher has done in conducting his or her study. Although qualitative and quantitative research studies approach the attainment of knowledge differently, the manner in which the results of the research is presented is similar. Here are some of the major headings that are often used when writing research manuscripts:

Abstract. A short summary of the article that is generally less than 100 words.

Review of the literature. This section provides a review of past research that has been completed in the area being studied and elaborates on the statement of the problem. The review can be as short as one page or as long as ten and should justify the research hypothesis or research question.

Research hypothesis or research question. Generally the hypothesis or research question can be found at the end of the review of the literature. The hypothesis or research question defines the variables, identifies the relationships among the variables, and defines the population to be studied.

Methodology. The methodology or procedures section is a description of how the study was conducted and includes a description of the participants; statements about instruments used, including their reliability and validity; the sources of data; procedures employed in conducting the study; and procedures used in collecting the data. An individual who reads this section should be able to replicate the study being presented.

Results. This section of the manuscript describes the types of statistical analysis or data synthesis that were used as well as an objective description in writing or through the use of charts, tables, and figures of results found.

Discussion, implications, and conclusions. This section describes how the results are related to the research question or hypothesis. Results should be related to past research, and possible reasons why the results were found should be discussed. Any methodological problems should be described in this section. Although authors have some liberty in this section to speculate about the results, they should do so tentatively. Often the author concludes this section with how the research might be applied to future studies.

References. Almost all educational and psychological publications require that manuscripts use the style of the *Publication Manual of the American Psychological Association* (APA, 2001e). If you learned referencing using a different style, this approach will initially seem foreign to you. However, generally the *Publication Manual* encourages simplicity in its approach, and you will quickly become used to its streamlined manner of citing and referencing. Without going into detail on how to reference, throughout all manuscripts, citations should be listed whenever statements need to be supported by past research, and all citations are referenced at the end of the manuscript.

Program Evaluation

The Purpose of Evaluation

Although many research concepts are used in evaluation, the purpose of evaluation is generally different from the purposes of research (Leary, 2001). Whereas research tends to examine new paradigms to expand understanding and knowledge and how such knowledge can be applied to practice, program evaluation has to do with whether or not a program has achieved its goals and objectives and has been shown to have worth and value (Halley, Kopp, & Austin, 1998; Leary, 2001; Sanders, 1994).

As a counselor you will be asked to evaluate the progress of your clients and the effectiveness of programs you will conduct. For instance, you may be asked to show evidence that clients have improved through counseling or demonstrate the efficacy of a self-esteem program, a classroom guidance program, a career development program, a parenting effectiveness program, or simply a program that explains the services of your agency to your clients. Program evaluation also has an important place in examining the effectiveness of job-related behaviors at your school or agency. The use of evaluation techniques is also an important step in the accountability process and assures the public and funding agencies that an agency is performing essential and effective services for its clients (Ohlsen, 1983). In order to improve the program while it is occurring or to improve it for the next time that it might be given, formative and summative evaluation measures should be undertaken.

Formative and Summative Evaluation

Sometimes called process and outcome evaluation, formative and summative evaluation have different purposes. Formative evaluation is concerned with the assessment of a program during its implementation in order to gain feedback about its effectiveness and to allow for change in the program as needed. On the other hand, summative evaluation involves assessment of the total training program in order to decide whether or not the program should be offered again. For instance, suppose I implement a new program that examines the effects of self-esteem training on job attainment. In an effort to better meet the needs of those involved in the program, I want to assess the effectiveness of the program while it is occurring. In addition, to determine if the program is worthwhile for future potential consumers, I want to evaluate the total effectiveness of the program when it is completed.

Formative Evaluation

When presenting a program, workshop, or conference, it is important to assess effectiveness through an ongoing evaluation process. Formative evaluation offers immediate feedback to staff who are running a program. Such evaluation is often informal and can be ongoing throughout the length of the program.

There are a number of ways to conduct a formative evaluation. Probably the most basic way is to ask for verbal feedback from your audience. In this case, the presenter needs to be open to feedback, especially any negative criticism, and be willing to change his or her program midway. A less threatening and sometimes more revealing method of

BOX 13.9

Outcome Evaluation of a Drug and Alcohol Training Program: Program Evaluation (N = 202)

Describe your reaction to each of the following statements in terms of this scale:

1. Never
2. Seldom
3. Sometimes
4. Usually
5. Always
6. Not applicable

Program Presenters:	Mean	Standard Deviation
1. were well prepared.	4.7	.3
2. delivered material in a clear, organized manner.	4.7	.2
3. stimulated intellectual curiosity.	3.9	.5
4. showed respect for questions and opinions of participants.	4.6	.3
5. allowed for relevant discussion when appropriate.	4.7	.3
6. were concerned that participants understood them.	4.6	.2
7. were accessible for individual and group concerns.	4.6	.1
8. offered information applicable to one's field.	4.0	.5
9. presented in a comfortable, conducive environment.	4.4	.2
10. provided a beneficial, educational experience.	4.1	.6

formative evaluation is to have participants write down reactions to the program while it is occurring. Doing this anonymously allows for participants to express their feelings openly, without fear of repercussion. Along these same lines, participants can be asked to complete rating forms during the program in order to offer ongoing feedback to the program facilitator. Data from rating forms can be easily collated and offer a quick and yet somewhat structured mechanism to obtain immediate feedback. The disadvantage to rating forms is that they do not allow for feedback outside of the questions being asked. Of course, rating forms could be created that include room for written feedback.

Summative Evaluation

As opposed to formative evaluation, summative evaluation is used to show the efficacy of a program in order to determine if it should be used for future clients and is a way of showing accountability to funding agencies and agency administrators. Summative evaluation is generally an involved and formal process that often assesses a large segment of the people who have been involved with the program. For instance, a few years back I received a federally funded grant to administer a program at a local school that would identify, assess, and intervene with students at risk for drug and alcohol abuse. In measuring its effectiveness, a couple of measures were employed. First, an objective test to measure knowledge obtained by the participants was developed and administered. Second, rating scales were used at the conclusion of the program to assess total program effectiveness (see Box 13.9).

In some cases, you might expect training programs to have some far-reaching effects, and this too can be an aspect of summative evaluation. For instance, in the drug and alcohol program just discussed, some of the long-term outcome measures that we hoped to see from this training included the reduction in alcohol and drug use by students, a decrease in the dropout rate (as chemical abuse has been shown to be related to dropout

TABLE 13.3

Differences in Formative and Summative Evaluation

	FORMATIVE EVALUATION	SUMMATIVE EVALUATION
Purpose	To improve program	To certify program utility
Audience	Program administrators and staff	Potential consumer or funding agency
Who should do it	Internal evaluator	External evaluator [sometimes internal evaluator]
Major characteristic	Timely	Convincing
Measures	Often informal	Valid/reliable
Frequency of data collection	Frequent	Limited
Sample size	Often small	Usually large
Questions asked	What is working? What needs to be improved? How can it be improved?	What results occur? With whom? Under what conditions? At what training? At what cost?
Design constraints	What information is needed? When?	What claims do you wish to make?

SOURCE: *Educational evaluation: Alternative approaches and practical guidelines* by Blaine R. Worthen and James R. Sanders, p. 36.

rate), and an increase in the age of first use of drugs or alcohol. To obtain information like this would be a major undertaking and would involve large-scale assessment of students. Though not an easy project, these behaviors are measurable and could be an indication that our program was effective.

Summative evaluation will sometimes involve the use of specific research designs. For instance, in employing survey research, a graduate counseling program might desire to survey all students who have graduated within the past five years, as well as their employers, in an effort to assess how effective they believe the counseling program was in preparing them to become counselors. Even experimental designs can be employed in summative research. For instance, one might develop a true experimental design to compare the effectiveness of two videotape programs that focus on the attainment of empathy skills for counselor trainees. Forty students could be randomly assigned to each videotape program. Each student could then view the videotape and then be asked to respond empathically to a role-played client. A statistical comparison on the empathy scores can then be completed using a T-test. Whatever technique is used in summative evaluation, you can see that it is often more involved than formative evaluation.

Although both formative and summative evaluation procedures share some similar goals and purposes, there are major differences, as noted above. Summarizing these differences, Worthen and Sanders (1987) offer the chart shown in Table 13.3.

Summarizing Quantitative Research, Qualitative Research, and Evaluation

Quantitative research, qualitative research, and evaluation all offer us different ways of expanding our knowledge base and help us understand what works and what needs to be improved. Table 13.4 summarizes some of the major points of quantitative and qualitative research and of evaluation.

TABLE 13.4

A Comparison of Different Types of Research and Evaluation

	QUANTITATIVE				QUALITATIVE		EVALUATION
	Experimental: True, Quasi, Single-subject	*Non-experimental: Expo Facto*	*Non-experimental: Correlational*	*Non-experimental: Survey*	*Ethnographic*	*Historical*	*Evaluation*
Focus	Cause and effect	Cause and effect	Corelation-ships among variables	Survey a population	Behavior of selected population	Conditions and events of past	Assess value of a product or program
Purpose	Show that X causes Y	Suggest that X causes Y	Describes relationship; predict one variable from another	To assess opinions, beliefs, and attitudes	Phenomeno-logical approach to understanding groups and cultures	To describe and analyze conditions and events from the past.	Determine relative value or merit
Hypotheses and questions	Hypotheses	Hypotheses	Hypotheses and questions	Hypotheses and questions; usually questions	Hypotheses and questions; usually questions	Hypotheses and questions; usually questions	Specific questions concerning viability of program
Population	Individuals or groups chosen for study	Groups in study	Groups being correlated	Population being surveyed	Group/culture identified for study	Event or group from past	Group obtaining services (e.g., workshop, guidance group)
Design	Use group or single subject; apply and manipulate treatment (X), test for outcome (Y)	Mostly group; test for Y; examine X (X is not manipulated)	Variables defined then correlated	Sampling population and admin-istering question-naires and instruments	Researcher decides how to optimize immersion in group	Researcher decides how to optimize gaining information from data sources	Informal, descriptive, sometimes true experimental quasi-experimental or ex post facto

Multicultural Issues

Bias in Research and Evaluation

> *If the computer package did not ask you your values prior to its analysis, it could not have considered your value system in calculating p's [probabilities], and so p's cannot be blithely used to infer the value of research results. Like it or not, empirical science is inescapably a subjective business.* (Thompson, 1993, p. 365)

Researchers choose to study specific issues because of their preferences and biases (Parham, 1993). They design studies based on their values. They include or exclude certain participants based on their biases, and they make conclusions that are at least somewhat a function of the prism through which they view the world. There is little getting

BOX 13.10

Female Genital Mutilation from a Qualitative Research Perspective

Recently there has been an uproar in many Western countries concerning the act of female genital mutilation, which occurs in some parts of Africa, the Middle East, and parts of Indonesia and Malaysia (Council on Scientific Affairs, 1995). The practice generally includes anything from a partial clitoridectomy to excision of the clitoris, the inner labia, and the skin of the outer labia. In some cases the remaining skin is stitched, leaving a tiny opening which makes it difficult to urinate, leaves the women prone to infections, and acts as a kind of chastity belt (Lightfoot-Klein, 1993; Walker, 1993). The procedure, which typically occurs at around age 7, symbolizes the induction into adulthood, reduces or eliminates sexual pleasure, and often results in painful sexual intercourse (Council on Scientific Affairs, 1995). With up to 200,000 American immigrants and 100 million women around the world having undergone this procedure, it is anything but rare (Lightfoot-Klein, 1993). To accommodate this cultural tradition, some hospitals in this country have allowed a small cut in the labia as a symbolic way of preserving this tradition. In helping us understand this ritual, Lightfoot-Klein (1993) notes:

> *. . . even educated women within the cultures that perform them [clitoridectomy's] may be among their staunchest advocates. This phenomenon becomes more comprehensible once it is understood that uncircumcised women have been historically associated with slaves, prostitutes and other non-male-protected women of low caste . . .* (p. 191)

If one were to examine this procedure from our Western perspective, undoubtedly we would find this procedure distasteful, sexist, without purpose, oppressive, and abusive. The qualitative researcher, however, would ask the following questions:

1. When does the event occur in the culture?
2. Who is involved in doing this event?
3. What does this event symbolize for the culture?
4. How do the participants in this event view it?
5. Are the meanings to the event viewed in the same manner by all of the participants?

around the fact that all research, to some degree, is biased as a result of the preferences of the researcher. This is especially true when doing cross-cultural research (Atkinson, 1993; Mio & Iwamasa, 1993; Parham, 1993).

Although quantitative research has brought us many advances, its so-called "purity" must be called into question when we realize that every decision a quantitative researcher makes in designing, implementing, analyzing, and interpreting a study is a reflection of his or her personal biases. The subject matter that is chosen, the population to be examined, the kinds of designs that are chosen, even the statistical analysis used can lead a researcher to certain conclusions. On the other hand, qualitative research offers us a unique opportunity to conduct research that focuses on the worldview of the participants. Such research seems like a natural fit for counselors who are used to taking on a phenomenological perspective when working with clients (Merchant & Dupuy, 1996).

Qualitative research allows us to peek inside the world of other groups and cultures in an effort to understand how individuals within that group or culture understand reality. For instance, examine Box 13.10, which discusses female genital mutilation, and see if you could approach this subject in an unbiased fashion. Then consider how a qualitative researcher might approach this topic.

Reading a qualitative researcher's study on female genital mutilation would offer a counselor a broad understanding of the issues involved; help the counselor have empathy for women who have undergone such a procedure; and, when counseling a woman who has undergone this procedure, assist the counselor in avoiding counseling her from a

Western perspective. Although few if any of us would ever approve of such a procedure, qualitative research can help us understand the circumstances around the procedure and how it has meaning to the individuals within the culture.

Although qualitative research can offer a unique perspective on events, let us not be misled into thinking that such research does not have its share of biases. It is the unique researcher who can enter a group or culture and truly leave his or her self behind. For this reason, qualitative research can surely be criticized as too subjective. Therefore, when conducting or reading quantitative or qualitative research, we must always keep in mind that even the seemingly purest of research studies will be biased by the researcher. We must both learn from research and question it.

White Researchers Conducting Multicultural Research: An Unnatural Fit?

From 1932 to 1972, the United States Public Health Services examined the effects of untreated syphilis on African American men in Tuskegee, Alabama. This appalling research, known as "the Tuskegee Experiment," was one of a number of abuses against minorities and women that have taken place in the name of research. Thus, it is not surprising that some researchers have questioned whether white researchers should even perform multicultural research (Atkinson, 1993; Mio & Iwamasa, 1993; Parham, 1993; Weinrach & Thomas, 1996). In an effort to reduce biases by white researchers, Parham (1993) suggests a number of prerequisites when conducting multicultural research. He concludes that white researchers should:

- Examine their worldview and consider whether it is compatible with doing multicultural research.
- Make sure that samples are representative of all groups.
- Consider conducting more qualititative research.
- Achieve a broader understanding of cultures in order to better understand how the research they conduct may, or may not, be relevant to a particular culture.
- Be less concerned about "finding significance" and examine how any research they conduct can have a positive impact on minority clients.

Ethical, Professional, and Legal Issues

Ethical Issues

ACA's ethical guidelines (ACA, 1995a) have a separate section on research and publication that emphasizes many important research issues (see Appendix A, Standard G). Summarizing a few of these, we find the following.

Research responsibilities: Research must be conducted in a manner that respects individuals from all cultures and takes reasonable precautions to avoid psychological, physical, or social injury to subjects.

Informed consent: Prior to consenting to participate in research, subjects must be told the purpose of the research, procedures, any potential risks involved, the potential benefits, alternative procedures to the research, any limits to confidentiality, and the fact that they can withdraw from the study at any point.

Deception: Deception in research can be used only if it can be shown that an alternative method is not available and the value of the research justifies the deception. If deception is involved, there must be extremely low risk, if any, of harm to subjects.

Confidentiality: All information obtained from research must be kept confidential, and the plans for keeping the research confidential must be explained to the subjects.

Professional Issue: Standards in Research

ACA and APA both set standards in conducting research through statements in their Codes of Ethics (ACA, 1995a; APA, 1992; see Appendix A). In addition, research and program evaluation is one of the eight core content areas designated by CACREP for counselor training programs. Thus, in order for programs to obtain accreditation, they must teach the specific areas identified by CACREP. Finally, although no one division of ACA specifically addresses research, all divisions are committed to research, as is reflected in each of their publications.

Legal Issues

Exclusion of Females and Minorities in Research

The National Institute of Mental Health and other agencies now require that females and minorities be included in all research unless there is a compelling reason not to include them (Swenson, 1997).

Institutional Review Boards

Federal legislation now requires that all organizations that conduct research supported by federal funds have a human subjects committee or institutional review board whose purpose is to assure that there is little or no risk to research participants. Today, many institutions have adopted human subjects committees even if they do not receive federal funds.

The Counselor in Process: Discovering New Paradigms

Whitson (1996) challenges all practitioners to come forth and risk leaping into the black hole called research. It's scary to dive in, but one comes out a scholar and a better counselor. Counselors must see themselves as conductors of research, readers of research, and publishers of research (see Thompson, 1995b). We cannot afford to be bound by our fears of research, because this keeps us stuck in our inert, former ways of understanding the profession of counseling. We must move forward toward new paradigms. Research and evaluation allow us to continually examine what we are doing, change what we have done, and adapt to new and better ways of working with clients. We need to stop criticizing research and embrace its process; we need to stop fearing statistics and learn how to use them; we need to realize that research is not a virus to avoid but a living process that offers us new directions for the future and new ways of defining who we are and how we work. Learn various ways of doing research and evaluation, apply them, and publish them. Become a true scholar in the helping professions. Give to both your clients and your peers.

Summary

This chapter examined research and evaluation. We noted that research and evaluation help us find answers to the questions we ponder, move us forward in our understanding of the world, help to show us that what we are doing is working, and offer us new ways of approaching our work. We noted that qualitative and quantitative research approach the process of attaining new knowledge differently, both offering an important perspective. We explained that although evaluation is not research, it will often employ research designs to complete its task.

Explaining the differences between quantitative and qualitative research, we noted that quantitative research assumes that there is an objective reality within which research questions can be formulated and reductionistic, scientific methods used in the pursuit of knowledge, while qualitative research holds that there are multiple ways of viewing knowledge and that the role of the researcher is to carefully observe and describe phenomena and to interpret them within a social context.

In examining quantitative research, we distinguished between experimental and nonexperimental research. Experimental research includes true experimental, quasi-experimental, and single-subject designs, all of which attempt to show cause and effect and manipulate the independent variable. Nonexperimental research includes ex post facto designs, correlational research, and survey research, and generally does not imply cause and effect; there is no manipulation of the independent variable.

In looking at qualitative research, we distinguished between ethnographic and historical research, although each type of research employs the case study method of probing or analyzing an event. Ethnographic research examines a phenomenon or event within its social context by having the researcher immerse him- or herself in the culture being studied, while historical research relies on the systematic collection of information in an effort to examine and understand past events within a contextual framework.

In discussing some of the statistics that are used with quantitative research, we noted that descriptive statistics are often used with survey research, while inferential statistics are generally used when one is examining group differences or relationships among treatment groups. On the other hand, when organizing results from qualitative research, one generally relies on a process called inductive analysis, which means that patterns and categories emerge from data. Thus the researcher examines data from observation, interviews, artifacts, records, and relics and looks through the information for salient patterns and ways of categorizing information.

In examining issues of quality when conducting research, we noted that quantitative research relies on an examination of a study's internal validity to show potential confounding variables and its external validity to show the ability of the research to generalize to other populations. Whereas quantitative research examines the kinds of strict control one has over internal and external validity, qualitative research is more concerned with whether or not there is congruency between the researcher's understanding of events and the actual events that have taken place. Standards of excellence are generally employed to assure such congruence.

Although qualitative and quantitative research are different in their approach to understanding knowledge, they both start with a problem statement, a review of the literature, and a hypothesis or research question. After a study is complete, researchers generally respond to the hypothesis or research question by publishing their results. Generally, a publication includes a literature review, the statement of the problem, the hypothesis or research question, the methods that were used to conduct the study, an objective reporting of the results, discussion about the results, and implications for future research.

Unlike research that examines new paradigms, program evaluation examines the value and worth of a program and the extent to which a program has achieved its goals and objectives. Whereas formative (process) evaluation is concerned with the assessment of a program during its implementation, summative (outcome) evaluation involves assessment of the total training program in order to decide whether or not the program was worthwhile and/or whether it should be offered again. Formative evaluation can include informal assessment procedures and is an ongoing process as long as a program is being conducted. Summative evaluation, on the other hand, may involve more formal assessment procedures and may use research designs to show the efficacy of a program. Both formative and summative evaluation techniques are becoming increasingly important in being accountable to administrators and funding agencies.

In this chapter we firmly stated that all research is biased. The subject matter that is chosen, the population to be examined, the kinds of design that are picked, and even the statistical analysis used can lean a researcher to certain conclusions. However, that does not mean that research is not important. On the contrary, research can offer much to our understanding of the world, but we need to know its limits. The strict controls of quantitative research provide us with answers to many questions, but its extremely focused results often limit its generalizability. On the other hand, the less rigid structure of qualitative research offers us a way of understanding the world of others but can be criticized for being too subjective.

We noted that a recent controversy has questioned whether white researchers should even perform multicultural research. We stated that white researchers should examine their biases, assure accurate samples, conduct more qualitative research, gain a better understanding of cultural differences, and focus more on how research can help minorities.

As we neared the end of the chapter we highlighted a number of ethical, professional, and legal issues related to research and program evaluation. We noted that researchers must respect all research participants and assure that no harm will occur to any person, assure that research participants give informed consent, avoid deception in research, and keep all information gained from research participants confidential. In speaking to standards in the profession, we noted that in addition to the ethical guidelines requiring adherence to high standards in research, CACREP requires that counseling programs address specific content issues in the area of research and program evaluation. Two legal issues we discussed were the necessity of institutional review boards in assuring that no harm occurs to research participants and the importance of including minorities and women in research.

Finally, we ended this chapter by noting the importance of diving into research, the importance of becoming a conductor of research, a reader of research, and a publisher of research. We must be active researchers if we are to remain alive and forward-thinking in our profession and if we are going to be helpful to our clients and add knowledge to the world.

INFOTRAC and Other Information Resources (e.g., ERIC and PsycINFO)

Note: When relevant, key words are in quotation marks.

1. Compare and contrast the role of "quantitative research" and "qualitative research" in counseling today.
2. Review the literature on "ethics and counseling research."
3. Through a literature review, study how "program evaluation" has been used in the field.

SECTION **VI**

Social and Cultural Foundations in Counseling

Overview

The tragedy of September 11, 2001, makes it clear that issues of class, race, ethnicity, and culture are some of the most pressing concerns of the 21st century. These issues weigh heavily on the counselor and the counseling profession and must be addressed. Thus, this section of the text offers two chapters that will examine the ever-important area of multicultural counseling.

The two chapters in this section are a natural complement to one another. Chapter 14 focuses on theory and concepts of multicultural counseling and thus offers you the foundational aspects of this important area. With this basic grounding intact, you are ready to move on to Chapter 15, which zeroes in on knowledge and skills necessary when working with diverse populations. Although the chapters differ in their general thrust, in both chapters I will present some statistics on diversity in the United States and around the world, and I will define basic terms in the field of multicultural counseling. In addition, in both chapters I will examine issues of discrimination, and prejudice and I will challenge you to look at your own cultural identity as well as the biases and stereotypes you have that could deleteriously affect the counseling relationship.

Both chapters will present multicultural counseling as one of the most pressing issues in the mental health profession. Called by some a "fourth force" in counseling, multicultural counseling represents a major new thrust for the profession. As you read through these chapters, consider the importance that a knowledge of multicultural issues has on you, our profession, our country, and the world.

CHAPTER **14**

Theory and Concepts of Multicultural Counseling

There is an old story. We are each of us told in its tale. A child went to a rabbi and asked why God started with just Adam and just Eve. The child asked why God had not made everyone at once. The rabbi answered that God had made only Adam and only Eve so that no one of us could ever turn to another person and say, "Your father is not my father, your mother is not my mother, and we are neither brother nor sister." So this can never be said. By any of us. To any of us.
(Author Unknown)

Growing up in New York was a world unto itself: the ethnic foods, the multicultured music, the people; oh, how I loved to watch the people. Walk down a Manhattan street, and you can watch an endless sea of people, a sea that seems to change color as it flows by you, a sea whose shape transforms constantly; and, if you flow with it long enough, you can visit every part of the world. There is no question that New York gave me a multicultural perspective that many people don't have an opportunity to obtain. However, despite this exposure to a variety of cultures and ethnic groups, I really never got below the surface. I could taste the foods, I could see the people, and I could listen to the music, but that experience alone was still from a detached perspective. Even though I might see the brightly colored clothes of the Nigerian, I still didn't know that person. Even though I could taste the sushi, I didn't understand the world of the Japanese. And even though I could listen to the Latino music, I didn't really understand the people.

This chapter is about differences, similarities, and understanding one another. We will begin the chapter by suggesting a number of reasons why issues related to multicultural counseling must take a prominent place in the counseling profession today. We will review important definitions in the field and examine continued patterns of discrimination and prejudice that exist in America. By exploring models of minority identity development and white identity development we will try to understand why large numbers of white counselors have a difficult time working with minority clients. The chapter will highlight the importance of counselors understanding their own attitudes and beliefs, having basic knowledge of many cultures, and of knowing cross-cultural counseling skills if they are to work effectively with culturally different clients. Near the conclusion of the chapter we will stress the importance of multicultural counseling training standards and examine some important ethical, professional, and legal issues.

What Is Multicultural Counseling?

The concept of multicultural counseling has changed over the years and continues to change today. Some have preferred a rather narrow definition that includes only those minority groups that have been most discriminated against (e.g., African Americans, gays, and lesbians) (Helms, 1994; Locke, 1990). In fact Helms (1994) suggests that too broad a definition obscures the critical importance of racial factors in the therapy process:

> *Nevertheless, a decided disadvantage of the all-inclusive, pluralistic, or multicultural perspective was that it permitted the mental health specialities to shift their attention away from an analysis of the impact of racial factors on the therapy process.* (Helms, 1994, p. 162)

Others, using a more inclusive definition, suggest that a multicultural counseling relationship is one in which individuals from differing cultures with different world views are brought together in a counseling relationship (Das, 1995; Pedersen, 1991a, 2000; Vontress, 1988). Still others consider multicultural counseling to be any therapeutic relationship in which there are differences in values (Niles, 1993). Some might argue that this broad a definition would include all counseling relationships.

I believe that all counseling relationships challenge counselors to work through cultural differences with each of their clients, even clients who are seemingly from the same cultural background. However, if we were to define multicultural counseling in such a broad context, we would be faced with a monumental task and detract from examining the important issues that face those clients who have already been greatly damaged by the counselor's lack of awareness of multicultural issues. Consider the analogy of the emergency room. A number of individuals come in at once, some with minor wounds, some with major. Whom do we treat first? Clearly, we treat the ones who most need immediate attention. And thus it is with multicultural counseling. Even though it would be important to attend to the needs of all groups, the counseling issues of those who have been most harmed by prejudice and discrimination in society are most pressing. Although I believe we can focus on more than just racial minorities, I also think we need to limit ourselves to those who have been clearly discriminated against. Therefore, borrowing from Axelson (1999), we will view multicultural counseling within the following context:

> *[Multicultural counseling] encompasses all the components of the many different cultural environments in a democratic society, together with the pertinent theories, techniques, and practices of counseling. In this regard, the approach takes into specific consideration the traditional and contemporary backgrounds and environmental experiences of diverse clients and how special needs might be identified and met through the resources of the helping professions.* (p. 22)

Why Multicultural Counseling?

Diversity in America

The most obvious answer to the question "Why multicultural counseling?" is that America is the most diverse country in the world—a country that is truly a conglomerate of ethnicities, races, cultures, and religions. Examine Table 14.1, and you will see individuals from every race/culture/ethnicity, individuals who have heritages from all parts of the globe, individuals with different sexual orientations and a wide range of religious diversity. We are a truly multicultural nation and thus are called to offer counseling services to individuals from many diverse backgrounds. We cannot idly sit by and ignore who we are. However, besides the sheer numbers of individuals from diverse backgrounds, there are numerous other reasons why multicultural counseling is critical to American society.

Counseling Is Not Working for a Large Segment of Our Population

If you were distrustful of therapists, confused about the counseling process, or felt worlds apart from a counselor you were seeing, would you want to go to or continue in counseling? Assuredly not. Unfortunately, this is the state of affairs for many minority clients. In

TABLE 14.1

Number and Percentage of Individuals from Select Racial, Ethnic, Religious, and Sexual Identity Backgrounds in the United States

ETHNICITY/RACE*	NUMBER (IN MILLIONS)	PERCENTAGE	RELIGION**	NUMBER (IN MILLIONS)	PERCENTAGE
White	211.5	7.1	Protestant	169	64
Black or African American	34.7	12.3	Baptist	56	21.1
Hispanic	35.3	12.5	Methodist	32	12.1
Asian	10.2	3.6	Lutheran	20	7.7
American Indian and Alaska Native	2.5	0.9	Presbyterian	12	4.5
Native Hawaiian and other Pacific Islander	0.4	0.1	Episcopalian	6	2.6
Some other race	15.4	5.5	Roman Catholic	66	25
Two or more races	6.8	2.4	Muslim	?	?†
			Jewish	5	2.3
SEXUAL ORIENTATION††			Eastern Orthodox	4	1.5
Gay	1–10		Other religions	5	2.0
Lesbian	2–6		No preference	18	16.7
Heterosexual	90–95				

*Figures from U.S. Census Bureau (2002)
The majority of Asians have the following ancestries: Chinese, Filipino, Indian, Vietnamese, Korean, and Japanese.
The majority of Hispanics have the following ancestries: Mexican, Puerto Rican, Cuban, and the Dominican Republic.
The majority of whites have the following ancestries: German, English, Irish, Slavic, French, Italian, Scottish, Scandinavian, and Dutch (Allen & Turner, 1988).
**Percentage of religions from *Comptons Encyclopedia* (1996).
†Muslims probably range in the millions, but most have not officially registered as a religious sect.
††Studies on percent of homosexuality range from 1% to 10%, with most from 3% to 6%. Number of bisexuals vary considerably based on study (see Singer & Deschamps, 1994).

fact, it is now assumed by many that when minority clients work with majority counselors, there is a strong possibility that the counselor will (1) minimize the impact of social forces on the client, (2) interpret cultural differences as psychopathological issues, and (3) misdiagnose the client (Mwaba & Pedersen, 1990; Yeh & Hwang, 2002).

Counseling is not working for many clients from diverse backgrounds. A large body of evidence shows that minority clients are frequently misunderstood, often misdiagnosed, find therapy less helpful than their majority counterparts, attend therapy at lower rates than majority clients, and tend to terminate therapy more quickly than majority clients (Garretson, 1993; Gonzales et al., 1997; Good, 1997; Lee & Mixson, 1995; McKenzie, 1999; Morrow & Deidan, 1992; Poston et al., 1991; Solomon, 1992; Wilson & Stith, 1991). In addition, clients from cultural backgrounds different from that of their counselor may experience the helping relationship more negatively than if the helper is of the same culture (Atkinson, 1985; Atkinson, Poston, Furlong, & Mercado, 1989; Phelps, Taylor, & Gerard, 2001). It is understandable that today we find minority clients underrepresented at mental health centers (Sue & Sue, 1999).

Why is counseling not working for a good segment of our population? Some have suggested the following reasons (Midgette & Meggert, 1991; Sodowsky & Taffe, 1991; Solomon, 1992; Yutrzenka, 1995):

1. *The melting pot myth.* Some believe this country is a melting pot of cultural diversity. However, this is not the experience of many minority clients, who find themselves on the fringe of American culture, view themselves as different from the mainstream, and cannot relate to many of the values and beliefs held by the majority. In truth, most cultures want to maintain their uniqueness and are resistant to giving up their special traditions. Thus, the counselor who assumes the client should fit into and conform to the values of the majority culture may turn off some clients. Probably, viewing American society as a cultural mosaic, a society with a myriad of diverse values and customs, more accurately represents the essence of diversity that we find today. The counselor who idealistically believes we are all the same may turn off the client who has been raised in a minority culture and has experienced it as quite different from the majority culture.

2. *Incongruent expectations about counseling.* The Western, particularly American, approach to counseling has a number of assumptions concerning the counseling process. For instance, it assumes that the counseling process should emphasize the individual; stress the expression of feelings; encourage self-disclosure, open-mindedness, and insight; and show cause and effect. In addition, most counselors are not bilingual, approach counseling from nonreligious perspective, and view the mind and body separately. However, many cultures do not place high value on these attributes, and clients from those cultures will therefore enter such a relationship with much trepidation, may face disappointment when a counseling relationship does not meet their expectations, and may even be harmed by the counseling relationship (Sodowsky & Taffe, 1991; Yutrzenka, 1995). For example, the Asian client who is proud of her ability to restrict her emotions may leave counseling feeling as if she disappointed her counselor who has been pushing her to express feelings.

3. *Lack of understanding of social forces.* Although counselors may be effective at attending to clients' *feelings* concerning how they have been discriminated against, abused, or affected by other "external" factors, the same counselors will often de-emphasize the actual influence these social forces have on clients. Counselors often assume that most if not all negative feelings are created by the individual, and they often have difficulty

BOX 14.1

An Ethnocentric World View

I went to college in the early 1970s. In my dorm was a student from Iran. At that time, students from Middle Eastern countries came less frequently to American colleges than they do now, and our understanding of Islam was much less than it is now. He seemed strange to us, and we treated him poorly. We made fun of him and ostracized him. Only later did I realize that he was not the strange one, we were. We were not used to his customs, and therefore assumed he was odd. We only understood our view of the world. Muhammad, I wish I knew where you were today so I could apologize to you.

understanding the power of social influences. By de-emphasizing social forces, counselors are likely to have a difficult time building a relationship with a client who has been considerably harmed by external factors. For instance, the client who has been illegally denied jobs due to his disability may be discouraged when a counselor says, "What have you done to prevent yourself from obtaining the job?"

4. *Ethnocentric worldview*. People who are not cross-culturally aware tend to view the world through the lens of their own culture (see Box 14.1). Ethnocentric counselors tend to falsely assume that their clients view the world in a similar manner or believe that when one presents a differing view of the world he or she is emotionally disturbed, culturally brainwashed, or wrong. Although the importance of understanding a client's unique worldview is always crucial to an effective helping relationship, this is particularly significant when working with minority clients whose experience of the world may be particularly foreign to our own. For instance, a counselor may inadvertently turn off a Muslim when she says to her client, "Have a wonderful Christmas."

5. *Ignorance of one's own racist attitudes and prejudices*. Of course, the counselor who is not in touch with his or her prejudices and racist attitudes cannot work effectively with minority clients and may indeed be harmful to those clients. Understanding our own stereotypes and prejudices takes a particularly vigilant effort, as oftentimes our biases are unconscious. For instance, the heterosexual counselor who unconsciously believes that being gay is a disease but consciously states he is accepting of all sexual orientations may subtly treat a gay client as if there is something wrong with him.

6. *Inability to understand cultural differences in the expression of symptomatology*. What may be seen as "abnormal" in the United States may be considered quite usual and customary in another culture. The counselor's lack of knowledge about cultural differences as they relate to the expression of symptoms can seriously damage a counseling relationship and result in misdiagnosis, mistreatment, and early termination of culturally different clients from counseling. For instance, whereas many individuals from Anglo-European cultures would show grief through depression, agitation, and feelings of helplessness, a Hispanic might present with somatic complaints.

7. *The unreliability of assessment and research instruments*. Over the years, assessment and research instruments have notoriously been culturally biased. Although advances have been made, one can still readily find tests that have cultural bias and research that does not control adequately for cultural differences. One common problem in the use of

assessment instruments is that individuals from other cultures may inadvertently be answering questions in a manner that would be considered "abnormal" by American standards when indeed they do not have an emotional disorder. For example, when an item

…s Hispanic client might answer "yes," …e in her culture. Although Americans …y that they "hear voices" because that

…acism is embedded in society and even …D'Andrea & Daniels, 1991, 1999), it is …ased and counselors will unknowingly …t clients. Examples are plentiful. For in… …e *DSM-IV-TR* have been shown to be …e been given precedence in the profes… …useless when working with clients from …ms have, until recently, not stressed … biased statements in this text of which

…unseling. Although still in its infancy, it …there has been an outcry by many in the …n multicultural counseling (Arredondo, 1999; Baker, 1995; Fukuyama, 1994; Lee, 1994; Sandhu, 1995; Sue, Arredondo, & McDavis, 1992; Sue & Sue, 1999). For culturally different clients, we hope that this call to the profession will result in (1) counselors having a better understanding of diversity, (2) counselors being able to make more accurate diagnoses, (3) a decrease in the dropout rate from counseling, and (4) an increase in satisfaction with the counseling process (Quintana & Bernal, 1995).

Some Definitions

In examining differences within American society, many have differentiated between such terms as *culture*, *race*, *minority*, *ethnicity*, *social class*, and *power* while highlighting how stereotyping, prejudice, racism, and discrimination have affected our clients and our work with them (Atkinson et al., 1998; Baruth & Manning, 1998). Understanding terms gives all of us a common ground with which to communicate. The following are brief definitions of some of these terms.

Culture

Shared values, *symbols*, *language*, *ways of being in the world* are some of the words and phrases I think of when reflecting on the word *culture*. Culture represents the common values, norms of behavior, symbols, language, and common life patterns that people learn and share with one another. For instance, despite great diversity in the United States, most Americans do have a similar cultural heritage because within this society there is a shared language, symbols that most of us recognize, and patterns of behavior with which most are familiar. Traveling throughout this country we find many symbols of a common culture (e.g., fast-food restaurants, music, laws, basic values, shared language). Yet, even as I acknowledge this common culture, I am acutely aware of the unique patterns of behaviors and values that distinguish many subcultures within our country. Examples of some subcultures include urban gays and lesbians; various racial, ethnic, and religious groups; subcultures based on gender; and subcultures based on the region of the country in which one lives (e.g., "the South") (Samovar & Porter , 2001). In attempting to delineate cultural identity, Whitfield, McGrath, and Coleman (1992) have identified 11 elements that can be used in helping to understand specific cultural patterns. They include how each culture:

- Defines its sense of self.
- Dresses and values appearances.
- Embraces specific beliefs and attitudes.
- Relates to family and significant others.
- Plays and makes use of leisure time.
- Learns and uses knowledge.
- Communicates and uses language.
- Embraces certain values and mores.
- Uses time and space.
- Eats and uses food in its customs.
- Works and applies itself.

Race

Genetic heritage, skin color, ambiguity are some of the words and phrases I think of when reflecting on the word *race*. Whereas the concept of culture has been based on such characteristics as shared learned traits, race has traditionally been defined biologically, with people of the same racial heritage being said to share similar genetic heritage (Krogman, 1945). However, this definition has been recently challenged. For instance, research on the human genome shows that humans share much more genetically than was at one time thought (Davies, 2001). In fact, genetic differences between any two people is only 0.2 percent. Behaviorally, there seem to be more differences within racial groups than among them (Atkinson et al., 1998). In addition, gene pools throughout the world, and especially in the United States, have become increasingly mixed due to migration, exploration, invasions, systematic rape as a result of wars and oppression of minorities, and intermarriage. With some sociologists saying there are no races, others saying there are three, and still others concluding that there are as many as 200, the issue of race is cloudy and perhaps doesn't matter. Because of the confusion concerning this term, some now advocate for discontinuing its use (Cameron & Wycoff, 1998). Generally, I agree with this stand, and for the most part I have instead used the words culture, ethnic background, or minority.

Ethnicity

Heritage, ancestry, and *tradition* are some of the words that come to mind when I reflect on the word *ethnicity*. More specifically, when a group of people share a common ancestry, which may include specific cultural and social patterns, they are sometimes said to be of the same ethnic group (Davis, 1978; Rose, 1964). Ethnicity, as opposed to race, is not based on genetic heritage but on long-term patterns of behavior that have some historical significance and may include similar religious, ancestral, language, and/or cultural characteristics. Therefore, Jews, who share religious and perhaps similar ancestral characteristics, may be considered an ethnic group but may not share the same culture (Jews live in many different cultures throughout the world). Similarly, people of Asian heritage, although considered a race by some, may not share the same culture or the same ethnic background.

Social Class

Money, power, status, hierarchy: These are the words that come to mind when I think of the term *social class.* Calling it the "missing dimension" in understanding diversity, Hannon, Ritchie, and Rye (1992) note that social class has been largely overlooked when examining issues of diversity. One's social class represents the perceived ranking of an individual within a society and is based on a number of dimensions, including the amount of money an individual has, the kind of status one holds (e.g., one's occupation, one's position in the community), and the amount of power an individual wields (see "power differentials," below) (Macionis, 2001). An individual's social class may cut across a person's ethnicity, cultural identification, or race (Ihle, Sodowsky, & Kwan, 1996). Therefore, even though individuals may share a similar culture, ethnicity, or race, they may have little in common with one another due to differences in social class. For instance, it is not unusual to find a poor African American who may have little in common with a wealthy African American.

Power Differentials

Potential abuse, force, control, and *superior/underling* are some of the words and phrases that come to my mind when I think of the term *power differential.* Power differentials may represent greater disparities between people than culture, ethnic group, race, or social class. Power can be a function of race, class, gender, occupation, and a host of other factors and can easily be misunderstood. Whether perceived or real, power can be abused. For instance, the professor may abuse his or her power by sexually harassing the student. An upper-management Mexican-American female who does not abuse her power may still be disliked because the workers believe that Hispanic females should not hold positions of power. And the white male may be given a leadership position in a management group, not because of his expertise, but because it is unconsciously believed by the other group members that white males have power.

Minority

A minority is any group of people who are being singled out due to their cultural or physical characteristics and are being systematically oppressed by those individuals who are in a position of power. Using this definition, a minority could conceivably be the numerical majority of a population, as was the case for many years for blacks in South Africa and as is the situation with women in the United States (Atkinson et al., 1998; Macionis, 2001).

Stereotypes, Prejudice, and Racism

Stereotypes are rigidly held beliefs about a group of people that assume that most or all of the group has certain characteristics, behaviors, or beliefs (e.g., Asians are intelligent people, American Indians are alcoholics) (Lum, 2000). Whereas the word *stereotype* refers to *specific* behaviors or beliefs of a group, prejudice is a positive or negative bias about a group as a whole (e.g., "I hate gays"). Whereas prejudice can be toward any group, racism is a specific belief that one race is superior to another (e.g., whites are better than blacks). Some authors have taken the position that racism is a disease noting that, like other mental disorders, racism is based on a distortion of reality (Skillings & Dobbins, 1991).

Discrimination

Whereas the words *stereotypes, prejudice,* and *racism* refer to attitudes held by people, discrimination is an active behavior, such as gay bashing or unfair hiring practices, that negatively affects individuals within ethnic or cultural groups (Lum, 2000).

What is the extent of prejudice and discrimination in America? A study by the Anti-Defamation League (ADL, 1992) found, in surveying American households, that many people felt that prejudice and discrimination were experienced by a wide variety of subcultures in this country. In particular, Americans felt that a considerable amount of discrimination was experienced by blacks (76%) and homosexuals (74%), while over 50% of Americans felt that Jews, Asians, Hispanics, and women experienced some discrimination. Unfortunately, the most recent hate crime statistics from the FBI (1999) indicate that we still we have much work to do in this country:

> *Of the 7,876 incidents, nearly 55 percent were motivated by racial bias; 18 percent by religious bias; 17 percent by sexual orientation bias; 11 percent by ethnicity/national origin bias; and less than one-half of one percent by disability and multiple biases.* (p. 5)

Political Correctness, or, Oh My God, What Do I Call Him or Her?

Hispanic, Latino, Latina, Chicano, Chicana, black, negro, African American, Afro-American, Oriental, Asian American, Chinese American, Japanese American, Native American, Indian, Eskimo, Inuit, Aleut, native, American Indian, Asian Indian, Jew, Hebrew, Jewish American, Protestant, WASP, Muslim, Moslem, Islamic, Born Again, Fundamental Christian, Christian, Catholic, white, Caucasian, European American, American, gay, homosexual, straight, heterosexual, bisexual, lesbian, transgendered, transsexual, transvestite, disabled person, individual with disability, handicapped person, physically challenged, and on and on. Did I offend anybody? I hope not, but in these days of political correctness, finding the correct term is often difficult. And, even once you find the correct term, you will offend somebody.

Although there is a great amount of variety concerning how individuals should be addressed, usually the following terms have been used. For Americans with African heritage, the term *African American* is generally used, although *black* is still acceptable in some circles. *Asian American* refers to any of a number of individuals with heritage from Asia and the Pacific Islands, including approximately 40 distinct subgroups that differ in language and cultural identity (Sandhu, 1997). *Hispanic* refers to Mexican Americans, Puerto Ricans, Cuban Americans, individuals with Central and South American heritage, and individuals with roots from Spanish-speaking countries in the Caribbean. However, not all individuals from these countries are comfortable with the term *Hispanic*, especially many Cuban Americans. Islam is a religion whose followers are called *Muslim* (less commonly called Moslem). Homosexuals today generally use the terms *gay* for men and *lesbian* for women. The term *straight* is becoming less acceptable to describe heterosexuals because of the implication that it is better than another type of orientation (e.g., "on the straight and narrow"). Individuals who have been born in this country and identify with their cultural or ethnic background often place the word *American* following their heritage. Therefore, it is not unusual for us to find individuals referring to themselves as Irish American, Italian American, Arab American, and so forth. Individuals who are naturalized citizens generally do not use the term "American" following their country of origin. For instance, a colleague of mine who was raised in Mexico and became a U.S. citizen refers to herself as "Mexican." Finally, rather than saying handicapped or disabled person, generally people now say "individual with a disability," although some prefer the term "physically challenged."

Although I cannot describe the politically correct term for individuals from every culture, ethnic, or minority group, I have attempted to use commonly accepted terms throughout Chapters 14 and 15. Of course, people vary in how they wish to be addressed. However, I believe that making an effort to use terms correctly shows our sensitivity to individuals from diverse cultures.

Conceptual Models for Working with Diverse Clients

Every person is like all persons, like some persons, and like no other person. (paraphrased from Kluckhohn & Murray, 1953, in Speight, Myers, Cox, & Highlen, 1991, p. 32)

Existentialists have noted that, in trying to understand individuals, we need to be aware of their uniqueness *(Eigenwelt)*, the common experiences held in groups and cultures *(Mitwelt)*, and shared universal experiences *(Umwelt)* (Binswanger, 1962, 1963). Keeping this in mind, we need to ask ourselves, "How can the counselor be effective with culturally different clients?" Using the above existential framework, one model of working with all clients assumes that each client has specific issues related to his or her culture, is unique unto him- or herself, and shares universal issues common to all people (Speight et al., 1991, p. 32) (see Figure 14.1). Each of these spheres represents a unique aspect of the individual. The overlap of the spheres suggests that we can only understand the totality of our clients' situation if we can understand the uniqueness of these three components.

Minority Identity Models

One conceptual way of understanding diverse clients is to determine whether they identify with their own culture or the majority culture. Such a model can assist the counselor in understanding how the minority client might respond to working with minority and majority counselors. One such model, by Bell and Evans (1981), offers four interpersonal styles of relating.

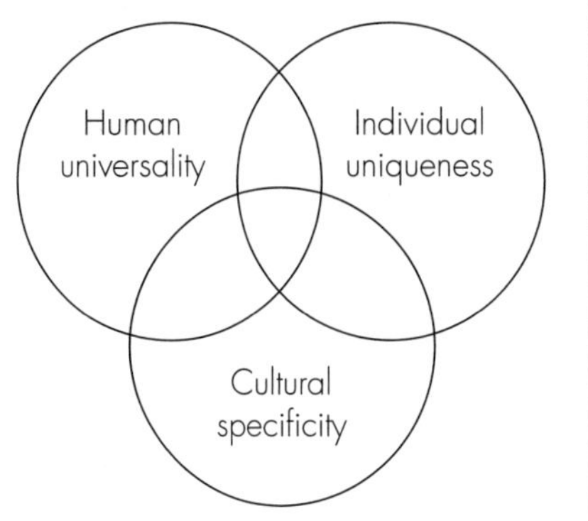

FIGURE 14.1
Each Sphere Represents a Unique Aspect of the Individual. The intersection where the spheres overlap suggests that we can only understand the totality of our clients' situation if we can understand the uniqueness of these three components.

SOURCE: From "A Redefinition of Multicultural Counseling," by S. L. Speight, J. Myers, C. F. Fox, and P. S. Highlen, 1991, *Journal of Counseling and Development*, *70*, 29–36. Copyright 1991. American Counseling Association. Reprinted by permission.

Bell's Interpersonal Model

THE ACCULTURATED INTERPERSONAL STYLE The acculturated individual rejects, on both conscious and unconscious levels, his or her racial/ethnic or cultural background in order to assimilate into the dominant culture. Uncomfortable with his or her own culture, this individual acts, sounds, and lives a life as if he or she is from the majority culture with the purpose of escaping the oppression of the dominant group. This person experiences self-hate and is uncomfortable with members of his or her own racial/ethnic or cultural group. Counseling around cross-cultural issues is particularly difficult for this person, and he or she is likely to be more comfortable with a counselor from the majority culture.

THE BICULTURAL INTERPERSONAL STYLE The bicultural individual feels comfortable in his or her cultural group as well as in the majority culture and can easily flow into and out of either culture. As opposed to the acculturated individual, this person has not rejected his or her culture but may at times feel a sense of split personality, being torn between the two cultures. Recognizing that all cultures have positive features, this person is often found seeking out experiences from many cultures. This individual feels at ease with a majority or minority counselor, and although the counselor feels comfortable with the bicultural client, at times he or she may not recognize the tension the client feels concerning living in both cultures.

THE CULTURALLY IMMERSED INTERPERSONAL STYLE Having rejected the majority culture, this individual is convinced that the majority's only goal is to oppress minorities. This person is often called radical, fundamentalist, or militant. A political activist, this person is often very intelligent and will blame society for social problems. This individual may be particularly guarded during counseling sessions, and such sessions will often deteriorate into power plays, especially if the individual is faced with a majority counselor. Counselors who work with culturally immersed clients must focus on why the client came to counseling as opposed to getting drawn into discussions around issues of societal oppression.

THE TRADITIONAL INTERPERSONAL STYLE Being deeply rooted in his or her cultural style, this individual is immersed in the symbols, customs, and traditions of his or her culture. This person does not accept or reject his or her cultural identity—this person knows only this cultural identity. Often, these individuals may be older than the individuals in any of the other three styles. This person is difficult to counsel cross-culturally, as his or her language or dialect may be foreign to the counselor, and the individual usually has little if any familiarity with the counseling process.

Atkinson's Developmental Model

In contrast to Bell and Evans's (1981) nonstage model, Atkinson and associates (1998) suggest that identity in many minority groups is developmental. Their five-stage model moves from complete immersion in the dominant culture, through complete emersion in the minority culture, to the final stage in which the individual has pride and acceptance of his or her cultural identity and is able to reject or accept values from other cultures.

Atkinson and associates (1998) note that this model can serve several purposes in that it can "sensitize counselors to (1) the role oppression plays in a minority individual's identity development, (2) the differences that can exist between members of the same

TABLE 14.2

Minority Identity Development Model

STAGES OF MINORITY IDENTITY DEVELOPMENT MODEL (MID)	ATTITUDE TOWARD SELF	ATTITUDE TOWARD OTHERS OF THE SAME MINORITY	ATTITUDE TOWARD OTHERS OF DIFFERENT MINORITY	ATTITUDE TOWARD DOMINANT GROUP
Stage 1—Conformity	Self-depreciating	Group-depreciating	Discriminatory	Group-appreciating
Stage 2—Dissonance	Conflict between self-depreciating and appreciating	Conflict between group-depreciating and group-appreciating	Conflict between dominant-held views of minority hierarchy and feelings of shared experience	Conflict between group-appreciating and group-depreciating
Stage 3—Resistance and Immersion	Self-appreciating	Group-appreciating	Conflict between feelings of empathy for other minority experiences and feelings of culturocentrism	Group-depreciating
Stage 4—Introspection	Concern with basis of self-appreciating	Concern with nature of unequivocal appreciating	Concern with ethnocentric basis for judging others	Concern with the basis of group depreciation
Stage 5—Synergetic Articulation and Awareness	Self-appreciating	Group-appreciating	Group-appreciating	Selective appreciation

SOURCE: Counseling American minorities: A cross-cultural perspective (5th ed.), by D. R. Atkinson, G. Morten, and D. W. Sue (Eds.), p. 35.

minority group with respect to their cultural identity, and (3) the potential that each individual minority person has for changing his/her sense of identity" (p. 33).

Table 14.2 examines the attitude that the culturally diverse client holds toward self, toward others of the same minority, toward individuals from different minority groups, and toward the dominant group as he or she transverses five stages of development. Using this model, consider how the counseling process might differ for minority clients at different stages of development. In addition, minority counselors may want to assess where they fall on a minority identity model, such as the ones we discussed.

Stages of White Identity Development

A number of models have been developed to assess the racial consciousness and developmental maturity of white counseling students in their ability to relate to and work with individuals from diverse backgrounds. As in Atkinson and associates' (1998) minority identity model, these models assume there is a stage progression in the development of racial consciousness that can be identified for white counseling students. Teachers and supervisors can facilitate movement of students through the stages by developing activities to support and challenge students' self-understanding. Research on white identity models suggests that development of white identity may be positively correlated with one's ability to work with diverse clients (Carter, 1990; D'Andrea & Daniels,1999; Helms, 1984, 1990, 1995; Ottavi et al., 1994).

In an effort to find common themes running through some of the more prevalent models in the literature, Sabnani and associates (1991) examined three models of white identity development. They subsequently formed a five-stage model incorporating the basic themes that ran through these models. The three models are listed in Table 14.3 and separated into the five stages as identified by Sabnani and associates. In addition to the three models, I incorporated into their table one additional model developed by D'Andrea and Daniels (1991, 1999), which has recently taken on some prominence. A description of the five stages identified by Sabnani and his colleagues is followed here by an examination of the four models and how they fit into the stages (see Table 14.3). Keep in mind that new graduate students will be found at each of these stages.

Stage 1, Pre-exposure. In this stage, white graduate students show naiveté and ignorance about multicultural issues. Sometimes these students believe that racism does not exist or, if it does, only to a limited degree. Racism is generally thought of as over, and students in this stage do not understand more subtle, embedded racism.

Stage 2, Exposure. Students enter this stage when first confronted with multicultural issues. Often this occurs when students take a course in multicultural counseling or encounter multicultural issues as a component of a class. Increasing awareness concerning how racism is embedded in society leads students in this stage to have feelings of guilt over being white, depression with this newfound awareness, and/or anger over the current state of affairs. This stage is often highlighted by a sense of conflict between wanting to maintain majority views and the desire to uphold more humanistically oriented nonracist and nonprejudicial views.

Stage 3, Prominority/antiracism. With movement into this stage, students often take a strong prominority stance, are likely to reject racist and prejudicial beliefs, and sometimes will reject their own whiteness in an effort to assuage the guilt felt in stage 2. Students in this stage tend to have an intense interest in diverse cultural groups and are likely to have an increasing amount of contact with individuals from different cultures.

Stage 4, Retreat to white culture. In this stage some white students tend to retreat into their own culture as they experience rejection from some minority individuals as they, of course, are dealing with their own identity issues (see Table 14.3). As students enter this stage, intercultural contact is ended because they feel hostile and fearful of minorities. The cozy home of the student's culture of origin is feeling quite safe at this point in time.

Stage 5, Redefinition and integration. Students who enter this stage are developing a world view of multiculturalism and are integrating this into their identity. Such students are able to feel good about their own identity and their roots, and simultaneously have a deep appreciation of the culture of others. Students in this stage are able to expend energy toward deeply rooted structural changes in society.

Sabnani and associates (1991) note that there are a number of variations in the ways students can move through the stages. A few examples are listed in Figure 14.2. For instance, Student A is stuck in stage 1. As the student is confronted with multicultural issues, perhaps in a course on multicultural counseling, he or she retreats back to stage 1 behavior, wanting to be in denial about racism and prejudice in society. The change process is too fearful for him or her. Student B moves through the first three stages, does not feel a strong need to retreat into his own culture in stage 4, and moves on to stage 5, in

TABLE 14.3 **Comparison of Models of White Racial Identity**

	WHITE IDENTITY DEVELOPMENT MODEL (HARDIMAN, 1982)	WHITE RACIAL CONSCIOUSNESS DEVELOPMENT MODEL (HELMS, 1984)	RACIAL CONSCIOUSNESS DEVELOPMENT MODEL (PONTEROTTO, 1988)	STAGES OF RACISM (D'ANDREA & DANIELS, 1991, 1999)
STAGE 1: PREEXPOSURE/ PRECONTACT	*Lack of social awareness** Presocialization stage marked by unawareness of social expectations and role Beginning awareness of racial differences *Acceptance:* Unconscious identification with whiteness Acceptance of stereotypes about own group and other groups	*Contact* Unaware of self as racial being Oblivious to cultural/racial issues Naiveté regarding the impact of race on self and others	*Preexposure* Little thought given to multicultural issues or to one's role as a white in an oppressive society Has not begun to explore own ethnic identity	*Affective-impulsive stage* Hostile, illogical ways of thinking Overt feelings of hostility and aggressiveness toward different racial/cultural/ethnic backgrounds Marginal impulse control
STAGE 2: CONFLICT	*Transition from acceptance to resistance* Reexamination of assumptions about whites Begin to face dissonant issues challenging accepted ideology and self-definition as white Guilt and anger	*Contact and disintegration* Forced to acknowledge that he or she is white Caught between white and black culture and between oppression and humanity	*Exposure* Forced to examine role as white member of U.S. society Examine his or her own cultural values Confronted with the realities of race and racism Guilt and anger	*Dualistic rational stage* Dualistic thinking Superficial politeness but underlying fear and negativity toward individuals from diverse backgrounds Impulse control over strong feelings—but feelings still persist
STAGE 3: PROMINORITY/ ANTIRACISM	*Resistance* Rejection of internalized racist beliefs and rejection of whiteness Guilt and anger at having conformed to socialization Anger at whites and whiteness Compassion and concern for minorities	*Disintegration* Overidentification with blacks Paternalistic attitudes toward blacks	*Zealot half of zealot-defensive* Taking on the minority plight Maintaining a prominority stance	*Liberal stage of racism* Beginning of multiple perspective taking Expression of liberal views Despite liberal views and multiple perspective taking, there is little follow-through. Avoidance of advocacy or risk-taking behaviors Apathetic relative to taking action
STAGE 4: RETREAT INTO WHITE CULTURE		*Reintegration* Antiblack, prowhite attitudes Anger, fear	*Defensive half of zealot-defensive* Retreating from multicultural contact and retreating to only same-race relations	
STAGE 5: REDEFINITION AND INTEGRATION	*Redefinition* Development of a white identity that transcends racism Defining whiteness in a way that is not dependent on racism Recognition that all races are unique Development of pride in ethnic group membership *Internalization* Integration of the new white identity into all other aspects of self	*Pseudo-independence* Intellectual acceptance and curiosity regarding blacks and whites Internalization of whiteness *Autonomy* Biculturally or biracially transcendent world view	*Integration* Greater balance in multicultural interest and endeavors Renewed interest, respect, and appreciation for cultural differences	*Principled stage of racism* Truly relativistic thinker. Mature understanding of social problems Greater awareness of inner experience and greater ability to express complex thinking re: racism Compelled to address social ills personally and professionally, but lack of commitment to work toward deeply rooted systemic change *Principled activistic stage of racism* All of qualities of principled stage person plus: willing to work toward systemic change; compelled to action; hopeful for social reform; tenacious and committed

SOURCE: Sabnani, Ponterotto, & Borodovsky, 1991.
*Italicized words in each model represent stages posited by the model.

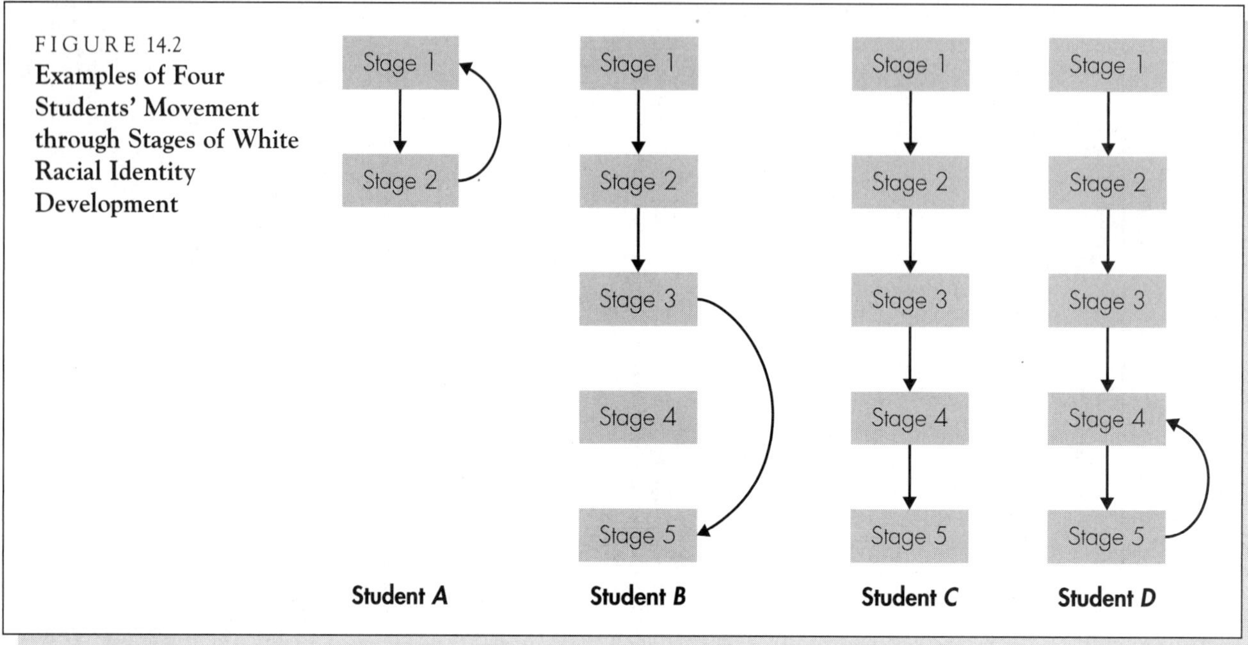

FIGURE 14.2
Examples of Four Students' Movement through Stages of White Racial Identity Development

which he or she can feel good about his or her own culture while having an understanding and appreciation for others. Student C, on the other hand, feels a need to retreat as he or she is rejected by some minority individuals (stage 4). This student becomes angry, upset, and discouraged; moves away from cross-cultural contact; and needs time to reflect on his or her experiences. This student does not understand that minority individuals are dealing with their own identity issues, which lead some of them to reject whites, even whites with good intentions. Some stage 4 students will eventually move out of their shells and have an easy transition to stage 5. Others, however, such as Student D, poke their heads out as they consider moving on to stage 5; but, because they continue to struggle with feelings of rejection and anger, will quickly move back to stage 4. Keep in mind that because this is a developmental model, it is assumed that any student, if given a conducive environment, can move to the higher stages.

The Helping Relationship and Cultural Diversity

In Chapter 1 it was suggested that the effective multicultural counselor should (1) be *multilingual*: have some working knowledge of the language of clients with whom they work, (2) have a *multicultural view*: understand their clients values and ways of living in the world, (3) be *multiculturally literate:* know about important works of art and writings from other cultures, (4) be *ethnically informed*: understand the unique customs and habits of people from various cultures, and (5) be *ecologically literate*: have knowledge of the environment from which the client comes and how it affects their way of living in the world (Whitfield, 1994).

Others have suggested that an effective multicultural counselor needs to (1) be aware of his or her attitudes and beliefs toward culturally diverse populations, (2) have a

BOX 14.2

Lack of Awareness of Own Biases and Prejudices

Robertiello and Schoenewolf (1987) note a number of mistakes that were made by helpers due to their lack of awareness of their own biases:

1. The liberal white therapist who refuses to deal with a black client's mistrustful and suspicious dreams of him due to the helper's denial of the tension in the relationship.
2. The feminist helper who blindly encourages her client to leave her husband because he is a batterer. The client leaves her husband but ends up in another battering situation because the helper did not examine the part the woman was playing in picking abusive men.
3. The helper who reassures her client that the client's homosexual feelings do not mean she is a lesbian. The helper does this out of fear of dealing with the client's sexuality and instead tries to ignore the subject. The client may or may not be homosexual, but reassuring her that she is not does not allow the client to explore her sexuality.
4. The helper who refuses to hear her client's atheistic views because they are contrary to her religious beliefs. This has the effect of cutting off meaningful conversations in other areas because the client loses trust in the helper.

knowledge base that supports his or her work with diverse clients, and (3) have the necessary skills to apply to clients with diverse backgrounds (Pedersen, Draguns, Lonner, & Trimble, 1996; Sue et al., 1982, 1992). Let's examine each of these skills.

The Culturally Skilled Counselor: Beliefs and Attitudes, Knowledge, and Skills

Attitudes and Beliefs

The effective cross-cultural counselor has an awareness of his or her own cultural background and has actively pursued gaining awareness of his or her own biases, stereotypes, and values. Although the effective cross-cultural counselor may not hold the same belief system as his or her client, he or she can accept differing worldviews as presented by the helpee. Being sensitive to differences and tuned into his or her own cultural biases allows the cross-cultural counselor to refer a minority client to a counselor of the client's own culture when a referral will benefit the helpee. Unfortunately, examples of how mental health professionals have failed culturally different clients as a result of their own biases and prejudices abound in the literature (Cayleff, 1986) (see Box 14.2).

Knowledge

The effective cross-cultural counselor has an awareness of sociopolitical issues in this country and the barriers that hinder culturally diverse clients from using social service agencies and has, or is willing to gain, a knowledge of the characteristics of specific cultural and ethnic groups (e.g., personality styles, customs, and traditions). At the same time, such a counselor does not assume that, just because a client comes from a specific cultural background, he or she necessarily has these characteristics. In other words, the counselor has knowledge of the group from which the client comes, yet does not jump to conclusions about the client's ways of being. Unfortunately, lack of knowledge of a cultural group can cause counselors and others to jump to incorrect conclusions (see Box 14.3).

BOX 14.3

Lack of Knowledge: Blackbirds Sitting in a Tree

A white female elementary school teacher in the United States posed a math problem to her class one day. "Suppose there are four blackbirds sitting in a tree. You take a slingshot and shoot one of them. How many are left?" A white student answered quickly, "That's easy. One subtracted from four is three." An African immigrant youth then answered with equal confidence, "Zero." The teacher chuckled at the latter response and stated that the first student was right and that, perhaps, the second student should study more math. From that day forth, the African student seemed to withdraw from class activities and seldom spoke to other students or the teacher. . . .

If the teacher had pursued the African student's reasons for arriving at the answer zero, she might have heard the following: "If you shoot one bird, the others will fly away." Nigerian educators often use this story to illustrate differences in world views between United States and African cultures. The Nigerians contend that the group is more important than the individual, that survival of all depends on interrelationships among the parts. . . . (from Sue, 1992, pp. 7–8)

Skills

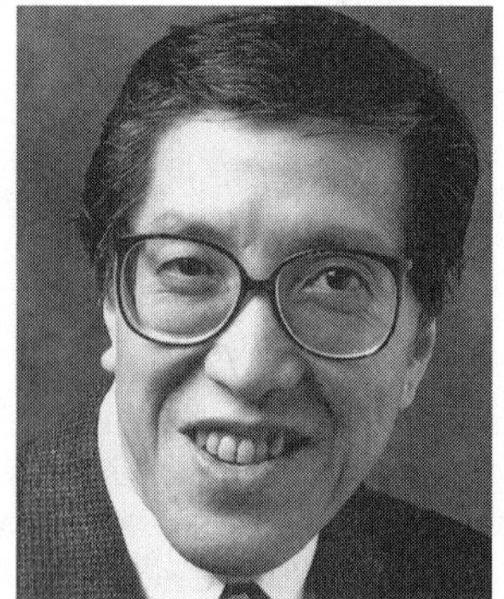

Derald Sue, one of the leaders in the area of multicultural counseling

The counselor who is effective with culturally diverse populations is able to apply generic interviewing and counseling skills, when appropriate, with culturally diverse populations while at the same time being aware of and able to employ specialized skills and interventions that might be effective with specific minority populations. In addition, the culturally sensitive counselor understands the verbal and nonverbal language of the client and can communicate effectively with the client. What happens when a counselor does not have the appropriate skills when working with a culturally diverse client? Most likely, the client will drop out of counseling early, feel discouraged and dissatisfied with counseling, and/or have little success in counseling (see Box 14.4).

As you can see by the examples in Box 14.4, there is a close connection between our beliefs about culturally diverse clients, our knowledge base of such clients, and our effective use of skills. Counselors who have a clear understanding of self, especially their own racial identity, are able to develop healthy attitudes and beliefs and the needed knowledge base to work with diverse clients and can implement the appropriate skills for clients who are culturally different.

Multicultural Issue: Multicultural Counseling as the "Fourth Force"

An article written by Essandoh (1996) raises the possibility that multicultural counseling may represent a new paradigm in the counseling profession—a "fourth force." The first three forces in our profession are identified as the development of psychoanalysis, behaviorism, and humanistic psychology, respectively. However, he warns that the process of applying theory to practice has been slow, and he calls us to be activists in pushing our professional associations and our colleagues to find new theories and adapt existing theories and concepts in their clinical practice:

BOX 14.4

Lack of Skills

A female [Asian] client complained about all kinds of physical problems such as feeling dizzy, having a loss of appetite, an inability to complete household chores, and insomnia. She asked the therapist if her problem could be due to "nerves." The therapist suspected depression since these are some of the physical manifestations of the disorder and asked the client if she felt depressed and sad. At this point, the client paused and looked confused. She finally stated that she feels very ill and that these physical problems are making her sad. Her perspective is that it was natural for her to feel sad when sick. As the therapist followed up by attempting to determine if there was a family history of depression, the client displayed even more discomfort and defensiveness. Although the client never directly contradicted the therapist, she did not return for the following session.
(Sue & Sue, 1990, p. 199)

If this counselor had the appropriate knowledge and skills, he would have known that for Asian clients physical complaints are a common means of expressing emotional problems. An appropriate response to this client would have been to focus on the somatic complaints and suggest physical treatments prior to working on emotional problems (Sue & Sue, 1990).

> *What is needed is more action in terms of applying these theories and concepts in clinical practice. When this happens on a large scale, multicultural counseling and therapy will have the legitimacy that the first three forces had, and this will open the door for more informed research to move multicultural counseling from a position of a fourth dimension to one of a fourth force.* (Essandoh, 1996, p. 136)

Multicultural counseling is changing the ways in which we understand the counseling relationship. It is changing many of the very paradigms that have driven the profession for the past 50 years. It may indeed be the fourth force that will be instrumental in transforming the profession in the current millennium.

Ethical, Professional, and Legal Issues

Increasing Emphasis on Multicultural Standards

Increasingly, multicultural counseling standards have filtered into every aspect of the counseling profession. For instance, today we find inclusion of multicultural issues within our ethical guidelines. And, recently, ACA has called for a close examination of these guidelines to assure that they do justice to multicultural issues (ACA, 2001b).

Also, for the training of counselors we have the *Multicultural Counseling Competencies and Standards* (Arredondo, 1999; Arredondo et al., 1996; Sue et al., 1992). These competencies, which represent minimum standards needed by counselors if they are to work effectively with diverse clients, delineate the attitudes and beliefs, knowledge, and skills in three areas: (1) counselor awareness of their own assumptions, values, and biases, (2) the world view of the culturally different client, and (3) intervention strategies and techniques (see www.counseling.org/multi_diversity/).

In addition to these standards, as noted in Chapter 12, the *Multicultural Assessment Standards* (Prediger, 1994) have been developed to address issues related to testing. Also, the APA offers *Guidelines for Providers of Psychological Services to Ethnic, Linguistic, and Culturally Diverse Populations* (APA, 1990), a guide for questions on diversity issues and accreditation (APA, 1997), and a whole Web site on diversity-related issues (see www.apa.org/pi/oema/onlinebr.html).

The standards are there, but perhaps the more important task lies ahead of us—can we implement the standards in such a manner that will make a significant difference in the ways in which we work with culturally different clients?

Training in Multicultural Counseling

Recognizing the importance of multicultural counseling, CACREP has included "Social and Cultural Issues" as one of their standards. Although CACREP is not specific about how programs should incorporate multicultural theory and practice, counselor training programs tend to either weave multicultural perspectives throughout their counseling program, offer separate course work in multicultural counseling, or do both (Das, 1995; Garcia, Wright, & Corey, 1991).

The integration of multicultural training into our graduate programs is critical if future counselors are to work effectively with culturally different clients (Fukuyama, 1994; Yutrzenka, 1995). One method of increasing the efficacy of training in multicultural counseling has been the development, dissemination, and implementation of the competencies, standards, and ethical guidelines noted earlier. To assure that training competencies are being met, Ponterotto, Alexander, and Grieger (1995) offer a checklist to assess whether or not programs meet minimum competencies and standards for training in multicultural counseling. Your professor may want to review these standards and discuss whether your program meets them.

In addition to training standards, new models to assist in the training of students in cross-cultural counseling will have to be developed if students are to work effectively with culturally different clients. One such model, developed by Pedersen (2001), suggests that a safe environment be created for the counselor to learn about the culturally different client. In this triad model, the client, the counselor, an anticounselor, and a procounselor all meet together during an interview with the function of the anticounselor being to highlight the differences in values and expectations between the client and counselor while the procounselor highlights similarities in values and expectations. The procounselor and anticounselor give continual and immediate feedback to the counselor in an effort to increase the counselor's ability to understand the client's perspective, recognize client resistance, recognize the counselor's defensiveness, and learn how to recover from mistakes that the counselor might make during the interview. Although Pedersen's model is a start, other models that find new and effective ways of training in cross-cultural counseling are sorely needed.

Association for Multicultural Counseling and Development

In an effort to supply leadership for helping professionals in the area of multicultural counseling, the Association of Multicultural Counseling and Development (AMCD), a division of ACA, provides workshops, graduate program training standards in multicultural counseling, and publications, such as the *Journal of Multicultural Counseling and Development*. If you have a particular interest in multicultural counseling, training, and research, you might consider joining AMCD (reach AMCD via www.counseling.org).

Knowledge of Legal Trends

In just about every chapter of this text you will find some legislative initiative that addresses multicultural concerns. And every year new laws will be passed, and old ones will be amended. Counselors need to have intimate knowledge of the law and how it affects the culturally different client if they are to (1) assist the client in advocating for his or her rights; (2) be an advocate for the client; (3) campaign for legislative initiatives on the local, state, and national level; and (4) protect themselves from potential malpractice suits.

The Counselor in Process: Working with Culturally Different Clients

Sue and Sue (1999) note that working with culturally different clients should be viewed as a constantly changing process. In this context, they note that the helping relationship "is an active process, that it is ongoing, and that it is a process that never reaches an end point. Implicit is recognition of the complexity and diversity of the client and client populations, and acknowledgment of our own personal limitations and the need to always improve" (p. 227).

One way that counselors can assure that they are continually improving their ways of interacting with clients from diverse backgrounds is through supervision. Although supervision is crucial throughout the counselor's professional life, with minority clients having higher dropout rates from counseling and being less satisfied with counseling (Quintana & Bernal, 1995), adequate supervision of cross-cultural counseling relationships becomes even more critical. Counselors must assure that they are reaching all of their clients. They cannot idly stand by and assume that their work with minority clients is as effective as their work with majority clients.

Summary

This chapter reviewed theoretical and practice issues related to multicultural counseling. We started the chapter by noting that over the years multicultural counseling has been defined in different ways, some insisting that multicultural counseling should focus only on those minority groups that have been most discriminated against, while others insist that all counseling relationships are of a multicultural nature. Taking somewhat of a middle-of-the-road approach, we defined multicultural counseling as a relationship with a helper and a client, where the client is from a different culture of the counselor.

We next discussed some of the reasons why multicultural counseling has become so important. We first noted that many clients from different cultures are misdiagnosed and dissatisfied with counseling and drop out of counseling at high rates. We then noted a number of reasons why minority clients are poorly served in counseling. We pointed out that some counselors (1) view this country as a melting pot instead of a cultural mosaic,

(2) have incongruent expectations about counseling, (3) lack an understanding of social forces, (4) have an ethnocentric worldview, (5) are ignorant of their own prejudices, (6) are unable to understand that the expression of symptomatology is often a function of culture, (7) have used assessment and research instruments that are biased and unreliable, (8) are unaware of how institutional racism affects the counseling process, and (9) are uninformed about how the counseling process only works well with certain kinds of clients.

In an effort to give us common ground on which to communicate, a number of terms were defined in this chapter. We defined the terms *culture*, *race*, *ethnicity*, *social class*, *power differentials*, *minority*, *stereotypes*, *prejudice*, *racism*, and *discrimination*. We noted that surveys have shown that discrimination is still quite prevalent in this society. We also discussed the politically correct terms that are generally used to describe various cultural groups in the United States.

In this chapter a number of conceptual models were offered to help us understand our work with clients from diverse backgrounds. Speight and associates (1991) offered us a model that helps us understand how each individual is unique *(Eigenwelt)*, shares experiences with a culture *(Mitwelt)*, and shares universal experiences *(Umwelt)*. Describing a model of minority development, Bell and Evans (1981) explained differences between four styles of relating to the world, which included the acculturated, bicultural, culturally immersed, and traditional interpersonal styles. Offering a developmental perspective, Atkinson and associates (1998) proposed a five-stage model of minority identity development, which included conformity, dissonance, resistance and immersion, introspection, and synergetic awareness and integration.

Whereas minority identity models help the counselor understand the culturally different client and assist minority counselors in understanding themselves, models of white identity development help the white graduate student in counseling understand how he or she might react to minority clients. Sabnani and colleagues (1991) found common themes running through three models of white identity development and subsequently developed a model that has five stages through which many white counseling students might pass as they attend graduate school. Their model includes the pre-exposure, exposure, prominority/antiracism, retreat to white culture, and redefinition and integration stages.

In order to work effectively with clients from diverse backgrounds, a number of authors have suggested that it is important that counselors understand their attitude and beliefs, have a basic knowledge of many of the cultures from which our clients come, and know the skills necessary to work with clients from diverse cultures.

Within this chapter the possibility was raised that multicultural counseling may represent a new paradigm in the counseling profession. However, the process of applying theory to practice has been slow, and we were called to challenge ourselves and our colleagues to develop new theories and adapt existing theories to the multicultural counseling setting. We asserted that counseling programs must integrate multicultural training standards if multicultural counseling is to become a fourth force.

We stressed in the chapter that training programs that follow the *Multicultural Counseling Competencies and Standards* and the CACREP standards offer us the best chance to help counselors understand themselves and apply their knowledge and skills within the cross-cultural counseling relationship. Besides training standards, it was stressed that new training models, such as Pedersen's (2001) triad model, need to be developed to assist students in becoming more effective cross-cultural helpers.

Near the end of the chapter we highlighted some of the important activities of the Association of Multicultural Counseling and Development (AMCD), a division of ACA.

We also stressed that many laws now affect minority clients, and counselors were called to have intimate knowledge of legal issues if they are to best service their clients and be advocates for multicultural issues.

Finally, we concluded the chapter by presenting Sue and Sue's (1999) belief that multicultural counseling is a constantly changing process that is active, ongoing, and never ending. As counselors, we must continually stretch ourselves to work with clients from many different cultures.

INFOTRAC and Other Information Resources (e.g., ERIC and PsycINFO)

Note: When relevant, key words are in quotation marks.

1. Research any of the minority identity models in more detail.
2. Examine the research on the "efficacy of counseling minorities."
3. Review the literature on theories of counseling when working with minorities.

CHAPTER **15**

Knowledge and Skills of Multicultural Counseling

You scorn us, you imitate us, you blame us, you indulge us, you throw up your hands, you tell us you have all the answers, now shut up and listen. (Lamar, 1992, p. 90)

I wondered about whether I should include a section of my book on some of the unique characteristics of culturally diverse people in the United States. My concern was that by highlighting differences, this chapter would promote differentness, and the reader might generalize to all members of a group from characteristics held by some of the group.

I continue to have this hesitance, and I urge each of you who read this chapter not to jump to conclusions when working with a culturally different client. However, when editing this chapter, I was taken by the important history and the cultural uniqueness of each group mentioned. Let me share a few points that stood out. For example, as I reread this chapter I was again astounded by the number of slaves who died coming over to this country and how Japanese were interned in America during the Second World War. I was reminded of the strong nationalism felt by many Hispanics and of the uniqueness of each American Indian tribe. I read again the fact that most gays do not live a "gay and lesbian lifestyle," and that there are some very distinct skills one may want to consider when counseling women and when counseling men. I was reminded of the many, many different religions across this land. And I remembered that each of us has special needs that can be addressed in the counseling relationship if the counselor wants to take the time to find out what those needs are.

We should not assume that, because a person comes from a minority group, he or she shares the characteristics of that group; however, having knowledge about different groups can assist us in understanding individuals who do share many of the characteristics of that group. The fact is that most of us are blind to the history and cultural values of many of the cultural/ethnic groups outside of our own sphere. Therefore, this chapter hopes to give you a taste of the history and culture of some of the people who share our society while stimulating your interest about multicultural counseling. We cannot touch on all diversity in America, for to do so would require much more than one small chapter. However, we can spend a little time focusing on some of the groups of people that have been most obviously discriminated against (although I'm sure some will argue with me about the inclusion of "men"). Finally, by noting special issues and identifying counseling strategies unique to the groups identified, we will attempt to offer you ways in which you can optimally work with clients from diverse groups.

After discussing a number of cultural/ethnic groups we will examine the debate in the profession concerning the importance of being knowledgeable about all cultures when doing counseling. Near the end of the chapter we will discuss the ethical guidelines of ACA, their relevance to cross-cultural counseling, and ethical decision making from a cross-cultural perspective. We will conclude the chapter by considering the future of cross-cultural counseling. But first let's start by examining just how diverse we are!

The Changing Face of America

America is the most diverse country in the world and is becoming increasingly more so. In fact, today, almost 30% of Americans are racial and ethnic minorities (U.S. Census Bureau, 2001a), and midway through this century minorities will constitute almost 50% of the American population (U.S. Census Bureau, 2001b). Some of these changes will include an increase in Native Americans from 0.9% to 1.1%, Asian and Pacific Islanders from 4.2% to 9.3%, Hispanics from 12.1% to 24.3%, and African Americans from 12.9% to 14.7%, and a decrease in white Americans from 71% to 52.8% (see Figure 15.1).

These changing demographics are a function of a number of factors, including higher birth rates of culturally diverse populations, the fact that most immigrants no longer come from Western countries, and because immigration rates are the largest in American history. With the great majority of immigrants now being Asian (39%) or Hispanic (43%) (U.S. Census Bureau, 2001c), as compared to past immigrants who were mostly white European,

FIGURE 15.1
Percent of Population by Race/Culture Over Time

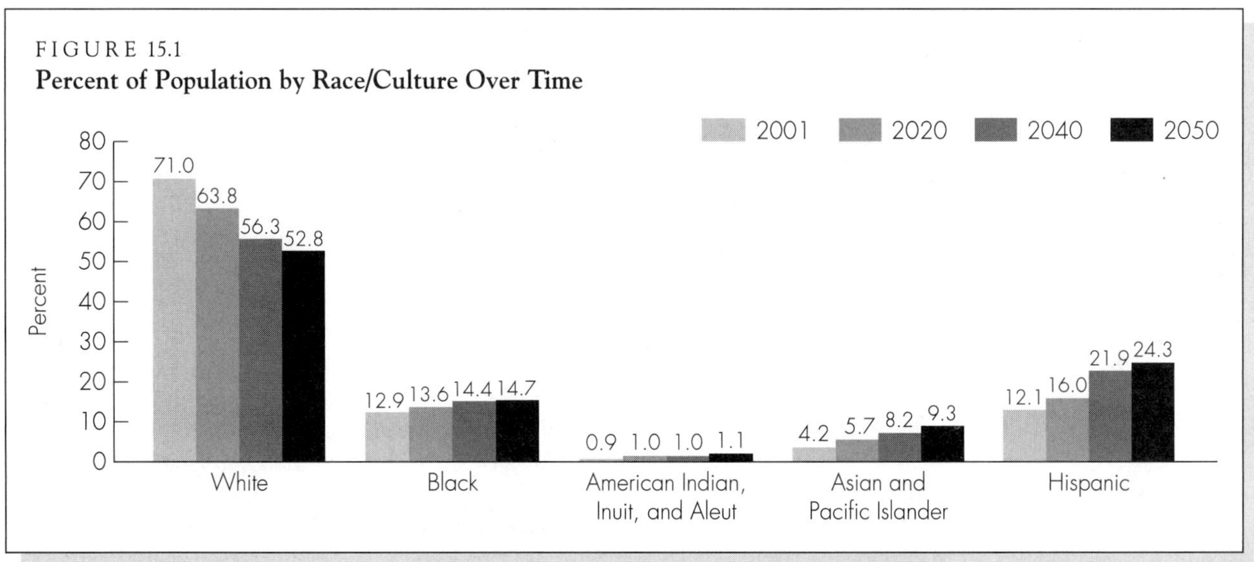

they have a greater tendency to want to assert their cultural heritage rather than be swallowed up by the Western-based American culture.

Changes in the racial, ethnic, and cultural backgrounds of Americans bring with them changes in the religious composition of the country. As increasing numbers of Asians, Hispanics, and people from the Middle East arrive at our shores, we will find religions that were previously rare in America. But diversity in religion is not only brought to us by our immigrants. Although America is a country that is largely Christian, diversity in Christianity in America is now greater than ever. From a multitude of Protestant faiths, to Roman Catholics who are increasingly varied in their beliefs, to Eastern Orthodox, Mormons, Christian Scientists, Seventh Day Adventists, Amish, Mennonites, and on and on, Christian religion in America is a religious mosaic in and of itself.

In addition to the changing ethnic, cultural, and religious diversity in America, today there are changes in sex-role identity. The macho male is no longer considered a model for maleness, while expectations concerning the woman's role in the workplace and as a child care provider have changed dramatically. Also, in America today we see increased awareness of the gay and lesbian subculture. Whereas in the past many homosexuals felt a need to hide their sexual preference for fear of discrimination, today we find an increasing number of gays and lesbians coming out. In addition, changes in federal, state, and local laws as well as a gradual move toward more tolerance of difference in our culture have given us an increased sensitivity and awareness of a number of special groups, including the physically challenged, older persons, the homeless and the poor, individuals who are HIV positive, the mentally ill, and others. Let's spend a little time examining all of these groups.

Understanding and Counseling Select Culturally Diverse Groups

The following are behaviors, values, and customs that some groups tend to embrace as well as some information that you might find interesting about these groups. It is hoped that this section will offer you valuable knowledge about how to work with individuals from these diverse groups. As noted in Chapter 14, when reading this section, remember that effective cross-cultural counselors (1) have examined their attitudes and beliefs, (2) are knowledgeable in that they are willing to learn about history and customs of various groups, and (3) have the skills and are open to learning specific counseling skills applicable to varying populations.

People from Varying Cultural/Racial Heritages

African Americans

Today there are approximately 35 million Americans of African heritage—about 12% of the population. Of these, nearly 90% are descendants from slaves. Conditions in the ships that brought the slaves were deplorable, and it is estimated that 6 to 10 million Africans died in passage (Allen & Turner, 1988). By 1790, 19% of the U. S. population was of African heritage, with this percentage dropping after slave trading was made illegal in 1809. By 1860, 90% of African Americans lived in the South and tended to remain there following the Civil War, becoming sharecroppers or working for white farmers. Restrictive work laws and lack of education made it difficult for blacks to leave the South. It wasn't until the early 1900s that blacks began to move to urban centers where there were hopes of better educational and career opportunities and to leave increasing violence toward blacks in the South. However, more recently there has been a reversal of this trend, with better educated blacks moving to the South to obtain higher-level jobs.

Laws restricting access to education, work, and recreational facilities and generally supporting segregation continued in some states until the early 1970s. With racism and prejudice being endemic throughout American society, it was necessary in 1991 to pass the Civil Rights Act to protect minority workers, particularly African Americans, from discriminatory practices in employment. There is no question that African Americans have been particularly oppressed in this country—and we are all still paying the price for this oppression.

Today, African Americans continue to have to fight racism and prejudice, although such attitudes now often exist in much more subtle, covert, and unconscious ways. In fact, 38% of all incidents of hate crimes are perpetrated against African Americans (FBI, 1999)! Although a large number of African Americans have now assimilated into middle-class America, there continues to be a large underclass of African Americans who have little opportunity for upward mobility in American society (Axelson, 1999). We must all take responsibility for the continued oppression and discrimination against African Americans in today's society and work collectively to end it.

Perhaps more than any other cultural group, African Americans' values are differentially affected as a function of their social class, experience with racism, and the degree to which they have been exposed to African heritage. However, some commonalities may exist among many African Americans. Generally, African Americans are group oriented and value cooperation and interdependence, especially in relationship to the extended family and the community. The extended family can be varied and is particularly important, and family matters tend to be kept within the family or extended family (McGoldrick et al., 1996). Exposure to racism may justifiably make some African Americans guarded, defensive, and minimally verbal with whites, including white counselors (Phelps et al., 2001). On the other hand, these same individuals may be open, expressive, and responsive with other African Americans. Recently, many African Americans have rediscovered some of the cultural values of their African heritage as is reflected in the commemoration of Kwanzaa, in which the principles of "unity, self-determination, collective work and responsibility, collective sharing, purpose, creativity, and faith" are celebrated (Axelson, 1999, p. 119).

Finally, African Americans vary widely in their connectedness to their culture, and one must assess the degree to which their culture affects them if one is to work effectively with a black client (see "Minority Identity Models," Chapter 14).

Hispanics: People of Central American, South American, and Caribbean Origin

Collectively, people of Central America, South America, and from various islands in the Caribbean are called Hispanic, sometimes Latino or Latina, although most Hispanics would likely state their country of origin when asked to describe their cultural heritage (Castex, 1998). Most Hispanics in this country have origins in Mexico, Puerto Rico, or Cuba, with lesser numbers from such countries as Haiti, Guatemala, Panama, the Dominican Republic, Brazil, Jamaica, and the West Indian islands (see Chapter 14, Table 14.1).

Because much of California was a northern province of Mexico, a large number of Mexicans became citizens of California when it achieved statehood in 1850. Other Mexican Americans first emigrated here in the middle 1800s, traveling north from Mexico to the Southwest and West, looking for gold in California, good grazing land for cattle, and economic prosperity. A second wave of Mexican immigrants arrived here in the late 1800s and early 1900s with many moving to California. Today over 50% of the Mexican American population live in California.

Most Puerto Ricans settled in the United States during the 20th century. In 1898, following the Spanish American War, Puerto Rico became a territory of the United States. In 1917 Puerto Ricans were given citizenship, and in 1952 Puerto Rico became a Commonwealth of the United States. Over the years many Puerto Ricans have moved to New York City, where there were hopes of a better life, and more recently there has been a large migration of Puerto Ricans west in search of better employment opportunities. Although Puerto Rico has one of the best economies of Latin America, it lags far behind the economy in the 50 states.

Most Cubans came to the United States in the late 1950s and early 1960s following Fidel Castro's overthrow of the Cuban dictatorship under Batista. Cubans came to the United States out of fear of persecution and imprisonment and out of ideological differences with the communist regime. The vast majority of Cubans settled in southern Florida, although there are sizable communities in New York, Chicago, and Los Angeles.

In America today there is a sizable number of Americans of Spanish descent who arrived here from Central and South America. Many of these people settled along the Rio Grande, although during the 1800s many of these individuals migrated to New Mexico, Arizona, and Colorado. Finally, from the 1960s until recently, due to political turmoil in their own countries of origin, many people from Central America have migrated to the United States.

Many Hispanics in the United States are poor and have had a difficult time acculturating and becoming upwardly mobile. A number of reasons account for this. For instance, many Hispanics have not established roots in this country due to the proximity of their countries of origin, the lack of economic opportunity as compared to past immigrants, the ability to make frequent trips back to their countries of origin, and the fact that shared common language with other Hispanics makes it easier to maintain a Hispanic culture (Axelson, 1999).

Although the term *Hispanic* is used to describe individuals with origins from a number of countries, there is great disparity in the culture of these individuals and, when working with Hispanics, it is best to have knowledge of the client's country of origin or ancestry. Mostly, the term *Hispanic* has been utilized "to further mutual interests or to resolve a problem, such as in education, employment, or social inequality" (Axelson, 1999, p. 121). There are certain values and customs, however, that are shared by most Hispanics. For instance, the extended family is emphasized and interdependence is valued over independence. Also, the Hispanic family tends to be patriarchal and follow traditional sex roles. In addition, in Hispanic culture, individuals are respected based on their age, socioeconomic status, gender, and the perception of the individual's importance. Finally, many Hispanics tend to deeply embrace traditional Catholic values while at the same time believing in cultural fatalism or the belief that life is out of one's control (Comas-Diaz, 1993).

When working with Hispanic clients it is important to recognize that they tend to feel a strong sense of nationality to their country of origin, and counselors should be careful to not lump all Hispanics together into one group. Therefore, it is crucial that the counselor understands the client's unique values, behaviors, symbols, and even language, all of which are functions of the client's country of origin. Although great differences will exist among Hispanic clients, based on their country of origin, it is still prudent to assess the degree to which some of the common qualities noted above may motivate the Hispanic client.

People of Asian and Pacific Island Origin

The majority of people of Asian and Pacific Island origin include fairly large numbers of Chinese, Filipinos, Japanese, Koreans, Asian Indians, Vietnamese, and native Hawaiians, and lesser numbers of Laotian, Thai, Samoans, and Guamanians. In 1965 major changes in the immigration law created more equity in who could immigrate to the United States and resulted in an increase in Asian and Pacific Island immigrants from all of the 25 countries that make up this part of the world.

To escape poverty, many Chinese immigrated to the United States during the Californian gold rush of the mid-1800s. However, whites ousted many Chinese from the mines, and a large number ended up taking low-paying farm and blue-collar jobs. Because of prejudice and poor working conditions, many Chinese dispersed to Midwestern and Eastern cities. In addition, the development of Chinatowns represented a haven for many of the Chinese. Today, many Chinese have moved out of the Chinatowns, and these areas now generally house the poorer Chinese.

In the late 1800s, a large number of Japanese, Asian Indians, and Koreans settled in California, and like the Chinese, took low-paying farm jobs. During the Second World War, many west-coast Japanese Americans were forcibly removed from their homes and placed in internment camps. In 1943, some of the Japanese who were interned were able to leave the camps if they promised not to live on the west coast. Many of these moved to the Midwest while others chose to remain in the camps to the end of the war when they were allowed to resettle on the west coast. Japanese Americans who were placed in internment camps recently won a monetary settlement from the government for their hardship.

Following the end of the Spanish-American War in 1898, the United States set up colonial rule in the Philippines. Although this takeover of the Philippines was not met calmly by the Filipino people, it did lead to a large influx of Filipinos to this country. Many went to Hawaii and worked as sugar growers. In the 1920s and 1930s many Filipinos moved to California and Alaska, some for low-paying jobs and others to pursue an education. In addition, until recently, Filipinos who enlisted in the armed services for a specified length of time could obtain citizenship, and many therefore relocated to naval cities such as Norfolk, VA.

Following the Korean and Vietnam wars, large numbers of Koreans and Vietnamese emigrated to this country. A sizable number of Korean immigrants were war brides, war orphans, and professionals, whereas many of the Vietnamese immigrants were refugees from the Vietnam War and were brought to this country following the fall of South Vietnam to the communists.

Although some general customs are shared among people of Asian and Pacific Island origin, as with Hispanics, there is great variability in the customs and traditions among the varying countries. A few of the similar values among people of this area include the fact that children tend to be obligated to parents and place them first, family members are highly interdependent, families are generally patriarchal and sons are highly valued, guilt and shame is used to control the behavior of family members, individuals are restrained and pride themselves on their ability to control their feelings, and formality in social relationships is the norm (Sue & Sue, 1998).

When working with an Asian client it is important to have knowledge about the client's country of origin. Differences in language, social behavior, economic development, and history are vast and should not be underestimated, because they greatly affect the Asian client's way of living in the world. On the other hand, a counselor should also assess the degree to which some common qualities, as noted above, may be embraced by the Asian client.

Native Americans

Native Americans consist of three major groups: American Indians, Aleuts, and Inuits (Eskimos). These groups have dramatically different histories and cultural values and should not be confused with one another.

Approximately 10,000 years ago, people from Siberia crossed over the Bering Strait land bridge to what is now Alaska. Some of these people headed westward toward the Aleutian Islands and are now called Aleuts, whereas others headed north and east and are now called Inuits (Eskimos). Alaska, which was owned by Russia, sent Russian Orthodox missionaries to bring Christianity to Alaskan natives. Today, there are approximately 57,000 Inuits and 24,000 Aleuts (U.S. Census Bureau, 2001d).

American Indians were numerous when Columbus landed in America; however, due to disease brought by the Europeans and the wars they initiated, today there are only about 1.9 million. With 150 to 200 tribal languages and close to 900 federal and state-recognized tribes and bands, American Indians are a diverse group (LaFromboise, 1998; Thomason, 1993). Although there are some commonalities among American Indians, differences among tribes are great.

Approximately one-half of all American Indians live on reservations where living conditions are not good and social problems, which can be traced back to the uprooting of their civilization, are great (Heinrich, Corbine, & Thomas, 1990). Social problems include poor health care, malnutrition, and high rates of unemployment, suicide, chemical dependence, illiteracy, and delinquency (LaFromboise, 1998). American Indians also have higher rates of emotional illness, most likely related to their serious social problems. Unfortunately, American Indians tend to underutilize available mental health services.

American Indians tend to view mental health problems from a spiritual and holistic perspective (LaFromboise, Trimble, & Mohatt, 1998). Such problems are seen as an extension of the community, and thus the community is often actively involved in the healing process. The use of ceremony, storytelling, and metaphor are important in understanding the individual, and often the American Indian's connection to the community is an important part of the healing process.

As with Hispanics and Asians, it is important to understand the unique language and cultural traditions of the tribe with which the Native American has been affiliated. In addition, as many Native Americans have acculturated, when counseling Native Americans it is important to assess how much their culture of origin continues to influence their lives.

Counseling Individuals from Different Cultures

Although cultural differences are great among African Americans, Asian Americans, Hispanics, and Native Americans, there are some broad suggestions that one can make when working with individuals from these cultures (Garrett & Pichette, 2000; Neukrug, 1994, 2002; Westwood & Ishiyama, 1990):

1. *Have the right attitudes and beliefs, gain knowledge, and learn skills.* Be prepared to work with clients with varying cultural heritages by embracing the appropriate knowledge, skills, and beliefs prior to meeting with them.
2. *Encourage clients to speak their own language.* Make an effort to know meaningful expressions of the client's language. When language becomes a significant barrier, refer to a counselor who speaks the client's language.
3. *Assess the cultural identity of the client.* Use the racial identity models in Chapter 14 to assist in knowing how to work with clients. For example, a client who has acculturated and has little identification with his or her culture of origin is very different from a client from the same culture of origin who is a new immigrant.
4. *Check the accuracy of your client's nonverbals.* Don't assume that nonverbal communication is consistent across cultures. Ask the client about his or her nonverbals when in doubt.
5. *Make use of alternate modes of communication.* Use appropriate alternative modes of communication, such as acting, drawing, music, story telling, collage making, and so forth, to draw out clients who are reticent to talk or have communication problems.
6. *Encourage clients to bring in culturally significant and personally relevant items.* Have clients bring in items to better understand them and their culture (e.g., books, photographs, articles of significance, culturally meaningful items, and the like).
7. *Vary the helping environment.* When appropriate, explore alternative helping environments to ease the client into the helping relationship (e.g., take a walk, have a cup of coffee at a quiet restaurant, initially meet your client at his or her home, and so forth).

Religious Diversity in America

The religious makeup of the American people has shifted dramatically since 1960, and there is every indication that those trends will continue in the future. In general, the nation has become less distinctly Protestant and more pluralistic in character (Gallup, 2001). As with racial and cultural background, the United States is truly a diverse country when it comes to religion. In the United States today there are close to 75 religious groups each having over 50,000 members (Bedell, 1996). Of the millions of Americans who report some affiliation with a religious group, approximately 64% of them are Protestant. But even in this religious tradition, there is considerable variability in beliefs and traditions as we find such diverse groups as Baptists, Methodists, Lutherans, Presbyterians, Episcopalians, and others. In addition to these diverse Protestant groups, a large number of Americans identify themselves as Roman Catholic and lesser numbers are Muslim, Jewish, and literally dozens of other religions (Gallup, 2001; http://www.adherents.com). With 65% of Americans claiming religious affiliation and 85% stating that religion is fairly or very important in their lives (Gallup, 2001), it is clear that understanding the diversity of religious beliefs in America is extremely important.

As one might expect, there is a relationship between religious affiliation and social class, culture, ethnicity, race, and political attitudes (Macionis, 2001), although one should be careful not to stereotype a person too readily based on his or her religious affiliation. For many within a specific cultural group, religion can be a unifying factor and offer a sense of community, direction, and strength (Locke, 1998). However, religion can also be divisive, such as when wars are started over religious differences and individuals are oppressed because of their religious beliefs. With the great diversity of religion in this country, and knowing that religious affiliation is closely aligned with cultural factors, it is a sad statement that in many texts and articles on multicultural counseling religion has little or no mention. With this in mind, we will examine, very briefly, five religions.

Christianity

Founded 2000 years ago on the teachings of Jesus of Nazareth, Christianity now represents close to 2 billion of the world's population. Starting as a Judaic movement, followers of Jesus believed him to be the Christ, "the chosen one," fulfilling God's promise of salvation. Although Judaism eventually rejected Jesus as the Christ/Messiah, Christianity was born, and the teaching of Jesus was consolidated into what we now call the New Testament. Over the centuries, interpretation of the Gospel (the "good news" of Jesus) has varied greatly as a function of the religious scholar or leader. Thus, throughout the world we have seen the development of many different Christian religious groups that have ranged from conservative to liberal in their interpretations of the Gospel. In fact, Bedell (1996) notes that there are a few hundred Christian sects, all of which espouse slightly different forms of Christianity:

> *A committee consisting of one member from each of: Episcopal, Jehovah's Witness, Methodist, Mormon, Presbyterian, Southern Baptist and Unity Church would probably fail to reach a consensus on almost any basic Christian belief or practice. In fact, some committee members would probably refuse to recognize some of the others as fellow Christians.* (Ontario consultants . . . , 1997)

Differences among Christian churches and between Christian religions and non-Christian religions have led to tensions among people throughout the world. On the other hand, Christianity has also brought people together in a common worship of Jesus as part of the Holy Trinity along with God the Father and the Holy Spirit. In addition it has also offered answers to questions about life's meaning and has been an important factor in focusing world attention on the importance of assisting those in need.

Buddhism

Founded around 525 B.C.E. in India by the Buddha, Gautama Siddhartha, Buddhism is based on the Tripaka, teachings of the Buddha, and the Sutras, which are comments about Buddha's teachings. These texts are philosophical in nature and speak to the monastic life. Four truths of Buddhism include (1) the truth of suffering; (2) the cause of suffering, which is desire; (3) the cessation of suffering, which is the renunciation of desire; and (4) the way that leads to the cessation of suffering (Bach, 1959). Related to these truths, Buddhists believe that reality is an illusion, that one lives and is reborn due to attachment to an illusory self, and that Nirvana is reached when, through meditation, you can transcend attachment to the illusory self. The actual practice of Buddhism varies greatly depending on the sect to which the person belongs. Although Buddhists represent 6% of the population of the world, in American culture Buddhism continues to be misunderstood and viewed as somewhat of an oddity.

Hinduism

Hinduism began to develop around 1500 B.C.E. when Aryan invaders of India intermixed their religious practices and beliefs with the native Indians. The sacred texts include the Veda, Upanishads, Bhagavadgita, Mahabharata, and Ramayana. These texts are mythological and philosophical commentaries about life. Although the religion speaks to many gods, heroes, and saints, Hindus believe in one divine principle, that many gods are aspects of a single divine unity. Hindus believe that people are born and reborn based on their *samsara,* or separation from the divine, and that one's *karma,* or total way of acting and being, can be improved through pure actions and meditation. Through these pure acts, one can eventually become closer to the divine. Hindus believe that reincarnation is the road to unity with the divine and that it answers many perplexing questions, such as why there are so many personalities in this world. Although Hindus represent 13% of the population of the world, like Buddhists, Hindus are misunderstood and considered strange by many Americans.

Islam

Fully 18% of the world is Islamic, and yet this mostly nonauthoritarian and egalitarian religion continues to be misunderstood by most Americans. Following the beliefs established in 622 by Muhammad, the Prophet, Muslims accept Allah (God) as the creator of the universe, merciful, kind, and all powerful. Humans are seen as the highest creation of God, good by their very nature, although they are capable of forgetting their true nature and can be misled by Satan. However, Muslims believe that if a person forgets his or her true nature, he or she can repent, return to a state of remembering, and go to Paradise. Two of the major texts of Muslims are the Quran, which is said to be the true word of God given by the angel Gabriel to Muhammad, and the Hadith. Muslims have five duties to which they should adhere: to profess their faith to Allah, to pray five times a day, to give regularly a portion of their material wealth to charity, to fast daily until sundown during the month of Ramadan, and to attempt to make at least one pilgrimage to Mecca.

In the United States, Muslims have obtained an undeserved negative reputation. This has been particularly so since the tragedy at the World Trade Center where some Americans view the majority of Muslims and Arabs as closed-minded terrorists. Certainly, the vast majority of Muslims are peace loving, and in sync with the teachings of Muhammad as purported in the Quran.

Judaism

Judaism is a monotheistic religion that began to coalesce around the year 1300 B.C.E. It is an evolving religious civilization whose purpose is to transform what is into what should be, which includes peace and cooperation, the love and acceptance of others, and a progressive view toward life. Judaism is based on the Hebrew Bible, which includes the five books attributed to Moses (called the Torah), the writings of the prophets, and the writings of the ancient historians, kings, and wisdom-teachers. Later writings called the Talmud, which are interpretations by teachers (rabbis) and judges of the early writings, are also used as a basis for knowledge and worship.

Adherence to Jewish laws varies from those who are very orthodox to those who are very liberal, although the majority of Jews in America are somewhere in between on this continuum. Some of the major holidays include Rosh Hashanah, the new year; Yom

Kippur, the day of atonement for one's sins; Hanukkah, the festival of lights; and Passover, which celebrates the liberation of Jews from slavery in Egypt and is symbolic of liberation in general. Finally, the Bar or Bat Mitzvah, a religious celebration of a child entering adulthood at age 13, is another major Jewish ceremony to which many Jews adhere.

Jews have faced a particularly long history of oppression. Despite the fact that the Jewish religion is a peaceful, forward-thinking religion, and that Jewish individuals have fully assimilated into American society, false stereotypes of Jews continue, and discrimination against Jews is still evident. In fact, 65% of Americans believe Jews are discriminated against, and 14% of all hate crimes have been committed against Jews despite the fact that they represent only 2% of the population (ADL, 1992; FBI, 1999).

Counseling Individuals from Diverse Religious Backgrounds

A client's religious background and current religious beliefs may hold the key to understanding the underlying values that motivate him or her. Some pointers to keep in mind concerning religion and the counseling relationship include (Faiver, O'Brien, & Ingersoll, 2000; personal communication with Dr. John Lanci, May 1, 2002; Zinnbauer & Pargament, 2000):

1. *Have the right attitudes and beliefs, gain knowledge, and learn skills*. Be prepared to work with clients of different religions by embracing the appropriate knowledge, skills, and beliefs prior to meeting with them.
2. *Determine the client's religious background early in counseling*. To assist in treatment planning, know the client's religious affiliation. Be sensitive to any client who may resist discussion of his or her religious background.
3. *Ask the client how important religion is in his or her life*. Assess the part religion plays in a client's life to assist in goal setting and treatment planning. Do not assume that clients know much about their religion because they present themselves as deeply religious, or know little because they are not religious.
4. *Assess the client's level of faith development*. Assess the client's faith development to determine how you will work with the client. For instance, a dualist would most likely work better with a fair amount of structure and the setting of firm goals, while an individual of higher faith development would be likely to feel more comfortable in a counseling relationship that values abstract thinking and self-reflection (see Chapter 9).
5. *Don't make false assumptions*. Don't stereotype (e.g., the counselor who assumes all Jews keep kosher homes). Don't project (e.g., the counselor who is Christian and assumes that people of all faiths are born with original sin) (see Box 15.1).
6. *Be familiar with your client's religious beliefs and important holidays and traditions*. Become familiar with your client's religion to show respect and understanding and to not embarrass yourself (e.g., a Muslim would not want to be offered food during the month of Ramadan).
7. *Understand that religion can deeply affect a client on many levels, including unconscious ones*. Understand that some clients who deny a religious affiliation (e.g., "lapsed Catholics") are still driven unconsciously by the basic tenets of the religious beliefs they were originally taught (e.g., a client may continue to feel guilty over certain issues related to the religious beliefs he or she was taught despite the fact that the client insists he or she is no longer affected by his or her religion).

BOX 15.1

Religion as Projection of Self

My wife was raised Catholic, and I was raised Jewish. We have two daughters, who are 7 and 2, and we consider them Jewish and Catholic. When my oldest child was still an infant I remember telling a therapist I had been seeing how Jewish my daughter seemed and that I thought my wife would see her in this light also. After reflecting on this for a moment, he gave me one of those looks like, "Yeah, get real—you best check this out," but said, "uh huh." As soon as I got home I asked my wife, "Do you see Hannah as Jewish?" She laughed and said, "No, I think she seems Catholic." I was quickly reminded how so much of our inner experience is projected onto the world.

Gender Differences in America

There are many differences in the demographic characteristics between men and women. For example, the labor force growth rate of women has doubled that of men; today more men take on child care as compared to the past (although women continue to do most of the child care); men own the vast majority of corporations in America; regardless of occupation, on average, women earn less than men; women outlive men; women are less likely to finish college; elderly women are less likely to commit suicide than elderly men, and on and on (Chandras, 1991; Taeuber, 1996; United Nations, 2000).

In addition to demographic variations, the evidence that personality differences exist between males and females is also great (Burnett, Anderson, & Heppner, 1995). Some authors have found that men and women encounter different developmental tasks (Horst, 1995), while others have suggested that the male reality may be different than the female reality (Gilligan, 1982; Miller, 1976; Schaef, 1981). Whether these differences are a function of genetics and/or social forces is still unclear; however, it is obvious that generally, the ways men and women approach life are different (Gray, 1998). For instance, evidence suggests that generally men are more restrictive in their ability to express emotion, less communicative, have more difficulty with intimacy, and are more competitive than women; whereas women are usually more nurturing, more concerned about how their actions affect others, and have more difficulty expressing anger than men (Basse & Greenstreet, 1991; DeVoe, 1990; Rabinowitz, 1991; Sharkin, 1993). Also, women may struggle more than men with issues of self-esteem, especially in light of the fact that it seems easier for men to survive in this world than women (Burnett et al., 1995).

Because men tend to be in positions of power in this society, it is generally agreed that their power is sometimes used to oppress women. This oppression is endemic in American society and, as with racism, is often unconscious. However, it also has some devastating effects on the lives of men as the oppression of others unconsciously damages men's psyches and harms their souls. In addition to how oppression of others affects the oppressor, men have their own issues with which to deal, issues that can cause a wide range of psychological and physical problems (Osherson, 1986, United Nations, 2000).

The good news is that there is some evidence that both men and women are beginning to take on new roles in relationships, in families, and in the world of work. This may indeed be a positive change as some research seems to indicate that individuals who take on multiple roles, including nontraditional sex roles, may be more satisfied in life than those who do not (Hammond & Fong, 1988).

Counseling Women

Women and men share much in common, but each also has unique issues that may be of concern in counseling. As women seek out counseling more frequently than men, and because they are sometimes misunderstood by counselors, it is particularly important that counselors attempt to know some of the unique concerns of women (Simon, Gaul, Friedlander, & Heatherington, 1992; Worell, 1980):

- Women are sexually harassed on the job and at other places.
- Women receive less money for the same work as men.
- Job opportunities and job advancement are less for women than for men.
- Women are physically abused by their spouses or partners at alarming rates.
- Single and divorced women and their children are found below poverty level at alarming rates.
- Assumptions about the abilities of girls and women prevent females from realizing their potential.
- Women tend to be more comfortable with expression of sad feelings, intimacy, and nurturing behavior and less comfortable with the expression of anger and assertive behavior.
- Women, on average, tend to be less comfortable in competitive situations.
- Women are more frequently misdiagnosed than are men when seeking mental health services.
- Women are sometimes torn between their roles as nurturer and child-care provider and their place in the world of paid work.
- Nearly all cases of complaints made against therapists for sexual exploitation are from women complaining about male therapists.
- Women have biological issues unique to them (e.g., premenstrual syndrome, breast cancer, pregnancy, ovarian cysts, ovarian cancer).

Because some mental health professionals were concerned with the ways that women were treated by counselors/therapists, the Division of Counseling Psychology (Division 17) of the APA developed 13 guiding principles for counselors and therapists when working with women (Fitzgerald & Nutt, 1998) (see Box 15.2).

Feeling that the guidelines have not gone far enough, some feminist therapists offer a more radical approach to working with women. Feminist therapists generally believe that issues brought by women to counseling relationships are inextricably related to oppression of women in society (Fitzgerald & Nutt, 1998; Gladding, 2000). They suggest that counseling offers women an opportunity to develop their female identity and argue that female therapists can usually be more productive in this process (McNamara & Rickard, 1989). This process involves helping female clients examine how their presenting problems may be related to sociopolitical issues. Psychodynamic and cognitive behavioral strategies are downplayed, and the therapist actively assists the client to move toward autonomy, self-sufficiency, and becoming an advocate for female issues. Downing and Roush (1985) offer one such model that includes five stages:

> *Stage I: Establish a relationship and demystify the counseling process.* Here counselors may downplay the "expert" role and encourage the women to trust themselves. Counselors may identify with client issues and self-disclose as a way of forming a close relationship. Counselors can assist in identifying social issues related to client problem(s) and use them to set goals.

BOX 15.2

Guidelines for Working with Women

I. Counselors/therapists should be knowledgeable about women, particularly with regard to biological, psychological, and social issues which have an impact on women in general or on particular groups of women in our society.

II. Counselors/therapists are aware that the assumptions and precepts of theories relevant to their practice may apply differently to men and women. Counselors/therapists are aware of those theories and models that prescribe or limit the potential of women clients, as well as those that may have particular usefulness for women clients.

III. After formal training, counselors/therapists continue to explore and learn of issues related to women, including the special problems of female subgroups, throughout their professional careers.

IV. Counselors/therapists recognize and are aware of all forms of oppression and how these interact with sexism.

V. Counselors/therapists are knowledgeable and aware of verbal and nonverbal process variables (particularly with regard to power in the relationship) as these affect women in counseling/therapy so that the counselor/therapist interactions are not adversely affected. The need for shared responsibility between clients and counselors/therapists is acknowledged and implemented.

VI. Counselors/therapists have the capability of utilizing skills that are particularly facilitative to women in general and to particular subgroups of women.

VII. Counselors/therapists ascribe no preconceived limitations on the direction or nature of potential changes or goals in counseling/therapy of women.

VIII. Counselors/therapists are sensitive to circumstances where it is more desirable for a woman client to be seen by a female or male counselor/therapist.

IX. Counselors/therapists use nonsexist language in counseling/therapy, supervision, teaching, and journal publication.

X. Counselors/therapists do not engage in sexual activity with their women clients under any circumstances.

XI. Counselors/therapists are aware of and continually review their own values and biases and the effects of these on their women clients. Counselors/therapists understand the effects of sex-role socialization upon their own development and functioning and the consequent values and attitudes they hold for themselves and others. They recognize that behaviors and roles need not be sex-based.

XII. Counselors/therapists are aware of how their personal functioning may influence their effectiveness in counseling/therapy with women clients. They monitor their functioning through consultation, supervision, or therapy, so that it does not adversely affect their work with women clients.

XIII. Counselors/therapists support the elimination of sex bias within institutions and individuals.

SOURCE: "The Division 17 Principles Concerning the Counseling/Psychotherapy of Women: Rationale and Implementation," by L. F. Fitzgerald and R. Nutt. In *Counseling diverse populations* (2nd ed.), by D. R. Atkinson and G. Hackett, pp. 229–261.

Stage II: Validate and legitimize a woman's angry feelings toward her predicament. Here counselors assist clients to understand how they have become victimized through sociopolitical forces. Counselors assist clients in combating feelings of powerlessness, helplessness, and low self-esteem. Counselors encourage participation in women's issues (books, seminars, women's groups).

Stage III: Provide a safe environment to express feelings as clients begin to form connections with other women. Here counselors validate feelings of fear and competition with other women that result from society's objectification of women. As these feelings dissipate, clients will move toward a strong and special connection to women. Counselors assist clients in understanding the difference between anger at a man and anger at a male-dominated system.

Stage IV: Help clients with conflicting feelings between traditional and newfound values. Here clients may feel torn between newfound feminist beliefs and values that do not seem congruent with those beliefs (e.g., wanting to stay home to raise the children). Counselors validate these contradictory feelings, acknowledge the confusion, and assist clients to fully explore their belief systems.

Stage V: Facilitate integration of client's new identity. Here counselors assist clients in integrating their newfound feminist beliefs with personal beliefs, even those personal beliefs that may not seem to be traditionally feminist. Clients are able to feel strength in their own identity development and no longer need to rely on an external belief system.

Counseling Men

You're just not allowed to have issues; you're just a white male.
(Kristina Williams-Neukrug)

Although concerns of men are generally quite different from those of women, they are no less important. As with women, men need to feel supported in therapy and not feel judged for having their own unique issues, issues that are common to the male experience and that cut across all racial, ethnic, and cultural groups. Men tend to seek counseling less frequently than women, attend counseling for fewer sessions than women, and seek counseling when in a state of crisis (Moore & Leafgren, 1990; NIMH, 1990; Scher, 1979, 1981); so it is particularly important to understand some of the unique concerns of men. For instance:

- Men tend to be more comfortable with angry feelings, aggression, and competitiveness, and less comfortable with sad feelings, collaboration, self-disclosure, and intimacy.
- Men are sometimes ostracized for expressing feelings, especially those considered to be traditionally feminine feelings, and yet criticized for not being more sensitive. Along these lines, men are sometimes torn between acting in the role of the strong male and being the sensitive, caring man.
- Men are criticized for being too controlling and made to feel inadequate if they do not take control.
- Men are socialized to be more aggressive and individualistic and are thus more prone to accidents, suicide, and acts of violence.
- Men are encouraged to be competitive and controlling (take charge), and yet these very behaviors lead to increased stress and are likely to play a factor in the shorter life expectancy of men as compared to women.
- Men are socialized to not be engaged in child rearing and yet are criticized for being distant fathers.
- Men have biological problems unique to them (e.g., prostate cancer, prostatitis, more tendency to stress-related diseases, testicular cancer).

Although the women's movement has led to numerous positive societal changes, including helping to sensitize men, it has also resulted in some therapists having taken on negative attitudes toward men and men's issues. These counselors will certainly not be effective with men in treatment. A counselor needs to be aware of men's issues and believe that they are real (Kelly & Hall, 1992; Osherson, 1986). A number of authors offer some ideas that can be incorporated into a set of guidelines when working with male clients (Osherson, 1986; Scher, 1981):

1. *Have the right attitudes and beliefs, gain knowledge, and learn skills.* Be prepared to work with men by embracing the appropriate knowledge, skills, and beliefs prior to meeting with them.
2. *Accept men where they are.* Accept men as they are in an effort to build trust. Men, who are often initially very defensive, will work hard on their issues once they can trust the counselor (Moore & Haverkamp, 1989; Scher, 1979).
3. *Don't push men to express what may be considered "softer feelings."* Don't push a man too quickly to express feelings, as you may push him out of the helping relationship. Men tend to be uncomfortable with certain feelings (e.g., deep sadness, feelings of incompetence, feelings of inadequacy, feelings of closeness), and more at ease with "thinking things through," problem solving, goal setting, and the expression of some other feelings, such as anger and pride.
4. *Early on in therapy, validate the man's feelings.* Validate a man's feelings, whatever they are. Remember that in order to protect their egos, men may initially blame others and society for their problems, which is often expressed through anger at others.
5. *Validate the man's view of how he has been constrained by male sex-role stereotypes.* Note, early in the therapy process, how the man is constrained by sex-role stereotypes and pressure in society (e.g., he must work particularly hard for his family). Validation of these views helps to build trust and establish the relationship.
6. *Have a plan for therapy.* Be clear with men that you want to develop a plan for therapy and collaborate with them on this plan. Men like structure and a sense of goal directedness even if it is changed later on.
7. *Begin to discuss developmental issues.* Introduce common male developmental issues so a man can quickly identify some concerns that may be impinging upon him (e.g., midlife crises) (Levinson,1985).
8. *Slowly encourage the expression of new feelings.* Reinforce the expression of these newfound feelings. Remember that men will begin to feel comfortable sharing what are typically considered to be more feminine feelings (e.g., tears, caring, feelings of intimacy) as trust is built.
9. *Explore underlying issues and reinforce new ways of understanding the world.* Explore underlying issues as they emerge (e.g., childhood issues, feelings of inadequacy, father–son issues). For example, how a father modeled for his son, distanced himself from him, and attempted to show his love to him and others in the family becomes the template for the male's relationships in the world, particularly his male relationships. The father relationship is a painful one to examine and the male client must learn how to "heal his wounded father" (Osherson, 1986):

   > *In order for us to be able to "hold" others as men, we have to imagine ourselves being held by our fathers, perhaps the first male we wanted to hold and be held by.* (Osherson, 1986, p. 213)

10. *Explore behavioral change.* Encourage men to try out new behaviors as insights into their old behaviors occur.
11. *Encourage the integration of newfound feelings, new ways of thinking about the world, and new behaviors.* Actively reinforce the expression of new feelings, newly gained insights, and new ways of acting in an effort to help the client integrate them into his way of living in the world.

12. *Encourage new male relationships*. Encourage new male friendships in which the client can freely express his feelings while maintaining his maleness. For instance, a men's group can offer men an opportunity to be build deeper, more intimate male relationships and also will challenge a man to change (Moore & Haverkamp, 1989; Williams & Myer, 1992).
13. *Say goodbye*. Be able to say goodbye and end the relationship. Although some men may want to continue in therapy, many will see it as time limited, a means to a goal.

Counseling Men and Women: A Final Viewpoint

Regardless of whether working with a man or a woman, an effective counselor needs to be aware of his or her own gender biases (Seem & Johnson, 1998). Knowledge of one's own biases can allow a counselor to be effective at what some have called gender-aware therapy (Good, Gilbert, & Scher, 1990). Such therapy considers gender central to counseling; views problems within a societal context; encourages counselors to actively address gender injustices; encourages the development of a collaborative and equal relationship; and respects the client's right to choose the gender roles appropriate for him- or herself regardless of their political correctness. Finally, we must always keep in mind that as many differences as there are between men and women, there is still much that we share in common. We must not overemphasize the differences, as we all share in the sea of humanity:

> *In general it is imperative that researchers learn to conceive of sex differences dialectically, constantly balancing the tendency to overemphasize differences with the tendency to underemphasize differences*. (Horst, 1995, p. 276)

Differences in Sexual Orientation

In his famous studies of the 1940s, Kinsey found that when examining male sexual preference 50% of men have had some sexual history with other males in their adult life, 13% had more homosexual than heterosexual experiences, 8% are exclusively homosexual for three years of their lives between the ages of 16 and 55, and 4% are exclusively homosexual throughout their lives (Kinsey, Pomeroy, & Martin, 1948; Kinsey, Pomeroy, Martin, & Gebhard, 1953). Kinsey also found that most individuals are not purely homosexual or heterosexual but rather fall on a continuum between homosexual and heterosexual feelings. Those who fall in the middle of the scale, Kinsey discovered, sometimes identify themselves as bisexual, but more often will identify themselves as either homosexual or heterosexual. Although some have questioned Kinsey's results (Cole, Gorman, Barrett, & Thompson, 1993), there is little doubt that a significant part of the population is gay, lesbian, bisexual, or not uniquely homosexual or heterosexual (see Table 14.1) (Singer & Deschamps, 1994). Regardless of the numbers of homosexuals or heterosexuals in society, the most current research suggests that sexual preference is determined very early in life, most likely related to biological and genetic factors, and has little if anything to do with choice (Finn, 1996).

Unfortunately, despite the fact that one is likely born homosexual (or heterosexual, or bisexual), homophobia, or fear of homosexuals, is still quite common (Gallup, 1999/2000). Like racism, homophobia can be seen as a distortion of reality, as the homosexual unconsciously represents a threat to the homophobic's understanding of sexuality.

BOX 15.3

Middle School Student Wins $900,000 in Gay-Bashing Case

Jamie Nobozny was spat on, subjected to a mock rape, urinated on, kicked in the stomach to the point where he needed surgery, and repeatedly beaten up at the middle school he attended in Eau Claire, Wisconsin. A student at the middle school said that Jamie was subjected to the violence because he "didn't act like we did . . . [and] was girlish." Suing in federal court, a jury found two male school administrators and a female principal guilty of failing to protect Jamie from the violence. The student accepted a $900,000 settlement from the school district. ("Student Wins," 1997, p. A8)

Homophobia leads to prejudice and discrimination, which, unfortunately, are still quite prevalent despite the fact that society in general seems to be a little more tolerant of lesbians and gays (ADL, 1992; Gallup, 1999/2000) (see Box 15.3). For instance, FBI hate crime statistics indicate that 17% of all hate crimes were perpetrated against individuals due to their sexual orientation, with 70% of those directed toward male homosexuals (FBI, 1999).

Attitudes toward homosexuality seem mixed. For instance, a poll of Americans found that 42% would object to having a gay elementary school teacher and 21% would object to having a gay doctor (Gallup, 1999/2000). When asked if homosexual relations between two consenting adults should be legal, 50% said they should, while 43% said they should not (7% had no opinion); and, when questioned if homosexuals should be able to marry, 62% said they should not, while 34% said they should. On the other hand, when asked if homosexuals should have equal right to job opportunities, 83% said they should, while the remainder either said they should not or had no opinion.

Unfortunately, stereotypes concerning homosexuality continue to flourish despite the fact that most gays and lesbians do not fit them. For instance, one falsehood is that sexual orientation is related to gender affiliation. Denouncing this misconception, Atkinson and Hackett (1998) point out that "gay men are men, and lesbian women are women" (p. 24) and that gay men and lesbian women exhibit the same range of gender-role behaviors as do male and female heterosexuals. Another persistent misconception is the confusion between transgenderism, intersexuality, transsexuality, transvestism, and homosexuality. *Transgenderism* is a term designating those who are not traditionally male or female, including transsexuals, transvestites, intersexuals, and the like. An intersexual, formerly called hermaphrodite, is one who was born with male and female sexual organs. A transsexual is an individual whose gender orientation does not fit his or her biological sex and thus feels trapped in his or her mismatched body. Transvestites are those who enjoy cross-dressing. All forms of transgenderism are not uniquely homosexual or heterosexual, and in actuality, transvestism is not too common among gay men (Moses & Hawkins, 1986).

Today, there is a mountain of evidence disputing the old notion that homosexuality and bisexuality are illnesses (Dean & Richardson, 1964; Dworkin & Gutierrez, 1989; Evans, 1970; Finn, 1996; Hammersmith & Weinberg, 1973; Hooker, 1957; Sang, 1989; Weinberg, 1970). In fact, since the early 1970s the American Psychological Association and the American Psychiatric Association have come out endorsing the belief that homosexuality is a sexual orientation, not an illness. Despite this fact, negative attitudes have persisted toward homosexuals on the part of some counselors and therapists. For instance, it was found that many counselors and therapists viewed homosexuality as not as healthy as heterosexuality, were uninformed about lesbian and gay issues, and have held distorted views toward the understanding and treatment of homosexuals (Casas, Brady, & Ponterotto, 1983; Davison & Friedman, 1981; Graham, Rawlings, Halpern, & Hermes, 1984). On a positive note, counselors and therapists generally have more liberal views toward homosexuality than does the general public.

Counseling Gay Men and Lesbian Women

A number of general guidelines to the counseling of gays and lesbians have been highlighted by some authors (Browning, Reynolds, & Dworkin, 1998; Pope, 1995; Shannon & Woods, 1998). In brief, they include:

1. *Have the right attitudes and beliefs, gain knowledge, and learn skills.* Be prepared to work with gay and lesbian clients by embracing the appropriate knowledge, skills, and beliefs prior to meeting with them.
2. *Adopt a nonhomophobic attitude and don't jump to conclusions about lifestyle.* The importance of adapting such an attitude cannot be stressed enough, as so many individuals (including counselors!) have embedded biases and stereotypes about gays and lesbians.
3. *Know community resources that might be useful to gay men and lesbian women.*
4. *Know identity issues.* Be familiar with the identity development of gay men and lesbian women, especially as it relates to the coming out process (e.g., see Cass, 1979).
5. *Understand the idiosyncrasies of religion toward homosexuality.* For example, some religions view homosexuality as sinful.
6. *Be tuned into domestic violence issues.* Be aware that domestic violence can occur in gay and lesbian relationships as it occurs in heterosexual relationships.
7. *Know about substance abuse treatment.* Understand substance abuse issues, as gay men and lesbian women have a greater tendency toward the use of substances as a method of dealing with the coming out process and the inherent prejudices in society (Dyne, 1990).
8. *Know about sexual abuse.* Be particularly cognizant that a large percent of lesbian women have been sexually abused before the age of 18 (38%, according to Loulan, 1987).

Other Diverse Populations

A number of special populations exist today that also demand our attention because individuals from these groups are misunderstood and/or discriminated against. Following is a brief overview of some of these populations (Atkinson & Hackett, 1998).

Individuals Who Are HIV Positive

It is now estimated that between 800,000 and 900,000 people in the United States are HIV positive; and, since AIDS was first identified, approximately half a million Americans have died of the disease (Centers for Disease Control, 2002). AIDS continues to spread in this country, and worldwide, more than 36.1 million children and adults are HIV positive or have AIDS (World Health Organization, 2001). Although the largest number of AIDS cases are in sub-Saharan Africa, the rate of increase of infection is great-

BOX 15.4

Legal Problems in Health Care Access

In an effort to maintain their patents, 39 of the world's major pharmaceutical companies sued South Africa, which was attempting to have other drug companies manufacture expensive AIDS drugs at a much reduced cost. The drug companies received so much negative press about their lawsuit that the lawsuit was dropped; however, the ability to manufacture the drugs is still in doubt due to legal issues and economic problems in South Africa (Jetter, 2001).

Meanwhile, in the United States, the Supreme Court denied an appeal that would have prevented insurance companies from dropping health insurance coverage for individuals with AIDS and other catastrophic illnesses. The obvious result of this decision is that many individuals who have serious illnesses may find themselves without medical coverage (Savage, 1992).

est in Asia. With some U.S. insurance companies dropping individuals who become chronically ill, and with drug companies fighting to ban easy access to AIDS drugs in Third World countries, it is clear that this epidemic has had a personal and economic cost to people throughout the world (see Box 15.4).

The response to the epidemic in the social service field has varied and includes programs that offer support and counseling groups for HIV-positive individuals and their families, needle exchange programs, programs for children who have AIDS, prevention and education programs in the schools, condom distribution programs, and hotlines to respond to questions about AIDS (Britton, 2000; Kain, 1989). Workshops and articles about the AIDS virus and how to counsel individuals who have tested HIV positive are now commonplace at conferences and in professional journals. No doubt, until a cure to this disease is found, AIDS will continue to have a major impact on America's health care system.

In the 21st century, the counselor will play an increasingly important role in offering education and prevention activities about the disease, as the deliverer of counseling services for those who are already infected, and as the supervisor of those many volunteers and paraprofessionals who are giving their time and humanity to assist in the caretaking of those infected, their families, and their friends (Britton, Rak, Cimini, & Shepherd, 1999; Viney, Allwood, Stillson, & Walmsley, 1992). As sexual activity with an HIV-positive individual is potentially life-threatening, counselors who are in a helping relationship with HIV-positive clients may very well be challenged with ethical dilemmas concerning confidentiality with their client versus the duty to warn those who may be recipients of the virus (Cohen, 1990) (see ACA ethical standards, section B.1.d in Appendix A).

COUNSELING INDIVIDUALS WHO ARE HIV POSITIVE A number of challenges face the counselor who works with an individual who is HIV positive or who has AIDS. A number of authors have highlighted Shannon and Woods's (1998) points to consider when counseling an individual who is HIV positive (Britton, 2000; Holt, Hout, & Romano, 1999; Shannon & Woods, 1998):

1. *Have the right attitudes and beliefs, gain knowledge, and learn skills.* Be prepared to work with HIV-positive individuals by embracing the appropriate knowledge, skills, and beliefs prior to meeting with them.

2. *Know the cultural background of the client.* Keep in mind that HIV-positive individuals are found in all cultures, races, and ethnic groups. Counselors need to remember that a client's background may change how the counselor works with him or her.
3. *Know about the disease and combat myths.* Knowledge helps fight fear. Armed with knowledge, counselors can become advocates for the HIV-positive person.
4. *Be prepared to take on uncommon counselor roles.* Realize that the counselor may need to be an advocate, caretaker, and resource person for the client, roles in which the counselor has not always been comfortable.
5. *Be prepared to deal with unique treatment issues.* Be prepared to deal with unique problems, including feelings about the loss of income from the loss of work or the high cost of medical treatment, depression and hopelessness concerning uncertain health, changes in interpersonal relationships when others discover the client is HIV positive (rejection, pity, fear, and so forth), the probability that the client will have friends and loved ones who are HIV positive or have died of AIDS if he or she is from a high-risk group.
6. *Deal with your own feelings about mortality.* Be able to deal effectively with your own feelings about a client's impending death and how those feelings may raise issues concerning your own mortality.

The Hungry, the Homeless, and the Poor

It is estimated that as many as two million Americans may be homeless in any one year (National Law Center on Homelessness and Poverty, 2001); and, despite a considerable increase in the homeless over the past 15 years, resources to serve these individuals have remained minimal. Although homelessness has always existed throughout history, today the homeless person is no longer the stereotypic hobo. The homeless today include children who have run away from home, single-parent families, intact families who have no place to live, poor single men and women, and the deinstitutionalized mentally ill. In addition, as compared to past years, the homeless of today are more likely not to have shelter, are younger, are less apt to find employment, and are heavily over represented by minorities.

In past years the poor were not necessarily at much greater risk of being homeless, but today, being poor is often one step away from not having a roof over one's head. The number of poor Americans is 32.3 million, or 11.8% of the population (U.S. Census Bureau, 2000a). About 12% of the poor work full-time and over 40% work some part of the year (U.S. Census Bureau, 2000b). In addition, a staggering 16.9% of all children in the United States live in poverty. Also, poverty is associated with race, as 23.6% of African Americans, 22.8% of Hispanics, 10.7% of Asians or Pacific Islanders, and 9.8% of whites are below the poverty level (U.S. Census Bureau, 2000c). Figure 15.2 shows that when you examine poverty rates, minorities are disproportionately represented (U.S. Census Bureau, 2000d).

Poverty is more prevalent in cities and the South and appears to be related to educational level, as the more educated have lower poverty rates than those less educated (U.S. Department of Commerce, 1992). Although the McKinney Act of 1987 provides job training, literacy programs, child care, and transportation funds and subsidizes counseling for the poor and homeless, the outlook for this section of society seems bleak (Waxman & Reyes, 1988).

FIGURE 15.2
Comparison of Poverty Rates of Select Racial/Ethnic Groups

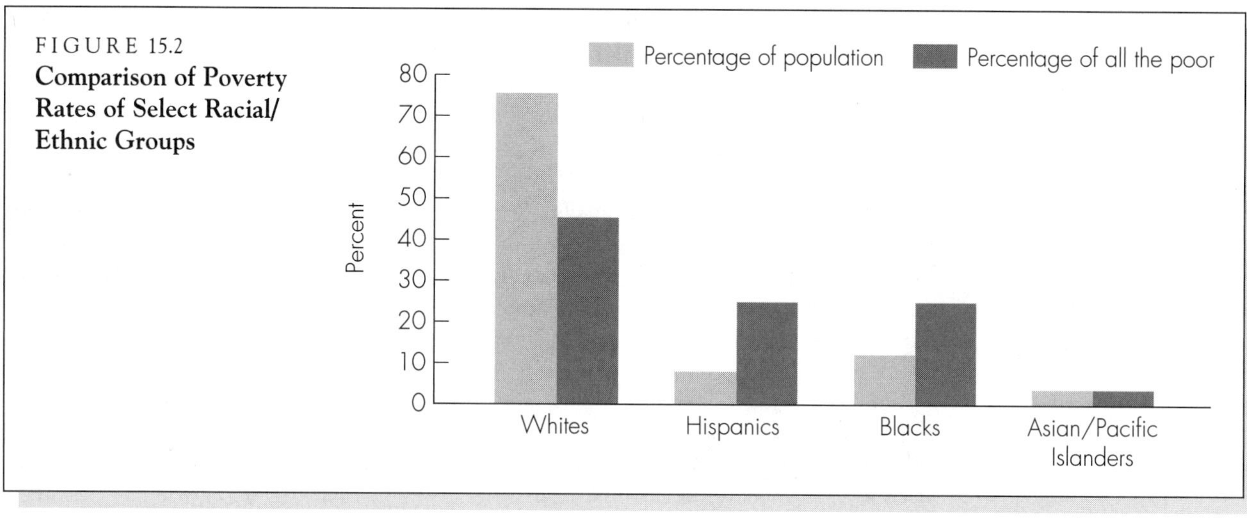

COUNSELING THE HOMELESS AND THE POOR A number of unique points should be considered when counseling the homeless and the poor (Axelson & Dail, 1988; Blasi, 1990; Rossi, 1990). Some of these include:

1. *Have the right attitudes and beliefs, gain knowledge, and learn skills.* Be prepared to work with the homeless and the poor by embracing the appropriate knowledge, skills, and beliefs prior to meeting with them.
2. *Focus on social issues.* Help clients obtain basic needs such as food and housing, as opposed to working on intrapsychic issues.
3. *Know the client's racial/ethnic/cultural background.* Be educated about the cultural heritage of clients, because a disproportionate number of the homeless and the poor come from diverse racial/ethnic/cultural groups.
4. *Be knowledgeable about health risks.* Be aware that the homeless and the poor are at much greater risk of developing AIDS, tuberculosis, and other diseases, and be able to do a basic medical screening and have referral sources available.
5. *Be prepared to deal with multiple issues.* Be prepared to deal with mental illness, chemical dependence, and other unique problems, because as much as 50% of the homeless are struggling with these problems.
6. *Know about developmental delays and be prepared to refer.* Know how to identify developmental delays and have potential referral sources, because homeless and poor children are much more likely to have retarded language and social skills, be abused, and have delayed motor development.
7. *Know psychological effects.* Be prepared to deal with despair, depression, and a sense of hopelessness as a result of being poor and/or homeless (Blasi, 1990).
8. *Know resources.* Be aware of the vast number of resources available in your community and make referrals when appropriate.

Older Persons

In 1900, 3% of the population of the United States was over 65 years of age. By 1960, this figure rose to 9.2%; and, in 2000, 12.7% of the population was over 65 (U.S. Census

Bureau, 2000e; U.S. Department of Commerce, 1991). It is estimated that, by the year 2030, fully 20% of the population will be over 65 years old (U.S. Census Bureau, 2000f).

Partly as a result of these changing demographics in the United States, there has been an increased focus on treatment for and care of the elderly. Across the country we have seen an increase in day-treatment programs for the elderly and in long-term care facilities such as nursing homes. In addition, housing that is specially designed for older persons, senior centers, and programs for the elderly offered through religious organizations and social service agencies are now prevalent around the country (Myers & Salmon, 1984). Of course, as America has become increasingly diverse, so has our aging population, and counselors will need to be familiar with both the unique concerns of older persons and the race/ethnicity/culture of their clients.

COUNSELING OLDER PERSONS Older persons have a number of problems and concerns that need to be addressed when they are counseled (Gibson & Mitchell, 1999; Schlossberg, Waters, & Goodman,1995; Schwiebert, Myers, & Dice; 2000). Below are just a few of the more prevalent concerns:

1. *Have the right attitudes and beliefs, gain knowledge, and learn skills.* Be prepared to work with older clients by embracing the appropriate knowledge, skills, and beliefs prior to meeting with them.
2. *Adapt your counseling style.* Adapt your counseling style to fit the needs of the older client. For instance, for the older person who has difficulty hearing, the counselor may use journal writing or art therapy. For clients who are not ambulatory, the counselor may need to have a session in the client's home.
3. *Build a trusting relationship.* Spend time building a trusting relationship. Remember that older persons seek counseling at lower rates than other clients (Hashimi, 1991), and those who do seek out counseling may be less trustful of therapy, having grown up in a generation when counseling was much less common.
4. *Know sources of depression and related treatment approaches.* Be knowledgeable about various treatment approaches as a function of the source of depression in the older client (e.g., loss of loved ones, lifestyle changes as the result of retirement, and changes in one's health).
5. *Know about identity issues.* Know that as individuals age, they once again face the issue of "Who am I?" Remember that many older persons had defined themselves based on their career, family, or roles in the community.
6. *Know about possible and probable health changes.* Be aware of the many potential health problems common to the elderly. Predictable changes in health can lead to depression and concern about the future. Unpredictable changes in health can lead to loss of income and a myriad of emotional problems.
7. *Have empathy for changes in interpersonal relationships.* Examine and have empathy for how each client may be affected by changes in his or her relationships. Aging inevitably brings the death of spouses, partners, and friends; changes in one's health status that prevent visits to and/or from friends; and relocations, such as to a retirement community, retirement home, or nursing home.
8. *Know about physical and psychological causes of sexual dysfunction.* Be aware of the possible physical and psychological causes of sexual dysfunction in the elderly. As individuals age, it is fairly common for both men and women to have changes in their sexual functioning. Remember that regardless of our age, we are always sexual beings.

With an increasing number of elderly in the United States and a concomitant increase in programs to service this population, it is evident that large numbers of counselors will be employed in community centers for the elderly, nursing homes, gerontological centers, and retirement communities (Myers, 1983; Myers, Loesch, & Sweeney, 1991). Counselors must be made aware of how to best work with the aging population.

The Chronically Mentally Ill

In 1955 there were 560,00 inpatients in psychiatric hospitals, while in 1995 this figure fell to 65,000 (Burger & Youkeles, 2000). Although there are fewer individuals now hospitalized for psychiatric problems, the number of psychiatric facilities that offer mental health services today is a staggering 4941 (U.S. Department of Commerce, 1991). Unfortunately, the reduction in the number of inpatients is not a result of increased mental health but the consequence of a number of important events since the 1950s.

First, the development of new psychotropic medications, such as antipsychotics (e.g., Haldol, Thorazine), antidepressants (e.g., Prozac, Zoloft, Elavil), and antianxiety agents (e.g., Valium, Tranxene, Xanax), has made the management of severe emotional conditions possible outside the inpatient setting. Second, the passage of the Community Mental Health Centers Act of 1963 funded the establishment of mental health centers and made it possible for those with severe emotional problems to obtain mental health services for free or at low cost (Burger & Youkeles, 2000). Third, the proliferation of social service programs introduced through the Great Society initiatives of the Johnson presidency created myriad social service agencies, many of which service the multiple needs of the chronically mentally ill. Finally, in 1975 the Supreme Court decision of *Donaldson* v. *O'Connor* stated that a person who is not dangerous to him- or herself or to others could not be institutionalized against his or her will at inpatient psychiatric hospitals (see Box 2.3 in Chapter 2).

These events have greatly shaped the delivery of mental health services in the country. Today, most individuals who are chronically mentally ill manage to maintain themselves through the use of medication, the support of friends and relatives, and a variety of services that are offered through community social service agencies.

Unfortunately, many of the chronically mentally ill find themselves on the streets and homeless, with some sources stating that anywhere from 20% to 60% of all homeless people may have severe psychiatric problems (Fisher, 1991; Mental illness and . . . , 1999). Counselors who will be working with the chronically mentally ill will need to understand psychiatric disorders, psychotropic medications, and the unique needs of the chronically mentally ill, such as dealing with homelessness, continual transitions, difficulty with employment, and dependent family relationships.

COUNSELING THE MENTALLY ILL Specific treatment guidelines when working with the chronically mentally ill include:

1. *Have the right attitudes and beliefs, gain knowledge, and learn skills.* Be prepared to work with the mentally ill by embracing the appropriate knowledge, skills, and beliefs prior to meeting with them.
2. *Help the client understand his or her mental illness.* Fully inform clients with up-to-date knowledge about their mental illness. Many do not have an understanding of their illness, the course of the illness, and best methods of treatment.
3. *Help the client work through feelings concerning his or her mental illness.* Help clients work through their feelings about being mentally ill. Mental illness continues to

be stigmatized in this society, and clients are often embarrassed about their disorder. Support groups and a nonjudgmental attitude can go a long way in normalizing the view clients have of themselves.

4. *Assure attendance in counseling*. Increase the chances of clients coming to counseling by calling the day before, having a relative or close friend assist the client in coming to counseling, or having counselors develop specific strategies to help clients remember to come in for their appointments (e.g., putting Xs on a calendar). Clients will miss appointments due to denial about their illness, embarrassment about seeing a counselor, problems remembering, or not caring.
5. *Assure compliance with medication*. Be vigilant about encouraging clients to continue to take their medication. Clients will discontinue medication due to forgetfulness, denial about the illness, the false belief that they will not have a relapse because they feel better (the medication is working), and because the medication is not helpful for the particular client or the dosage is too small or too large.
6. *Assure accurate diagnosis*. Accurately diagnose clients to assure proper treatment planning and the appropriate choice of medication. Accurate diagnosis can be assured through testing, clinical interviews, interviews with significant others, and appropriate use of supervision.
7. *Reevaluate the client's treatment plan and do not give up*. Be committed to working with clients and reevaluate treatment plans as often as is necessary. The mentally ill are some of the most difficult clients with whom to work. Progress, if any, is slow, and it is easy to become discouraged.
8. *Involve the client's family*. Assure adequate family involvement and have the family understand the implications of the client's diagnosis. Families can offer great support to clients with mental illness and can be a window into the client's psyche.
9. *Know resources*. Have a working knowledge of resources, as the mentally ill are often involved or need to become involved with many other resources in the community (e.g., Social Security disability, housing authority, support groups).

People with Disabilities

Today, nearly 1 in 8 individuals identify themselves as having a disability and 1 in 5 see themselves as having a severe disability. Of the 53 million Americans who consider themselves as having a disability, 5 million are under 15 years old, and only 1 in 6 of these individuals were born with their disability (U.S. Census Bureau, 2001e).

Some of the most common forms of disabilities include mental retardation, learning disabilities, emotional problems, and speech impairments, while some other disabling conditions include hearing impairment, visual impairment, orthopedic impairment, multiple disabilities, and other health impairments. Individuals with disabilities are discriminated against in many ways. For instance, some illegally are denied job opportunities, illegally receive inferior educational opportunities, and illegally are denied access to business and recreational facilities. But as disturbing as the above are, perhaps the worst mistreatment of people with disabilities is the reaction many get from others, for many individuals with disabilities are feared, ignored, stared at, infantilized, treated as intellectually inferior, accused of faking their disability, or pitied.

A number of federal laws have had an impact on the ability of individuals with disabilities to receive services. The Education for All Handicapped Children Act of 1975 (PL94-142) and the subsequent Individuals with Disabilities Education Act (IDEA) assure the right to an education within the least restrictive environment for all children who are identified as having a disability that interferes with learning. The Rehabilitation Act of 1973 assures access to vocational rehabilitation services for adults with disabilities who are in need of employment. The Americans with Disabilities Act of 1992 updated these laws and assures that qualified individuals with disabilities cannot be discriminated against in job applications procedures, hiring, firing, advancement, compensation, fringe benefits, job training, and other terms, conditions, and privileges (U.S. Department of Labor, 1993).

COUNSELING INDIVIDUALS WITH DISABILITIES As federal laws have increasingly supported the right to services for individuals with disabilities, the counselor has taken an increasingly active role in the treatment and rehabilitation of such individuals (Lombana, 1989). Some treatment guidelines when working with the individual who has a disability include:

1. *Have the right attitudes and beliefs, gain knowledge, and learn skills.* Be prepared to work with clients who have a disability by embracing the appropriate knowledge, skills, and beliefs prior to meeting with clients.
2. *Have knowledge of the many disabling conditions.* To be effective, a counselor should understand the physical and emotional consequences of the disability of the client.
3. *Help clients know their disabilities.* Inform clients of their disabilities, the probable course of treatment, and the prognosis. Such knowledge allows them to be fully involved in the counseling process.
4. *Assist the client through the grieving process.* Help clients pass through stages of grief as they deal with their loss and move toward acceptance. Similar to the stages of bereavement (Kubler-Ross, 1969), it is usual for a client to experience denial, anger, negotiation, resignation, and acceptance.
5. *Know referral resources.* Be aware of potential resources in the community (e.g., physicians, social services, physical therapists, experts on pain management, vocational rehabilitation). Individuals with disabilities often have a myriad of needs.
6. *Know the law and inform your client of the law.* Know the law to assure that the clients are receiving all necessary services and not being discriminated against. In addition, clients often feel empowered when they know their rights.
7. *Be prepared to do, or refer for, vocational/career counseling.* Be ready to either do career counseling or to refer a client to a career counselor. Often, when faced with a disability, clients are also faced with making a career transition.
8. *Include the family.* Whenever possible and reasonable, include the client's family in the treatment process, as they can offer support, assist in long-term treatment planning, and help with the client's emotional needs.
9. *Be an advocate.* Advocate for clients by knowing the law, fighting for clients' rights, and assisting clients in fighting for their own rights. Individuals with disabilities are faced with prejudice and discrimination.

Multicultural Issue: Is All Counseling Multicultural?

First counselor asserts: *"All counseling is multicultural, for everyone has different values and just because you're black, or Asian, or Hispanic doesn't mean you're any different from the white person I counsel who has different values than me."*

Second counselor retorts: *"You have no understanding of the plight of minorities. You cannot understand what it's like to be culturally different. To assert that all counseling is multicultural just shows your ignorance and borders on racism."*

In a nutshell, the above represents the current debate regarding the focus of multicultural counseling. Some assert that being a culturally sensitive and culturally appropriate counselor by gathering specific knowledge of ethnic/minority groups has inherent problems (Patterson, 1996). They warn that (1) it tends to generalize and stereotype people; (2) it leads to a self-fulfilling prophecy, whereby clients end up acting in a certain manner because we believe they should respond that way (e.g., we have a low expectation of self-disclosure from a client and thus do not offer the client ample opportunity to talk); (3) there is no evidence that increased knowledge of cultures will lead to more effective counseling; and (4) modifying some traditional counseling approaches in order to meet culture-specific stereotypes can lead to failure in counseling (e.g., we are not empathic because we believe a more directive approach should be used with a particular minority group).

On the other hand, others assert that knowledge of a client's cultural background is essential if we are to be effective. For instance, McFadden (1996) notes that not incorporating knowledge of the client's culture "contributes to retardation of the developmental process of those populations" (p. 232). Others state that we can no longer believe that all people will respond to our Western-based counseling approaches in the same ways and that we must adapt our counseling style to the individual and his or her culture (Ivey, Simek-Morgan, & Ivey, 1997).

What is the answer? Should we learn about all of the differences between people or does that lead to unnecessary stereotyping and potentially poor counseling? The answer probably lies somewhere in the middle. Is it necessary to know about cultures? Yes, if we are to have empathy and understanding of others, we need to be inside our client's world. Can knowledge of varying cultures lead to stereotyping and generalizing? Yes, we need to be vigilant in our efforts not to stereotype, so that when we work with the acculturated minority client who has no knowledge of his or her culture we will not make false assumptions. Perhaps the answer lies in the following quotation from Pedersen (1996b):

> *Although there may indeed be a problem of overemphasizing cultural diversity and differences in some of the multicultural literature, it is equally serious to ignore diversity and thereby deprive cultural groups of their identity.* (p. 236)

Ethical, Professional, and Legal Issues: Making Wise Ethical Decisions

As noted in Chapter 3, the ethical code of ACA (1995b) includes many statements that focus on diversity, and you are encouraged to review them. However, some suggest that there are limitations to the code, stating that it is somewhat based on the views of the dominant culture and tends to be somewhat technique oriented (Corey et al., 1998;

Pedersen, 1996a; Welfel, 1998). Indeed, ACA is now soliciting feedback specifically to improve how the code handles multicultural issues (ACA, 2001b).

Rather than using ethical codes, some have suggested using the moral foundation of ethical codes when making ethical decisions. They suggest using principles such as, do no harm to others, promote the good of society, act in a fair manner, and promote client freedom of choice (Kitchener, 1984). However, others even question the use of underlying moral principles, stating that how one person defines the good of society may be drastically different from how another person defines it. Where does this leave us?

Clearly, ethical decision making is complex. On the one hand, we must be careful when using the ethical guidelines, as they might hold some inherent bias. On the other hand, using a moral model may also be biased. At the very least, when making ethical decisions we must make careful, wise decisions based on all of the evidence (Ibrahim, 1996).

The Counselor in Process: The Ongoing Process of Counseling the Culturally Different

Despite the fact that throughout this text we have stressed specific methods of working effectively with clients, it should be emphasized that counseling is not fixed. This is particularly true in the realm of multicultural counseling, as new approaches to working with clients from diverse backgrounds are quickly finding their way into the professional literature. For instance, international counseling theories, which have been largely ignored by American counselors and psychotherapists and which approach counseling in very different ways than we are used to, are now finding their way into the literature (Locke, 1992). This is particularly important because, as Usher (1989) noted, "It is widely acknowledged that current counseling theories are products of Western culture and, as such, are not universally applicable to cross-cultural counseling situations" (p. 62). Other examples abound in the literature as we find new ways of counseling men, women, gays and lesbians, and individuals from many diverse backgrounds. As counselors, we must continue to find the best ways to assist all individuals in their emotional needs. We must continue to examine new treatment approaches, explore new counseling theories, and be open to an expansive view of counseling all individuals. Perhaps we can learn from Romano (1992), who wisely noted:

> *Not ours, not theirs; no one way of counseling surpasses another . . . As cultures differ, so must counseling.* (Romano, 1992, p. 1)

Summary

In this chapter we examined the changing face of America and noted that the United States is becoming increasingly more diverse. Highlighting a few minority groups, we presented some background information about African Americans, Hispanics, Asian Americans, and Native Americans. In addition, while encouraging the reader not to overgeneralize, we examined some common customs, values, and behaviors held by many individuals within each of these groups. Also, we highlighted important issues that should be addressed in the counseling relationship with these minority groups and presented specific suggestions for working with individuals from these groups.

In addition to examining the four minority groups noted above, we also explored a number of other groups because of their unique needs and their tendency to face discrimination. We discussed diversity in religious affiliation and differences between women and men and gays and lesbians; and the special issues of individuals who are HIV positive, the homeless and the poor, older persons, the mentally ill, and individuals with disabilities. No doubt, other groups with unique needs could have also been highlighted.

For each diverse group discussed, we highlighted some of the major issues that individuals within that group are likely to face. For instance, we discussed the importance of recognizing the differences among religions in the United States and throughout the world; the sociopolitical and psychological differences between men and women; some of the myths about and biases against gays and lesbians; the physical and emotional needs of individuals who are HIV positive; the unique characteristics and needs of many individuals who are homeless and/or poor; the interpersonal, psychological, and physical changes that face many older persons; the changes in the treatment of the mentally ill over the years; and the emotional, physical, psychological, and legal concerns of individuals with disabilities. For each of the groups discussed, we stressed that the counselor must be aware of the unique needs and issues that face the culturally different client if he or she is to counsel such a client effectively.

As we neared the end of this chapter, we noted that there has been a debate in the field concerning the definition of multicultural counseling. Some assert that being a culturally sensitive and culturally appropriate counselor by gathering specific knowledge of ethnic/minority groups has inherent problems, such as leading to stereotyping and gross generalizations. Others assert that knowledge of a client's cultural background is essential if we are to understand and work effectively with that client. We concluded that in order to gain empathy for the culturally different client it is important to learn about cultures. However, we also warned the counselor not to stereotype and generalize as a result of the knowledge he or she has gained.

We also noted that a controversy exists around the use of the ACA ethical guidelines, with some stating that, despite recent changes in the code, they are inherently biased because they are based on Western values. We suggested that a moral-based model might be used as an adjunct to the ethical guidelines. However, we noted some potential problems with that model also and suggested that being wise and careful when faced with ethical dilemmas is crucial. We noted that perhaps one day we will have an ethical decision-making model that is based on identified universal values.

Finally, we concluded the chapter by noting that the theories and skills important to the multicultural counseling relationship will continue to change in the future. However, in contrast to the rest of the counseling field, this change is expected to occur more rapidly, and the counselor must stay abreast of it if he or she is to remain effective.

INFOTRAC and Other Information Resources (e.g., ERIC and PsycINFO)

Note: When relevant, key words are in quotation marks.

1. Review the literature on counseling any of the populations listed in this chapter or another diverse population of your choice.
2. Review the literature on skills needed for "effective multicultural counseling."

SECTION VII

Your Future in the Counseling Profession: Choosing a Specialty Area, Finding a Job, and Trends in the Future

Overview

Each chapter in this last section of the text examines possibilities for your future. Chapters 16, 17, and 18 look at three potential counseling specialty areas that you might choose to enter. Chapter 19 discusses applying to graduate school, applying for jobs, and trends in the future.

In Chapters 16, 17, and 18, I use the same basic format when discussing the specialty areas of school counseling, community agency and mental health counseling, and student affairs practice in higher education. In each specialty area I will first give a broad definition of what the specialty area encompasses, and then I will offer an overview of the history of the specialty area. Next I'll give some examples of where the counselor in that specialty area might work and present an overview of some of the typical functions and roles of counselors in each of the specialty areas. I also will provide an explanation of some possible theoretical approaches that might work best in each specialty area and discuss some special concerns that counselors might face in each of the specialty areas. Near the end of each of these chapters I will provide approximate salaries for counselors in these specialty areas. Finally, I will present an overview of multicultural, ethical, professional, and legal concerns unique to each specialty area.

In Chapter 19, I will look at changes that are likely to take place in the profession and choices you will have in your future relative to choosing a graduate program or finding a job. Specifically, I will discuss medical breakthroughs in the areas of genetic research and genetic counseling, the use of psychotropic medications, and the mind–body connection. I will also look at the changing nature of counseling as a result of managed care and computers and technology. In addition, I will offer some suggestions on applying to graduate school and finding a job, and I will explore how multicultural issues, accreditation, credentialing, standards of care, and the professional associations are likely to change and impact the profession in the 21st century. The chapter will conclude with a wellness model that you can use to assess your level of overall health as you move into this sometimes stressful profession.

CHAPTER **16**

School Counseling

I remember the first day I started my job as a high school counselor. I had been in private practice, worked in agencies, taught counseling, even done some testing in the schools, but I had never worked as a school counselor. Despite having taught for years that what you do as an agency counselor or a college counselor was basically the same as what you do as a school counselor, I now had my doubts. Had I been giving the party line for all of these years, or were there significant differences, differences that might suggest that school counseling is quite a different ball of wax than agency or college counseling?

Well, I must admit that my part-time school counseling job was not quite the same as the full-time counselors'. I had more time to do counseling than they did. Nevertheless, here I was, part of the counselors' team.

I'll never forget the first time a student came to see me. I closed my door, and suddenly this all seemed very familiar. I was doing counseling. The setting was different, but I was using my same basic skills, I was involved in a counseling relationship.

I learned over the next year that there were many differences between what the school counselor did and what it was like being an agency counselor. The amount of time with my clients was shorter, the paperwork was different, and many of the daily activities were not the same. But, whenever I would sit one-to-one with a student, I was back in that counseling relationship.

I also found many activities similar to what I had done before. I had responsibilities around consultation, I had to contend with the same basic ethical issues, I had someone evaluating me, and in some fashion I used all of the skills I learned in graduate school. And, although at times I did administrative activities, taught, advocated for clients, worked with data and testing, and made referrals, I was not an administrator, not a teacher, not a school social worker or school psychologist, not a resource assistant. I was a counselor with the unique identity that counselors have.

This chapter will explore the world of the school counselor. We will first give some brief definitions of school counseling and then offer a synopsis of the history of school counseling. This will be followed by a description of the functions and roles of the school counselor and some of the theoretical models from which the school counselor works. Next we will examine some of the similarities and differences between elementary, middle, and secondary school counseling. We will then discuss some special issues in school counseling and offer approximate salaries of school counselors. The chapter will conclude by discussing multicultural, ethical, professional, and legal issues in school counseling.

What Is School Counseling?

- A student is sent to the counselor by his teacher with a note that reads: "Sam hasn't been himself. He's not getting his work completed and doesn't seem to be paying attention. Would you please talk with him and see what might be going on?"
- Some fourth graders are immersed in a self-esteem group.
- A third-grade teacher approaches the counselor about a student and says, "Jeremiah is so disruptive. No matter how much positive attention I give him, he still blurts out answers, can't wait his turn, and says the most inappropriate comments at the worst possible times! I don't know what to do!"
- A twelfth-grade student asks her counselor to write her a college recommendation.
- Two fifth-grade students who were arguing on a school bus begin to push and shove one another. The bus driver tells them to go to the counselor or get disciplined. The counselor has them see a peer mediator who is trained and supervised by the school counselor.
- A seventh-grade student requests to see the counselor to talk about a problem in one of her classes. In the middle of her talk she blurts out that her parents have just separated, and she begins to sob.
- The parent of an eighth grader comes to see the counselor with concerns over the violence in her community and how it might affect her son. The counselor suggests that she should help start a community advocacy group to stop the violence.
- A tenth grader is confused about how to approach a job search. He comes to his counselor and asks for advice.
- A group of eleventh-grade girls come to the school counselor concerned about sexually transmitted diseases.
- A teacher asks the counselor how to interpret the achievement test scores of her classes.
- A first-grade student gets a happy face sticker from her counselor for behaving in class.

As you can see from the above, school counseling is many things. One moment a school counselor might be chatting with a student about his college application, and the next moment she is engrossed with a sobbing student threatening to kill herself. Who is the school counselor? The American School Counseling Association (ASCA, 1999), states that the school counselor is

> *. . . a certified/licensed educator who addresses the needs of students comprehensively through the implementation of a developmental school counseling program. School counselors are employed in elementary, middle/junior high, senior high, and post-secondary settings. Their work is differentiated by attention to age-specific*

> *developmental stages of student growth and the needs, tasks, and student interests related to those stages. School counselors work with all students, including those who are considered "at-risk" and those with special needs. They are specialists in human behavior and relationships who provide assistance to students through four primary interventions: counseling (individual and group); large group guidance; consultation; and coordination.* (¶ 1)

School counselors are employed at the elementary, middle, and high school levels. Some states offer a generic K-through-12 school counseling credential, while others have separate credentialing for elementary, middle, and secondary school counselors. In some states school counselors are required to have been certified as teachers, although the trend has been to eliminate this prerequisite. In order to become a school counselor, one must have a master's degree in school counseling. Such degrees are generally very similar to master's degrees in other counseling specialty areas and include a few distinctive courses in school counseling as well as practicum and/or internship experiences in the schools.

Although school counseling is commonplace today, this was not always the case. Let's review the history of school counseling and then take a more extensive look at the roles and functions of school counselors at the elementary, middle, and secondary levels.

A History of School Counseling

At the beginning of the 20th century, the first school counselors were a response to an increased need for vocational guidance. Society was becoming more complex, and individuals struggled to find their place in this increasingly changing world.

Recognizing the need to train experts in vocational guidance, Frank Parsons organized the Boston Vocational Bureau in 1908, which trained teachers and others in vocational guidance. Parsons, who developed the trait-and-factor approach to vocational guidance, believed that successful vocational choice was based on (1) an understanding of self (e.g., abilities, interests, basic personality dynamics), (2) knowledge of the principles of success and of occupational information, and (3) the ability to make a reasoned choice between one's understanding of self and one's knowledge of the world of work (Davis, 1969).

Parsons (1909) was very concerned about the counseling process, and many of his ideas were ahead of his time. For instance, Parsons believed that counselors should have:

1. A practical working knowledge of the fundamental principles and methods of modern psychology.
2. An experience involving sufficient human contact to give them an intimate acquaintance with human nature in a considerable number of its different phases; they must understand the dominant motives, interests, and ambitions that control people's lives, and be able to recognize the symptoms that indicate the presence or absence of important elements of character.
3. An ability to deal with young people in a sympathetic, earnest, searching, candid, helpful, and attractive way.
4. A knowledge of requirements and conditions of success, compensation, prospects, advantages, and disadvantages, etc., in different lines of industry.
5. Information relating to courses of study and means of preparing for various callings and developing efficacy therein.

6. [Knowledge of] [S]cientific method analysis and principles of investigation by which laws and causes are ascertained, facts are classified, and correct conclusions drawn. (Parsons, 1909, pp. 94–95)

Widely recognized as the "Founder of Vocational Guidance," Parsons' pioneering efforts helped to identify and launch a new profession, guidance counseling. His work greatly influenced American education and was the impetus for the spread of vocational guidance to school systems around the country (Aubrey, 1977) (see Chapter 2). Although Parsons died at a relatively young age in 1908, his efforts were responsible for the first school counselors, who were teachers that became half-time vocational counselors in the schools. Counseling, at least vocational counseling, was establishing itself in the schools.

On the heels of the vocational guidance movement came developments in the area of assessment (Baker, 1996). Soon, psychometrics was to become a crucial piece of vocational guidance, as it was the vehicle to help students and others identify their abilities and interests. In 1932, the Wagner O'Day Act legitimized and expanded vocational counseling by establishing the U.S. Employment Service and making vocational guidance commonplace in America. Vocational counseling was now embedded into the fabric of the United States, and the role of school counselors, with their vocational counseling emphasis, was strengthened.

As vocational guidance became common on the American landscape, individuals began to advocate for a broader approach to school counseling that attended to a large variety of students' psychological and educational needs (Aubrey, 1982). For instance, advocates like John Brewer (1932) suggested that guidance be seen in a total educational context and that guidance counselors be involved in a variety of functions in the schools, including adjustment counseling, assistance with curriculum planning, classroom management, and, of course, occupational guidance. During the 1930s and into the 1940s school guidance was shaped by one of the first comprehensive approaches to counseling, which became known as the Minnesota Point of View of E. G. Williamson. This largely directive approach promoted setting goals, overcoming obstacles, and achieving a satisfactory lifestyle (Baker, 1996).

During the 1940s the directive approach of E. G. Williamson was to be overshadowed by the nondirective, relationship-oriented, humanistic approaches of Carl Rogers and others (Aubrey, 1977; Beale, 1986). The humanistic philosophy was to affect all of counseling, and it soon seeped into the training of school counselors. The days where school counselors were seen as only providing vocational counseling within a directive and didactic framework were clearly gone. Now, within a humanistic framework, they would provide a broad spectrum of counseling services that included mental health counseling, consultation, coordination of services, and, of course, the more traditional guidance functions.

As school counseling expanded, we saw the development of professional associations. In 1953 the American School Counselor Association (ASCA, see www.schoolcounselor.org) became the fifth division of the American Personnel and Guidance Association (today, ACA). Over the years, ASCA has shaped the direction of school counseling through discussion, debate, conferences, and the publication of role statements, journals, position papers, and ethical standards. Also during the 1950s the Association for Counselor Education and Supervision (ACES) and the National Career Development Association (NCDA), two other ACA divisions, were founded. These associations have significantly contributed to the development of school counseling by highlighting school counseling issues, developing interest networks, establishing accreditation procedures, offering program sessions at conferences, supporting legislative initiatives, and collaborating with ASCA (Paisley & Borders, 1995).

In 1958 the Soviet Union launched the first earth satellite, Sputnik I. Suddenly, Americans were jolted into believing there was a great need for more trained scientists so we could beat the Russians to the moon. There was public criticism of education and its failure to supply trained individuals for careers identified as vital to national well-being. As a direct result, the National Defense Education Act (NDEA) of 1958 was passed to help create and define counseling positions within the public schools. This act allocated funds for training institutes to quickly graduate secondary school counselors. Those counselors were then charged with the task of identifying young people who had math and science talent and to encourage these students into further studies in the sciences. Although the goal of the NDEA was to train vocational counselors, the humanistic and mental health orientation of school counseling was firmly embedded into counselor training, and it was not long before these guidance counselors were doing many other things besides vocational counseling.

In the middle and late 1960s school counseling expanded further, with the passage of the Elementary and Secondary Education Act and Vocational Education Act Amendments. These acts focused on the implementation of specialized programs beyond the traditional college-bound and vocationally oriented students to include services for the poor, school dropouts, and those having severe academic problems (Minkoff & Terres, 1985). These acts and others directly stimulated growth in many other areas of the school counseling profession, including performance standards for school counselors, criteria for the development of the credentialing of school counselors, and the strengthening of accrediting bodies such as those established by state departments of education. All of these developments launched what became known as the new era in the guidance and counseling profession (Gibson & Mitchell, 1999).

During the 1960s, 1970s, and 1980s the school counseling profession saw a gradual but consistent broadening of the services it provided to students. During these decades graduate programs in counseling, and subsequently school counselors, gave greater notice to developmental theories and how school counselors can have an impact on the predictable stages of development experienced by all students (Havighurst, 1972). Today, school counselors offer comprehensive services within a developmental framework from prekindergarten through high school. Included in these services are individual and group guidance, individual and group counseling, consultation, and coordination of a wide range of activities (Borders & Drury, 1992; Gerler, 1992).

Recently, a new trend in school counseling has emerged. Spurred on by a number of grants given to counselor education programs by the Dewitt Wallace–Reader's Digest Fund, the funding is specifically focused on transforming school counseling programs so that there is an increased emphasis on advocacy, consultation, community involvement, use of technology, and the taking on of leadership roles by counselors so that they can help lessen the achievement gap that exists for minorities in the schools (see pp. 437–438).

Within the past 20 years, school counseling has sought to define its parameters by establishing professional codes and standards of accountability. Thus, we have seen CACREP establishing accreditation for school counseling programs, all states requiring a master's degree in school counseling to be a school counselor, a professional code of ethics developed by ASCA, professional organizations advocating and lobbying for legislative initiatives, and the establishment of credentialing for school counselors. More recently, in an effort to increase the viability of the school counseling profession, ASCA developed a set of National Standards for school counseling (ASCA, 2001a). The standards, which will be discussed in more detail later in the chapter, will go far in standardizing what school counselors do and will help school administrators understand the purpose, roles, and functions of school counselors. The standards are:

- Help school systems identify what students will know and be able to do as a result of participating in a school counseling program.
- Establish similar goals, expectations, support systems and experiences for all students.
- Serve as an organizational tool to identify and set priorities among the elements of an effective school counseling program.
- Provide an opportunity to discuss the role of counseling programs in school to enhance student learning. (¶ 2)

The profession of school counseling has grown dramatically over the years. From its meager beginnings at the turn of the century, to its slow inclusion in the schools over the years, to its rapid expansion as a result of Sputnik and the NDEA, to its broader humanistic, developmental and comprehensive focus in recent years, school counseling is an established profession. Whereas in 1964 there were 327 colleges and universities supporting counselor preparation programs, by 1999 there were 542 institutions offering close to 1000 graduate programs, with a large percentage of graduating students working as school counselors (Hollis & Dodson, 2000). With more states requiring elementary school counseling and increased numbers of students expected in our schools in the coming years, the field of school counseling is likely to continue to grow.

Roles and Functions of School Counselors

As we've learned, school counseling has evolved and changed dramatically over the last century. From its origins in early vocational guidance, the profession now encompasses comprehensive programming that addresses specific developmental needs and issues. Today the school counselor does a myriad of activities, and although the roles and functions of elementary, middle, and secondary school counselors are different, they can all be described under the terms of counseling, large group guidance, consultation, and coordination (ASCA, 1999).

Large Group Guidance

ASCA defines large group guidance as:

> *. . . a planned, developmental program of guidance activities designed to foster students' academic, career, and personal/social development. It is provided for all students through a collaborative effort by counselors and teachers.*
> (ASCA, 1999, ¶ 3)

The term *guidance* stems back to the activities of the vocational guidance counselor at the turn of the last century. However, today guidance activities include a wide range of what the counselor does and cover much more than vocational guidance. Guidance today generally includes (Borders & Drury, 1992; Schmidt, 1991):

- A specific focus or topic to be discussed.
- Activities that are counselor-centered; that is, the topic to be discussed is chosen by the counselor and discussion is led by the counselor.
- The dissemination of materials that are primarily informational in nature.
- Discussions that are reactive or preventive and developmental in nature (e.g., a discussion on suicide following the death of a student would be reactive, a career counseling module to discuss future career concerns would be preventive and developmental).
- The facilitation of student discussion by the counselor and a de-emphasis of "counseling."

Group guidance focuses on providing information in a largely didactic mode. Generally, group guidance is a preplanned activity based on the identified developmental needs of students. In some cases, teachers may assist in running group guidance sessions. In addition, it is not unusual for school counselors to divide large groups into smaller work groups to more intensively discuss specific issues. Some examples of topics for group guidance include how to get along with others, at the elementary school level; understanding your interests, at the middle school level; college planning, at the high school level; or family life education, which can be offered at all levels. Group guidance is an effective method of using the school counselor's time wisely.

Individual and Group Counseling

ASCA (1999) defines counseling as:

> *. . . a confidential relationship in which the counselor meets with students individually and in small groups to help them resolve or cope constructively with their problems and developmental concerns.* (¶ 2)

In providing counseling, the counselor works to establish a trusting, confidential, supportive environment for the child. Building on this foundation, the child will be able to increase his or her problem-solving and decision-making skills, examine and work on his or her ability to form healthy interpersonal relationships, and become more aware of his or her abilities, interests, and general personality style. Such beneficial changes will have a positive effect on learning (O'Bryant, 1991). Because counseling in the schools is almost always short-term, it is generally distinguished from therapy. Counselors will often refer to other helping professionals when they discover, through a counseling relationship, that a student needs more in-depth work. Counseling can occur either individually or in small groups.

Individual Counseling

Individual counseling in the schools is a one-on-one personal interaction between the student and the counselor, focusing on a particular topic or issue the child may present. Individual counseling in the school presents a number of unique problems that are generally not faced in other settings. For instance, in most cases, school counselors cannot guarantee children that what they say is confidential, as parents generally have the right to counseling information about their child (Attorney C. Borstein, personal communication, July 1, 2001; Davis & Mickelson, 1994; Hubert, 1996; Huey, 1986; Lawrence & Kurpius, 2000).

In addition, because of the large number of students generally assigned to a counselor, the limited attention span of many students, particularly younger ones, and the limitation of students' counseling time by classroom time, individual counseling in the schools is often very brief, usually lasting 20 or 30 minutes. Also, recently, many school systems no longer allow long-term counseling, believing that whenever a student is seen for more than a few sessions, he or she should be referred to outside resources.

Small-Group Counseling

Small-group counseling involves interactions between the counselor and four to eight students who meet for a set number of times to explore a common issue. These sessions give students an opportunity to discuss related concerns, brainstorm solutions to presenting problems, give and receive feedback, receive support from others, and practice new behaviors. These groups typically focus on both personal and academic issues, such as self-esteem, anger management, motivation, or decision-making. The nature of small group work enables the counselor to more efficiently serve the needs of a greater number of students.

Consultation

ASCA (1999) defines consultation as:

> *. . . a collaborative partnership in which the counselor works with parents, teachers, administrators, school psychologists, social workers, visiting teachers, medical professionals, and community health personnel in order to plan and implement strategies to help students be successful in the education system.* (¶ 4)

This cooperative process involves the counselor working with a teacher, administrator, parent, or other professional who shares concerns about a child in an effort to explore new ways of working with the child so that the child can achieve at his or her level. Consultation helps school counselors acquire more knowledge and skills for addressing the problems of students, and it assists them in becoming objective and self-confident when dealing with children's concerns (Hall & Lin, 1994; O'Bryant, 1991). This intervention can occur in a variety of ways, including individual meetings and group conferences or through staff development activities. Consultation has been championed by some as the most efficient way to respond to the needs of the increasing number of students a counselor may be responsible for serving (Coy, 1991; Fall, 1995; Hall & Lin, 1994).

Coordination

ASCA (1999) defines coordination as:

> *. . . a leadership process in which the counselor helps organize, manage, and evaluate the school counseling program. The counselor assists parents in obtaining needed services for their children through a referral and follow-up process and serves as liaison between the school and community agencies so that they may collaborate in efforts to help students.* (¶ 4)

Coordination involves the counselor assuming a leadership role in managing indirect services that could benefit students. This can occur in many ways. For instance, all counselors assist in the coordination of services between the school and community agencies. Most counselors will assist with the coordination of services of a child study team for students with learning disabilities. Many counselors might assist in the development of a parent education program by coordinating presentations, and some counselors might coordinate the delivery of an in-service training for teachers on such concerns as the interpretation of tests or family life education. Other examples include arranging for special events, locating speakers for career fairs, developing an orientation for new students, and developing a network of services for students who are in transition to the next school level.

Theory and Process of School Counseling

Although school counselors are trained in the same theoretical approaches as other types of counselors, it is likely that many practice a theoretical approach that lends itself to short-term or brief-treatment modalities. Therefore, behavioral, cognitive, and reality therapy approaches, which tend to be shorter-term than other traditional approaches, as well as some of the newer brief-treatment approaches, tend to be used by school counselors (Neukrug & Williams, 1993). Despite the fact that many school counselors use these briefer-treatment modalities, it is usual to find them also integrating basic person-centered skills in their repertoire of techniques, as such skills are essential to building relationships with students.

Whatever theoretical orientation the counselor adopts, it can be integrated into a comprehensive model for school counseling. Today, a comprehensive developmental counseling and guidance model is generally suggested for use in the schools (ASCA, 1997).

Comprehensive Developmental School Guidance and Counseling

The American School Counselor Association suggests that school counselors implement a comprehensive developmental counseling and guidance program at all educational levels (ASCA, 1997). This model urges counselors to be proactive and primarily focuses on how developmental issues affect learning and secondarily focuses on special problems and issues that students face (Gysbers & Henderson, 2000; Myrick, 1997). In this model, offering guidance, counseling, and consultation services and conducting coordination activities are the primary methods for providing comprehensive services. Counselors will also implement their own theoretical orientation while providing services. Comprehensive guidance and counseling programs are based on the following major premises (Hughey, 2001):

1. They support learning, actively involve teachers, and thus help to develop a positive total learning environment for all students.
2. They are an important part of the child's total educational process, from prekindergarten through adulthood, and work to encourage proactive involvement through planning and goal setting.
3. They are developmental and preventive and, by their very nature, can be carefully planned and include the total school community.
4. They often offer remedial programs that could include the total school community and other community resources.
5. They provide individual counseling, small-group interactions, group guidance, consultation, and coordination as integral components of the program.
6. They are driven by a fundamental belief in an appreciation for the unique abilities of each child that, when properly nurtured, can assist the child in reaching his or her potential.

A Developmental Guidance and Counseling Model

A visual representation of a comprehensive developmental counseling and guidance model was advanced by Neukrug and associates (1993). This conceptual model offers a way of understanding the roles and functions of the school counselor (e.g., guidance, counseling, consulting, and coordinating) as he or she interacts with teachers, parents, administrators, and students in an attempt to address developmental tasks and special issues (e.g., crises, situational issues) that face children in schools (see Figure 16.1).

Neukrug and his colleagues go on to describe how to develop a comprehensive guidance and counseling program. They suggest the following steps:

1. *Plan the program*. This involves obtaining support from administrators, teachers, parents, and the community; forming a steering committee to assist in the overall planning; and performing a needs assessment of the client population.
2. *Design the program*. This involves developing goals and objectives that are based on the needs assessment; developing approaches and strategies for each objective; securing appropriate resources, such as qualified counselors, appropriate facilities, materials and supplies, and clerical assistance; and developing both qualitative and quantitative evaluation methods.
3. *Implement the program*. The final step involves evaluating and changing the program as a result of newly identified needs of the total school community and the results of the evaluation methods.

Knowledge of the roles and functions of the school counselor, having a theoretical orientation, and applying a comprehensive developmental counseling and guidance model are the foundations for the school counselor offering effective counseling services in the schools today.

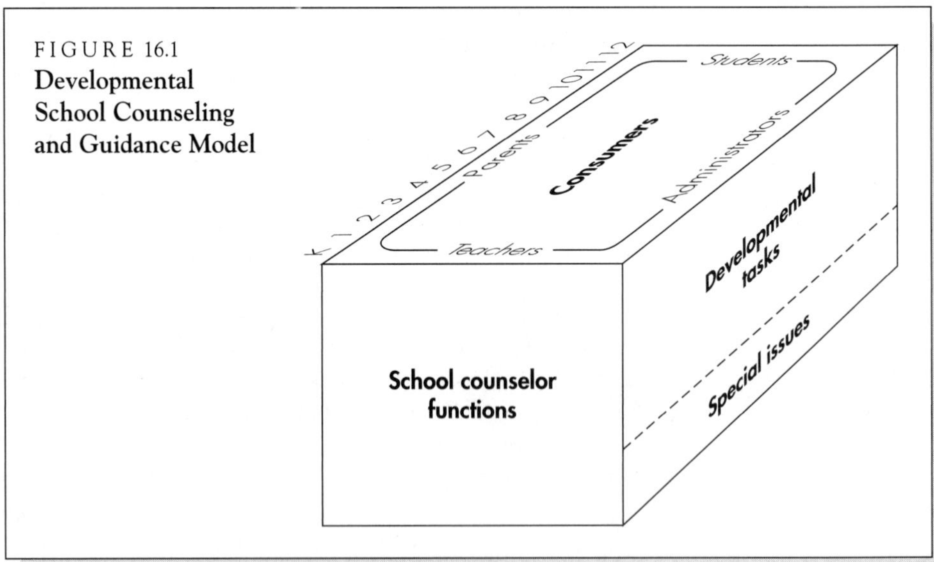

FIGURE 16.1
Developmental School Counseling and Guidance Model

Where Do You Find School Counselors?

Although there is much in common in the training of elementary, middle, and secondary school counselors, there are some major differences in actual job functions. For instance, looking at the distribution of services in Table 16.1, we find that, as compared to elementary school counselors, middle school and secondary school counselors do increasingly less guidance activities and group counseling and much more administrative, clerical, and nonguidance activities. On the other hand, the percentage of time doing testing, professional development, consultation, resource coordination, and individual counseling remains fairly constant.

Today, student/counselor ratios at all levels of school counseling tend to range from a low of 150 to 1 to a high of 1000 to 1, with most states requiring ratios closer to 500 to 1. The law of parsimony, or how to serve the greatest number of students effectively, often dictates the manner in which counseling and guidance services are delivered and is a common challenge to all counselors. Although individual and group counseling, guidance activities, and consultation make up the bulk of a school counselor's day, counselors are involved in a wide range of activities (see Table 16.1). Let's take a closer look at what the three types of school counselors do.

Elementary School Counselors

The elementary years of school life comprise the formative phase of child development. During this time, the tasks of school performance, such as the acquisition and mastery of reading, math, and science skills, provide the focus of cognitive growth. Equally significant

TABLE 16.1

What the School Counselor Does

	ELEMENTARY		MIDDLE/ JUNIOR HIGH		SENIOR HIGH	
ACTIVITY	M%	*SD*	M%	*SD*	M%	*SD*
Testing, appraisal	6.29	6.70	7.27	5.39	6.68	4.02
Guidance activities	24.19*	21.16	13.18[a]	11.75	11.47[a]	8.23
Individual counseling	27.31	18.99	28.60	13.91	30.96	16.56
Group counseling	11.21	8.19	12.44	11.94	8.77	6.26
Professional development	3.64	2.92	3.78	2.70	4.55	2.98
Consultation	12.10	6.45	13.50	8.11	11.32	6.24
Resource coordination	5.43	4.58	6.38	5.39	6.11	3.30
Administrative and clerical	7.02[a]	7.42	11.83[a]	10.16	17.27*	13.06
Other, nonguidance activities	4.43	12.99	5.08	5.31	3.98	7.18

[a]Means are significantly lower than means marked with an asterisk (*). $p < .05$

SOURCE: From R. L. Partin, "School counselors' Time: Where Does It Go?" *School Counselor*, 40(4), 1993, p. 278.

BOX 16.1

Anne: An Elementary School Counselor

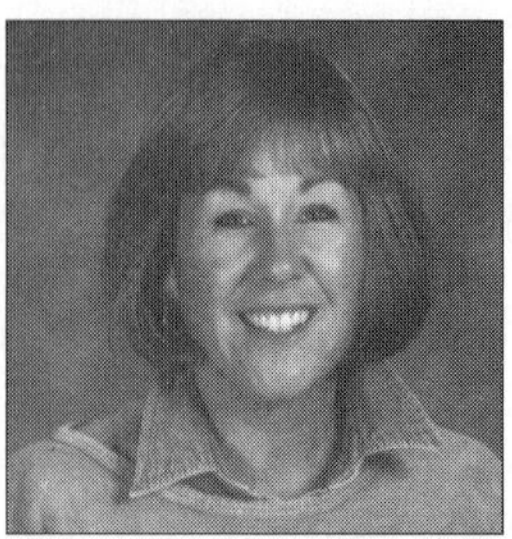

I started my career path as an art teacher in a small rural school in Vermont. After five years of teaching, I began to work on my masters in education at the Bank Street School in New York City. I wanted to become more involved with curriculum development and decided to work toward classroom certification. The foundations used for curriculum considered the developmental stages of students and integrated the academic, social, and emotional components into the learning process. During my third year as a head teacher, I decided, for personal reasons, to move back to my hometown in Virginia where I was hired to teach third grade in a public school in Norfolk. The children had so many needs! I felt torn between addressing those needs, which created road blocks to their readiness to learn, and trying to meet with the requirements of the curriculum. I became pregnant and took some time off from teaching.

After two years at home with my son, I began to seriously consider how to return to professional life. I volunteered as a facilitator for a parent support group. The group helped parents develop constructive disciplinary strategies and understand developmental issues and examined parenting styles. I quickly saw the impact I could have on parents and ultimately the happiness of their children. It was then that I decided to enroll in a counseling program in graduate school. I found the environment stimulating, as the requirements encouraged self-awareness through an integration of concepts. As I neared the completion of the program, I was hired as a part-time elementary counselor. After graduation, I moved into a full-time position.

What do I do? Well, my days vary considerably. Typically, I start the day off before students arrive, preparing to see students, calling parents, and consulting with teachers. When students do come to school, I might be on hall duty. I usually run two groups in the morning: a behavior control group or a self-esteem group. I might have time to also see one or two students individually. Before lunch I write down case notes, and after lunch I do classroom guidance, perhaps on peer relationships or decision making. I often see a couple of students individually, and I may sit in on a child study team. At the end of the day, I often walk the kids out to the bus. After they leave, I write down more case notes and prepare for the next day, which can take a couple of hours.

I love being an elementary school counselor. I feel I now have the luxury to address the needs I had observed through my professional career. Additionally, I am constantly learning more and more about human nature and the ways individuals express, cope, and develop. It's an unpredictable, challenging, and very rewarding job!

at this stage are children's acquisition and fine-tuning of basic social skills and learning how to make friends, solve problems, and manage conflicts. Through this socializing comes the development of an individual identity. This sense of self is based on the successes or the failures of the child's interactions with his or her environment and with others. Research has shown that the development of a positive self-image is related to the child's ability to do well in school (Lee, 1993; Lewis, 1984).

Elementary school counseling programs today have developed what is called an integrative focus, which attempts to address the complexity of issues related to all the developmental areas faced by elementary-aged children. This approach uses a wide variety of counseling and guidance activities to foster child growth in an effort to improve learning.

In elementary schools, individual counseling is generally short-term and responsive to personal or social concerns such as a conflict on the bus, a problem with a friend, death of a pet, or situational problems at home (Partin, 1993). Problems that require more in-depth interventions are generally considered beyond the scope of the school setting, and in these cases, in consultation with parents, counselors will then often refer to outside sources. (See Box 16.1.)

BOX 16.2

Second Grade Sample Divorce Group Counseling Plan: Session Two of Eight

Name of Activity: Some changes caused by divorce.

Objectives: To help students develop a feeling word vocabulary in order to understand feelings and emotions related to divorce; to explore the family unit, and to review changes in the family and examine how new consistent relationships can be formed.

Materials: Drawing paper, markers, house shapes, glue, chart paper, strips of paper, book *My Mother's House, My Father's House.*

Procedures:

1. Review group purpose and promises from last session. Stress confidentiality or "keeping what is said, in group." As a warm-up, distribute strips of paper and ask each student to write down one change he or she has experienced since the divorce. Fold these and place in a small container or cup. Have each child pull a strip from the cup and read the change. Ask others if they have experienced this change and to think about feelings they might have experienced as a result.
2. Explain that often one of the biggest changes as a result of divorce is that parents now live apart. Acknowledge that this can be difficult and children can have lots of different feelings about this. Read the book, *My Mother's House, My Father's House.*
3. Ask students to think about their families. Distribute drawing paper, house shapes and markers. Ask students to draw the family members and different homes. Give the following as examples:
   a. Mother in home, with or without child(ren).
   b. Father in another home, with or without child(ren).
   c. Mother and grandmother in a home with child(ren).
   d. Older brother or sister at home.
4. Have students share their drawings. Stress that family members can remain a family and care about each other even if they live in different houses.
5. Process by asking the following questions:
   a. How do the new living arrangements feel to you?
   b. How are your feelings the same or different from other group members?
   c. What is one thing you've learned or noticed about your feelings?

Small-group counseling is one of the most effective ways of meeting the needs of a large school population. After consulting with teachers, counselors will form special topic groups to address the needs of four to six students. Groups such as these will typically meet six to eight times and focus on the affective, behavioral, and cognitive components of the student. Some examples of topics discussed in small groups include divorce, self-esteem, conflict resolution, motivation, study skills, and peer relationships (see Box 16.2).

Group guidance activities make up the third major component of an elementary school counseling program. Developmental in nature, these groups address key issues for students at each grade level. Group guidance is presented in a didactic, structured manner and is generally presented in the classroom. There is usually an attempt to present topics that are related to the curriculum topics being covered by the teacher. Some typical guidance topics include self-esteem, study skills, friendship, respect and responsibility, peer relationship issues, and decision making. The importance of group guidance activities should not be underrated as they have been shown to be related to increased achievement in schools (Lee, 1993; Lewis, 1984).

Consultation, the last major component of elementary school counseling, takes many forms. For instance, elementary school counselors can be found consulting with teachers concerning a problem student, consulting with parents concerning their child, consulting with administrators concerning ways of providing a wide range of counseling and guidance services, and consulting with professionals in the community concerning possible referrals or to discuss a student.

Implicit in all aspects of elementary school counseling is the desire to provide a supportive, safe environment for all children that will help them learn in school. This early foundation prepares the child for future challenges that will be encountered during the middle and high school years.

Middle School Counselors

During the 1970s, the perception of the age at which children reached maturity was lowered. As a result, educators increasingly supported the concept of middle schools (grades 6–8) rather than junior high schools (grades 7–9) in the belief that children would be better matched for developmental tasks with these new groupings. Working with children ages 10 through 14, the middle school counselor focuses on the unique developmental tasks that face children who are quickly growing into young adults. Some of these developmental tasks faced include a general increase in autonomy, especially from parents; establishment of a sense of identity through comparison of self with others; an increased concern about peer relationships; and dramatic physical and emotional changes (see Box 16.3).

BOX 16.3

Joyce: A Middle School Counselor

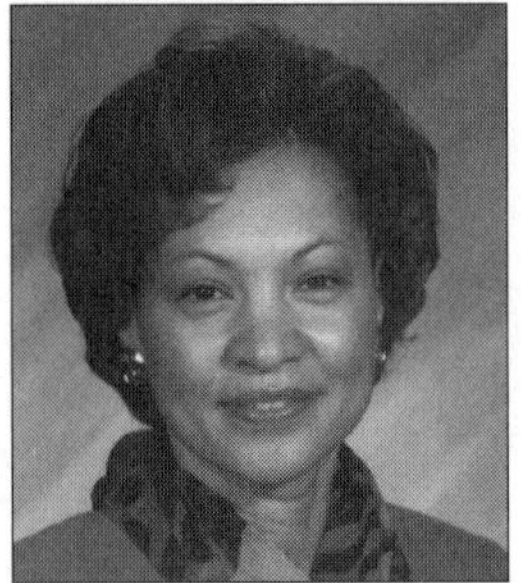

My interest in school counseling began early in my teaching career. As a teacher of educable mentally retarded students on the middle school level, my teaching duties often included providing information or community resources to parents while providing support to their children as they struggled with adolescent concerns and issues related to their developmental disabilities. Those years helped me to realize the very important role that teachers play in supporting children as they try to reach their maximum potential.

The second event that encouraged my interest in counseling was a new educational trend called teacher advising (TA). This educational component required teachers to facilitate "child focused" discussion groups, with topics ranging from such things as peer pressure to study skills. I loved the interchange that occurred between the students and myself. I loved being able to relate to the students as we learned how to respect and value each others' ideas. I knew then that if TA could provide me with such a feeling of self-worth, surely being a school counselor would do the same.

I obtained my degree in school counseling and started at my current middle school as a counselor in 1988. Each day was full of opportunities to support, advocate for, and guide students. And every day was different. I loved the uniqueness of the job. In 1991, when I was appointed chair of the guidance department, I decided to change the focus of the program. It was oriented toward mental health and was not meeting the needs of many of the school's minority populations. With its new focus, the guidance program helped students to identify their strengths and to believe in their abilities. The students' self-esteem was enhanced, and we assisted students in learning how to succeed in the world.

It is now several years later, and I have found evidence that the change in focus of the guidance program was worthwhile. Today, the students at my school have risen to a higher level of academic success. I see students believing that they can achieve and being successful in and out of school. I know that it is the variety of guidance activities that has helped this become a reality. Yes, I still do counseling, but my role as a school counselor includes much more than that. Perhaps most importantly, the guidance department is now seen as an integral part of the total school environment, as opposed to an ancillary service. I feel proud to be part of the success that has taken place in my school.

The middle school child is no longer in the safe confines of the elementary classroom, because students often find themselves switching rooms for subjects and independently maneuvering the hallways, being responsible for organizing and managing class assignments, and being independently involved with some extracurricular activities.

The middle school counselor is faced with a myriad of tasks in his or her attempt to meet the unique developmental challenges of middle school students. In many ways the middle school counselor is truly in the middle, often doing many of the same activities of the elementary school counselor, while frequently involved with many of the activities of the high school counselor. Some of the activities of the middle school counselor include:

- Counseling students individually and/or in small groups to assist with personal growth, self-understanding, and maturity (see Boxes 16.4 and 16.5).
- Providing individual and group guidance activities appropriate to the middle school child's developmental stage.
- Providing career guidance activities to help students identify interests and to have them begin to look at what they are good at.
- Helping students make appropriate educational choices as they ready for high school.
- Working with administrators in the placement of students in appropriate courses, programs, and grade levels.
- Assisting in identifying and referring students with special needs.
- Consulting with the school psychologist, social workers, parents, school staff, and other pupil personnel specialists to plan strategies for helping students.
- Serving as a consultant to parents and school staff on the growth and development of students.
- Helping parents become aware of resources available within and outside the school system.
- Interpreting data from cumulative records for teachers, administrators, parents, and other professionals.
- Providing support services for students with academic difficulties.

BOX 16.4

The Pain of Developing: Reggie and Sam

Reggie and Sam have come to the counseling office for the third time to participate in a conflict mediation session. For the past three months, Sam has been continually teasing Reggie about his size, and Reggie recently started a fight over it. After 10 minutes of discussion, which was more like bantering back and forth, Sam offers an apology to Reggie, and states he won't tease any longer. Shaking his head in disbelief, Reggie says, "You've said this before! What did I ever do to you?" Reggie looks dejected, perhaps on the verge of tears. "What do you think is going on, Sam?" the counselor asks. Slowly, Sam replies, "Kids have been teasing me about being learning disabled, and I can take it, why can't he!" The counselor spends a few moments having Reggie and Sam discuss their feelings, and a resolution occurs when Reggie and Sam shake hands and agree to leave each other alone. How long this resolution will last is not clear.

This exchange demonstrates the changes that begin to unfold during the middle school years and how some students respond to them. Faced with many transitions, the middle school years can leave children harboring great feelings of anger and/or hurt. The middle school counselor needs to expect to mediate disputes as a function of these transitions but can also provide preventive measures to attempt to ward off some of these predictable problems.

BOX 16.5

Sixth Grade Sample Self-Esteem Group Counseling Plan: Session Two of Eight

Title: The different parts of me.

Objective: To understand that each person is made up of many different parts.

Procedures:

1. Briefly review last week's session, especially members' names and group purpose.
2. Stimulate discussion so the students identify the different parts of themselves, such as "likes and dislikes," "interests," "abilities," "behaviors," "feelings," and "values." List each "part of self" on poster board.
3. Have each student complete the "Different Parts of Me" worksheet, below.
4. Process: Have members share their worksheets. Facilitate discussion by asking members for specific examples related to their responses.
5. Conclusion: Check for clear understanding regarding the different parts of self.

Different Parts of Me

Interests:

Something I like to do when I'm not in school is ______________________.

I am very curious about ______________________.

My favorite movie or TV show is ______________________.

Abilities:

I am really good at ______________________.

When I try hard, I am able to ______________________.

Likes/Dislikes:

My favorite food is ______________________.

My favorite school subject is ______________________.

Behaviors:

When I am in school, I usually act ______________________.

My family would describe me as ______________________.

My friends think that I am ______________________.

Feelings:

Something that makes me angry is ______________________.

The last time I cried was ______________________.

People know I'm happy when I ______________________.

Values:

______________________ is really important to me.

I really care about ______________________.

- Assisting with the coordination and interpretation of standardized tests, staff-development presentations, and other professional activities.
- Sitting on special education teams to assist in the development of individual education plans for students with learning disabilities.

Secondary School Counselors

The original school counselors, high school counselors, have a long history dating back to the turn of the 20th century. Like their predecessors, high school counselors of today are working with students who are concerned about future vocational, career, and educational decision making. Therefore, it is probably not surprising to find that high school counselors focus a large percentage of their counseling time on educational and career counseling as compared to personal and social issues (Partin, 1993). However, the high school counselor of today is involved with much more (Baker, 1996; Moles, 1991; Sears, 1993). For instance, high school counselors:

- Provide individual counseling for students with personal problems.
- Provide assistance with scheduling of classes for students.
- Administer and interpret interest inventories and aptitude tests for career counseling.
- Assist students with college applications.
- Have family conferences regarding behavioral and academic problems.
- Assist students in planning for college and work roles.
- Supervise the giving of aptitude tests such as the SATs and ACTs.
- Respond to crises.
- Provide group counseling for personal concerns.
- Provide group guidance for developmental concerns such as vocational guidance, occupational guidance, and interpersonal relationships.
- Provide prevention programs on such things as sexually transmitted diseases and suicide.
- Consult with teachers, administrators, and other professionals regarding student concerns and developmental issues.
- Perform needs assessments to determine what programs are most needed by students and teachers.
- Evaluate programs that they conduct.
- Sit on special education teams and assist in the development of individual education plans for students with learning disabilities.

Clearly, the role of the high school counselor has broadened greatly since its early days. However, high school counselors, more than other school counselors, seem to continue to get bad raps. Perhaps this is because they focus so much of their time on vocational and career counseling due to the immediate needs of the students. Perhaps it is because they are inundated with administrative and clerical work, which is at least partly a function of assisting in scheduling and in college applications (Monson & Brown, 1985). Perhaps they are not proactive enough in insisting that their role should be focused more on a comprehensive developmental model. Whatever the reason, high school counselors are continually struggling to prove themselves. They are criticized until they are needed (see Boxes 16.6 and 16.7).

BOX 16.6

Randy: A Secondary School Counselor

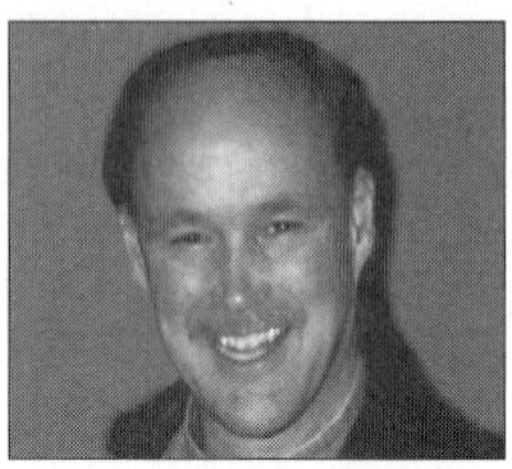

In 1977–78, while attending Loyola University, I interned in the primarily African American suburb of West Woodlawn in south Chicago, working in high schools and a community center. I returned home to South Bend, Indiana, to work in residential counseling at the local runaway shelter where my primary responsibilities were group and individual counseling. I next worked with the Big Brother and Big Sister agency as a caseworker helping to select children and adults for the program. Family counseling, school-based counseling, and tending to families on ADC were all components of the Big Brother program.

Then in 1988 I began work as a substitute teacher in the Virginia Beach school system. I loved the interaction with the students and began to think about a career as a school counselor. Elementary and middle school counseling didn't appeal to me because too much time was spent discussing discipline and not enough time was allocated for individual and group counseling. I decided to obtain my master's degree in counseling, with secondary school certification.

My secondary school work was in full swing in 1992 when I became a high school counselor. It was my duty to interpret transcripts of incoming students and to counsel individuals and families. I became the liaison for all career testing, military, and classroom-based career programs. I used the computer-based Discover program with the 11th graders to have each of them input information relating to job skills. The culmination of this career program was a Career Day held at the high school. That one day saw 1800 students participate, as well as 125 corporate representatives who offered information on over 100 different career opportunities. In 1995, I was given the opportunity to open up a guidance department at a new school. The first few months were taken up with processing academic records from the feeder schools and registering students for classes. With a minimum number of staff in the new department, my core program areas were increased. I continued work in the career field and represented our department as the military liaison. In addition to being responsible for NCAA clearinghouse data, I coordinated financial aid and testing. The latter program included SAT, PSAT, Advanced Placement tests, Tests of Achievement and Proficiency, and the ASVAB test. I also did individual counseling and ran small groups.

When I transferred to a technical and career center in 1997, I became the guidance director with responsibilities in many areas: financial aid, college placement, testing, military liaison, career counseling, scholarship committee, special education, vocational education, and personal counseling. My job includes selecting the most appropriate students to fill the 28 courses in such areas as auto body repair, culinary arts, cosmetology, child care, drafting, printing, and nursing. I screen over 1000 applicants in order to place 670 students in the school by early April. Workshops on scholarships, financial aid, and test-taking strategies for students as well as parents have been offered at the center in the evening. Outside presenters have helped us with staffing these. I organized the city-wide College Night in the fall, which was attended by 1600 students and parents, with over 165 colleges and training schools represented.

Individual, family, and group counseling continue to be the focus of my responsibilities. But a new area has become one of my duties as director. This is the in-service training for teachers through workshops. Recently, I organized a workshop on parent–teacher conferencing, which was to help the teachers understand the importance of an effectual conference. Teachers are interested in being trained to select students for their classes. They are given training in reading applications and cumulative records, along with how to interpret test data. My role as a high school guidance counselor and director has been to help the teachers take ownership of the selection process. As you see from this description of my work, high school counseling at the beginning of the 21st century involves many areas. I wear different hats for different jobs, but I immensely enjoy and take great satisfaction in all of them.

BOX 16.7

Death and Its Aftermath

It was a "normal" day at the high school. I had seen a few students for some personal concerns, consulted with a special education teacher, and run some guidance groups. I thought about some of the more difficult students I was seeing—students with emotional problems, those with severe ADHD. Suddenly, a fellow counselor called me aside and to ask me if I had "heard." One of my student–clients who was ADHD and a problem student had been killed in a horrible bus accident. Having stuck his head out of the window when the bus was about to leave, his head smashed into a telephone pole, killing him instantly. Death is something that children should not have to deal with, yet are increasingly being asked to do so. I thought about what I could do to help the students through this horrible experience. I came up with a plan, hardly realizing that deep down inside I had to deal with my own feelings about this student's untimely death. I quickly set up a room where students could come in small groups and talk about this young man. Other counselors and I offered individual counseling. Out of this, we soon found emerging, from the students, an idea for a memorial service. We helped to facilitate this for them. We were helping them to grieve this loss. It was a very long day; I went home and cried.

Special Issues in School Counseling

Transforming School Counseling in the 21st Century

School counselors may be on the verge of undergoing a major shift in how they do business. Arguing that school counselors are not trained for the 21st century, some have suggested that counselor education programs must change the way they train school counselors (The Education Trust, 2002). In an effort to transform school counseling, the Dewitt Wallace–Reader's Digest Fund has given major grants to a number of universities across the country to help them develop plans and implement change in their school counselor training programs (Guerra, 1998). The new model would have a much stronger emphasis on training counselors as educational leaders who can become advocates for all students as they focus on fostering academic achievement and career aspirations. Table 16.2 presents the new vision of the school counselor and compares it to how school counselors have been trained in the past.

The National Standards for School Counseling Programs

As noted earlier in the chapter in an effort to standardize and publicize the roles an[illegible] tions of the school counselor, ASCA has pushed for the development of *Natio[illegible] dards for School Counseling Programs* (ASCA, 2001a). One hopeful benefit of the [illegible] is to inform school administrators about the important roles and functions of [illegible] counselor. The *Standards* are centered around three broad areas, academic d[illegible] career development, and personal/social development. These three areas are [illegible] into nine standards as noted below.

Academic Development

Standard A. Students will acquire the attitudes, knowledge, and[illegible] ute to effective learning in school and across the lifespan.

TABLE 16.2

Transformation of Role of School Counselor (specifics on role change due to transformation)	
PRESENT FOCUS	NEW VISION
Mental health providers	Academic/student achievement focus
Individual student's concerns/issues	Whole school and system concern/issues
Clinical model focused on student deficits	Academic focus, building on strengths
Service provider, one-on-one and small groups	Leader, planner, program developer
Primary focus on personal/social	Focus on academic counseling, learning and achievement, supporting student success
Ancillary support personnel	Integral members of educational team
Loosely defined role and responsibility	Focused mission and role identification
Record keepers	Use of data to effect change
Sorters, selectors in course placement process	Advocates for inclusion in rigorous preparation for all—especially poor and minority youth
Work in isolation or with other counselors	Teaming and collaboration with all educators in school in resolving issues involving the whole school and community
Guardians of the status quo	Agents for change, especially for educational equity for all students
Involvement primarily with students	Involvement with students, parents, educational professionals, community, community agencies
Little or no accountability	Accountable for student success, use of data, planning and preparation for access to wide range of post secondary options
Dependence on use of system's resources of helping agencies as well as school system's resources	Brokers of services for parents and students from community resources and families
Postsecondary planners with interested students	Champions for creating pathways for all students to achieve high aspirations

Standard B. Students will complete school with the academic preparation essential to choose from a wide range of substantial postsecondary options, including college.

Standard C. Students will understand the relationship of academics to the world of work and to life at home and in the community.

Career Development

Standard A. Students will acquire the skills to investigate the world of work in relation to knowledge of self and to make informed career decisions.

...ndard B. Students will employ strategies to achieve future career success and ...tion.

... Students will understand the relationship between personal qualities, ...d training, and the world of work.

...al Development

...ndard A. Students will acquire the attitudes, knowledge, and interpersonal skills ...o help them understand and respect self and others.

Standard B. Students will make decisions, set goals, and take necessary action to achieve goals.

Standard C. Students will understand safety and survival skills.

Working with Troubled Youth

The shock of hearing about children being shot in schools has awakened many to the problems that many of our youth face today. One result of this increased awareness is that school counselors are increasingly being asked to play a role in working with troubled youth (Hughey, 2000; McAuliffe, 2001). A few of the many roles that the counselor takes on in this capacity include facilitating positive values and character building in students, assisting school staff in dealing with student behavior and discipline, assisting in developing safety programs in the schools, and doing bereavement counseling for students, families, and school staff.

Salaries and Job Outlook of School Counselors

Employment of school counselors in the near future is expected to grow "faster than average" according to the *Occupational Outlook Handbook* (2000–2001b). The increase in the number of jobs is the result of retirements, increased enrollments in the schools, and expanded roles of school counselors. Salaries of school counselors are almost always based on the salaries of teachers who have masters' degrees. Starting salaries in most communities these days range from $25,000 to $35,000. The mean salary of school counselors in 1998 was around $40,000.

Multicultural Issue: Creating a Multicultural School Environment

Americans, and American schools, are becoming increasingly diverse (D'Andrea & Daniels, 1995; Lee, 2001). As a result of these changing demographics, and with the increased focus on multiculturalism in the country, school counselors will increasingly be challenged to make the schools sensitive to diversity (Coleman, 1995; Hobson & Kanitz, 1996; Johnson, 1995; Pedersen & Carey, 1994; Whitledge, 1994). In particular, they will be expected to help *all* children develop a healthy self-concept, respect diversity, and develop a positive and confident attitude toward academic success. In addition, school counselors will be expected to promote a multicultural atmosphere in the schools by:

- Helping schools broadly define diversity to include individuals with disabilities, religious differences, and diverse sexual orientations, as well as older people.
- Finding ways of dealing with increasing numbers of students who have difficulty speaking English.
- Assuring the use of culturally sensitive textbooks.
- Offering workshops and programs to assist students, teachers, and administrators in becoming multiculturally sensitive.
- Evaluating guidance materials to assure that they are not biased.

BOX 16.8

Black or White?

My wife is an elementary school counselor. She used to work in a school that was all African American. One day, while running a small group counseling session, one of the girls in the group alluded to the fact that "Ms. Williams is white." One of the other girls in the group said, "No she's not, she's black." A discussion ensued about my wife's race. My wife is white, and it is not surprising that when a counselor connects with another person race becomes unimportant and indeed in some cases, nonexistent!

- Providing parents from culturally diverse backgrounds with materials they are able to understand and opportunities to feel included in the educational experience of their child.
- Constantly examining how the cultural backgrounds of students, in interaction with the total school environment, affect how that student interprets his or her circumstances.
- Finding ways of establishing a comprehensive counseling and guidance program that is developmental and multiculturally sensitive.
- Assisting schools in developing mechanisms for hiring individuals from diverse backgrounds.
- Becoming a multiculturally adept school counselor (see Box 16.8).

Ethical, Professional, and Legal Issues

Ethical Issues

ASCA's Code of Ethics

As a division of ACA, ASCA recognizes the school counselor's commitment to the ethical standards of ACA. However, in an effort to narrowly define some unique issues faced by school counselors, ASCA has developed a separate set of ethical standards for school counselors, which you are strongly encouraged to read (ASCA, 1998). The guidelines cover the following seven sections: Responsibility to Students, Responsibility to Parents, Responsibilities to Colleagues and Professional Associates, Responsibilities to the School and Community, Responsibilities to Self, Responsibility to the Profession, and Maintenance of Standards.

Tips for Counselors

In addition to the guidelines, in an effort to synthesize some of the major points of the guidelines, ASCA has developed *Tips for Counselors* (ASCA, 2001b) (see Box 16.9). Also, numerous resources are available through ASCA to assist the school counselor in becoming knowledgeable about ethical and professional issues (see www.schoolcounselor.org).

BOX 16.9

Tips for Counselors

1. Act in the best interests of the clients at all times. Act in good faith and in absence of malice.
2. Inform clients of possible limitations on the counseling relationships prior to beginning the relationship.
3. Increase awareness of personal values, attitudes, and beliefs; refer when personal characteristics hinder effectiveness.
4. Actively attempt to understand the diverse cultural backgrounds of the clients with whom you work, including your own cultural/ethnic/racial identity and its impact on your values and beliefs about the counseling process.
5. Function within the boundaries of personal competence.
6. Be able to fully explain why you do what you do. A theoretical rationale should undergird counseling strategies and interventions.
7. Encourage family involvement, where possible, when working with minors in sensitive areas that might be controversial.
8. Follow written job descriptions. Be sure that what you are doing is defined as an appropriate function in your work setting.
9. Read and adhere to the ethical standards of your profession. Keep copies of the ethical standards on hand, review them periodically, and act accordingly.
10. Consult with other professionals (colleagues, supervisors, counselor educators, professional associations ethics committee, and the like). Have a readily accessible support network of professionals.
11. Join appropriate professional associations. Read publications and participate in professional opportunities.
12. Stay up-to-date with laws and current court rulings, particularly those pertaining to counseling with minors.
13. Consult with a knowledgeable attorney, when necessary. In questionable cases, seek legal advice prior to initiating action.

Professional Issues in Counseling

The American School Counseling Association (ASCA)

With more than 12,000 members, ASCA is one of the largest and most active divisions of ACA. Some of the many things that ASCA does include the sponsoring of conferences and professional development workshops, the development of ethical standards, developing position statements on a number of important issues that face school counselors, assisting in accreditation and credentialing initiatives, advocating for legislative initiatives, supporting evaluation and research, sponsoring liability insurance, and publishing a newspaper, the *ASCA Counselor*, and a journal, *The Professional School Counselor*.

ASCA, in or out of ACA?

During the 1990s, ASCA considered leaving ACA (Hubert, 1995). As we moved into the 21st century, many of ASCA's leadership continued to feel that ASCA has not received its fair share of benefits from the umbrella organization. They felt that ASCA could better address some of the unique needs of school counselors with their own separate association. Although this would take a vote on the part of ASCA's membership, the issue is an important one. Perhaps it is time for us to consider how similar or different we are and at least entertain the idea that ACA may not be able to serve the needs of all counselors. Whether ASCA or other divisions disaffiliate from ACA, any unity among us can only come through an acceptance of our differences.

Specialty Certification in School Counseling

Although school counseling certification or licensure on the state level has been around longer than any other counselor credential, national certification was not initiated until 1992 when the National Certified School Counselor (NCSC) credential became established (Paisley & Borders, 1995). In 1994 this certification became affiliated with NBCC so school counselors now have to first attain the National Certified Counselor (NCC) credential prior to becoming an NSCS.

In addition to the NCSC, ASCA is supporting the development of a new certification offered through the National Board for Professional Teaching Standards (NBPTS). At this time, it is unclear when this certification will come to fruition and how it will compete with the existing certification offered through NBCC.

Select Legal Issues in School Counseling

Confidentiality, Privileged Communication, and the Law

Generally, school counselors do not have privileged communication, the legal right to keep information confidential from the courts. Therefore, if they are requested to reveal such information by the courts, they must comply. Although it is important to have a healthy respect for one's ethical guidelines, remember that the "law takes precedence over your ethical code and employer policies. Violating the law, even with the best intentions, or even if directed to do so by a superior, is a criminal act" (Tompkins & Mehring, 1993, p. 340). Ultimately, the counselor as the decision maker must make wise decisions taking into account the client's situation, the work situation, the ethical guidelines, and the legal system (Isaacs & Stone, 1999).

Child's Right to Confidentiality/Parents Rights to Confidential Information

Although ethical guidelines generally support a student's right to confidential counseling, the law has not (Attorney C. Borstein, personal communication, July 1, 2001; Davis & Mickelson, 1994; Hubert, 1996; Huey, 1986). Even though some states partially or fully protect student disclosure to counselors (Swenson, 1997), generally it is the counselor's legal obligation to reveal information about counseling sessions if a parent requests such information. Whenever reasonable and possible, school counselors are urged to collaborate with parents regarding counseling (Remley, 1988). Generally, most parents will respect the confidentiality of the counseling relationship if they are assured that the counselor is looking out for the best interests of the child and the family.

Public Law 94-142, IDEA, Section 504, and the ADA

Passed in 1975, PL94-142 has greatly affected the role of the counselor. This federal law assures the right of students to be assessed, at the school system's expense, if the student is suspected of having a disability that interferes with learning. PL94-142, along with the recent Individuals with Disabilities Act (IDEA), which expanded PL94-142, asserts that schools must make accommodations, within the least restrictive environment, for any student from age of 3 through age 21 with learning disabilities; that is, students must be taught in regular classrooms whenever possible. School counselors play an active role in the implementation of this law by referring students for testing, consulting with parents and teachers, and sitting on special education teams. These teams develop individual education plans (IEPs) specific to the educational goals of the student. PL94-142, the IDEA, along with section 504 of the 1973 Rehabilitation Act and parts of the Americans with Disabilities Act (ADA) are all important laws that aid children with disabilities to gain an education within the least restrictive environment.

Parental Rights to School Records (FERPA: The Buckley Amendment)

The Family Educational Rights and Privacy Act (FERPA), passed in the mid-1970s, allows parents to have access to the educational records of their children. Although it is unclear as to whether counseling records are "educational records," it is generally suggested that school counselors should assume that parents do have such rights.

Suspected Child Abuse

Virtually every state in the country now has a law that requires school counselors and others to report child abuse (Sandberg, Crabbs, & Crabbs, 1988). Although the laws vary to some degree, and each counselor needs to be aware of the specifics of the laws in his or her state, generally they require the reporting of *suspected* child abuse.

The Hatch Amendment

The Hatch Amendment, which addresses only those programs that receive federal funds, states that children cannot participate in research or experimental programs involving psychological examinations without the informed consent of their parents or legal guardians.

The School Counselor in Process: Adapting to the 21st Century

School counselors must be comfortable with change. They must be willing to examine some of their "sacred cows." (Terrill, 1990, p. 87)

The evolution of school counseling has been dramatic. From a vocational guidance focus to a comprehensive developmental counseling and guidance orientation, school counseling today covers a wide range of services (Paisley & Borders, 1995). And the school counselor of tomorrow is expected to see even more changes. Increased interactions with culturally different students, greater use of technology, increased career options for students, and increased involvement of families are a few of the challenges facing the school counselor of tomorrow. Thus, counselors will need to become increasingly adaptable as their roles and functions continue to change and expand. This will require each counselor to examine what he or she is doing and how he or she can respond to the everyday needs of students, parents, teachers, administrators, and community members while being able to handle crises that will occur on a frequent basis. The counselor who is comfortable with change will survive into the new millennium.

Summary

This chapter discussed the unique specialty area of school counseling. We began by briefly defining school counseling, noting that its purpose is to help students at all grade levels learn by assisting them with their educational, social, career, and personal concerns. We noted that today school counseling is developmental and the services the school counselor offers are interwoven throughout the school's total educational program.

We offered some background information on the emergence of school counseling, noting that its origins date back to the beginning of the 21st century, and the resulting need for vocational guidance. We noted that Frank Parsons and others were instrumental in defining vocational guidance and that teachers during this period were the first counselors, being one-half time teachers and one-half time vocational guidance counselors. Although the school counseling profession was slow to expand, during the 1930s, with influences from such individuals as E. G. Williamson and John Brewer, and the passage of the Wagner-O'Day act, the profession diversified and began to more clearly define itself.

During the 1940s the humanistic psychology and education movement was to shift the focus of school counseling from a directive, didactic approach to an approach that focused more on the importance of the relationship between the student and counselor and was more facilitative than directive. In addition, school counseling at this time was to take on a greater mental health focus.

The decade of the 1950s, with the launch of Sputnik and the subsequent passage of the National Defense Education Act (NDEA), saw a great increase in the need for school counselors. The 1960s saw continued expansion of school counseling and was the decade that brought a developmental focus to the profession. Increased professionalism and diversity were the major thrusts of school counseling in the 1970s and 1980s; and, as we moved into the 1990s, school counseling with a comprehensive developmental integrated focus was popularized.

We highlighted in this chapter that all school counselors do large guidance, individual and group counseling, consultation, and coordination. We also noted that although elementary, middle, and secondary school counselors all do guidance, counseling, consultation, and coordination, how they apply them can vary dramatically. We stated that, by necessity, school counselors today must take on a theoretical perspective that can be applied in a brief treatment form. We also noted that counselors apply their skills within a comprehensive developmental framework. We presented a framework for carefully planning, designing, and implementing a comprehensive developmental program.

Highlighting some of the differences among elementary, middle, and secondary school counselors, we noted that the developmental tasks of students vary considerably as a function of age and that the school counselor must adapt accordingly to how he or she responds to students. We noted some possible changes that may take place in school counseling as we move deeper into the 21st century, including an increased focus on helping all children achieve in the schools, a lessening of the mental health model as a focus of school counseling, and the importance of the development of standards in school counseling if administrators and others are to fully understand the role of the school counselor.

In this chapter we highlighted some of the unique challenges school counseling presents us relative to multicultural issues. We suggested that school counselors should particularly focus on lessening language barriers, advocating for minority students, sensitizing the total school community to multicultural issues, helping parents of minority children feel included, assuring that educational materials are not biased, striving to understand how students interpret their environment, and establishing a comprehensive developmental counseling and guidance program.

In this chapter we highlighted ASCA's ethical standards and gave tips for how school counselors can act ethically. In addition, we highlighted how the following legal issues have affected the role of the school counselor: the limits of privileged communication; the child's right to confidentiality and the parents' rights to confidential information; and how PL94-142, the IDEA, the ADA, the Rehabilitation Act, the Buckley Amendment, child abuse laws, and the Hatch Amendment have affected the role of the school counselor.

As we neared the conclusion of this chapter we emphasized the important role that ASCA has played in promoting school counseling. We also examined the debate among some leaders in ASCA to disaffiliate from ACA. We noted that today school counselors can become nationally certified through the National Board for Certified Counselors (NBCC) and that a new certification through the National Board for Professional Teaching Standards (NBPTS) may be on the horizon. Finally, we ended the chapter by highlighting the importance of school counselors remaining flexible in the face of the many changes that will occur in the schools as we move into the next century.

INFOTRAC and Other Information Resources (e.g., ERIC and PsycINFO)

Note: When relevant, key words are in quotation marks.

1. Review the literature related to "comprehensive developmental counseling and guidance."
2. Examine a counseling skill that may be effective with school children (e.g., "play therapy").

CHAPTER 17

Agency and Mental Health Counseling

I'm working at a crisis center, and a client tells me he's being followed by the Mob. They want to kill him, he states. He asks me what to do. I say, "Why don't you call the FBI, or the State Police?" He calls the State Police, and they want to see him. I drive him out to the State Police barracks, thinking along the way, "This guy is paranoid." We get there. The cops talk with him for half an hour. They come out and tell him to lie down in the back of my car so no one will see him. My heart drops. "He's not paranoid???" I think. "Oh my God!" They tell me to take the back roads back to the crisis center!

I'm working at a mental health center with a client who had been hospitalized for depression a few years back. I've been seeing her for a few months and have built a fairly solid relationship with her. At the end of the session she tells me, "You know, when I was hospitalized, one of the staff molested me."

I'm at the same mental health center. I've been seeing a client for about a year. She's been psychotic, on and off, for a number of years and is pretty stiff in the way she interacts with people. She's on some heavy-duty antipsychotic medication. She sees me once every three weeks for a check-in. Suddenly, at the end of a session she looks at me and tells me she had an abortion ten years ago. Her psychotic episodes started about ten years back. This certainly seems to be an interesting coincidence. I decide to see her weekly. She begins to share her guilt about the abortion, and within a couple of months she's practically off her medication. Now, I wouldn't have said she was back to normal, but she certainly was doing better! What a success! A month later, she dies in the middle of the night!

I'm in private practice, and it's a Friday afternoon. I'm seeing one of my last clients of the day, looking forward to going away on a weekend trip to the country. He's a 15-year-old I've been seeing for a while. At the end of the session, he blurts out that he was molested when on a recent vacation. There goes my weekend trip, as I have to deal with his parents, the law, and him.

My girlfriend and I have just broken up. It's my birthday. I'm very depressed. I go to my part-time job at a small counseling center. A new client walks in. She immediately tells me it's her birthday and that she and her husband have just split up. Is this a coincidence, or what? I wonder if I can get through the session.

So, you want to work at a community agency. It can be fun. It can be boring. It can be scary. It can be sad, and it can be exhilarating. It's the best of jobs and the worst of jobs. Let's see what it's all about.

This chapter is about working in agency and mental health counseling. We'll start by defining *agency* and *mental health counseling*. We'll then offer a brief overview of the history of this specialty area in counseling. This will be followed by an overview of some of the places you can find agency and mental health counselors. We will examine some of the theories used by counselors in these settings and some typical roles and functions of the agency and mental health counselor. We'll present some special issues currently impinging on the agency and mental health counselor and then offer some salary information. We'll end the chapter by exploring multicultural, ethical, professional, and legal issues in the area of agency and mental health counseling.

What Are Agency Counseling and Mental Health Counseling?

On the surface, this may seem like a relatively easy question. In actuality, defining agency and mental health counseling is not an easy task. In clarifying these terms, one might look to the Council for Counseling and Related Educational Programs (CACREP), which has distinguished, through the accreditation process, community counseling (which I call "agency counseling") and mental health counseling. CACREP views community counseling programs as mental health counseling programs that train counselors to work in any of a variety of agencies, whereas mental health counseling programs are 60-credit-hour programs that train counselors to work either in agencies or in private practice. However, this differentiation is often lost when we see that many individuals who go through 48-credit-hour programs eventually go into private practice, while many who go through the mental health counseling programs maintain careers in agencies. To make things even more confusing, since the majority of counseling programs are not CACREP accredited and may not even require 48 credit hours for the master's degree, we also find individuals with these degrees working in agency settings or picking up the additional credits and supervision that would make them eligible to work in private practice.

The bottom line is that any individual who receives a master's degree in counseling with a specialty in working in agencies can find employment at many agency settings and is generally eligible to apply for licensure as a professional counselor, if additional requirements are met. In fact, even individuals with closely related degrees, such as school counseling and student development counseling in higher education, can generally make the shift to working in agencies or working in private practice (see Box 17.1).

For the purposes of this text, I have combined mental health counseling and agency counseling into one chapter. I consider any agency or private practice in which mental health services are offered to be a subcategory of agency and mental health counseling. Others will argue with this position, saying that there are unique characteristics to specific agency work and that some types of agency counselors and/or private practitioners should be separated out from this chapter. In many ways I agree with this position. On the other hand, I believe the similarities are so great that one can justify lumping all counselors who work in agencies or private practice settings into one chapter. After finishing the chapter, you be the judge!

BOX 17.1

What a Long Strange Road It's Been

I received my master's degree in 1974 with a focus on counseling in higher education settings. My internship was at a college-affiliated crisis center. Subsequent to obtaining my master's degree, I worked at a drug and alcohol abuse funded store-front crisis center. A couple of years later, I obtained a job as an outpatient therapist at a community mental health center. After obtaining my doctorate in counselor education, I taught counseling and later worked part-time as an associate school psychologist and as a school counselor in New Hampshire. During this time I obtained clinical supervision and eventually obtained licensure as a psychologist in Massachusetts and in New Hampshire. Moving to Virginia, I applied for licensure as a psychologist. The psychology licensure board denied me such licensure saying my field was counseling not psychology. I then applied for and obtained licensure as a professional counselor. Thus, despite my original degree in college student development counseling, I was able, with some additional training, to freely move into a number of different settings and obtain a variety of different credentials. Although it has become increasingly more difficult to obtain certification and licensure in closely related fields like psychology or school psychology, still today, with some additional training, one can move fairly easily from one counseling specialty area to another.

A History of Agency Counseling and Mental Health Counseling

As noted in Chapter 2, the fields of psychiatry and clinical psychology arose around the turn of the 20th century. It was at that time that individuals began to link one's psychological state with one's emotional state and placed less emphasis on physical or demonic causes of emotional problems. Freud's psychoanalytic approach led to this new way of viewing emotional problems and drastically changed the manner in which mental disorders were conceptualized and treated. It was also during this period that sanitariums began to experiment with more humane methods of hospitalization (Smith & Robinson, 1995).

The early 1900s saw the beginning of vocational guidance. This movement, along with the development of the first assessment instruments, was to have an impact on the eventual role of counseling in the mental health field. Besides being a natural fit, vocational guidance and testing shared something else in common: They both were concerned about differences in people, and highlighting differences was soon to become the hallmark of counseling and psychotherapy in general.

During the 1930s the federal government began to earmark small amounts of money for mental health treatment, especially research in mental health. As the decade continued, one could see a new mindset sprouting in America. Influenced by psychoanalysis, the counseling movement, vocational guidance, an increasingly humane attitude toward mental illness, and existential philosophers (many of whom emigrated from Europe), America was now beginning to accept the concept that mental health services were a necessary and important aspect of living in a civilized world. However, traditional psychoanalysis was seen as too long-term and mostly used by the rich; vocational guidance was seen as too short-term and too directive in its approach; and existential philosophy was viewed as too ethereal. However, a merging of these three approaches seemed just right.

As the 1940s neared, a new approach to counseling and psychotherapy evolved, one that encapsulated many of the precepts of psychoanalysis, counseling, existentialism, and American take-charge philosophy. This approach was optimistic and relatively short-term as compared to psychoanalysis and had as its core belief that if people worked hard enough, they could change. Not surprisingly, it was during this time that we saw the beginnings of self-help groups like Alcoholics Anonymous and groups to assist new immigrants adjusting to American life, groups that affirmed the idea that individuals can change.

As a byproduct of the Second World War, evaluation techniques to determine who was emotionally fit to enter the military became much more sophisticated. In addition, the recovery rates of individuals who had emotional problems that resulted from the war was very high. Mental health providers were suddenly becoming more assured about their ability to successfully treat individuals (Hershenson, Power, & Waldo, 1996). It was on the heels of these successes that the National Mental Health Act was passed in 1946, which gave states funds for research, training, prevention, diagnosis, and treatment of mental health disorders.

During the late 1940s the National Institute of Mental Health (NIMH) was created by Congress. NIMH supported increased research and training in the mental health field and was the impetus for the 1955 Mental Health Study Act. This act established the Joint Commission on Mental Illness and Health, which made a number of far-reaching recommendations around increased funding and services for mental health and mental illness. Partly as a result of this act, the 1950s saw the expansion and acceptance of mental health services around the country. It was also at this time that we began to see the widespread use of psychotropic medication. During the late 1950s and continuing into the 1960s a number of new, and at the time revolutionary, approaches to counseling began to take shape.

The 1960s saw great upheaval in American society. There was unrest in the ghettos and a country in bitter turmoil over the Vietnam War. The civil rights movement was growing in momentum. Out of this turmoil came landmark civil rights, economic, and social legislation (Kaplan & Cuciti, 1986). One such legislative initiative was the 1963 Community Mental Health Centers Act, which funded the establishment of nationwide mental health centers that would provide short-term inpatient care, outpatient care, partial hospitalization, emergency services, and consultation and education services. This made it possible for individuals with a wide range of mental health concerns to obtain free or low-cost mental health services. In fact, approximately 600 community-based mental health centers could trace their origins to this act (Burger & Youkeles, 2000).

The late 1960s and early 1970s saw a number of federal laws passed that expanded the scope of community mental health centers and funded substance abuse treatment. In 1975 the Supreme Court decision in *Donaldson* v. *O'Connor* led to the deinstitutionalization of tens of thousands of state mental hospital patients who had been hospitalized against their will and who were not in danger of harming themselves or others. Many of these former patients would receive services at the newly established local community mental health centers. The 1970s also saw the passage of a number of important legislative acts that would have a direct impact on individuals with disabilities. One major legislative initiative was the Rehabilitation Act of 1973, which ensured access to vocational rehabilitation services for adults if they met three conditions: having a severe physical or mental disability, having a disability that interferes with their ability to obtain or maintain a job, and having feasibility of employment with their disability. This act increased the need for highly trained rehabilitation counselors.

With the election of President Carter in 1976, there was an increased focus on the importance of mental health treatment. In the late 1970s President Carter authorized the continuation and expansion of mental health services. Near the end of this decade we saw the establishment of the American Mental Health Counseling Association (AMHCA), ACA's first division to be focused solely on mental health counseling and mental health concerns. Although legislative actions of the 1970s brought with them increased diversification of the counseling field and resulted in large numbers of counselors settling into a variety of community counseling agencies, the boon of the 1970s was soon to end with the election of Ronald Reagan.

Carter's defeat by Reagan in 1980 led to the elimination and reduction of some mental health programs and a move toward federal block grants. Block grants had the effect of allowing the states to decide which programs to fund and resulted in less money for some programs, particularly mental health centers (Hershenson et al., 1996). Despite this temporary setback, the 1980s and 1990s saw a slow but steady expansion and diversification in the field of counseling and a settling-in phase in our profession. Counselors during these decades could be found in almost any mental health setting. In addition, it was during these decades that we began to see counselors working in settings where they had not been found before: family service agencies, prisons, gerontological settings, hospitals, and in business and industry.

Beginning in the 1990s and into the 21st century we have seen dramatic changes in the delivery of mental health services. This is widely a function of changes in our health care system as health maintenance organizations (HMOs) have increasingly become the primary insurance providers (Medical Economics Staff, 2001; Raymond, 1994). HMOs have resulted in fewer services for mental health problems as well as increased overseeing of mental health providers. Although providing mental health services serves an important need in American society, it has become clear that receiving government and charitable funding for such services and payment from insurance companies are becoming increasingly more difficult.

As the mental health field has become more diversified and mental health agencies more prevalent, so have counseling programs that offer degrees in agency counseling and mental health counseling. Whereas 20 years ago most students graduating from counseling programs specialized in school counseling, today 49% of graduate programs offer a degree in community and agency counseling and 24% offer a degree in mental health counseling (Hollis & Dodson, 2000). Of students who complete these programs, those in agency counseling and those in mental health counseling, respectively, find jobs in the following areas: managed care, 9% and 12%; private practice/agency, 13% and 21%; public agency, 58% and 52%; other, 4% and 3%; schools of higher education, 6% and 3%. Most of the remaining students (10% and 9%) pursue doctoral degrees. It is clear that the agency and mental health counselor have become core parts of the counseling profession.

Where Do You Find Agency and Mental Health Counselors?

With the spread of the community mental health movement, many agencies have arisen that offer mental health services and provide employment for agency and mental health counselors. The following is a brief description of some of these agencies.

Community Mental Health Centers

Counselors have been found working in mental health centers since they were first established more than 30 years ago (West, Hosie, & Mackey, 1987). Although a major function of the community mental health center is to assist individuals with severe emotional problems, the kinds of services they offer vary greatly. Today, many community mental health centers offer twelve types of services, and counselors can be found working in any of them. They include:

1. Short-term inpatient services.
2. Outpatient services.
3. Partial hospitalization (day treatment).
4. Emergency services.
5. Consultation and education.
6. Special services for children.
7. Special services for the elderly.
8. Preinstitutional court screening.
9. Follow-up care for mental hospitals.
10. Transitional care from mental hospitals.
11. Alcoholism services.
12. Drug abuse services.

Because community mental health centers offer such a wide range of services, they often employ hundreds of clinicians, including psychiatrists, psychologists, counselors, social workers, psychiatric nurses, and human service professionals. The responsibilities of clinicians at mental health centers vary and include such things as clinical assessment, consultation, referral, retention and education, and individual, group, and family counseling. Because there are a variety of different kinds of clinicians at mental health centers, it is not unusual for clinicians to work as a team (Male, 1990). For instance, for a new client who enters the system, one clinician might conduct the intake interview, the psychiatrist might meet with the client for a medication assessment, and the case might be presented at a team meeting in order to determine which clinician might work best with the particular client.

As federal money for mental health centers has dried up, mental health centers have had to go elsewhere to secure funding. Thus, we see mental health centers obtaining grants from organizations like the United Way, and we have seen them increasingly rely on third-party billing for reimbursement of services. Since licensing is generally needed for insurance reimbursement, mental health centers have increasingly had to hire individuals who are licensed and who are eligible to receive third-party reimbursements. As counselors have lagged behind social workers and psychologists in getting licensure laws passed and in being included in third-party reimbursement laws, this has become problematic for counselors in some states.

Although mental health counselors may be members of a variety of professional associations, AMHCA is the association to which many counselors who are employed at mental health centers belong. AMHCA is one of the largest divisions of ACA and has a long history of advocacy for mental health issues and legislation (see www.AMHCA.org).

Rehabilitation Agencies

With as many as 48 million adults and 5 million children having disabilities (U.S. Census Bureau, 2001e), the kinds of disabilities with which counselors work can vary dramatically and include such categories as mental retardation, learning disabilities, emotional problems, speech impairment, hearing impairment, visual impairment, orthopedic impairment, multiple disabilities, and other health impairments. Counselors who work at rehabilitation agencies are known as rehabilitation counselors. Usually, their function is to assess the client's disability and to develop a rehabilitation plan that will assist the client in obtaining a job, continue his or her education, or pursue a career path (Garfield & Beaman, 1996; Leahy & Szymanski, 1995; McCormack, 1990). Schumacher (1983) distinguishes twelve major functions of rehabilitation counselors:

1. Personal counseling.
2. Case finding.
3. Eligibility determination.
4. Training.
5. Provision or restoration.
6. Support services.
7. Job placement.
8. Planning.
9. Evaluation.
10. Agency consultation.
11. Public relations.
12. Follow-along.

In providing these services, the rehabilitation counselor works with the personal, social, and medical needs of clients, provides individual and group counseling, and coordinates community services for clients. Because of the wide range of disabilities with which the rehabilitation counselor works, it is important that a team approach is taken when working with clients.

The three most common rehabilitation agencies are state departments of vocational rehabilitation, Veteran Administration (VA) hospitals, and private rehabilitation agencies. Although VA hospitals and state agencies obtain federal and/or state funding, private agencies mostly rely on insurance reimbursement, worker's compensation, and other client-related methods of payment.

The rehabilitation counselor straddles two professional associations. The American Counseling Association has a division called the American Rehabilitation Counseling Association (ARCA), which many rehabilitation counselors join (reach ARCA via www.counseling.org). In addition, some rehabilitation counselors may decide to join the National Rehabilitation Counseling Association (NRCA), which is not affiliated with ACA (see www.nationalrehab.org/website/divs/nrca.html). In 1987, ARCA and NRCA jointly developed a code of professional ethics for rehabilitation counselors (NRCA, 2002). Recently, these two associations signed an agreement to join and form one group, although the specifics have yet to be worked out (Simmons, 2001).

Whereas accreditation for community agency counseling programs is offered by CACREP, the Council on Rehabilitation Education (CORE) is the accrediting body for rehabilitation counseling programs. Although the curriculum in many ways parallels the curriculum of CACREP-approved programs, rehabilitation counseling programs naturally have more of a focus on such things as vocational evaluation, occupational analysis, medical and psychosocial aspects of disability, legal and ethical issues in rehabilitation, and the history of rehabilitation counseling. An individual who has a degree in rehabilitation counseling can become a Certified Rehabilitation Counselor (CRC) and/or a Nationally Certified Counselor (NCC).

BOX 17.2

Kathy: A Rehabilitation Counselor

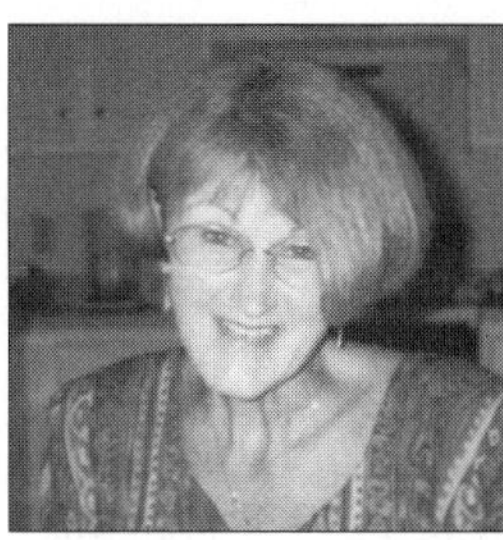

My desire to help people probably goes back to my childhood. In fact, reflecting on my life, I now realize that a number of significant events were precursors to my work as a rehabilitation counselor. Some of these included: the death of my father as the result of a brain injury caused by an auto accident, growing up with a cousin who was mentally retarded, working at a camp for children with disabilities, and an inclination to be a nurse at a very young age. As I grew older, I continued to want to be a helper. I was accepted into nursing school, but I didn't take well to science, so I switched my major to law enforcement and correction.

With a degree in law enforcement, I took a job in probation and parole. I found myself working with ex-offenders, helping to assess their transferable skills. I found it particularly satisfying to help someone with a barrier find suitable employment. Later, I had the opportunity to go back to school and major in rehabilitation counseling. This seemed to meet all of my desires; it was in the medical field, I was a helper, and it was an area that I had interest in—disabilities. After graduation, I obtained a certificate in medical assisting and worked with a pediatric cardiologist and a surgeon to monitor clients' physical therapy programs and help them return to functional employment. I eventually decided to go get a master's degree in counseling and obtain my credential as a Certified Rehabilitation Counselor (CRC). I then worked at a psychiatric hospital as a substance abuse counselor. Many of the patients were in chronic pain and had a secondary diagnosis of narcotic abuse. This led to my next job at a pain management and industrial rehabilitation program. Here, I gained knowledge of Federal and State Workers' Compensation Law as I assisted clients in managing their pain and in getting back to work.

Legislation, particularly the Americans with Disabilities Act, has greatly impacted the field of rehabilitation counseling. As a result of these laws, I found that my job began to change, and I started going to job sites to measure the physical activities of jobs to see how reasonable accommodations might be made to assist an individual with a disability in finding employment. Today, as a by-product of many of these laws, I am often involved with testifying as an expert in disputed workers' compensation claims.

Today, I find my role as a rehabilitation counselor to be multifaceted in that I need to have an understanding of such things as physiology, disabilities, the law, medicine, and insurance claims. I have come a long way from my early visions of being a nurse—but in many ways I'm doing what I always wanted to do.

As new medical procedures make it possible for individuals to live longer with disabling and chronic health conditions, it is likely that we will see an increase in the number of individuals with disabilities. This will result in the need for additional services in which we will likely find the rehabilitation counselor taking an active role (Garner, 2001). (See Box 17.2.)

Private Practice Settings

As licensure criteria for professional counselors have been adopted by most of the 50 states, there has been a concomitant rise in the number of licensed professional counselors, many of whom go into private practice. Generally, with licensure comes legislation that grants third-party reimbursement, allowing licensed counselors to obtain payments for their work from insurance companies. Private practice counselors usually provide a full range of mental health services, although additional training in psychopathology and assessment is often needed if a licensed counselor is to work with those who are seriously impaired. (See Box 17.3.)

BOX 17.3

Mike: A Licensed Professional Counselor in Private Practice

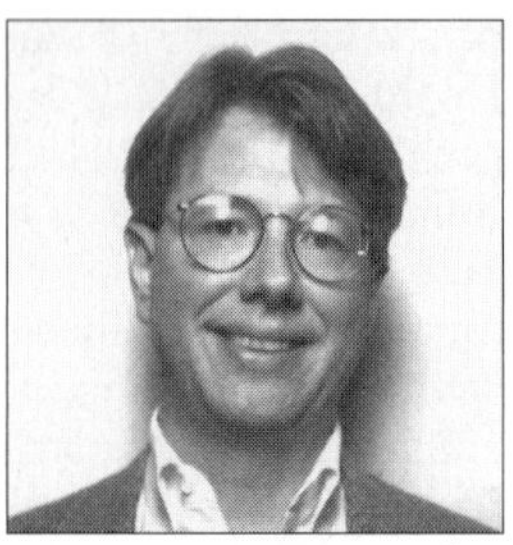

My interest in private practice began at 15 when I attended a weekend encounter group at a YMCA retreat. For the first time in my life I was exposed to peers who were open, honest, sensitive, and introspective. I was able to express myself and was rewarded by appreciation, approval, and regard. That weekend retreat was a turning point in my life.

In college I focused on competitive swimming and chose psychology as a major. In my junior year, a number of stresses led me to have panic attacks. As I struggled to understand this traumatic turn in my life, I sought counseling at the college clinic. There, I encountered a compassionate counselor who enabled me to cope during that very disturbing time. I worked with dreams from a Gestalt perspective and learned to understand some of the underlying dynamics of my life. The experience of finding someone who could guide me through such a disturbing time in my life filled me with wonder and respect, and I resolved to become such a counselor.

After I received my degree in psychology, I tried to find a meaningful job in the field. When I was unable to do so, I applied to graduate school and eventually completed my master's degree in psychology. Licensure did not exist in Virginia for master's-level psychologists, but I did eventually find a job doing psychological assessment at a psychiatric hospital. Under the supervision of a clinical psychologist, I administered and interpreted psychological tests to children and adults who had a wide range of mental health problems. I was diligent and enjoyed the challenge of integrating the various data obtained from the evaluations. However, I decided to get licensed in order to practice independently. I returned to school, completed additional courses in a master's program in counseling, and underwent 4000 hours of supervised work experience. When I passed the counselor licensure exam, I became a Licensed Professional Counselor (LPC). After nervously exploring various options, I signed a contract to work as an independent contractor at a small private practice.

Since that leap of faith over a decade ago, I have achieved my goal. I have helped countless people to varying degrees. I, too, have grown by walking along the paths of my clients, each of whom teaches me a little more about the person I am. I have contributed to my profession through many hours of service to clinical counseling associations, and I have survived the shrinking reimbursements that have been one result of managed care. I am happy with and grateful for my professional life and look forward to further service and growth. Finally, I have come to believe what I only glimpsed at the age of 15—that we are all a work in progress as we struggle to create our own reality!

Although most individuals think of private practice counselors as doing mostly individual, group, and family counseling, in point of fact they may take on many other roles. For instance, many private practice clinicians may be found doing such things as marital and divorce mediation, parent education, consultation to business and industry, stress management and biofeedback, educationally oriented workshops, supervision, evaluations for adoption and custody, and professional writing (Bertram, 1996).

With the cost of mental health services skyrocketing, insurance companies have increasingly cut back on the mental health services they provide (Adair, 1999; Huber, 1997; Wylie, 1995). This has affected the ability of licensed clinicians to earn a living and some suggest it reduces the quality of services (Janesick & Goldsmith, 2000). In an effort to contain the cost of mental health services, many employers now provide medical coverage through Health Maintenance Organizations (Medical Economics Staff, 2001). In addition, Employee Assistance Programs (EAPs) are now offered as an additional cost-reduction effort. HMOs are managed health care systems that limit accessibility to providers while strictly overseeing diagnosis and treatment. EAPs are programs run by business and industry in order to provide primary prevention and early referral for treatment.

Managed mental health programs maintain low costs by referring only to providers who agree to the terms of the HMO, by providing peer review of proposed treatment plans, through early detection and treatment, by preauthorization for admissions to hospitals, and by overseeing case management of clinicians (Foos, Ottens, & Hill, 1991). Although such vigilant review of clinicians' work may provide some cuts in the cost of mental health treatment, clinicians are increasingly feeling overwhelmed by the mountain of paperwork, and many are angry about the ever-looming presence of HMOs in their practice (Daniels, 2001; Wylie, 1995).

HMOs, PPOs, and EAPs

Ironically, although HMOs and EAPs have cut into the ability of private practitioners to make a living, they have provided another possible place of employment for agency and mental health counselors (Bloom, 1987; Hayes & Paisley, 1996). For instance, some HMOs have designated clinicians for whom they provide office space, and subscribers must see one of these clinicians unless they receive special authorization to see someone else. HMOs such as these will often hire master's-level counselors. Other HMOs will select specific private practices to which they will refer, and counselors are often one of the many kinds of clinicians that may be found in these practices. Finally, due to the overseeing of clinicians' work that generally takes place by HMOs, some will hire counselors to review the casework of other clinicians.

Preferred provider organizations (PPOs), which are a type of HMO, are another source of employment for counselors. PPOs are providers that organize to provide discounted rates to members. With PPOs there are gatekeepers who will refer clients to designated providers, although a client can go outside the PPO with the PPO paying a portion of the services.

Some businesses now hire counselors as part of their employee assistance programs. EAP counselors provide education and prevention on such topics as substance abuse and stress reduction, do assessment of employee problems, and sometimes provide short-term counseling. EAP counselors will often provide referrals to a wide range of community services such as mental health centers, substance abuse agencies, lawyers, and private practice clinicians (Hayes & Paisley, 1996; Todd & Bohart, 1999).

Gerontological Settings

As the population of individuals over 60 years old continues to rise, so does their need for increased mental health services (Cohen, 1984). Whereas older persons have traditionally been less amenable to counseling than younger people, as the baby boomers age, this trend is likely to end (Myers, 1983). It is therefore not surprising that across the country we have seen an increase in day-treatment programs for the elderly at community mental health centers, long-term care facilities such as nursing homes, housing settings that are specifically geared toward older persons, senior centers, and programs for the elderly offered through religious organizations and social services agencies (Myers & Salmon, 1984).

When working with older persons, both prevention and treatment become important, and counselors will often be found assisting the elderly with developmental challenges and with situational crises such as loss of a spouse (Fry, 1992; Gladding, 1997). Counselors often have to assist the elderly in dealing with the negative stereotypes placed on them by society as well as the psychological and physiological changes they face as a

BOX 17.4

Needs of Older Americans

In an effort to understand some of the needs of older Americans, I visited a local community center that had organized senior services. This included meals at reduced prices; educational activities, such as guest speakers on a variety of topics; and social activities, such as movies, travel to local theater productions, and so forth. At the Center I had lunch with Irving, Lasard, Izzi, Jeanette, Max, Joe, and some other senior citizens, with their average age being about 80 years old. We had an informal discussion about a number of issues facing older Americans. Although there was some debate concerning the amount of federal subsidies that should be given to seniors, some of their major issues seemed clear. For instance, all felt that seniors were entitled to safe and secure housing, access to good medical care, having their transportation needs met, having access to healthy meals. and having federal assistance in the delivery and implementation of these programs. Most of this group felt that they had spent a lifetime of hard work and now deserved something back in return.

Finally, it was clear that many of these seniors were dealing with losses in their lives. losses of spouses, of friends, and relatives. This psychological component, clearly, was not being attended to by any of the existing available services.

result of aging. Issues of loneliness, physical illnesses, loss and bereavement, and expected developmental changes of growing older are some of the things that counselors will face when working with older clients (see Box 17.4). Although both individual and family counseling can be means of treatment, some suggest that group counseling may be particularly effective when working with the elderly (Gladding, 1997; Robinson, 1990; Thomas & Martin, 1998).

With some graduate programs offering emphasis areas in the counseling of older persons (Myers, 1983; Myers et al., 1991), it is clear that this area of counseling has gained quite a bit of importance. Individuals who have an interest in gerontological settings often join the division of ACA known as the Association for Adult Development and Aging (AADA) (you can reach AADA via www.counseling.org).

Substance Abuse Settings

With nearly 15 million Americans using illicit drugs, 45 million binge drinkers, and 12 million heavy drinkers, it is clear that substance abuse services are necessary (U.S. Department of Health and Human Services, 2000). Drug and alcohol abuse today can be found in the inner cities and in middle-class America. It not only affects the users but has a great impact on family members and on society. Estimates suggest that as many as 1 out of 7 Americans are children of alcoholics (COAs) (Black, 1979; Woititz, 1983), and substance abuse is related to many of the problems facing our nation, including violent crime, problems on the job, and changing morals. Thus, the widespread abuse of substances, unfortunately, provides an array of places for counselors including hospital detoxification (detox) units, halfway houses, and drug and alcohol treatment centers (Field, 2000).

Counselors who work in substance abuse treatment centers provide individual counseling, group counseling, and periodic family therapy. In addition, educational programs may be a part of this counselor's role as he or she attempts to bring increased awareness to the client and his or her family concerning the role that drugs and alcohol may play in their lives. The International Association of Addictions and Offender Counselors (IAAOC) is the ACA division that many individuals with a focus on substance abuse will join (reach IAAOC via www.counseling.org).

Correctional Facilities

In 1999 there were 6.3 million people in jail, on probation, or on parole—over 3% of all U.S. adult residents—and of these, an extremely large number were minority males (U.S. Department of Justice, 2001). With most prisoners being undereducated, abused as children, abusers of drugs and alcohol, and coming from dysfunctional families, the need for counseling is paramount. It is not surprising that counselors today find themselves in multiple roles when working with those who are incarcerated. Some of these roles include counseling, assessment, crisis intervention, consultation, vocational training, assisting with day-to-day adjustment problems, and making referrals to outside agencies when the incarcerated individual is released from prison (Helwig, 1996; Hershenson et al., 1996).

With so many incarcerated individuals having been found to be addicted to drugs and alcohol, it is no wonder that the same association that focuses on addictions, the IAAOC, also focuses on work with incarcerated people.

Youth Services Programs

Today many state-assisted youth services programs employ master's-level counselors. Such programs range from counselors who work with foster children, to counselors who work in residential treatment centers for delinquent youth, to those who are employed in state correctional systems with juvenile offenders. Youth counselors provide a full range of services, including intake interviewing, assessment, guidance activities, consultation and referral with other mental health professionals, and individual, group, and family counseling (Helwig, 1996; Male, 1990). With the tragic recent rash of youth violence in the schools, counseling services to youth has become paramount (McAuliffe, 2001).

Family Service Agencies

Because of a historically strong emphasis on family issues and community advocacy, many family service agencies were originally established by social workers. As a result of this link, for many years family service agencies tended to hire only social workers. However, as counselors began to include family therapy in their repertoire of skills, they have increasingly been hired by such agencies (Wittenberg, 1997). These agencies often receive partial funding through such organizations as United Way and through government grants. In addition, these agencies also receive payments via clients' insurance companies or directly from clients on a fee-for-service basis. Although many of these agencies have a religious affiliation (e.g., Catholic or Jewish Family Services), religion usually does not play a major role in acceptance of clients for counseling (Male, 1990). Counselors who work in such agencies have a full range of responsibilities, including conducting intake interviews, providing case management, offering consultation and education, and providing individual, group, and family counseling. In addition to AMHCA, individuals who work for family service agencies are often members of the International Association of Marriage and Family Counseling (IAMFC, reached through www.counseling.org), a division of ACA, and/or the American Association of Marriage and Family Therapy (AAMFT, see www.AAMFT.org).

Employment Agencies

Counselors today can be found in both state employment offices and private agencies that offer employment counseling. Such counselors typically will assist individuals in "choosing an occupation, changing a career, or adjusting to a work environment" (Helwig, 1996, p. 75). Usually, such work involves the assessment of clients' interests and aptitudes and helping to bring self-knowledge to clients concerning their career development process. Besides AMHCA, individuals who work in these settings often join the National Career Development Association (NCDA) and/or the National Employment Counseling Association (NECA), both divisions of ACA. (Reach NCOA and NECA via www.counseling.org.)

The Military

The military is a unique work setting that offers a wide range of counseling opportunities. The primary role of the military counselor is to assist military personnel with the identification of educational or training opportunities that will assist them in their careers in the military (Helwig, 1996). Sometimes, such counselors will also assist military personnel in their shift to civilian jobs. In addition, military counselors can be found providing primary prevention programs, individual counseling, group counseling, and family counseling to the military or their dependents. Such counselors may work for a military family service center or at the outpatient department of a military hospital or clinic.

Residential Treatment Centers

Increasingly, we are finding counselors working in residential treatment centers. Such centers tend to have a rehabilitative focus, provide a live-in setting for the duration of treatment, and provide counseling services. Today, residential treatment centers service many different people, including those who are incarcerated, individuals with physical disabilities, individuals with mental illness, the developmentally delayed, substance abusers, delinquent youths, and individuals with eating disorders, to name just a few (Lynch & Lynch, 1996).

The focus of such settings varies but often includes individual and group counseling, vocational counseling, assistance with reentry into the community, and consultation and referral to other professionals when the individual is ready to reenter the community. Because of the wide range of clients who may be served in residential treatment centers, as with vocational rehabilitation settings, a team approach involving a number of specialists and group treatment planning is often used.

Pastoral, Religious, and Spiritual Counseling Agencies

Some counselors who obtain a degree in agency/mental health counseling are interested in working in settings that have a religious and/or a spiritual orientation. In fact, spirituality seems to be an increasingly important aspect of counseling for many counselors (Miller, 1999; Stanard, Sandhu, & Painter, 2000). This is evidenced by the fact that the Association for Spiritual, Ethical, and Religious Values in Counseling (ASERVIC, reached via www.counseling.org), a division of ACA, is one of the most rapidly expanding associations (Gladding, 1997).

Some who do pastoral counseling are ministers who do not have a degree in counseling. Some of these ministers will go on to obtain a master's degree in counseling. Others who have a strong religious orientation will obtain a degree in counseling and then seek out employment in a setting that fosters their particular point of view (e.g., Chris-

BOX 17.5

Bill: A Pastoral Counselor

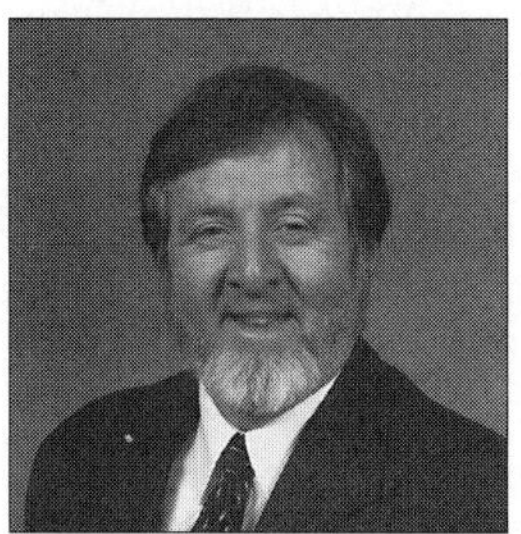

After being a church pastor for a number of years, I became increasingly aware of my lack of counselor training when interacting with some of my parishioners. It was then that I decided I needed training as a pastoral counselor.

When I went back to school for my doctorate in pastoral counseling, I had the opportunity to do counseling under supervision at an alcoholic unit of a psychiatric hospital. I learned much and realized the importance of advanced training in counseling for clergy who work with the personal issues of their parishioners. I realized that I wanted to dedicate my life to pastoral counseling.

Years later, when I became a Licensed Professional Counselor, I was required to have 4000 hours of counseling under close supervision and to take course work in nine academic core areas. Although some states license pastoral counselors separately from LPCs, my state only licenses LPCs. I have the same kind of training as any LPC, and I also have my specialty training in pastoral work. Thus, I see myself as both a Licensed Professional Counselor *and* a Pastoral Counselor. Pastoral counselors can become members of the American Association of Pastoral Counselors (AAPC). This organization certifies pastoral counselors. Those who are certified take courses in specific areas of religious foundations, core clinical theory, pastoral counseling theory, specialized technical studies, and practicum. Certification also requires endorsement as a minister of good standing in a recognized religious body, and you must present an audio- or videotape or a case study of a counseling session, as well as an interview with the Regional Certification Committee.

Today I do counseling at a church that provides an office for me free of charge. They view my work, and that of my colleagues, as part of the congregation's outreach and community service. The main office staff is responsible for arranging appointments and filing insurance papers for the various clients. Once a week a staff meeting is held and group supervision is obtained. The agency has close ties to local religious organizations and training courses are offered for clergy.

In 1992 a Gallop Poll found that 65% of those seeking counseling would prefer a therapist who represented spiritual values, and 81% preferred a therapist who could assist a client in integrating his or her spiritual values into the counseling process. Although I do not talk about God and spiritual values unless the client does, I enjoy being a pastoral counselor as I believe the core issue for most clients are problems of a spiritual nature.

tian counseling agencies). These individuals tend to integrate the basic precepts of their religious viewpoints with what they've learned in graduate school. Obviously, at times this makes for some interesting ethical dilemmas, such as the pro-life Christian counselor whose counselor education training has taught him or her to respect the client's right to make decisions for herself, including those clients who might want to have an abortion. Besides pastoral and religious counselors, an increasing number of counselors have integrated a spiritual viewpoint into their counseling orientation. These counselors tend not to be driven by religious convictions but believe that spiritual issues are primary to understanding one's search for meaning in life. (See Box 17.5.)

Pastoral counselors who are affiliated with a church, synagogue, temple, or mosque can often be found ministering at these settings. Religious counselors are often found in private practice groups that offer their particular religious bent, while counselors with a spiritual orientation can be found in all kinds of agency/mental health settings. Pastoral counselors, religious counselors, or counselors with a spiritual orientation might join the Association for Spiritual, Ethical, and Religious Values in Counseling (ASERVIC), a division of ACA, and/or the American Association of Pastoral Counselors (AAPC, see www.AAPC.org).

Other Settings

In addition to the settings listed above, counselors can be found at many other community agencies, including crisis centers, psychiatric hospitals, hospices, group homes, battered women's shelters, and departments of social services, to name just a few (Baxter, Toch, & Perry, 1997; Collison & Garfield, 1996; Garner, 2001). A degree in counseling is versatile and provides the counselor with a wide range of opportunities for employment. In fact, one might find the counselor in any setting where helping others is crucial (see Eberts & Gisler, 1998). If you are considering a job in counseling, review the agencies listed above, but keep your options open.

Roles and Functions of the Agency and Mental Health Counselor

One can see by the diversity of agencies in which agency and mental health counselors are found that their roles vary dramatically. Let's see if we can, however, generate a list of roles common to most agency and mental health counselors.

Case Manager

All agency and mental health counselors are involved in some kind of case management. Whether working in a mental health center, residential treatment center, or religious-affiliated counseling setting, the counselor has the responsibility to understand client needs, create treatment plans, and follow through on treatment goals.

Appraiser of Client Needs

Whether it is through a formal clinical interview, the use of the *DSM-IV-TR*, the use of tests, or an informal session with a new client, the agency/mental health counselor is assessing client needs and making some kind of determination about the disposition of the case.

Counselor

All agency and mental health counselors, of course, do counseling. Although some counselors may be using brief-treatment approaches while others will be doing long-term therapy, and some will be doing individual or group counseling while others practice family counseling, there is little question that the major role of the agency/mental health counselor is to assist the client through the counseling process.

Consultant

One of the most important roles of agency and mental health counselors is that of consultant. If we remember from Chapter 8, consultation for the agency and mental health counselor can be consulting outward or inward. The focus of outward consultation is on assisting individuals who have some mental health concerns but are not clients directly involved with the agency, such as the parents and teachers of a client. Inward consultation happens when the counselor works to assist the agency in the successful functioning of that agency and ultimately the effective treatment of its clients. Consulting with other clinicians about a client would be an example of inward consultation.

Supervisor and Supervisee

Remember from Chapter 8 that supervision is crucial to a client's growth, as it is designed to facilitate the therapeutic competence of the counselor (Loganbill et al., 1982). From a practical standpoint, supervision is also important because most states require a minimum of two years of clinical supervision as one aspect of obtaining licensure as a professional counselor.

A Professional Who Is Accountable

These days, accountability is a major function of all counselors. One way of showing accountability is through good record keeping. For instance, all counselors should be taking case notes, almost all counselors will be writing intake interviews and/or intermittent summary reports, and most counselors will be filling out paperwork for insurance companies or funding sources. Counselors are also accountable in other ways, such as when they complete needs assessments of their client population and when they evaluate the success of the counseling they do and the programs they run.

Other Roles

Although all agency and mental health counselors take on the roles listed above, there are other roles that are taken on by many counselors, some of the time. They include:

- *Outreach worker*, such as the counselor who goes on home visits to assure the well being of his or her clients.
- *Broker*, such as the counselor who assists his or her clients in using other social service resources.
- *Advocate*, such as the counselor who champions and defends clients' causes and clients' rights.
- *Evaluator*, such as the counselor who assesses the worth of client programs and shows that agencies are accountable for the services they provide.
- *Teacher/educator*, such as the counselor who tutors, mentors, and models new behaviors for clients.
- *Behavior changer*, such as the counselor who uses reinforcement contingencies when working in group homes.
- *Mobilizer*, such as the counselor who organizes client and community support in order to provide needed services.
- *Community planner*, such as the counselor who works with community members in designing, implementing, and organizing new programs.
- *Caregiver*, such as the counselor who offers direct support, encouragement, and hope to clients.
- *Data manager*, such as the counselor who develops systems to gather facts and statistics as a means of evaluating programs.
- *Administrator*, such as the counselor who runs, manages, and supervises community service programs.
- *Clinical assistant*, such as the counselor who works closely with and may be supervised by more highly trained professionals in an effort to assist in client growth (Neukrug, 2000; SREB, 1969).

Finally, Gladding (2000) offers another method of categorizing the work of the agency/mental health counselor. He suggests that the counselor distinguish whether his or her role is one of primary prevention, secondary prevention, or tertiary prevention. Those who focus on primary prevention concentrate on prevention of emotional problems and the promotion of a wellness outlook. Secondary prevention focuses on the control of nonsevere mental health problems, while tertiary prevention concentrates on the control

FIGURE 17.1
Comparison of the Focus of Counselors Who Provide Primary, Secondary, or Tertiary Prevention

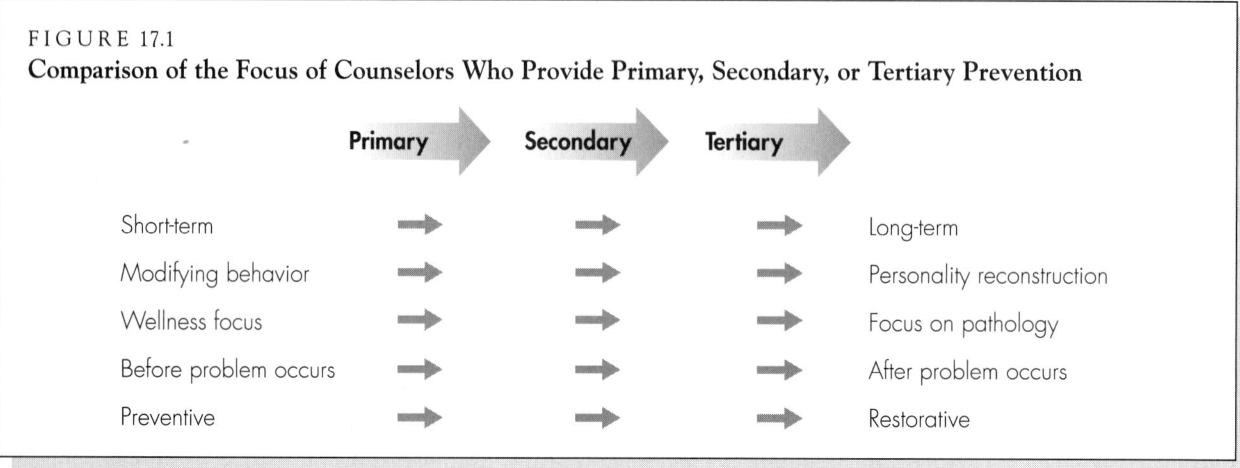

of serious mental health problems. A continuum exists whereby those who practice primary prevention focus less on assessment and diagnosis and more on presenting educationally oriented materials to ward off potential problems. Those involved with secondary and tertiary prevention respectively become increasingly involved in diagnosis, long-term treatment, and working with psychopathology (see Figure 17.1).

Theory and Process of Agency and Mental Health Counseling

Because there are so many different settings, roles, and functions of agency and mental health counselors, it is not a simple process to talk about a theoretical orientation for the agency/mental health counselor. In fact, sometimes a counselor's theoretical approach is driven by the type of agency in which he or she works. For instance, the counselor who works in an agency that mandates short-term counseling must resort to brief-treatment modalities. This leaves the counselor with a handful of theoretical approaches from which to choose. The counselor who works mostly with families must obviously have training in family therapy; and, again, this counselor must choose from the existing family therapy approaches. Similarly, the rehabilitation counselor who mostly conducts career counseling must choose from the career development approaches. Therefore, to attempt to define a general theoretical approach taken by most agency/mental health counselors would be impossible.

Although we might not be able to identify a general theoretical approach, there are some broad principles we can identify that are common to many counselors who work in these settings. For instance Hershenson and colleagues (1996) suggest that the following six principles govern the ways in which counselors deliver services at all agencies:

1. Respect for the client is a crucial element to any counseling process.
2. Clients will make progress if given a facilitative environment.

3. Counseling requires active participation on the part of the client and will result in learning and change.
4. Counseling should focus on the clients' strengths, not their weaknesses.
5. Counseling should seek to help the client define realistic goals and develop resources to reach those goals.
6. The counselor should use techniques that have been shown to be valid through prior research if he or she is going to be successful in helping the client reach his or her goals.

Special Issues in Agency and Mental Health Counseling

Changes in the Health Care Delivery System

The spread of HMOs has affected almost all agency/mental health counseling settings (Danzinger & Welfel, 2001). Whereas clients previously had choice as to the type and place of counseling-related services they desired, today HMOs carefully monitor which services are allowable and the specific providers a client may see (Huber, 1997; Raymond, 1994). In addition, HMOs often carefully monitor the number of allowable counseling sessions. The rise of HMOs and possible changes in Medicare and Medicaid all may dramatically affect the ways in which mental health services are delivered and whether or not they are accessible at all.

Deinstitutionalization

The 1975 Supreme Court decision in *Donaldson* v. *O'Connor* resulted in hospitals no longer being able to keep individuals hospitalized against their will unless they were likely to cause harm to themselves or others. Almost all community/mental health agencies are now dealing with the impact of this decision, and many of them now provide services for those individuals who are chronically mentally ill and/or their families.

Whereas counselors had been seen as mostly working with individuals who had developmental and adjustment problems, the increase in the numbers of nonhospitalized chronically mentally ill has forced agency/mental health counselors to have a working knowledge of diagnosis and treatment of those with severe emotional problems. Thus, knowledge of *DSM-IV-TR*, psychopathology, and medications used with this population have practically become a necessity in almost any community/mental health agency today.

DSM-IV-TR and the Agency/Mental Health Counselor

A 1988 survey by West, Hosie, and Mackey found that one area in which counselors seemed most lacking was knowledge of *DSM-III* (*DSM-IV-TR's* predecessor). Perhaps this is not surprising, since still today major coursework in abnormal psychology or psychopathology is not required by CACREP and is not offered by many counseling programs. Although counselors have been the last holdouts in the adoption and use of the *DSM-IV-TR*, it appears that the use of this diagnostic manual is now a necessity if one is to work at most agency/mental health settings. From a practical standpoint, counselors are in-

TABLE 17.1

Drawbacks and Benefits of *DSM-IV-TR*

DRAWBACKS	BENEFITS
Objectifies and depersonalizes the person, as we view him or her in a dispassionate manner, much like watching a rat in a maze.	Offers us a way of understanding the person more deeply, as we are challenged to make a thorough assessment of the client.
Labeling can lead to a self-fulfilling prophecy whereby the individual is seen as the diagnosis, is treated in a manner consistent with that diagnosis, and therefore is reinforced for that diagnostic label.	By understanding the diagnostic label and by knowing the research in the field, we can better match treatment plans and use of medication with the diagnosis, thus leading to better therapeutic outcomes.
Provides clinicians with a common language that enables them to discuss clients as if they were not real people with real concerns.	Offers clinicians a common language by which they can consult with one another and jointly come up with more effective treatment decisions.
Creates artificial categories that we "buy into," and thus we believe such diagnoses exist. In fact, such diagnoses are a social construction and are thus a function of the values of society.	Provides clear-cut diagnostic categories from which research designs can be generated and new treatments found.

creasingly coming to the realization that, in order to receive insurance payments, they must submit a diagnosis to the insurance company, a diagnosis from *DSM-IV-TR*.

Although some agencies receive payment for services from sources other than insurance companies, such as charities or grants, even those agencies are now acknowledging the importance of *DSM-IV-TR*. This is true for a number of reasons. For instance, *DSM-IV-TR* has given clinicians a common language from which to understand clients. In addition, it offers a system by which counselors can understand the nature of client problems and can thus provide possible treatment strategies geared specifically for identified diagnoses. Also, for counselors who work with children with learning disabilities, *DSM-IV-TR* offers us a way of identifying and understanding such disabilities.

Although the argument will continue to be made that *DSM-IV-TR*, or any diagnostic classification system, will tend to objectify and label the individual, we must not "throw the baby out with the bathwater," for *DSM-IV-TR* may be able to offer us some new ways of understanding our clients and provide possible avenues for treatment planning. Table 17.1 provides some of the benefits and drawbacks of the use of *DSM-IV* in clinical settings.

Psychotropic Medication

Closely related to the use of *DSM-IV-TR* is the willingness, or lack thereof, on the part of counselors to use psychotropic medication. With increasing evidence that some emotional disorders are genetically linked (Neukrug, 2001), and with research now showing that the treatment of some problems, such as depression, is best facilitated through a combination of therapy and psychotropic medication, it is becoming evident that counselors will need to learn how to use such medications (Conte et al., 1986; Norden, 1996). Not to do so will undoubtedly find the counselor out of sync with the rest of the mental health field. In addition, it may leave the counselor open to ethical misconduct charges and possible malpractice suits, as in some cases not to use medication may be viewed as practicing incompetent therapy.

Salaries of Agency and Mental Health Counselors

As you can see, the settings in which you find the agency/mental health counselor vary dramatically. Generally, the employment of counselors is expected to be strong, as reported by the Occupational Outlook Handbook (2000–2001b). Although salaries too might vary as a function of the setting or the region in which you live, generally, entry-level salaries for agency and mental health counselors are between $25,000 and $35,000, with most counselors starting in the mid- to upper 20s. Because advancement in many of these agencies is possible, counselors can often earn up to $50,000 or $60,000. Counselors in private practice who are well networked and established can earn up to $100,000 or more (Baxter et al.,1997; Collison & Garfield, 1996).

Multicultural Issues

Broad Issues Hindering Multicultural Counseling at Agencies

Gladding (1997) denotes a number of primary multicultural issues that face community agency/mental health counselors. They include that (1) most counseling theories are Western-based and might be dissonant with some minority cultures' values and attitudes; (2) some agency and mental health counselors may not have the sensitivity or the training necessary to work with minority clients; (3) many agency/mental health counselors have an ethnocentric world view; and (4) minority clients do not have access to effective counseling services because of the biases held by the majority culture. Agency and mental health counselors must take heed of these concerns if they are to work effectively with the increasingly larger numbers of minority clients we will see in the next century.

Assessment of Clients at Agencies

When assessing clients through testing, it is of particular importance to understand the nature of bias in tests and to remember that a counselor's bias can lead to misinterpretation of tests, even when they are designed to be cross-culturally fair (Hershenson et al., 1996).

When assessing a client for a clinical diagnosis, counselors must remember that a diagnosis is, to some degree, culturally predisposed, thus leading to the likelihood that individuals from some cultures will be misdiagnosed. To a limited degree, *DSM-IV-TR* attempts to control for this by listing approximately 25 "culture-bound syndromes." These syndromes may represent normal behavior within the culture or abnormal behavior that is specific to the culture and for which there is no corresponding *DSM-IV-TR* classification. For instance, some African Americans and European Americans from the South may undergo what is called a spell, in which they communicate with deceased loved ones or spirits while undergoing dramatic personality shifts, which may be misconstrued as a psychotic episode (APA, 2000). And, if you remember from Chapter 10, we discussed the south and east Asian disorder known as "koro," which is characterized by intense anxiety because the individual is fearful that his penis, or, in the case of a female, her vulva and nipples, will recede into the body and possibly cause death (APA, 2000). Clearly, when conducting a clinical assessment counselors must be extra careful to eliminate cultural bias.

Limited Numbers of Minority Counselors

One problem that has an impact on all of us is the limited number of individuals from diverse backgrounds who become counselors. If agencies are to offer services to clients from minority backgrounds, it is clear that more minority counselors are needed, for research consistently shows that minority clients work best with minority counselors (Atkinson, 1985; Atkinson et al., 1989, McKenzie, 1999; Phelps et al., 2001). It is all of our responsibility to encourage agency administrators to hire minority counselors and to assure that minority clients are treated with respect and in culturally sensitive ways. Of course, counselor education programs need to take strong steps to increase the numbers of minority graduate students who enter their programs.

Ethical, Professional, and Legal Issues

Ethical Complaints Made against Licensed Professional Counselors

One manner in which we can assess the kinds of ethical difficulties agency/mental health counselors may be facing is by examining the kinds of ethical complaints made against licensed professional counselors. Although many agency and mental health counselors are not LPCs, it is likely that most agency/mental health counselors face similar ethical dilemmas to LPCs. In surveying 45 licensing boards Neukrug and associates (2001) found that 24% of complaints were made for inappropriate dual relationship; 17% for incompetence in the facilitation of a counseling relationship; 8% for practicing without a license or other misrepresentation of qualifications; 7% for having a sexual relationship with a client; 5% for breach of confidentiality; 4% for inappropriate fee assessment; 1% for failure to inform clients about goals, techniques, rules, and limitations of the counseling relationship; and 1% for failure to report abuse. Another 33% of the ethical complaints were listed in an "other" category, with many boards indicating that drug abuse and felony or misdemeanor conviction was the cause. Although ethical complaints do not necessarily translate into ethical violations, it is likely that trends in ethical violations can be deduced by this data.

Table 17.2 examines the ethical complaints noted by Neukrug and associates (2001) and compares them with the specific ethical guidelines of ACA (1995) and of the AMHCA (2000). Please note that these are only excerpts from the ethical codes, and other portions of these ethical guidelines may also hold relevance to the ethical complaint presented.

Professional Associations and Credentialing

Because agency/mental health counseling is not specific to one type of agency or even one type of counseling, ACA does not have a division that focuses solely on agency/mental health counseling (Hershenson & Berger, 2001). However, a large percentage of agency/mental health counselors join AMHCA, one of the largest divisions of ACA. Many AMHCA members are interested in becoming nationally certified through the National Board of Certified Counselors as clinical mental health counselors (CCMHC) or masters addictions counselors (MAC). Becoming an NCC is the first step toward obtaining these certifications. Of course, many agency/mental health counselors also want to become licensed professional counselors (LPCs), as this will allow them to obtain

TABLE 17.2

Complaints Against Licensed Counselors and Corresponding Ethical Guidelines

COMPLAINT	ACA (1995a) GUIDELINE	AMHCA (1990) GUIDELINE
Inappropriate dual relationship	***Section A.6.a. The Counseling Relationship: Dual Relationships*** a. *Avoid When Possible*. Counselors are aware of their influential positions with respect to clients, and they avoid exploiting the trust and dependency of clients. Counselors make every effort to avoid dual relationships. . .	***Principal 1: Welfare of the Consumer*** *F) Dual Relationships* Mental health counselors are aware of their influential position with respect to their clients and avoid exploiting the trust and fostering dependency of the client. 1.Mental health counselors make every effort to avoid dual relationships with clients that could impair professional judgment or increase the risk of harm. Examples of such relationships may include, but are not limited to: familial, social, financial, business, or close personal relationships with the clients. . . .
Incompetence	***C.2.a. Professional Competence*** a. *Boundaries of Competence*. Counselors practice only within the boundaries of their competence, based on their education, training supervised experience, state and national professional credentials, appropriate professional experience. Counselors will demonstrate a commitment to gain knowledge, personal awareness, sensitivity, and skills pertinent to working with a diverse client population.	***Principle 7: Competence*** The maintenance of high standards of professional competence is a responsibility shared by all mental health counselors in the best interests of the public and the profession. Mental health counselors recognize the boundaries of their particular competencies and the limitations of their expertise. Mental health counselors only provide those services and use only those techniques for which they are qualified by education, techniques or experience. . . .
Practicing without a license or other misrepresentation of qualifications	***Standard C.4.a. Professional Responsibility: Credentials*** a. *Credentials Claimed*. Counselors claim or imply only professional credentials possessed and are responsible for correcting any known misrepresentations of their credentials by others. . . .	***Principle 12: Private Practice*** *B)* . . . mental health counselors should advertise the services in such a manner so as to accurately inform the public as to services, expertise, profession, and techniques of counseling in a professional manner. . . . Mental health counselors advertise the following: highest relevant degree, type and level of certification or license, and type and/or description of services or other relevant information. Such information should not contain false, inaccurate, misleading, partial, out of context, descriptive material or statements.
Sexual relationship with client	***Section A.7.a. The Counseling Relationship: Sexual Intimacies with Clients*** *a. Current Clients*. Counselors do not have any type of sexual intimacies with clients and do not counsel persons with whom they have had a sexual relationship. *b. Former Clients*. Counselors do not engage in sexual intimacies with former clients within a minimum of two years after terminating the counseling relationship. . . .	***Principal 1: Welfare of the Consumer*** *G) Sexual Relationships* Sexual relationships with clients are strictly prohibited. Mental health counselors do not counsel persons with whom they have had a previous sexual relationship. *H) Former Clients* Counselors do not engage in sexual intimacies with former clients within a minimum of two years after terminating the counseling relationship. . . .

(continued)

TABLE 17.2

Complaints against Licensed Counselors and Corresponding Ethical Guidelines *(continued)*

COMPLAINT	ACA (1995a) GUIDELINE	AMHCA (1990) GUIDELINE
Breach of confidentiality	***Section A.3.a. The Counseling Relationship: Client Rights*** a. *Disclosure to Clients*. . . . Clients have the right to expect confidentiality and to be provided with an explanation of its limitations . . . ***Section B.1.a. Confidentiality: Right to Privacy*** *a. Respect for Privacy*. Counselors respect their clients' right to privacy and avoid illegal and unwarranted disclosures of confidential information.	***Principle 3: Confidentiality*** Mental health counselors have a primary obligation to safeguard information about individuals obtained in the course of practice, teaching, or research. Personal information is communicated to others only with the person's written consent or in those circumstances where there is clear and imminent danger to the client, to others or to society. Disclosure of counseling information is restricted to what is necessary, relevant and verifiable. . . .
Inappropriate fee assessment	***Section A.10.a. The Counseling Relationship: Fees and Bartering*** *a. Advance Understanding*. Counselors clearly explain to clients, prior to entering the counseling relationship, all financial arrangements related to professional services . . .	***Principle 1: Welfare of the Consumer*** *L) Fees and Bartering* 1. Mental health counselors clearly explain to clients, prior to entering the counseling relationship, all financial arrangements related to professional services, including the use of collection agencies or legal measures for nonpayment. 2. . . . In the event that the payment of the mental health counselor's usual fees would create undue hardship for the client, assistance is provided in attempting to find comparable services at an acceptable cost. 3. Mental health counselors ordinarily refrain from accepting goods or services from clients in return for counseling service . . .
Failure to inform client about rules of counseling relationship	***Section A.3.a. The Counseling Relationship: Client Rights*** a. *Disclosure to Clients*. When counseling is initiated, and throughout the counseling process as necessary, counselors inform clients of the purposes, goals, techniques, procedures, limitations,, potential risks and benefits of services to be performed. . . .	***Principle 1: Welfare of the Consumer*** *A) Primary Responsibility* . . . 3. Mental health counselors fully inform consumers as to the purpose and nature of any evaluation, treatment, education or training procedure and they fully acknowledge that the consumer has the freedom of choice with regard to participation.
Failure to report abuse (child, elderly, spouse)	***Section B.1.a. Confidentiality: Right to Privacy*** *a. Exceptions*. The general requirement that counselors keep information confidential does not apply when disclosure is required to prevent clear and imminent danger to the client or to others or when legal requirements demand that confidential information be revealed.	***Principle 3: Confidentiality*** . . . The protection of a child, an elderly person, or a person not competent to care for themselves from physical or sexual abuse or neglect requires that a report be made to a legally constituted authority. The mental health counselor complies with all state and federal statutes concerning mandated reporting. . . .

third-party reimbursement. Most states require a master's degree and a minimum of 60 credits for licensure. In addition, usually, two years of post-master's supervision and the passing of a licensing exam are also required. While some states use the NCC or CCMHC for their licensure exam, other states have devised a separate licensing exam.

Increasingly, as other specialty areas become more popular, we will see additional certifications arise. For instance, already today we can also find certification as a sex counselor, employee assistance counselor, and as a pastoral clinical supervisor.

The Agency and Mental Health Counselor in Process: Growing, Changing, Accepting

Probably more than any other counseling specialty area, the field of agency and mental health counseling has been undergoing dramatic changes in recent years, and it is likely to continue do so in the foreseeable future (Seiler, 1999). The ever-increasing acceptance of diagnostic tools such as *DSM-IV-TR*, the dramatic shifts in the health care delivery system, the increase in the kinds of counseling services offered, the ever-increasing knowledge of multicultural issues and their effects on client treatment, and the development of new ways of treating individuals with various emotional problems are just a few of the many issues that currently face the agency/mental health counselor. Thus, the agency/mental health counselor must not hide his or her head in the sand and continue to operate as usual. He or she must change with the times, attend conferences and continuing education opportunities, and be flexible enough to adapt to new ways of working with clients from all backgrounds.

Summary

This chapter examined the unique characteristics of the agency and mental health counselor. Exploring the history of the agency/mental health counselor, we noted that this counseling specialty area had its origins with the development of psychoanalysis, the testing movement, and vocational guidance at the turn of the century. Over the years the field was greatly influenced by existentialists from Europe and the Western philosophy of taking charge of one's life. The profession was launched into modern-day America through a series of legislative acts in the 1940s, 1950s, and 1960s. As a result of this legislation, research uncovered innovative therapeutic treatment modalities and new psychotropic medications that were to vastly change the way counseling was delivered. In addition, this legislation funded mental health centers and other counseling-related services, and soon counseling became more acceptable in America.

The spread of varying types of agencies that offered various counseling services was enormous during the 1960s and 1970s. Very quickly we began to see mental health centers emerge in almost every community in America. In addition, other agencies, such as substance abuse centers, family service agencies, and vocational rehabilitation agencies, became part of the American landscape. Today, we see counselors working in just about every agency where counseling services are offered.

Because counselors can be found in just about every setting where counseling takes place, it would be impossible to list every agency where we might find counselors today.

However, some of the more common settings we highlighted included community mental health centers, rehabilitation agencies, private practice settings, HMOs, PPOs, EAPs, gerontological settings, substance abuse settings, correctional facilities, youth service programs, family service agencies, employment agencies, the military, residential treatment centers, and pastoral, spiritual, and religious counseling agencies.

Although we noted that the roles and functions of agency and mental health counselors vary dramatically based on the setting, we did highlight some common roles taken on by most counselors. These include the roles of case manager, appraiser of client needs, counselor, consultant, supervisee and supervisor, and a professional who is accountable. In addition, we highlighted other roles taken on by many counselors. These included the roles of outreach worker, broker, evaluator, teacher/educator, behavior changer, mobilizer, community planner, caregiver, data manager, administrator, and clinical assistant. In addition, we noted that counselors' roles might vary based on whether they practiced primary, secondary, or tertiary prevention.

Because there are so many different settings, roles, and functions of an agency/mental health counselor, the theories used by such counselors vary dramatically. However, we were able to identify some broad principles that underlie the counseling process of agency and mental health counselors. These included respect for the client, creating a facilitative environment for client growth, encouraging active participation on the part of the client, focusing on the strengths of the client, defining realistic goals and developing resources, and using up-to-date techniques.

In this chapter we next highlighted a few issues that have particularly affected the delivery of counseling services of agency and mental health counselors. These included the recent changes in the health care system, particularly the increased popularity of HMOs; how deinstitutionalization has led to an increase in the numbers of individuals with severe emotional problems who use a wide range of counseling services; the role that *DSM-IV-TR* and diagnosis now play in treatment and insurance reimbursement; and how the use of psychotropic medication has become an important part of treatment for many clients at most community agencies.

Within this chapter we examined some primary issues related to multicultural counseling and the agency/mental health counselor. We noted that most counseling theories are Western-based and may not be effective with some minority clients, that some agency and mental health counselors may have little sensitivity or training in working with diverse clients, and that many agency and mental health counselors may have an ethnocentric world view. We also stressed that the agency/mental health counselor needs to be aware of bias in testing when doing assessments of minority clients, in diagnosing minority clients, and when doing an assessment of minority client problems. We noted that sometimes what appears to be pathology may be culturally normal behavior. Finally, we stated the importance of having more minority counselors in agency and mental health settings.

Examining some of the more prevalent ethical, professional, and legal issues, we noted some specific ethical concerns that are likely to be impinging on agency and mental health counselors. Specifically, we reported that ethical complaints were more likely to be made for inappropriate dual relationship, incompetence in the facilitation of a counseling relationship, practicing without a license or other misrepresentation of qualifications, or having a sexual relationship with a client. Other complaints were made for breach of confidentiality; inappropriate fee assessment; failure to inform clients about goals, techniques, rules, and limitations of the counseling relationship; failure to report abuse; drug abuse; or because the counselor had a misdemeanor or felony charge.

We stated that many agency and mental health counselors belong to AMHCA, and those who are rehabilitation counselors usually join ARCA or NRCA. However, we also noted that because of the varied types of agency and mental health counselors, there are many professional associations to which they belong. We stated that many agency and mental health counselors obtain an NCC, with some subsequently acquiring the CCMHC and/or licensure as professional counselors. We also noted that there are other certifications for agency and mental health counselors with two of the more popular ones being certifications in rehabilitation (CRC) and master addictions counseling (MAC). Finally, we noted that since funding sources have become less common for community agencies, it has become increasingly important for counselors to become licensed so the agency can obtain third-party reimbursement.

The chapter concluded by noting that agency and mental health counseling has probably undergone more changes in recent years than any other counseling specialty area and that the astute agency or mental health counselor must keep up with these changes if he or she is to work effectively with all clients.

INFOTRAC and Other Information Resources (e.g., ERIC and PsycINFO)

Note: When relevant, key words are in quotation marks.

1. Research the effects of "managed care" on community agency counseling.
2. Examine "quality assurance" and "evaluation" in community agencies.
3. Research the kinds of "ethical issues" that are of most concern to "mental health counselors."

CHAPTER 18

Student Affairs Practice in Higher Education

It was 1974, and I was obtaining my master's degree in counseling, thinking I was going eventually to work in an agency setting. However, somehow in my ignorance, I found myself in a counseling program that stressed counseling in higher education settings. Up until being admitted to that program I had wrongly believed that the attainment of a counseling degree meant that you became a school counselor or an agency counselor. I had a lot to learn. Suddenly, I was learning about the development of identity in college. My professors kept talking about this man named Chickering. Well, I figured that since I was already in the program, I might as well continue. I was 23, and identifying with much of what this guy Chickering said. "Maybe there's something in this for me," I thought.

Well, it didn't take long for me to realize that the college experience was crucial in the development of the individual. In fact, I realized that a lot of change had taken place for me as I had pursued my bachelor's degree. Suddenly I was rather interested in learning about this student affairs master's degree and the impact that a student affairs practitioner could have on the development of the college student. I began to see this as an option for my career.

I learned, through my program, that the history of student affairs practices is long and illustrious, and that student affairs practitioners, counselors being among them, are some of the most important individuals shaping the lives of college students. Today, it is common to find these student affairs practitioners working in many different college campus settings that focus on student development. Therefore, this chapter will examine those settings and look at the kinds of services that the counselor who works in those settings can offer college students.

In this chapter we will discuss the history of student affairs practices and the various ways in which the practice of student affairs has affected the development of the emerging adult. We will explore models and theories of student development, the settings in which we find student affairs counselors, the roles and functions of the student affairs practitioner, and the unique multicultural, ethical, professional, and legal issues that impinge on the work of the counselor in higher education settings. But first let us find out what exactly this specialty area is all about.

What Is Student Affairs?

First of all, there are a lot of names for this specialty area. It can be called student affairs, student affairs practices, college student development, student development in higher education, and college student personnel, and I've probably left out a few. So bear with me if throughout this chapter I use all of these names at different times.

Student affairs entails a broad range of services that includes, but is not limited to, recruitment activities, admissions, registration, orientation, residence life, counseling, and advising. Ideally, offices of student affairs provide programs and services to enhance the college experience of all students, whether they are the 18-year-old first attending college, the 35-year-old married father of two returning to college, the 60-year-old grandmother attending college for the first time, or the minority student who feels threatened by a seemingly hostile environment. Student affairs practitioners help to facilitate students' learning and knowledge of self by offering services directly to students, collaborating with faculty and administration, and being proactive in making changes in the institution.

The History of Student Affairs

Student affairs practices have a long history dating back to some of the earliest American colleges in the 1700s (Rentz, 1994). These colleges were almost exclusively religiously affiliated and had as their major goal the development of moral men for the clergy. Early college faculty believed that students were immature and in need of guidance if they were to develop morally. Not surprisingly, student affairs practices at this time were governed by the philosophy of *in loco parentis*, or the concept that college faculty would take on the role of parenting and guiding students. During these early years, the faculty took on most of the roles in which we find student development specialists today. For instance, it was usual at that time to find faculty doing informal counseling, involved in the discipline of students, assisting with admissions and registration, and being moral and religious mentors for students. During these times the educator was charged with developing the intellectual, personal, physical, and spiritual aspects of the student.

During the early part of the 19th century there was a movement away from faculty being involved with the moral and religious development of students and toward an increasingly academically oriented relationship. In the latter part of the 19th century, perhaps as a backlash to a century in which there was little concern about the emotional and spiritual aspects of students, there was a shift back to an emphasis on the personal development of students. It was at this time that many colleges began to hire deans of students who were charged with overseeing a broad range of student development concerns such as enrollment, admissions, and the moral development of students. In addition, this part of the century saw the first specialized student affairs staff, such as counselors, being hired. Student affairs was evolving as a profession.

As with community agencies and with schools, the emergence of psychoanalysis, testing, and the vocational guidance movement at the beginning of the 20th century were to have an impact on the role that colleges played in the development of the student. Thus, the early part of the century saw a psychological and humanitarian focus toward students and the use of intelligence and aptitude testing for both vocational guidance and for psychological services. At this time some of the first student affairs associations were developed, including the National Association of Women Deans and Counselors (NAWDAC), the National Association of Student Personnel Administrators (NASPA), and the American College Personnel Association (ACPA, see www.acpa.nche.edu).

The depression of late 1920s and the 1930s brought cutbacks in counseling and guidance and other support services and a resurgence of colleges solely focusing on the intellectual development of students. With declining college enrollment, and the focus of student affairs being the development of the whole student, administrators viewed student affairs as an unnecessary expense (Carpenter, 1996). However, as the country moved out of the depression and into the 1940s, there was a resurgence of student affairs practices with what became known as the student personnel point of view (American Council on Education, 1994). This was largely fueled by the GI bill at the end of World War II, which gave financial assistance to veterans to go to college. Thus, we saw extremely large numbers of individuals going to college, many of whom needed academic guidance and personal support services. This trend continued well into the 1950s.

The 1960s brought with it civil rights rallies and antiwar protests on college campuses. As one might expect, it was during this period that the concept of *in loco parentis* changed, as students increasingly insisted that they were not to be dictated to by any individuals in positions of authority. During the late 1960s there was increased federal aid for students and an increasingly diverse campus environment. Theories of development that focused on identity issues were introduced during the 1960s and increasingly applied during the 1970s, as student development specialists attempted to offer educationally oriented activities focusing on smoothing out developmental changes. This decade also saw a rise in proactive interventions on campus, such as the establishment of crisis centers, women's centers, and substance abuse centers. The decades of the 1960s and 1970s also saw counseling centers that offered a wide range of counseling-related services becoming more popular.

The 1980s saw increased refinement and application of developmental theories as well as the emergence of student services that offered assistance to individuals with disabilities, minorities, women, nontraditional students, and other students with special needs. This broadening of services was ironically happening during the same decade that funding cutbacks became more prevalent, thus forcing many student services offices to downsize. This decade also saw a number of legislative initiatives that would affect the implementation of student services, such as affirmative action, laws concerning sexual harassment, and laws affecting the rights of students (e.g., freedom of speech).

The early 1990s saw continued state and federal cutbacks to colleges, which often resulted in reduced services for students. Increasingly, colleges attempted to maintain academic programs while trying to reduce the cost of student services without eliminating them totally. This decade also saw a call within the profession to examine the effectiveness of student development theory. As the second half of the 1990s saw an economic upswing in the country, colleges and universities began to feel more solvent, and the place of student services was once again secure. Today, student affairs is an integral part of the college organizational structure, and the services offered have an impact on every college student.

Where You Find Student Affairs Specialists

There are a multitude of career opportunities in student affairs settings (Garner, 2001). Although the majority of counselors have the expectation of doing counseling once they obtain their degree, many settings within the postsecondary environment exist where the counselor can find work doing advising, consulting, supervising, and offering preventive educational workshops. The following represent some of the many places where you might find the student affairs specialist.

Counseling Centers

Today, most colleges and universities have counseling centers staffed by counselors and/or psychologists. Less frequently, social workers may also be found at these centers. Counselors at counseling centers work with students who are experiencing adjustment problems and normal developmental concerns. Some college counselors may work with students with severe problems, while others are likely to refer such students to private practitioners or community agencies. Counselors work with students on a wide range of issues, such as concerns over academic success, self-esteem, relationship problems, test anxiety, stress, sexuality and sexual concerns, depression, suicidal thoughts, substance abuse, eating disorders, and career development concerns (Collison & Garfield, 1996). In addition, staff

BOX 18.1

Bruce: The Path to Becoming a College Counselor

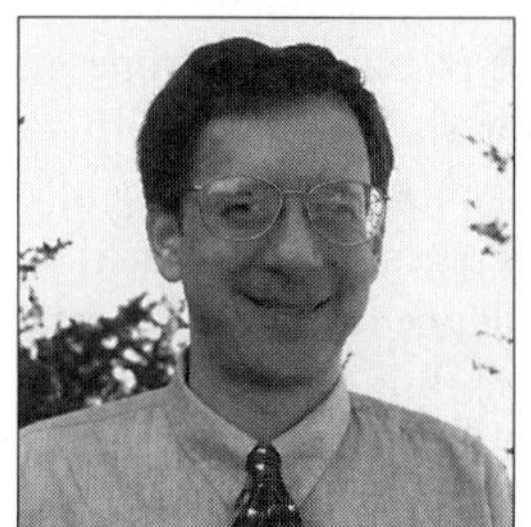

I work as a counselor in a university counseling center. Being able to have a positive influence on young adults during a time when they are experiencing many potentially stressful changes is an aspect of the job I enjoy. Providing time-limited personal counseling, doing outreach presentations in the residence halls or to other groups on mental health or academic skills topics, supervising graduate counseling students in training, assisting students with study skills or in choosing a major, doing intake assessments and making referrals to community mental health resources, and collaborating with coworkers are among my diverse duties.

Growing up with two parents who were compassionate, had worked as teachers, and had overcome stressful events in their lives helped me develop a sensitivity to underdogs and taught me how to gain satisfaction from helping others. Being an only child, I was drawn to various group activities that exposed me to both conflicts and solutions that occur in group settings. Volunteering for a crisis hot line and majoring in psychology were additional choices that influenced my career path. After college, I worked at an inpatient psychiatric unit of a hospital. Here I matured both personally and professionally as I experienced first-hand the capabilities and limitations of mental health professionals when working with a severely disturbed population.

I eventually obtained my PhD in counseling psychology with an eye toward working with clients who had less severe/long-term concerns and with a desire to offer preventive interventions. The course work, practica, and internships at a community mental health center and college counseling center prepared me for my career at a college counseling center.

I find college students a diverse and challenging population. Many are examining how they were affected by their family system, experiencing stressful developmental issues, or facing other crises in their lives. As students reach their counseling goals, I see them build a foundation for more effective relationships and better life skills for their future. The severity of concerns that students present at counseling centers has increased in recent years, and being able to refer some students for longer-term counseling is another important task. In addition to the counseling part of my job, I find it rewarding to engage in other roles that help promote positive development and mental health in the university community.

often will provide remedial and preventive assistance by offering workshops, courses, or support groups on campus. Often, such centers offer testing as an adjunct to counseling. Increasingly, counselors at large universities are required to have a doctorate in counseling or psychology, while smaller colleges and community colleges will often hire master's-level counselors.

Career Development Services

Almost all colleges have an office that provides career development services. Although some of these offices are part of the counseling center, today they are more frequently found separate from it. Career development services tend to include a wide range of activities. Some of the major services often include individual counseling related to career choice, testing and assessment relative to career decision making, access to career resource materials, and computerized career development programs to assist in choice of major, choice of careers, and job placement. In addition, most career development centers provide assistance with resume writing, job interviewing skills, cooperative education programs (e.g., internships), finding employment, and obtaining graduate assistantships.

Residence Life and Housing Services

The office of residence life and housing services generally provides a wide range of services related to student living. Some residence life staff will live in student housing, oversee the day-to-day living of students, and assist with any housing-related problems that may arise. Other staff will assist students with their educational, social, and developmental concerns and may conduct preventive workshops on such things as stress management, time management, communication skills, diversity issues, and other living skills concerns. In addition, staff will often be found assisting students who are having problems adjusting to college, struggling with personal problems, or dealing with interpersonal concerns with roommates and other students. Although staff who work in residence life may have a variety of degrees related to student affairs, clearly a master's in counseling is ideal, as many of the issues that face such staff are of a personal nature. (See Box 18.2.)

Office of Disability Services

Counselors who work for an office of disability services provide a wide range of services, including short-term counseling, running support groups, assuring compliance of the university with the Americans with Disabilities Act, assisting faculty in understanding how they can support individuals with disabilities in their academic pursuits, arranging transportation when appropriate, and assisting individuals with disabilities with campus housing. The range of disabilities with which the counselor works varies greatly. Some of the more common disabilities include the physically challenged, learning disabled, hearing impaired, and visually impaired.

Multicultural Student Services

Today, most colleges and universities have an office of multicultural student services that focuses on issues unique to minorities, women, men, and gays, lesbians, and bisexuals. Staff who work in such offices will often have a degree in counseling or in student affairs and

BOX 18.2

Kevin: Becoming the Director of Residence Life

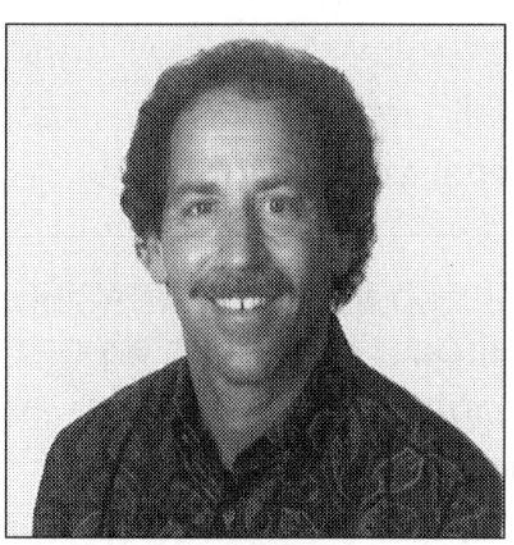

When my mother introduces me to her friends she says, "This is my son the college professor." This would be fine if I was a professor, but I'm not. I am a college administrator—a director of residence life. My mother still does not grasp what I do for a career, nor do the vast majority of people that I meet after I tell them my job title.

So, how does somebody get into a career about which so little is known? Well, typically a college student will start out as a residence hall assistant. If he or she enjoys this, the student may decide to go into a career working with college students. This generally requires a master's degree in counseling or a related field, with a focus on college student personnel work. While working on the master's degree, the student may work and/or do an internship as a residence hall director or in some other capacity in student affairs. Most graduate students will also get involved in regional and national conferences, as these conferences tend to focus on cutting-edge issues and are a good source for mentoring and networking. After graduate school, if the student remains interested in pursuing a career in residence hall life, he or she will continue up the organizational food chain to positions such as assistant director of residence life, associate director of residence life, and eventually director of residence life.

My path to being a director of residence life, however, was not quite as traditional. While working on my master's degree in counselor education, I did a practicum with the assistant dean of minority affairs. I enjoyed this experience intensely and thought it would be a great career. So, after completing my degree, I packed my bags for my first national college administrators' conference in search of an assistant dean of students position. The place was chaotic. There were more than a thousand candidates and employers attempting to interview them. Unfortunately, there wasn't an abundance of assistant dean jobs just waiting for me. Rather, almost all of the entry-level positions were working in residence hall positions. Because I had limited residence hall experience, I discovered that I wasn't as marketable as I had thought. Thankfully, one employer was willing to take a chance on a neophyte graduate and give me a job as a residence hall director.

To my astonishment, I really liked residence hall work. It provided me with an opportunity to have a positive impact on the growth and development of college students. My career from there followed the traditional career path I described earlier. Then one day 17 years ago, I finally became a Director of Residence Life. And here I am—perhaps if I my mom reads this, she'll better understand what I do!

will provide a variety of services that includes offering workshops for campus administrators, faculty, and staff to educate them on diversity issues; providing a supportive office where students from diverse backgrounds can feel welcome; assisting in providing a safe and accepting campus-wide atmosphere; serving as advocates for individuals from diverse backgrounds; and educating the campus community on relevant laws. (See Box 18.3.)

Student Activities Services

Often administered by the office of the dean of students, the office of student activities services is responsible for ensuring the smooth functioning of student organizations, advising student government, scheduling campus activities, publishing student handbooks, enforcing student regulations, supervising student media (e.g., newspaper and radio), running intramural and recreational activities, and organizing social, cultural, and educational activities. As with many student affairs offices, a degree in counseling or student affairs is often needed to obtain a position with student services.

BOX 18.3

Carreta: Director of Multicultural Student Services

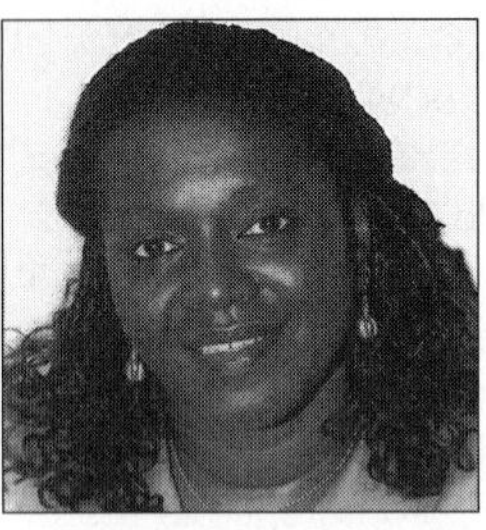

I was always curious. I also wondered about people, and I grew up in a city where race, ethnicity, and class defined who you were. A wonderfully ethnic place, Detroit had kosher delis, Black Muslims, Polish bakeries, Italian and Soul food restaurants, and world-famous museums.

Emigrating from the South, my father, a Korean War veteran, finished mortuary science school, married my mom, and settled in Detroit. I was lucky—my parents were able to afford me a life that was rare for an African American child growing up during the civil rights era. Ballet, voice, and piano lessons, dressup social occasions, and private education were experiences that might have left me unaware of the fast-changing world around me. However, my parents helped educate me. At a time when black history was a paragraph in history books about Lincoln freeing the slaves, I was being told about Denmark Vesey, Nat Turner, Harriet Tubman, and the contributions that African Americans made and were making in this country. I was a small child during the March on Washington but vividly remember the pride on my father's face as I sat on his lap and we watched it on television. I also remember not being able to use the bathroom in Tennessee, and looking at the signs that said "White Only" in Maryland as we drove to visit my relatives in the South. I guess that's why we always drove from Detroit to Sumter, South Carolina, in a day! I find it an honor to be part of a people who have endured and survived.

An International Relations major in college, I was determined to be the first African American and female ambassador to China. I thought I would go on to law school. However, as an intern in the admissions office in college, I was fascinated by work in student services. Besides, my older sister was studying for the bar exam, and it scared the hell out of me! So, upon graduating I began work as a financial aid counselor at a small Catholic college that had a diverse student body. I loved the college environment and decided China could wait—for a while anyway.

I came to multicultural student services still searching for my career in international relations. Accepting a position as Assistant Director for Minority Student Services at a large university near Washington, D.C., I thought I could obtain a job at an international agency and move closer toward my goal of becoming a diplomat. However, I soon realized that I loved the work I was doing. After a racial incident on campus, I started pulling people together to have frank discussions about difference, "isms," to share perceptions. I found myself energized.

Well, it's almost 20 years since my graduation, and I'm not the ambassador to China, but I have served more diverse groups than a career diplomat. Today, I am director of multicultural student services at a large university. As an administrator, I am inundated with administrative minutia and paperwork, which I don't like. However, I love working with the student community around issues of diversity. I love meeting people who have issues about race, ethnicity, and difference. I try to help them to better understand themselves and ultimately to heal.

I want to finish my doctorate and move into a consulting role. But I will always be committed to diversity in the higher education setting. Whether it be speaking about the impact of diversity on college campuses, assisting faculty with infusing diversity issues into their curriculum, helping administrators deal with changing demographics, or helping people heal, I will never stop being that curious child—wanting to know the how and why of it all and, along the way, helping others and learning about myself.

The one thing grander than the sea is the sky.
The one thing greater than the sky is the spirit of the human being.

Office of Human Resources

The office of human resources is involved with overseeing benefit packages for faculty, administrators, and staff and running preventive educational programs such as workshops on drug and alcohol abuse, stress management, communication skills, and financial management. Some human resource staff may be involved with hiring staff and assisting new faculty in their transition to the university or helping faculty who are leaving the university find new jobs and/or move to a new area of the country. Some staff may also be involved in providing workshops and advice on sexual harassment issues and on affirmative action laws. Some human resource offices may have employee assistance programs that provide educational workshops, crisis intervention, short-term counseling, and referral to community agencies. Individuals who work for a human resource office may hold a degree in counseling or student affairs.

Health Services

Many universities have their own health services that provide health care and preventive educational programs to students, faculty, staff, and administrators. Although many health services are run by physicians, nurses, nurse practitioners, and physicians' assistants, some university health services also offer counseling services. In these cases, the counseling center is often seen as part of the health services, although, in some rarer cases, counseling services may be offered at both the counseling center and at health services. In addition, counselors will often be hired by health services to offer educational and preventive programs on such things as AIDS awareness, stress management, and living a healthy lifestyle.

Academic Support Services

There is a wide range of academic support services offered at many colleges these days, and it is common to find a counselor working at many of these settings. Some of them include academic advising, learning resources centers for students with special needs, and tutoring services. The kinds of services offered students at these centers include assistance with scheduling, time management, study skills, stress reduction, and consulting with faculty concerning the special needs of these students.

Other Student Services Offices

The degree in counseling with a specialty in student services is versatile, and such individuals can be found in almost any setting on a college campus. Besides the ones listed above, some of the more prevalent offices include the admissions office, financial aid office, commuter services, and the office of the registrar. Although traditional counseling is not offered at these offices, individuals with a background in counseling are often hired because of the heavy emphasis on advising at these offices. Counselors, with their training, make excellent advisors. In addition, many graduates will obtain jobs in these offices as a stepping-stone to other student services positions, positions that might have a more involved counseling role, more status, and better pay.

Roles and Functions of Student Affairs Specialists

As you might expect, the roles and functions of the student development practitioner will vary dramatically depending on the setting and the kind of job within that setting. Despite this wide variance, Delworth and Hanson (1991a) define four major roles in which you are likely to find the student affairs practitioner, regardless of the setting. They include the administrator, who designs and manages programs; the counselor, who guides, supports, and advises students; the specialist, who fosters intellectual and personal growth; and the campus ecology manager, who creates a climate on campus for successful student development. Let's take a brief look at each of these roles.

The Administrator: Designing and Managing Programs

For each of the many offices in which one finds student affairs specialists, there is an administrator who must assure its smooth functioning. Although many student services management models have evolved over the years, all models have to attend to the same essential elements needed for the successful functioning of student services programs (Ambler, 1991). They include:

Students. Ever since the inception of student services, the commitment to the educational, psychological, and physical well-being of students has been the core of its existence. Ultimately, it is the administrator's responsibility to assure that the needs of students are being assessed in order to meet this commitment. However, administrators also have to walk a precarious balance between meeting student needs and meeting the needs of the institution, which are sometimes in conflict, such as when a financial crisis causes a reduction in student services.

Services and programs. Once an administrator has assessed student needs, services and programs must be developed to meet these needs. It is the responsibility of the administrator to develop, implement, and assess the worthwhileness of these services and programs.

Structure. For student services to function effectively, there must be an organizational structure that allows for clear lines of communication within each student service office and between student service offices. It is the responsibility of the administrator to assure that this healthy communication occurs.

Staff. Effective programming requires well-trained and satisfied staff who are clear on their roles and functions. The administrator is responsible for assuring that job descriptions are clear and for monitoring the working relationships among staff.

Sources. Whether it is funding sources or ways of obtaining free resources (e.g., interns working at a counseling center), student service administrators must be able to handle budgets and resources to assure the successful functioning of student service offices.

The Counselor: Guiding, Supporting, Advising Students

Although all student development practitioners do not do counseling, they all are committed to a counseling approach of working with students, which includes (Forrest, 1991):

1. A belief in the importance of the emotional, physical, spiritual, and interpersonal aspects of the student; a belief in the "whole" student.
2. A belief that every student is unique.
3. The importance of the affective domain in the student's development.
4. The importance of a developmental perspective in understanding the needs of students.
5. The importance of the personal characteristics of the helper in facilitating student growth.
6. A belief that counseling can be of value to students and ultimately to universities.

As is evident by the above basic assumptions, the student affairs practitioner is a counselor, even though he or she may not always be doing counseling. In the role of counselor, the student affairs practitioner will be a role model to students, provide direct support to students, develop and provide preventive psychological programs, facilitate groups, make referrals to mental health experts, request psychological expertise from clinicians, and advocate for change in the system to foster student growth (Forrest, 1991).

The Educator: Fostering Intellectual and Personal Growth

The student development practitioner is an educator who fosters both the intellectual and personal growth of the student. To do this, the practitioner must be able to assess the developmental needs of students, help students define goals, design and implement programs, and evaluate student progress (Brown, 1991). In helping students reach their goals, there are a number of educational roles the practitioner may take on. They include the roles of:

Advisor. The student development practitioner is able to understand the developmental needs of the student and advise him or her on a course of academic and personal study and growth that will meet the specific needs of that student.

Mentor. The practitioner mentors, advises, counsels, and guides students (Cross, 1976). He or she is involved in ongoing relationships with students that can be transforming experiences for them.

Curriculum builder/instructor. The student development practitioner can assist in curriculum building in a number of ways, including assisting faculty in developing their coursework to have an impact on the whole student, influencing curricula at the university level, offering courses through departments, offering workshops throughout the university, and referring to educational workshops in the community that have an impact on the whole person.

Evaluator-assessor. The student affairs practitioner evaluates the students' progress toward stated goals and offers feedback to students on how successful they have been at reaching the goals.

Scholar-researcher. The effective student development practitioner is willing to pursue research ideas and measure the value of the programs he or she is running (Steenbarger & Smith, 1996). If the programs are shown to be ineffective in helping students reach their goals, they need to be disbanded. If new programs are implemented that show promise of helping students reach their goals, they need to be published.

The Campus Ecology Manager: Creating a Successful Student Development Climate

As manager of the campus ecology, the student development practitioner focuses on how the total campus environment can affect the physical, emotional, spiritual, and educational needs of the student and challenges the traditional view of student services, which focuses solely on the individual student (Banning, 1991). This approach can be applied in four ways:

1. *Creating an organizational framework.* If student services staff are to work as a team in changing the total university environment, it is crucial that there be a

clear organizational framework that allows the various student services offices to work together on specific issues. For instance, if one were to address the issue of increasing tolerance of diversity on campus, a clear organizational structure must be present that allows all student services to come together and discuss how they can jointly make changes to create greater tolerance on campus.

2. *Studying specific groups*. The ecological model assumes that different groups on campus have different needs, and, if a problem is to be addressed, an acknowledgment and understanding of these varying groups is crucial. Thus, if we are to look at the issue of diversity, how faculty, staff, traditional students, nontraditional students, administrators, and so on approach diversity must be known, and a plan that takes into account these differences and includes all student services must be developed.
3. *Examining the unique contribution of each student services department*. Each student services office must examine how it can uniquely address identified issues. Thus, how residence life will address issues of diversity will be different and must be coordinated with how the counseling center will address the same issue.
4. *Studying events and issues*. A broad understanding of how specific events are affected by the total campus environment must be examined if changes in the way student services are delivered will be effective. Thus, relative to our issue of diversity, it would be important to have knowledge of how various student services in the past dealt with issues of diversity and to measure the effectiveness of what they have done.

The role of manager of campus ecology is relatively new for the student services worker and offers much promise in changing the way that student services are delivered and the effectiveness of what student services does.

Theories of Student Development

The driving force behind student affairs is the concept that, as students attend college and graduate school, they develop in predictable ways, and that student affairs offices can assist in facilitating this development. Pascarella and Terenzini (1991) note that fostering student development leads to growth and change in the individual as a result of physical maturation and how the individual interacts with the environment. Ultimately, such growth, they state, moves an individual toward greater cognitive complexity. Many of the theories of developmental growth that occur in students have already been discussed in Chapter 9. Thus, it is not unusual for student affairs experts to talk about changes in moral development as noted by Kohlberg (1969) and Gilligan (1982), or interpersonal development as noted by Erikson (1963, 1968), or constructive/cognitive development as noted by Kegan (1982). It is not surprising, therefore, that individuals who study student development generally spend much of their time understanding various developmental theories and their impact on the college student. Although a chapter such as this cannot touch on all of the developmental theories that may have an impact on students, two that have been consistently used to describe changes in students over time are Chickering's seven vectors model (Chickering, 1969; Chickering & Reisser, 1993), and Perry's scheme of intellectual and ethical development (1970).

Chickering's Seven Vectors of Student Development

In 1969 Chickering identified seven vectors that he believed were crucial in the development of college students. These vectors have become the standard in the profession for understanding college student development. He postulated that students can mature along each vector, increasingly developing a more complex identity, and that, through knowledge of these vectors, student affairs specialists can foster student development. The vectors include:

Achieving competence. Chickering believed that each student's ability at successfully developing his or her intellectual, physical, and interpersonal competence is crucial during the college years and that such growth ultimately leads one to a sense of self-worth.

Managing emotions. As students develop into adulthood they increasingly struggle with finding ways of managing emotions, especially anger and emotions related to their sexuality, both of which become ever more salient in the college years. The task for students is to establish new, more mature ways of managing all of their emotions.

Developing autonomy. The developing college student is increasingly faced with issues of autonomy as he or she disengages from his or her family of origin and develops a separate sense of self.

Establishing identity. As students become autonomous, self-sufficient adults, they are better able to understand their intellectual, physical, and interpersonal competence and strive to more effectively manage their emotions. In this process students begin to examine who they are within these domains and establish a sense of self, an identity.

Freeing interpersonal relationships. As individuals increasingly become more aware of their own identity, they are better able to form relationships with others and ultimately become more tolerant of differences.

Developing purpose. Perhaps one of the most important vectors, developing purpose relates to how individuals make meaning out of their lives. Deciding what is purposeful can only be accomplished if an individual has a clear sense of who he or she is—has established his or her identity.

Developing integrity. A strong sense of purpose, a belief in personally held values, and a sense that one's life is governed by a well-thought out internal belief system lead one to a sense of integrity.

The challenge for student affairs specialists is to find ways they can stimulate and facilitate growth along each of these vectors and thus assist in the healthy development of identity for all college students.

Perry's Scheme of Intellectual and Ethical Development

Perry's cognitive development scheme asserts that there are developmental stages that reflect a logical and sequential manner in which students develop their cognitive processes. Thus, for the student affairs practitioner, it would be crucial to identify the probable stage of development from which most students operate in order to understand how they make meaning of the world. Equipped with such knowledge, interventions could be designed that would facilitate higher-level meaning making. Although we have discussed Perry in previous chapters, below is a brief recap of his theory. Perry set forth a theory that identified nine positions interspersed through three stages. Below are descriptions of the three stages.

Dualism

Students who are dualists tend to view truth categorically, as right or wrong, and have little tolerance for ambiguity. Such students might see the professor, professional documents, texts, and the like as holding the truth to knowledge in their field. They believe that there is one right answer to questions and have difficulty with uncertainty, ambiguity, or the unknown. These students tend to like to be told "the truth" and will regurgitate such knowledge in class, on an exam, or in conversation. As students reach the latter position in dualism, they approach what some call multiplicity or transition (Magolda & Porterfield, 1988), in which a beginning recognition of the limits of authority occurs. These students are moving toward relativism.

Relativism

Relativists are able to think more abstractly and allow for differing opinions. In relativism, a student comes to understand that there may be many ways of constructing reality and of defining truth. They become more comfortable with ambiguity and realize that knowledge is relative and that there are limits to what we know. They are more comfortable sharing information and thoughts with one another and value not only the knowledge of experts, but also the knowledge of their peers.

Commitment to Relativism

Generally this stage is only reached by individuals who are older (have lived life) and who have a number of years of education behind them (Lovell, 1990). Individuals who have reached this stage have the capacity to maintain their relativistic outlook and are also able to commit themselves to specific behaviors and values. For example, the committed relativist may make a specific religious or job commitment while at the same time recognize the possibility that new information may modify that choice (Widick, 1977). Although most adults do not reach the higher levels of this development (Lovell, 1990), these models suggest that if afforded the right opportunities, most can do so. Some research suggests that such development is universal across cultures (Snarey, 1985).

Although students develop in all areas as they go through college, and even though it is difficult to arbitrarily separate out one's intellectual development from one's interpersonal, spiritual, and even physical development, few would argue that the most important aspect of the college experience is the development of one's cognitive processes. This is why Perry's scheme has been given particular attention over the years.

Other Theories of Development

Chapter 9 presented a number of developmental theories, perhaps all of which can be examined when we are interested in understanding changes in college students. Whereas Chickering's seven vectors model and Perry's scheme of intellectual and ethical development are two of the most prevalent models that are used by student development practitioners, there is little arguing that moral development (e.g., Kohlberg, 1969; Gilligan 1982), constructive/cognitive development (e.g., Kegan, 1982), lifespan development (e.g., Erikson, 1963, 1968; Levinson, 1985, 1996), psychosexual development (e.g., Freud, 1969), faith development (e.g., Fowler, 1995), and racial identity development (Atkinson et al., 1998; D'Andrea & Daniels, 1992) are all crucial aspects of the developing college student. Thus, it is important that the student development practitioner has a working knowledge of many developmental theories as he or she works with students and develops programs to facilitate their growth.

Special Issues in Student Development Counseling

Barriers to Academic Excellence of Underrepresented Students

In recent years the number of minority students, women, and nontraditional students attending college has dramatically increased. This is a function of greater tolerance of diversity in our society as well as laws that have demanded equal access for all. However, rapidly increasing numbers of diverse college students have led to an artificial barrier between these new students and many traditional faculty (Delworth & Hanson, 1991b; Fenske & Hughes, 1991). Differences in language, ways of meaning making, perceptions of racial and ethnic conflict, and general cultural differences have made it difficult for underrepresented students to adjust to and achieve in college (Ancis, Sedlacek, & Mohr, 2000; Schwitzer, Griffin, Ancis, & Thomas, 1999). The student affairs practitioner must face the changing demographics of higher education and work with all individuals within the university to lessen this gap so that all students will have an equal opportunity to achieve in all majors.

In Loco Parentis: A New View

Until the 1960s, colleges were largely seen as taking on the role of parents *in absentia*. Students were thus responsible to and to a large degree ruled by the institution they attended. With the unrest of the 1960s and an increasingly more diverse and older student population in the 1970s, 1980s, and 1990s, students demanded and, in many respects, were given freedom from the former parental relationships they held with colleges. Recently, however, this relationship has again become an issue, but in a new way. A number of lawsuits initiated by students have suggested that colleges may have a duty to protect students from physical harm that might occur through such things as sexual attacks, psychological problems such as suicidal ideation, sports-related injuries, and substance abuse (Gibbs & Szablewicz, 1994; Swenson, 1997). Whereas *in loco parentis* was formerly seen as protecting student moral development, this new *in loco parentis* suggests that there is a duty of colleges to protect students from harm. Student affairs practitioners will need to pay special attention to these and other issues as they move into the 21st century.

Defining the Role of Student Affairs

Although student affairs practice is very much alive on campuses today, how it defines itself within the many different kinds of college and university environments is still very much in question. Should student affairs solely support academics? Should student affairs support all aspects of the person's development? Should student affairs be a global unit of interacting offices, or separate offices, each dealing with its own issues? These are some of the questions that student affairs specialists are now asking. In the 21st century a unifying philosophy of student affairs must be found if these lingering questions are to be answered (Knock, Rentz, & Penn, 1994; Whitt, Carnaghi, Matkin, Scalese-Love, & Nestor, 1994).

Salaries of Student Affairs Practitioners

Because of the diversity of student affairs practitioners on college campuses, salaries vary considerably within any one institution. In addition, colleges and universities vary dramatically on how much they pay student affairs practitioners. This tends to be a function of the geographical location of the college, whether it is a private or public institution, the financial stability of the institution, and the value the institution places on the specific student affairs job. For instance, Baxter and associates (1997) note that the salaries for career counselors generally range from $19,000 to $34,000 but are sometimes much more. Similarly, deans and vice presidents of student affairs may earn anything from $40,000 to $95,000, while directors of major programs can earn from $30,000 to as much as $80,000. Unfortunately, entry-level positions tend to range in the low to mid-$20s (Collison & Garfield, 1996).

Multicultural Issues

With up to one-third of all college students being ethnic minorities in the 21st century, multicultural issues are playing an increasingly important role in student affairs practices. Although offices of multicultural student services can be traced back to the 1960s, as more minorities and women attend colleges, addressing multicultural issues can no longer be the sole responsibility of multicultural student services. All student services offices and student affairs practitioners will need to learn how to effectively deliver services in this increasingly diverse population (Fenske & Hughes, 1991; Palmer & Shuford,1996; Stage & Downey, 1999). The following summarizes some of these ways.

Addressing the Student–Faculty Barrier

As noted earlier, a major multicultural issue facing student affairs staff today is the increasing number of minority students, women, and nontraditional students attending college and how such diverse populations have led to an artificial barrier between some faculty and many of these new college students. One role that student affairs practitioners can play is to work with faculty to assist them in feeling more comfortable with all students.

Applying Student Development Theory to Minority Students

Student affairs practitioners must increasingly assure that the theories they use are cross-culturally appropriate. In addition, all student affairs practitioners should be current on minority identity models if they are to work effectively with minority students (see Chapter 14).

Implementing a Cultural Environment Transitions Model

All student affairs practitioners must take part in helping universities transform their total university environment into one that embraces diversity. It is crucial that student affairs practitioners jointly develop a model that will assist universities that operate mostly from a white Eurocentric perspective to transition to one that embraces all cultures.

Becoming a Cultural Broker

Student affairs practitioners can actively assist all parts of the university in implementing specific changes that can move the university toward increased cultural sensitivity. Some select examples might include:

1. Helping administrators see how the use of culture-specific terms like Christmas vacation might be offensive to some non-Christians and to some cross-culturally sensitive Christians.
2. Helping orientation leaders to assess the needs of minority students in order to better address their specific issues during orientation.
3. Assisting in the recruitment of staff that better reflects the diversity on campus.
4. Encouraging the use of nonsexist language by the campuswide community.
5. Offering diversity workshops for students, staff, faculty, and administrators.

Ethical, Professional, and Legal Issues

Ethical Concerns

Ethical Guidelines

The American College Personnel Association (ACPA) offers ethical guidelines for student affairs practitioners, and the American College Counseling Association (ACCA), a division of ACA, applies the ACA ethical guidelines for student affairs practitioners. Although the ACPA ethical guidelines are more specific to higher education settings, both guidelines are important for addressing ethical issues.

Confidentiality and Duty to Warn

Although confidentiality is an issue that faces all counselors, it has been particularly focused upon in college settings with a landmark case that has become known as the "Tarasoff rule" (Corey, 2000a; Swenson, 1997) (see Chapter 4, Box 4.7). This case, which examined the liability the university holds when an individual is at danger of harming another, has far-reaching implications for mental health professionals who work in a college setting.

Confidentiality, Informed Consent, and the Breaking of Rules

Because student affairs specialists are working for both students and the institution, they are sometimes faced with the dilemma of deciding to whom they owe their allegiance (Winston, 1991). Thus, students will sometimes come to advisors with confidential information that the advisor may be obligated to pass on to the institution. An example of this might be a student revealing to an advisor that he or she has cheated or knows of someone who has cheated. Thus, the student affairs practitioner must be clear on the limits of confidentiality when working with students and must obtain informed consent from the client for any advising or counseling that will take place under the limitations.

Professional Issue: Diversity of the Profession

Reflecting the broad diversity in the field of student affairs are the numerous professional associations. Today, the American College Counseling Association (ACCA, reached via www.collegecounseling.org), which is a division of ACA and the American College Personnel Association (ACPA, see www.acpa.nche.edu/) are the two associations joined most frequently by counselors who work in student affairs. ACPA generally attracts those who identify with student affairs in general, while individuals who work in a counseling capacity in higher education generally join ACCA (Dean & Meadows, 1995). Another important association that focuses the work of administrators is the National Association of Student Personnel Administrators (NASPA, see www.naspa.org). Also, many who work in student development offices will join other associations specific to their field of interest. For instance, we often find those working in career services joining the National Career Development Association (NCDA) and those working in counseling centers joining the American Mental Health Counselors Association (AMHCA). (Reach NCDA and AMCHA via www.counseling.org.)

Legal Issue: Liability Concerns

Student affairs practitioners face many liability concerns that many other counselors do not. Barr (1991) has identified some of the more common ones.

Negligence

Some of the more prevalent negligence concerns include the responsibility of the institution to assure that, with reason, situations do not exist that can cause danger to a person on campus (Schuh, 1999). For example, such issues as sexual assault, accidents, and theft on campus can all be potential concerns for liability.

Alcohol Abuse

When a university has condoned the use of alcohol, which subsequently becomes the reason for an accident or death, the university may be found to be at fault. Certainly, not being vigilant about addressing underage drinking or allowing alcohol at events, resulting in a car accident, may be two examples.

Defamation and Libel

When written or oral materials are used with the intention of defaming a person, a university may be held liable. Thus, student affairs specialists who work with student organizations or media on campus must be knowledgeable about how such organizations might defame a person.

Civil Rights Liability

Universities are increasingly being challenged to protect the rights of all people. Thus, when rights are in some way violated, the university may be held liable.

Contract Liability

Numerous publications are initiated by a university, many of which are viewed as a contract (e.g., the university catalog). Thus, student affairs specialists who are involved in the development of such publications must be keenly aware of potential liability concerns.

The Buckley Amendment (The Family Educational Rights and Privacy Act: FERPA)

The Buckley Amendment assures all individuals the right to inspect their educational records and to request a formal hearing if they believe the record to be false. Parents do not have rights to student records at postsecondary institutions unless their child is a dependent according to the tax code.

The Counselor in Process: The Student Affairs Practitioner

Colleges and universities have historically been known to be on the cutting edge; they are our nation's laboratories, where we experiment for the future. They exist to provide and expand our knowledge base. Any individual who wants to work at such an institution must be a forward thinker, take risks, test out new paradigms, and provide new ways of offering services. The student affairs practitioner must be willing to move forward with the changes that will inevitably take place in our universities and later be reflected in society. Whether it be women's centers, multiculturalism, political correctness, or new student development models to be tested, the student affairs practitioner is ever moving and ever changing. As Rentz (1996) so succinctly stated:

> *Student affairs' future role, its mission and goals continue to be the subject of considerable debate, now as they have been since the early 1900s, 'twas ever thus, and just perhaps, that is not a bad thing after all.* (p. 53)

Summary

This chapter examined the scope of student affairs practice. We began by highlighting that student affairs offices provide services that will enhance the college experience of all students. We noted that the main purpose of the student affairs practitioner is to help facilitate student learning and increase knowledge of self by offering services directly to students, collaborating with faculty and administration, and by being proactive in making changes in the institution.

The history of student services, we noted, dates back to the early colleges. These colleges were mostly religiously oriented and had as their purpose the development of moral persons. These early colleges stressed the concept of *in loco parentis*, and faculty often filled the role that is today taken by student affairs practitioners. The 19th century saw many changes in the delivery of student services, and in the latter part of this century there increasingly was a shift toward working with the whole person. The field of student services became firmly established during the 20th century, and with an exception during the depression, this focus has generally remained on the whole person. The end of World War II saw extremely large increases in the number of college students and a concomitant rise in student affairs practices. This trend continued well into the 1950s. The 1960s saw an emphasis on the application of developmental theories, and this focus remains today. The 1970s saw an expansion of student affairs practices that leveled off during the 1980s. The 1980s saw increased refinement and application of developmental theories and an increased focus on nontraditional and minority students. As we moved into the 1990s, we saw an increased emphasis in student affairs on promoting academic success and an attempt to find ways of reducing the cost of student services without eliminating them totally. The latter part of the 1990s saw an economic upswing in this country that led to increased solvency on the part of student services. Over the years, with the development of the student affairs profession, we saw the establishment of a number of professional associations, including: the American College Counseling Association (ACCA), which is a division of ACA; the American College Personnel Association (ACPA); and the National Association of Student Personnel Administrators (NASPA).

In this chapter we identified some of the student affairs offices where one is likely to find individuals who hold a degree in counseling. These included counseling centers, career development centers, residence life and housing services, disability services, academic support services, multicultural student services, the office of student activities, the office of human resources, and health services. Although the roles and functions of the student development specialist will vary dramatically depending on the setting and the kind of job within that setting, we were able to identify four major roles in which you are likely to find the student affairs practitioner, regardless of the setting. They included the role of administrator, who designs and manages programs; the counselor, who guides, supports, and advises students; the specialist, who fosters intellectual and personal growth; and the campus ecology manager, who creates a climate for successful student development.

Within this chapter we noted that developmental theories are a driving force behind student affairs practice. We noted that many of the theories of developmental growth that we discussed in Chapter 9 can be applied to student affairs practice, and that two theories in particular, Chickering's seven vectors model (Chickering, 1969) and Perry's scheme of intellectual and ethical development (1968), have been particularly used by student affairs practitioners. Chickering believed that students mature along seven vectors and that knowledge of these could help facilitate student affairs practices. These vectors included achieving competence, managing emotions, developing autonomy, establishing identity, freeing interpersonal relationships, developing purpose, and developing integrity. Perry, on the other hand, examined changes in cognitive development as a function of college experience, noting that individuals tend to move from a dualistic, rigid way of viewing the world to a relativistic, more open manner of understanding the world.

Some special issues that seem to affect student affairs practices today include the establishment of an artificial barrier that has been formed between some faculty and some minority students as a function of the changing demographics at the university; the changing view of *in loco parentis* from one that has viewed the university as a surrogate parent to one in which the university is seen as needing to be responsible for creating a safe environment for students; and the fact that still, today, the philosophy behind the practice of student affairs continues to be challenged and may change as the new millennium unfolds.

We noted that because there are so many types of student affairs practitioners, the salaries of such staff can vary dramatically. However, we were able to identify entry-level salaries as often starting in the mid-20s and directorships in some offices going as high as $100,000.

Noting that college campuses are becoming increasingly diverse, we highlighted a few issues that student affairs practitioners should address if they are to be advocates for a more tolerant multicultural environment. They included the importance of becoming familiar with minority identity development models, the role that student affairs practitioners play in assisting in the development of a campuswide model that advocates for tolerance of diversity, and the importance of becoming cultural brokers; that is, being able to work with individuals throughout the university setting in assisting the change toward increasing tolerance of diversity.

Two major ethical issues we identified included concerns over confidentiality, especially in reference to our responsibility toward an individual who may be in danger of harm, and the conflict that sometimes exists between confidential information we receive from clients and our responsibility of reporting such information to our supervisors or the institution at large.

Some liability issues that student affairs practitioners face today include concerns over negligence, such as when students may be exposed to a dangerous situation on campus; concerns over the university's potential role in alcohol abuse on campus; the responsibility of the university to prevent defamation of character; the responsibility of the university to protect the civil rights of all students; the contractual role of publications; and the right of students to inspect their records, as noted in the Buckley Amendment.

Finally, we concluded by noting that the student affairs practitioner of today must be willing to move forward with the changes that will inevitably take place in our universities and later be reflected in society. Noting that the mission and goals of student affairs will continually be debated, we highlighted the fact that it is positive to challenge and examine what we are doing and whether or not it is working.

INFOTRAC and Other Information Resources (e.g., ERIC and PsycINFO)

Note: When relevant, key words are in quotation marks.

1. Research one or more "theories of college student development."
2. Research important ethical and legal issues in college student development counseling.

CHAPTER **19**

A Look Toward the Future

I've had a lot of jobs in the helping profession. Changing jobs was stimulating and afforded me new opportunities. Sometimes I still think about changing jobs. I think, "Why should I remain here, at this school, in this city, when I have a whole world I could explore?" It sounds so exciting to move on. But I don't do it. Underneath, I must love the security of my current place in the world. I must love the stability of my job, my home, and my family.

In my 25 or so years in the counseling profession I've seen a lot of changes. For instance, I've seen a greater focus on ethics and multiculturalism, changes in the popularity of different counseling theories, and a great expansion of the field. Each change was not without controversy.

Change brings with it a kind of disequilibration. While it opens up a whole new world of possibilities, it necessitates letting go of something familiar.

*T*his chapter looks toward future changes—changes in the profession and changes in you. There are no giant leaps in this chapter. Most likely, the changes we will discuss will sound like common sense to you. Specifically, we will examine how the counseling relationship will be affected by medical breakthroughs, the increasing use of managed care, the expansion of computers and the information superhighway, the impact of multicultural issues, the future of accreditation and credentialing, the likely increased focus on standards of care, and some probable changes in the organizational structure and the purpose of professional associations. In addition, we will look at your immediate future, whether it is finding a graduate school, if you are not already in one, or finding a job. Finally, we will conclude the chapter by examining a wellness model that could help alleviate the stress that results from working in a difficult profession.

Medical Breakthroughs

In recent years we have seen some incredible breakthroughs in science that will likely impact the practice of counseling in the future. Three areas in particular—genetic research and genetic counseling, the use of psychotropic medications, and research on the mind–body connection—seem particularly important.

BOX 19.1

Huntington's Disease

Huntington's is a severe, progressive, neurological disease in which neurons rapidly shed in the caudate nuclei of the brain. Average age of onset is 36. The disease progresses through roughly four 5-year stages. At first, small losses of muscular coordination come, then changes in personality, making victims angry, hostile, depressed, and sexually promiscuous (probably due to loss of neurons from the frontal lobe). The second stage brings slurred speech, grotesque facial distortions, constant muscular jerkiness, clenching and unclenching of fists, staggering, falling, and involuntarily flailing of the limbs. . . . The third stage brings incontinence, severe mental deterioration, and dependence on others at home or in institutions. In the last stage, victims stare blankly ahead and never move. (Pence, 1990, p. 306)

Genetic Research and Genetic Counseling

As the causes of various health and mental health problems are discovered, genetic counseling promises to be an important aspect of what the counselor does. In the future, researchers will increasingly be able to identify individuals who are likely to acquire a serious disease or mental disorder (Nova, 2000). In many cases, the identification of the gene that causes a disorder, or that carries a predisposition to a disorder, will precede the actual treatment of the disease. For instance, as a result of genetic research, individuals now have the ability to know whether or not they have the gene for Huntington's, a debilitating disease that usually appears in early adulthood and is always fatal (see Box 19.1).

Huntington's is one of many genetic diseases. Some forms of diabetes, certain types of cancers, Alzheimer's disease, some types of heart disorders, bipolar disorders, schizophrenia, and perhaps even tendencies toward depression or anxiety disorders may be just a few of the disorders to which we may discover a genetic link. The ability to identify whether or not one carries a gene for a disorder raises a number of issues. For instance, individuals may struggle with whether they should be tested for a disease, how they should live out their lives if a disease gene is present, whether or not they should have children if they are not tested or if they discover the gene is present, and whether they should share the knowledge that they carry a gene for a particular disease with family and friends. These are difficult personal decisions with which a well-trained counselor might assist.

As genetic links to disorders become apparent, counselors will need to be knowledgeable concerning the procedures for working with individuals who are struggling with these issues and the legal and ethical ramifications specifically related to genetic counseling (Benkendorf, Callanan, Grobstein, & Schmerler, 1994; Lupton, 1994; Pencarinha, Bell, Edwards, & Best, 1992; Pence, 1990).

Psychotropic Medications

> *[We] stand at the threshold of a new era in brain and behavioral science[research]. . . . And we will be able to use this knowledge to develop new therapies that can help more people overcome mental illness.* (U.S. Department of Health and Human Services, 1992)

Understanding the biochemical activities of the brain has, over the years, helped us discover new medications that can assist in the treatment of mental illness and day-to-day

BOX 19.2

Medication and an Ad in *Time Magazine*

Psychotropic medication used to be the treatment of last resort, given out carefully by trained psychiatrists and occasionally by family practitioners. Now such medication is advertised in *Time Magazine* and prescribed regularly by family practitioners, and psychologists are now vying for the right to prescribe such medication. The following excerpt was taken from an ad in *Time Magazine* (Ask your doctor about Effexor tablets, 1995). In fact, the excerpt even has a footnote stating that the questionnaire was partially based on *DSM-IV:*

> *If you or someone you care about answers yes to five or more of these questions (including questions #1 or #2) . . . and if the symptoms described have been present nearly every day for 2 weeks or more, you should consider speaking to a health care professional about different treatment options for depressions, including Effexor (venlafaxine HCL).**
>
> *Yes No*
>
> ☐ ☐ 1. *Do you or they feel a deep sense of depression, sadness, or hopelessness most of the day?*
>
> ☐ ☐ 2. *Have you or they experienced diminished interest in most or all activities?*
>
> ☐ ☐ 3. *Have you or they experienced significant appetite or weight change when not dieting?*
>
> ☐ ☐ 4. *Have you or they experienced a significant change in sleeping patterns?*
>
> ☐ ☐ 5. *Do you or they feel unusually restless . . . or unusually sluggish?*
>
> ☐ ☐ 6. *Do you or they feel unduly fatigued?*
>
> ☐ ☐ 7. *Do you or they experience persistent feelings of hopelessness or inappropriate feelings of guilt?*
>
> ☐ ☐ 8. *Have you or they experienced a diminished ability to think or concentrate?*
>
> ☐ ☐ 9. *Do you or they have recurrent thoughts of death or suicide?*
>
> *Other explanations for these symptoms may need to be considered.*
>
> *Adapted from the *American Psychiatric Association: Diagnostic and Statistical Manual of Mental Disorders,* Fourth Edition. Washington, DC: American Psychiatric Association; 1994.

psychological problems. Although modern-day psychotropic medications have been used for more than 50 years, recent advances in brain research and the subsequent development of new medications will continue to greatly affect the counseling profession. Today, there are promising new medications that can be beneficial in the treatment of psychoses, depression, anxiety, attention deficit disorder, dementia, and other related illnesses. Literally millions of Americans now take medication as a partial or full treatment of a psychological disorder (see Box 19.2). To treat an individual without knowledge of the effectiveness of these medications in today's world would be incompetent practice. All counselors need to be aware of the effects of various medications and be in touch with the development of new medications (see Chapter 10 for an overview of psychotropic medications).

The Mind–Body Connection

The connection between the mind and the body continues to be vastly misunderstood and is often not examined as a source of health or disease (Chopra, 1999). Today, research clearly shows that there is a connection between how we think and act and our physical and emotional states. For instance, evidence suggests that meditation and other mind-altering experiences can reduce levels of stress, have a positive effect on recovery from mental health problems, and alleviate physical symptoms associated with a large range of stress-related illnesses (Fava & Sonino, 2000; Ryff & Singer, 1996). Conversely, many illnesses may be confused as psychological disorders, and counselors should be knowledgeable about the client who may present as having a psychological disorder but may indeed have a physical ailment.

If counselors are to be effective, they need to be acutely aware of the mind–body connection. In the future counselors will have to know how to (1) screen for medical problems that might be confused for psychological problems, (2) screen for medical problems that might cause psychological problems, and (3) teach techniques, such as stress reduction and meditation, to help people reduce stress and the potentially damaging effects it can have on the body (Benson & Klipper, 2000; Pollak, Levy, & Breitholtz, 1999).

HMOs, PPOs, Uh Oh, and the Changing Nature of Therapeutic Practice

The discussion ranges over lawyers and legal liability, advertising brochures and corporate logos, data bases and form letters, niche marketing and high-tech, multi-feature phone systems. Unhappy about their experience with managed care companies—the intrusive micromanagement of their work, rigid time limits, endless paperwork, and the struggle to get reimbursed—they [seven therapists] have decided, like thousands of other therapists in America, to pool their talents and find a way to do together what is increasingly hard to do independently: practice their profession with a reasonable degree of freedom, autonomy, and integrity and still make a living. (Wylie, 1995, pp. 20–21)

The health care system in the United States is changing. The cost of health care, particularly mental health services, skyrocketed in the second part of the 20th century and apparently will continue to do so in this century (Janesick & Goldsmith, 2000; Smith, 1999). As a result, health insurance companies are offering fewer services for mental health treatment, require stricter documentation of the services they do provide, require evidence that treatment is progressing, and have an expectation that most treatment will be brief (Granello & Witmer, 1998).

In an effort to lower the cost of health care, many businesses have opted to join managed care organizations such as HMOs (health maintenance organizations) and PPOs (professional provider organizations). Such organizations limit the choices of individuals in selecting their providers (e.g., physicians and therapists), limit the number of counseling sessions, and require large amounts of paperwork in an effort to control the health care system and lower costs. Despite the fact that most mental health providers have negative feelings about managed care, evidence seems to suggest that HMOs and PPOs are here to stay (Danzinger & Welfel, 2001).

With the changes in the health care system, our usual ways of offering counseling will need to change as we progress through the 21st century. Counselors are faced with a dilemma. A counselor can continue to offer traditional counseling services, knowing that insurance companies are likely to limit the number of counseling sessions and force the counselor to either (1) offer services for free, (2) offer services at a reduced fee, or (3) terminate services in the middle of treatment. Or the counselor can become knowledgeable about brief-treatment approaches, treatment approaches that until recently have rarely been taught in traditional counseling programs. Both counselors and counseling programs will need to face this dilemma head on if we are to survive in the 21st century (Daniels, 2001).

Computers and the Information Superhighway

In the United States today, 61% of homes have a computer, and 42% have Internet access (U.S. Department of Commerce, 2000). In business, these numbers are even higher. These are truly amazing statistics, especially in light of the fact that only 20% of households had a computer in 1992, only 20% had Internet access in 1998, and the first PCs were sold just over 20 years ago.

Counselors and other mental health professionals have quickly adapted to the use of computers (Guterman & Kirk, 1999; Wilson, 1995). For instance, counselors now use computers and other technologies such as interactive videos and CD-ROMs in case management, record keeping, clinical assessment and diagnosis, personality assessment of clients, comprehensive career counseling, documentation of client records, billing, marketing, and assisting clients in the learning of new skills (e.g., parenting skills, assertiveness training, and vocational skills for specific jobs).

Computers have also been shown to be successful in training counselors and other helping professionals (Casey, 1999; Haney & Leibsohn, 1999; Hohenshil, 2000; Neukrug, 1991). But perhaps the greatest change in the use of technology has been the expansion of the Internet. The Internet has brought us home pages for our professional associations, e-mails to colleagues, distribution lists and listservs of professionals who have common interests, video streaming for professional conferencing, Web-based courses, search engines for research, downloadable files on just about any counseling-related subject you might think of, and the controversial topic of counseling on-line (see Box 19.3). In fact, ACA has now adopted *Ethical Guidelines for Internet On-Line Counseling* (ACA, 1999). The Internet holds much potential, and the counseling profession has not lagged behind in getting on-line (Granello, 2000; Sampson, Kolodinsky, & Greeno, 1997; Wilson, 1995).

Your Future: Choosing a Counseling Program/Finding a Job

When making an informed decision about going on to graduate school, one should examine whether or not the program is accredited, the kinds of counseling specialties and degrees offered, philosophical orientation, entry requirements, size, faculty–student ratios, the cost and number of available scholarships, location, and job placement (Baxter et al.,

BOX 19.3

Advantages and Disadvantages of Counseling on the Internet

Summarizing some of the advantages of delivering counseling services on the Internet, Sampson, Kolodinsky, and Greeno (1997) point out that such a mechanism may

> *(a) improve client access to counseling in remote areas; (b) improve client orientation to the counseling process; (c) facilitate completion of assessment instruments and homework assignments; (d) enhance record keeping and monitoring of client progress; (e) enhance counseling referrals; (f) expand access to assessments and support for test interpretation; (g) reduce scheduling complications in couples and family counseling; (h) encourage individuals to seek counseling via self-help resources; (i) increase options for supervision and case conferencing; and (j) enhance the collection of research data.* (p. 211)

On the other hand, noting some disadvantages, they point out that the Internet will likely:

> *(a) limit the confidentiality of the counseling relationship; (b) deliver invalid information; (c) lack necessary counselor intervention; (d) be misused by inadequately trained or overworked counselors; (e) limit counselor awareness of important location-specific counseling variables; (f) restrict equality of access to counseling resources; (g) limit needed privacy for counseling; and (h) encourage service delivery by counselors without appropriate credentials.* (p. 211)

1997). Similarly, the job seeker should know the kinds of minimum credentials needed for the job, the philosophical orientation of the setting, the number and type of clients one is expected to see, and the possibilities for job advancement.

The Application Process

When applying to graduate schools or for a job, one should do the following: (1) Meet all application deadlines. (2) Complete all necessary forms. (3) Take any appropriate tests (e.g., GREs for graduate schools, personality tests for some jobs). (4) Write a *great* essay or statement of philosophy. (5) Find out if an interview is required and prepare for it. (6) Find out about faculty members' research or be knowledgeable about your employer's background and find an opportunity to ask questions about what they have accomplished. (7) Provide a well-written resume. (8) Consider submitting a portfolio. (9) Be positive, focused, and prepared. (10) Don't be negative or cynical.

The Resume

Some programs and most potential employers will ask you to submit a resume. Good resumes often present a broad picture of who you are, so it's usually a good idea to submit one even if it is not asked for. When submitting a resume, make it is readable, attractive, grammatically correct, and to the point. Don't be overly concerned about length. Don't give too much detail, and don't make it too wordy or too chaotic. For a more detailed look at resumes, get a good book on resume writing, such as *The Job You Want: A Guide to Resumes, Interviews, and Job-Hunting Strategy*, by Donaho and Meyer, 1990, and *Job Resumes: How to Write Them, How to Present Them, Preparing for Interviews*, by Biegeleisen, 1991.

The Portfolio

In addition to a good resume, other materials may increase your chances of being admitted to graduate school or obtaining a wanted job. For instance, a paper or Web-based portfolio can furnish the prospective employer or graduate program with a broad survey of your knowledge and skills (French, 1993; Cobia, Carney, & Shannon, 2000). Portfolios may include such things as transcripts, papers you have written, statements about your counseling philosophy, and outlines of workshops you presented (Baltimore, Hickson, George, & Crutchfield, 1996).

Locating a Graduate Program/Finding a Job

You're ready to apply to a program or find a job. So where do you look? Well, there are some specific places you can contact to find the graduate program of your choice, and there are ways to increase your chances of obtaining your dream job.

Finding a Graduate Program

A number of resources are available to assist potential graduate student in locating a graduate school (see Baxter et al., 1997; Collison & Garfield, 1996; Garner, 2001). Some of these include the following:

- *For lists of master's and doctoral programs in counseling:*
  Council for Accreditation of Counseling and Related Educational Programs (CACREP)
  5999 Stevenson Avenue
  Alexandria, VA 22304
  Phone: (703) 823-9800 5999 Web site: www.counseling.org/cacrep
- *For detailed information on master's and doctoral-level graduate programs in counseling:*
  Hollis, J. W., & Dodson, T. A. (2000). *Counselor preparation 1999–2001: Programs, faculty, trends* (10th ed.). Philadelphia: Taylor & Francis.
  Phone: 1-800-222-1166 Web site: www.taylorandfrancis.com/
- *For a list of doctoral programs in counseling psychology:*
  American Psychological Association (APA)
  750 First Street NE
  Washington, DC 20002
  Phone: (202) 336-5500 Web site: www.apa.org/ed/doctoral.html
- *For information on accredited rehabilitation counseling programs:*
  National Council on Rehabilitation Education
  Rehabilitation Counseling Program, California State University–Fresno
  5005 North Maple Avenue, M.S. 3
  Fresno, CA 93740-8025
  Phone: (559) 278-0325 Web site: www.nchrtm.okstate.edu/ncre
- *For information on accredited marriage and family therapy programs:*
  Commission on Accreditation for Marriage and Family Therapy Education
  1133 15th Street, N.W., Suite 300
  Washington, DC 20005-2710
  Phone: (202) 452-0109 Web site: www.aamft.org/about/COAMFTE/aboutCOAMFTE.htm
- *For accredited clinical pastoral programs:*
  Association for Clinical Pastoral Education, Inc.
  1549 Clairmont Road, Suite 103
  Decatur, GA 30033
  Phone: (404) 320-1472 Web site: www.acpe.edu

BOX 19.4

Randy: Getting Networked, Getting Involved, and Getting a Job

Randy was a former student of mine who was enthusiastic about the counseling field. He joined his professional associations, he worked with me on research, and he participated in professional activities whenever possible. Because Randy was so involved, he had the opportunity to co-present a workshop with me at a state professional association conference. His enthusiasm and knowledge so impressed one of the participants that at the end of one workshop she offered him a job—right there.

- *For accredited graduate programs in social work:*
  Council on Social Work Education
  1725 Duke St., Suite 500
  Alexandria, VA 22314
  Phone: (703) 683-8080 Web site: www.cswe.org
- *For accredited art therapy programs:*
  American Art Therapy Association
  1202 Allanson Road,
  Mundelein, IL 60060
  Phone: (847) 949-6064 or (888) 290-0878 Web site: www.arttherapy.org

Finding a Job

NETWORKING You've finished your training and now are ready to find a job. What do you do? Well, if you wanted to get a head start on the process, you would have joined your local, state, and national professional associations prior to finishing your training. Networking in this manner, is one of the most widely used and best methods of obtaining a job (see Box 19.4).

GOING ON INFORMATIONAL INTERVIEWS You have your resume and have developed a portfolio, you're networked, you look good and sound good—now what do you do? Well, you've probably identified a few different types of jobs in the counseling field. Now it's time to find some people who have these jobs and go on some informational interviews. These interviews will allow you to get a closer look at exactly what people do and will help you make a decision regarding whether or not you really want to pursue a particular job. In fact, sometimes people will let you shadow them on the job, and sometimes informational interviews can lead you to a specific job opening.

RESPONDING TO ADS IN PROFESSIONAL PUBLICATIONS Today, there are a number of professional publications that list jobs locally, statewide, and nationally. An active counseling association in your community or state may have a job bank and list jobs in its newsletter. *Counseling Today*, the monthly ACA newspaper, lists a variety of counseling-related jobs throughout the country. So does the APA newspaper, *The Monitor*. Similarly, the *Chronicle of Higher Education* lists jobs nationally, although most of the listed jobs are confined to the area of student affairs or doctoral-level jobs.

INTERVIEWING AT NATIONAL CONFERENCES Often, the large national conferences, such as the annual counselor conference sponsored by ACA, will offer a process whereby individuals who are looking for jobs can interview with a prospective employer at the conference. Although this is generally focused on doctoral-level counselor educator jobs, some master's-level jobs are also available.

COLLEGE AND UNIVERSITY JOB PLACEMENT SERVICES Job placement services and career management centers at colleges and universities will often have a listing of local community agencies that can be helpful when doing a job search. Sometimes these placement services will have job listings and offer job fairs that are relevant for graduate students in counseling.

OTHER JOB-FINDING METHODS Remember the tried-and-true methods for finding jobs—such as applying directly to an employer, responding to a newspaper ad, contacting a private or state employment agency, and placing an ad in a professional journal. These methods sometimes do work!

Being Chosen, Being Rejected

Counselor educators avoid saying a person is "rejected" from a program or a job, saying instead that the individual was denied admission or given other opportunities. Nevertheless, most people who are not admitted to their first-choice school or not offered their dream job do feel rejected. If you are denied admission or not given a desired job, ask for feedback about your application and/or the interview process. Although it is sometimes hard not to take a denial personally, take the opportunity to discover what you can do to improve your application. Once you know what was amiss, you can strengthen your future opportunities.

Multicultural Issues: Increased Emphasis on Multicultural Counseling

It is no longer possible for counselors to ignore their own culture or the culture of their clients. (Pedersen, 1991b, p. 11)

Multicultural counseling is a hot topic. It is one of the most frequent topics discussed in the *Journal of Counseling and Development* (Williams & Buboltz, 1999), and issues surrounding multiculturalism are often presented and debated at conferences. Yet, when surveyed about their experiences in counselor education programs, many students indicated that they were dissatisfied with their training in multicultural counseling (Holcomb-McCoy & Myers, 1999).With almost 30% of Americans now racial and ethnic minorities (U.S. Census Bureau, 2001a) and the prospect that 60% of Americans will be minorities by 2050 (U.S. Census Bureau, 2001b), dissatisfaction with multicultural training is not acceptable.

Because our profession has always prided itself on showing tolerance toward others, it seems evident that we will and must see increased training in multicultural counseling, new theories and models of multicultural counseling, as well as increased research on the efficacy of varying counseling approaches with diverse clients (Hanna, Bemak, & Chung, 1999; Holcomb-McCoy & Myers, 1999).

Ethical, Professional, and Legal Issues: The Future?

Expansion of Accreditation

Slowly, but assuredly, more counseling programs are moving toward CACREP accreditation, and such accreditation is increasingly being seen as essential to the field (Sweeney, 1995). Today, of the 500 institutions that have a graduate program in counseling, 150 have at least one CACREP-accredited program (CACREP, 2000). Although accreditation of programs undoubtedly raises standards, there are drawbacks. For instance, smaller programs will have a more difficult time becoming accredited as the standards require a minimum number of faculty and type of facilities that smaller programs sometimes do not have. Also, standardization of programs leaves less flexibility for creativity in curriculum development. However, most agree that the time for accreditation of programs is past due and that the benefits outweigh the drawbacks. As many in our profession note, "Would you want to go to a physician who did not go through an accredited medical school? Then why would we expect any less from our profession?"

Proliferation of Credentials

As with accreditation, it is likely that the future will see an increase in the numbers of counselors becoming credentialed (Neukrug, Milliken, & Walden, 2001). It now appears that the lobbying efforts to require licensure in all the states will succeed. In addition, it is more than likely that the number of counselors obtaining national certification and specialty certification will continue to swell. As credentialing becomes increasingly important for obtaining and maintaining jobs, for obtaining third-party reimbursement, and as way of demonstrating that counselors are providing high standards of care, there is little doubt that most counselors will seek licensure or certification.

Increased Emphasis on Standards of Care

To be helpful to clients, avoid malpractice, and be accountable to insurance companies, funding sources, and employers, counselors will increasingly be asked to show adequate standards of client care. In considering what are acceptable standards of practice, the courts generally look at what is regarded as the "minimal acceptable practice" in the profession. To demonstrate that counselors offer adequate care, some suggest that in the future counselors will increasingly have to (1) offer professional disclosure statements, (2) develop sound treatment plans, (3) take good clinical progress notes, (4) conduct formative (ongoing) evaluations of counselor effectiveness, (5) conduct outcome research of counselor effectiveness, (6) consult, be supervised, and make appropriate referrals, (7) ensure their own mental and physical health, (8) be aware of legal and ethical concerns, (9) be multiculturally asttute, and (10) obtain appropriate credentials and partake in continuing education (Anderson, 1992; Granello & Witmer, 1998).

After Changes upon Changes, We Are More or Less the Same

During the 1990s the American College Personnel Association (ACPA), one of ACA's largest divisions, disaffiliated from ACA. Also, the boards of two of ACA's largest divisions, the American Mental Health Counselors Association (AMHCA) and the

American School Counselors Association (ASCA), asked their members to vote on disaffiliation. Both votes were defeated. This decade also saw the formation of three divisions: the International Association of Marriage and Family Counselors (1990) (IAMFC) in 1990, the American College Counseling Association (ACCA) in 1992, and the Association for Gay, Lesbian, and Bisexual Issues in Counseling (AGLBIC) in 1997. More recently we saw the formation of an ACA organizational affiliate, Counselors for Social Justice (CSJ). Also, the American Rehabilitation Counseling Association (ARCA) and the National Rehabilitation Counseling Association (NRCA) have recently signed an agreement to merge and become one organization (Simmons, 2001).

Due to a by-law the ACA Governing Council placed into effect in 1998, a professional can now join any of six divisions and one organizational affiliate without joining ACA (C. Neiman, personal communication, June 15, 2001). Two of these divisions, AMHCA and ASCA, handle their own memberships and hardly acknowledge the existence of ACA on their Web sites.

It is clear that in recent years the state of ACA has been, to say the least, in flux. Some might decry these changes, while others might welcome them (Myers, 1995), but the bottom line is that ACA continues to be an organization that is willing to change with the times. We could be impatient and become irritated with these changes. But, perhaps like a client who is constantly changing, we need to accept the fact that organizations do change and realize that this may actually be a sign of good health!

A Wellness Model for Counselors

Unfortunately, stress, cynicism, and burnout are likely to be major concerns of counselors in the 21st century. Hans Selye and others (Selye, 1956, 1974; Pritts et al., 2000) have noted that stress can be an adaptive response that enables individuals to handle new and/or highly charged situations. Others are quick to point out that too much stress is associated with myriad psychological and physical problems (Fava & Sonino, 2000). What can a counselor do to prevent too much stress? Some have suggested that effective counselors must be ever-vigilant in attending to their physical, emotional, behavioral, interpersonal, and attitudinal domains if they are to minimize stress in their lives (Kahill, 1988a,b).

One method of assessing your level of health is through what Myers, Sweeney, and Witmer (2000) describe as the Wheel of Wellness. This model, although originally intended for client use, is easily applied to counselors, asking individuals to assess their level of health in the areas of spirituality, work and leisure, friendship, love, and self-direction, which is further divided into twelve subtasks (see Figure 19.1). You may want to complete an informal assessment on each of the tasks and subtasks to determine what areas you believe you should work on. For instance, score yourself from 1 to 5 on each of the tasks and subtasks, with 5 indicating the greatest need to focus on that area. Then write down ways you can better yourself in any area where you gave yourself a score of 3, 4, or 5. (For a more involved analysis, see Myers et al., 2000.) Examine the total of your scores and reflect on whether you are living a relatively healthy life.

Finally, Carl Whitaker (1976) suggests a number of ways to keep oneself healthy. The following list combines his points and a few thoughts of my own:

1. Place yourself as a priority.
2. Learn how to love.
3. Listen to your impulses.
4. Listen to your inner voice, as well as to others.

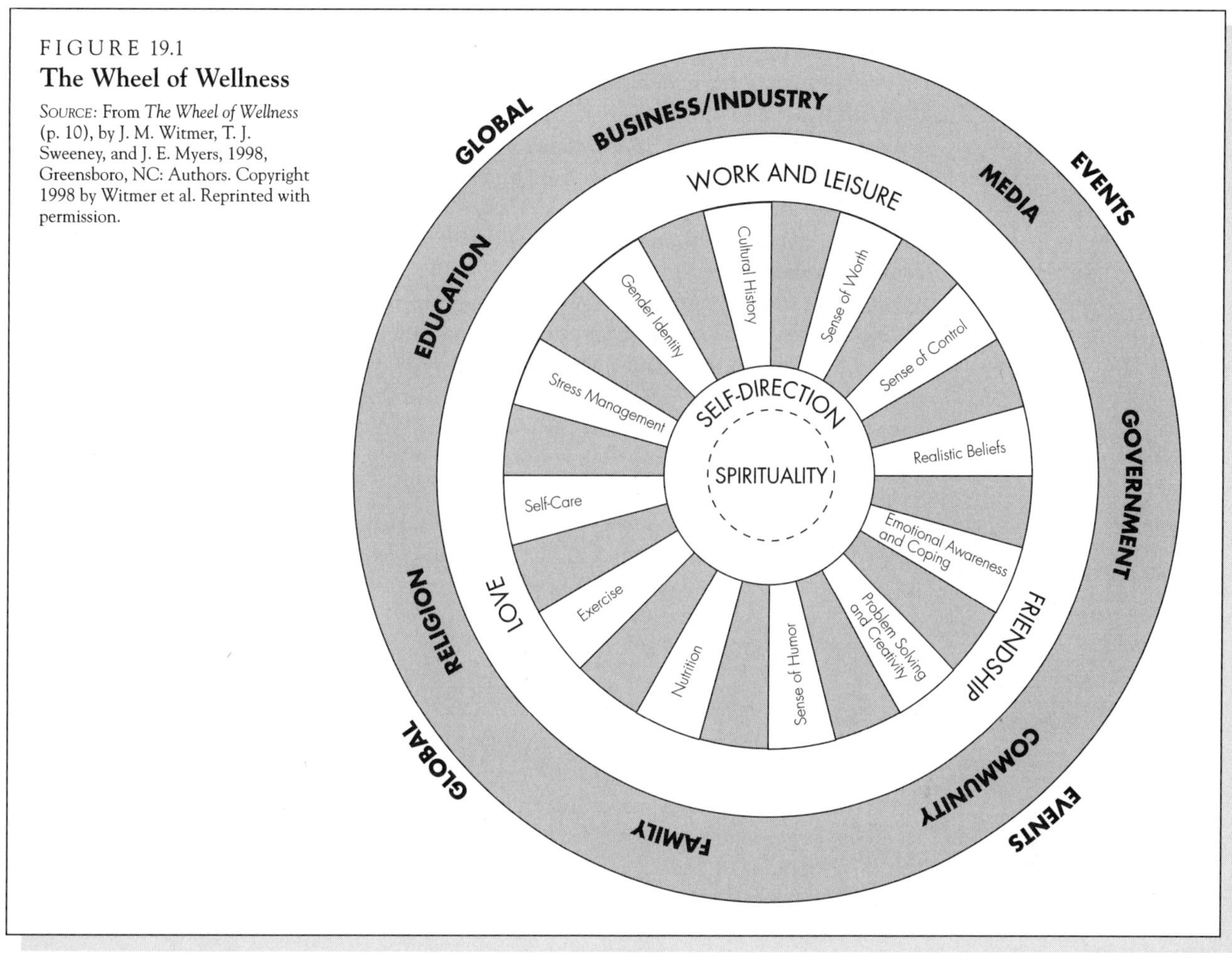

FIGURE 19.1
The Wheel of Wellness

SOURCE: From *The Wheel of Wellness* (p. 10), by J. M. Witmer, T. J. Sweeney, and J. E. Myers, 1998, Greensboro, NC: Authors. Copyright 1998 by Witmer et al. Reprinted with permission.

5. Enjoy your significant other more than anyone else.
6. Fracture role structures and challenge authority.
7. Challenge yourself—you're not always right.
8. Build long-term relationships so you feel safe and grounded enough to express your feelings.
9. Act "crazy" and whimsical.
10. Face the fact that you must grow until you die.

The Counselor in Process: Remaining Behind or Moving Forward?

Change can be painful. It requires giving up a former way of living in the world and accommodating to a new way. Even when the past way is not working, it is our security blanket. It is what we know, and often it feels safer to stick with the familiar than to take the risk of moving into unknown territory. After all, if people weren't afraid of change, they would hardly need counselors.

The 21st century brings many challenges to our profession and to our usual ways of doing things. Our skills will come into question, new theories will be offered, new lines will be drawn in the sand over professional rivalries, new technology will change the way we counsel, and numerous other changes that are as yet unknown will occur. We have a choice. We can continue to do business as usual, never facing the upcoming challenges, or we can be risk takers and try out new theories, new skills, new technology, and whatever else comes along.

There is something to be said for sticking with what has worked. It's like our favorite old armchair. We can rely on it to be comfortable and faithful to us. We can always fall back on it. There is something to be said for taking risks. Like roller blading for the first time, it's exhilarating. Once in a while you may fall, but generally you end up on your feet.

As you move into your career as a counselor, are you feeling comfy in your armchair or are you going roller blading? Those who get too comfortable at some point will be lost in the past. And those who move too fast will at some point fall. Perhaps we need both—the stability of our past and the innovations of the future. Yes, both might do just fine. Go roller blading, and then relax in your chair!

Summary

This chapter examined the future of the counseling profession and your future in the profession. We started by exploring some medical breakthroughs that might change the face of counseling. We first discussed the implications that innovations in genetic testing, with its ability to predict diseases, will have on the counseling relationship. Next, we noted that the development of new psychotropic medications has changed and will continue to change how we do counseling. We noted that in the future counselors must better understand the mind–body connection and be able to screen for medical problems that might be mistaken for psychological problems, screen for medical problems that might cause psychological problems, and teach techniques to help reduce stress and its damaging effects.

We next discussed changes in the health care system and how they have altered, and will continue to alter, the delivery of mental health services, particularly as a result of the growth of managed care organizations. In general, we are likely to see fewer services for mental health treatment, stricter documentation of the services, and an increased focus on providing evidence that treatment is progressing. Counselors will increasingly be asked to provide brief treatment counseling.

Next, we noted that technology, especially through the use of the computer, will increasingly be used in clinical practice for a wide range of activities. For instance, we will see the increasing use of e-mail, distribution lists, listservs, video streaming, Web-based courses, search engines for research, downloadable files, home pages, and counseling online. We noted that ACA has developed *Ethical Guidelines for Internet On-Line Counseling*.

As we move into the future we will be faced with career choices. Thus we talked about applying to graduate schools and finding jobs. We highlighted some points to address in the application process, whether it be to a school or a job. We then listed a number of organizations that can be contacted when applying for graduate school. We noted numerous ways of finding a job, including networking, going on informational interviews, interviewing at conferences, responding to ads, and using employment services and university placement services.

In the 21st century there will be a continued focus on multicultural issues in counseling. We will likely see counseling programs increase their training in multicultural counseling, more research on the efficacy of varying counseling approaches with diverse clients, and the development of new theories of multicultural counseling.

The 21st century will undoubtedly bring an increased focus on standards in the profession, including a proliferation of accredited counseling programs and an expansion of credentialing for counselors. Future counselors will be asked to offer professional disclosure statements, develop sound treatment plans, take good clinical progress notes, conduct formative clinical evaluations, conduct clinical outcome evaluation and research, ensure their own physical and psychological health, be aware of legal and ethical issues, be multiculturally astute, obtain appropriate credentials, continue their education, and be supervised, and make appropriate referrals.

We noted that in recent years there have been a number of changes in the status of divisions among professional organizations. A number of new divisions were formed. One division, ACPA, disaffiliated, and two divisions, AMHCA and ASCA, considered disaffiliation. We noted that it is now possible to join six divisions without joining ACA, and that two of these divisions, AMHCA and ASCA, handle their own memberships and hardly mention ACA on their Web sites. In addition, we pointed out that ARCA and NRCA have signed a preliminary agreement to become one organization. Finally, we asked you to reflect on whether or not changes such as these are dysfunctional or part of the healthy life cycle of an organization.

Unfortunately, the field of counseling will continue to be a high-stress profession, and stress can result in both psychological and physical ailments. Thus, we offered a wellness model and some suggestions that might help you reduce stress and live a healthy life.

Finally, we asked you to consider whether you are the kind of person who sits back and watches things change or a risk taker who initiates change. We noted that perhaps a balance between the two is healthy. As you reflect on your new career in the counseling profession, are you comfy sitting back and watching or are you out there being a risk taker?

INFOTRAC and Other Information Resources (e.g., ERIC and PsycINFO)

Note: When relevant, key words are in quotation marks.

1. Review the literature on “stress,” “burnout,” and “wellness” in the mental health professions.
2. Examine how new “technologies” might be applied to the mental health profession.
3. Research, in depth, any of the subjects you found interesting within this chapter.

References

AAC (Association for Assessment in Counseling). (1987). *Responsibilities for the users of standardized tests*. Retrieved June 1, 2001, from the World Wide Web: http://aac.ncat.edu/documents/rust.html.

AAC (Association for Assessment in Counseling). (1992). *Multicultural assessment standards*. Retrieved June 1, 2001, from the World Wide Web: http://aac.ncat.edu/documents/mcult_stds.htm.

AAC (Association for Assessment in Counseling). (2001). *Rights and responsibilities of test takers: Guidelines and expectations*. Retrieved June 1, 2001, from the World Wide Web: http://aac.ncat.edu/documents/ttrr.html.

AAMFT (American Association of Marriage and Family Therapists). (2001a). *Marriage and family therapy licensing & certification*. Retrieved June 5, 2001, from the World Wide Web: http://www.aamft.org/resources/boardcontacts.htm.

AAMFT (American Association of Marriage and Family Therapists). (2001b). *AAMFT code of ethics*. Retrieved June 1, 2001, from the World Wide Web: http://www.aamft.org/about/RevisedCodeEthics.htm.

AAMFT (American Association of Marriage and Family Therapists). (2001c). *AAMFT overview*. Retrieved June 1, 2001, from the World Wide Web: http://www.aamft.org/about/aamft.htm.

AAPC (American Association of Pastoral Counselors). (2001). *Training programs in pastoral counseling*. Retrieved June 1, 2001, from the World Wide Web: http://www.aapc.org/training.htm.

ACA (American Counseling Association). (1995a). *Code of ethics and standards of practice* (rev. ed.). Alexandria, VA: Author. Retrieved June 1, 2001, from the World Wide Web: http://www.counseling.org/resources/codeofethics.htm.

ACA (American Counseling Association). (1995b). *ACA history: 1995*. Alexandria, VA: Author.

ACA (American Counseling Association). (1999). *Ethical standards for Internet on-line counseling*. Retrieved June 1, 2001, from the World Wide Web: http://www.counseling.org/gc/cybertx.htm.

ACA (American Counseling Association). (2001a). *Mission and vision statements*. Retrieved June 5, 2001, from the World Wide Web: http://www.counseling.org/join_aca/mission.htm.

ACA (American Counseling Association). (2001b). *Special message: The ACA ethics committee to examine ACA code of ethics for its multicultural content and sensitivity*. Retrieved June 1, 2001, from the World Wide Web: http://www.counseling.org/urgent/special111599.html.

ACA (American Counseling Association). (2001c). *Liability insurance program*. Retrieved June 1, 2001, from the World Wide Web: http://www.acait.com/html/rates.html.

ACA (American Counseling Association). (2001d). *State licensure chart (online)*. Retrieved June 1, 2001, from the World Wide Web: http://www.counseling.org/resources/licensure_summary.htm.

ACES (Association for Counselor Education and Supervision). (1990). Standards for counseling supervision. *Journal of Counseling and Development*, *69*, 30–36.

ACES (Association for Counselor Education and Supervision). (1993). *Ethical guidelines for counseling supervisors*. Retrieved June 1, 2001, from the World Wide Web: http://www.siu.edu/~epse1/aces/documents/ethicsnoframe.htm.

ACES (Association for Counselor Education and Supervision). (1995). Ethical guidelines for counseling supervisors. *Counselor Education and Supervision*, *34*, 270– 276.

Ackerman, N. W. (1958). *The psychodynamics of family life*. New York: Basic Books.

Ackerman, N. W. (1966). *Treating the troubled family*. New York: Basic Books.

ACLU (American Civil Liberties Union). (2001). *Using the freedom of information act: A step-by-step guide*. Retrieved June 1, 2001, from the World Wide Web: www.aclu.org/library/foia.html#basics.

ACT Discover Center. (1998). *Discover, colleges and adults*. Hunt Valley, MD: Author.

Adair, A. (1999). *Impact of capitation on clinical judgment in suicide risk assessment* (Doctoral dissertation, University of Tennessee, 1999). Dissertation Abstracts International: 60, 8-B, AAG9944227

Addams, J. (1910). *Twenty years at Hull House*. New York: Macmillan.

Adler, A. (1959). The progress of mankind. In K. A. Adler & D. Deutsch (Eds.), *Essays in individual psychology* (pp. 3–8). New York: Grove Press.

Albee, G. W., & Ryan-Finn, K. D. (1993). An overview of primary prevention. *Journal of Counseling and Development*, *72*, 115–123.

Alford, C. F. (1989). *Melanie Klein and critical social theory: An account of politics, art, and reason based on her psychoanalytic theory*. New Haven, CT: Yale University Press.

Allen, E., & Gottfried, W. (Eds.). (1984). *Home environment and early cognitive development*. New York: Academic Press.

Allen, J. P., & Turner, E. J. (1988). *We the people: An atlas of America's ethnic diversity*. New York: MacMillan.

Allen, T. W. (1967). Effectiveness of counselor trainees as a function of psychological openness. *Journal of Counseling Psychology*, *14*, 35–40.

Altekruse, M. K., & Wittmer, J. (1991). Accreditation in counselor education. In F. O. Bradley (Ed.), *Credentialing in counseling* (pp. 81–85). Alexandria, VA: Association for Counselor Education and Supervision.

Amaranto, E. A. (Ed.). (1972). Glossary. In H. I. Kaplan & B. J. Sadock, *The origins of group psychoanalysis* (pp. i– xlix). New York: Jason Aronson.

Ambler, D. A. (1991). Designing and managing programs: The administrator role. In U. Delworth & G. Hanson (Eds.), *Student services* (2nd ed., pp. 247–264). San Francisco: Jossey-Bass.

American Council on Education. (1994). The student personnel point of view. In A. Rentz (Ed.), *Student affairs practice in higher education* (2nd ed., pp. 66–78). Springfield, IL: Charles C Thomas. (Originally published 1937)

American Psychoanalytical Association. (June 5, 2001). *About psychoanalysis* [online]. Available: http://apsa.org/pubinfo/about.htm.

Americans with Disabilities Act. (1992, July). Americans with disabilities act. *The Resource*, p. 1. Norfolk, VA: Old Dominion University Office of Personnel Services.

AMHCA (American Mental Health Counselors Association). (1987). *Code of ethics for mental health counselors*. Alexandria, VA: Author.

AMHCA (American Mental Health Counselors Association). (2000). *Code of ethics of the American Mental Health Counselors Association: 2000 revision*. Retrieved June 1, 2001, from the World Wide Web: http://www.amhca.org/ethics.html.

Anastasi, A. (1985). Mental measurement: Some emerging trends. In J. V. Mitchell, Jr. (Ed.), *The ninth mental measurements yearbook* (pp. xxiii–xxix). Lincoln, NB: University of Nebraska Press.

Anastasi, A. (1992). What counselors should know about the use and interpretation of psychological tests. *Journal of Counseling and Development, 70*, 610–615.

Anastasi, A., & Urbina, S. (1997). *Psychological testing* (7th ed.). Englewood Cliffs, NJ: Prentice Hall.

Ancis, J. R., Sedlacek, W. E., & Morh, J. J. Student perceptions of campus cultural climate by race. *Journal of Counseling and Development, 78*, 180–185.

Anderson, C. A., Lepper, M. R., & Ross, L. (1980). Perseverance of social theories: The role of explanation in the persistence of discredited information. *Journal of Personality and Social Psychology, 39*,1037–1049.

Anderson, D. (1992). A case of standards of counseling practice. *Journal of Counseling and Development, 71*, 22–26.

Andrews, H. B. (1995). *Group design and leadership: Strategies for creating successful common theme groups*. Boston: Allyn & Bacon.

Anthony, E. J. (1972). The history of group psychotherapy. In H. I. Kaplan & B. J. Sadock, *The origins of group psychoanalysis* (pp.1–26). New York: Jason Aronson.

Anti-Defamation League (ADL). (1992). *Anti-defamation league survey on anti-Semitism and prejudice in America*. 823 United Nations Plaza, New York.

APA (American Psychiatric Association). (1981). *The principles of medical ethics with annotations especially applicable to psychiatry*. Retrieved June 1, 2001, from the World Wide Web: http://www.psych.org/apa_members/ethics_princpl.cfm.

APA (American Psychiatric Association). (1994). *Diagnostic and statistical manual of mental disorders* (4th ed.). Washington, DC: Author.

APA (American Psychiatric Association). (2000). *Diagnostic and statistical manual of mental disorders* (4th ed., text revision). Washington, DC: Author.

APA (American Psychological Association). (1954). *Technical recommendations for psychological tests and diagnostic techniques*. Washington, DC: Author.

APA (American Psychological Association). (1988). *Code of fair testing practices in education*. Retrieved, June 1, 2001, from the World Wide Web: http://www.apa.org/science/fairtestcode.html.

APA (American Psychological Association). (1990). *APA Guidelines for providers of psychological services to ethnic, linguistic, and culturally diverse populations*. Retrieved June 1, 2001, from the World Wide Web: http//www.apa.org/pi/oema/guide.html.

APA (American Psychological Association). (1992). *Ethical principles of psychologists and code of conduct*. Retrieved June 1, 2001, from the World Wide Web: http://www.apa.org/ethics/code.html#General principles.

APA (American Psychological Association). (1994). *Publication manual of the American Psychological Association* (4th ed.). Washington, DC: Author.

APA (American Psychological Association). (1997). *Diversity and accreditation*. Retrieved June 1, 2001, from the World Wide Web: http://www.apa.org/pi/oema/diversity/book3/book3.html#over.

APA (American Psychological Association). (February 6, 1998). *Guidelines for providers*. Internet: http://www.apa.org.pi/guide.html.

APA (American Psychological Association). (1999). *Standards for educational and psychological testing*. Retrieved June 1, 2001, from the World Wide Web: http://www.apa.org/science/standards.html.

APA (American Psychological Association). (2001a). *Society of clinical psychology*. Retrieved June 5, 2001, from the World Wide Web: http://www.apa.org/divisions/div12/about.shtml.

APA (American Psychological Association). (2001b). *Ethics code of psychologists* (draft). Retrieved June 1, 2001, from the World Wide Web: http://anastasi.apa.org/draftethicscode/draftcode.cfm#intro.

APA (American Psychological Association). (2001c). *Program consultation and accreditation*. Retrieved June 1, 2001, from the World Wide Web: http://www.apa.org/ed/accred.html.

APA (American Psychological Association). (2001d). *APA public interest: Ethnic minority brochures online*. Retrieved June 1, 2001, from the World Wide Web: http://www.apa.org/pi/oema/onlinebr.html.

APA (American Psychological Association). (2001e). *Publication manual of the American Psychological Association* (5th ed.). Washington, DC: Author.

APNA (American Psychiatric Nurses Association). (2001). *Association overview*. Retrieved June 5, 2001, from the World Wide Web: http://www.apna.org/overasso.htm.

Appignanesi, R. (1990). *Freud for beginners*. New York: David McKay Company.

Arbuckle, D. S. (1965). *Counseling: Philosophy, theory and practice*. Boston: Allyn & Bacon.

Arbuckle, D. S. (1975). *Counseling and psychotherapy: An existential-humanistic view*. Boston: Allyn & Bacon.

ARCA (American Rehabilitation Counseling Association). (2000). *Code of professional ethics for rehabilitation counselors*. Retrieved June 1, 2001, from the World Wide Web: http://www.crccertification.org/html/code_of_professional_ethics.html.

Argyle, M. (1975). *Bodily communication*. London: Methuen.

Arredondo, P. (1999). Multicultural counseling competencies as tools to address oppression and racism. *Journal of Counseling and Development, 77*(1), 102–108.

Arredondo, P., Toporek, R., Brown, S. P., Jones, J., Locke, D. C., Sanchez, J., & Stadler, H. (1996). Operationalization of the multicultural counseling competencies. *Journal of Multicultural Counseling and Development, 24*(1), 42–78.

ASCA (American School Counseling Association). (1997). *Position statement: The professional school counselor and comprehensive school counseling programs*. Retrieved June 1, 2001, from the World Wide Web: http://www.schoolcounselor.org/pdf/counsel.pdf.

ASCA (American School Counseling Association). (1998). *Ethical standards of school counselors*. Retrieved June 1, 2001, from the World Wide Web: http://www.schoolcounselor.org/ethics/standards.htm.

ASCA (American School Counseling Association). (1999). *Role statement: The role of the professional school counselor*. Retrieved June 1, 2001, from the World Wide Web: http://www.schoolcounselor.org/role.htm.

ASCA (American School Counseling Association). (2001a). *National standards*. Retrieved June 1, 2001, from the World Wide Web: http://www.schoolcounselor.org/national.htm.

ASCA (American School Counseling Association). (2001b). *Ethical issues: Tips for school counselors*. Retrieved June 1, 2001, from the World Wide Web: http://www.schoolcounselor.org/ethics/ethicaltips.htm.

ASGW (Association for Specialists in Group Work). (1992). Professional standards for the training of group workers. *The Journal for Specialists in Group Work, 17*(1), 12–19.

ASGW (Association for Specialists in Group Work). (1998a). *Best practices statement*. Retrieved June 1, 2001, from the World Wide Web: http://asgw.educ.kent.edu/.

ASGW (Association for Specialists in Group Work). (1998b). ASGW best practice guidelines. *Journal for Specialists in Group Work, 23*, 237–244.

ASGW (Association for Specialists in Group Work). (1998c). *Purpose*. Retrieved June 1,

2001, from the World Wide Web: http://asgw.educ.kent.edu/.

ASGW (Association for Specialists in Group Work). (2000). *Professional standards for the training of group workers*. Retrieved June 1, 2001 from the World Wide Web: http://asgw.educ.kent.edu/.

"Ask your doctor about Effexor tablets" (1995, November 13). *Time*, insert.

Associations Unlimited (June 1, 2001a). *American Psychological Association [On-line]*. Available on-line through most libraries.

Associations Unlimited (June 1, 2001b). *American Psychiatric Association [On-line]*. Available on-line through most libraries.

Associations Unlimited (June 1, 2001c). *National Association of Social Workers [On-line]*. Available on-line through most libraries.

Associations Unlimited (June 1, 2001d). *American Psychiatric Nurses Association [On-line]*. Available on-line through most libraries.

Associations Unlimited (June 1, 2001e). *American Association of Marriage and Family Therapists [On-line]*. Available on-line through most libraries.

Associations Unlimited (June 1, 2001f). *National Organization of Human Service Education [on-line]*. Available on-line through most libraries.

Assouline, M., & Meir, E. I. (1987). Meta-analysis of the relationship between congruence and well-being measures. *Journal of Vocational Behavior, 31*, 319–332.

ASWB (Association of Social Work Boards). (2001). *Licensing information*. Retrieved June 1, 2001 from the World Wide Web: http://www.aswb.org/licensing/license.html.

Atkinson, D. R. (1985). A meta-review of research on cross-cultural counseling and psychotherapy. *Journal of Multicultural Counseling and Development, 13*, 138–153.

Atkinson, D. R. (1993). Who speaks for cross-cultural counseling research? *The Counseling Psychologist, 21*(2), 218–224.

Atkinson, D. R., & Hackett, G. (1998). *Counseling diverse populations* (2nd ed.). Boston: McGraw-Hill.

Atkinson, D. R., Morten, G., & Sue, D. W. (Eds.). (1998). *Counseling American minorities: A cross-cultural perspective* (5th ed.). Boston: McGraw-Hill.

Atkinson, D. R., Poston, W. C., Furlong, M. J., & Mercado, P. (1989). Ethnic group preferences for counselor characteristics. *Journal of Counseling Psychology, 36*, 68–72.

Aubrey, R. F. (1977). Historical development of guidance and counseling and implications for the future. *Personnel and Guidance Journal, 55*, 288–295.

Aubrey, R. F. (1982). A house divided: Guidance and counseling in twentieth-century America. *Personnel and Guidance Journal, 61*, 198–204.

Axelson, J. A. (1999). *Counseling and development in a multicultural society* (3rd ed.). Pacific Grove, CA: Brooks/Cole.

Axelson, L. J., & Dail, P. W. (1988). The changing character of homelessness in the United States. *Family Relations, 37*, 463–469.

Axthelm, P. (1978, December 4). The emperor Jones. *Newsweek*, pp. 54–60.

Bach, M. (1959). *Major religions of the world: Their origins, basic beliefs, and development*. New York: Abington Press.

Bailey, W. R., Deery, N. K., Gehrke, M., Perry, N., & Whitledge, J. (1989). Issues in elementary school counseling: Discussion with American School Counselor Association leaders. *Elementary School Guidance and Counseling, 24*, 4–13.

Baker, E. L. (1985). Psychoanalysis and psychoanalytic psychotherapy. In S. J. Lynn & J. P. Garske (Eds.), *Contemporary psychotherapies: Models and methods* (pp. 19–67). Columbus, OH: Merrill.

Baker, S. (1995). Becoming multiculturally competent counselors. *The School Counselor, 42*, 179.

Baker, S. B. (1996). *School counseling for the twenty-first century*. Englewood Cliffs, NJ: Merrill.

Baker, S. B. (2000). *School counseling for the twenty-first century* (3rd ed.). Upper Saddle River, NJ: Merrill.

Ballenger, J. C. (1998). Benzodiazepines. In A. F. Schatzberg & C. B. Nemeroff (Eds.), *Textbook of psychopharmacology* (2nd ed., pp. 271–286). Washington, DC: American Psychiatric Press.

Baltimore, M. L., Hickson, J., George, J. D., & Crutchfield, L. B. (1996). Portfolio assessment: A model for counselor education. *Counselor Education and Supervision, 36*, 113–121.

Bandura, A. (1969). *Principles of behavior modification*. New York: Holt, Rinehart & Winston.

Bandura, A. T. (1977). *Social learning theory*. Englewood Cliffs, NJ: Prentice Hall.

Bandura, A. T., Ross, D., & Ross, S. A. (1963). Imitation of film-mediated aggressive models. *Journal of Abnormal and Social Psychology, 67*, 3–11.

Banning, J. H. (1991). Creating a climate for successful student development: The campus ecology manager role. In U. Delworth & G. Hanson (Eds.), *Student services* (2nd ed., pp. 304–323). San Francisco: Jossey-Bass.

Barker, P. (1998). *Basic family therapy* (4th ed.). Baltimore MD: University Park Press.

Barr, M. J. (1991). Legal issues confronting student affairs practice. In U. Delworth & G. Hanson (Eds.), *Student services* (2nd ed., pp. 80–111). San Francisco: Jossey-Bass.

Barry, V. C. (1982). *Moral aspects of health care*. Pacific Grove, CA: Brooks/Cole.

Baruth, L. G., & Huber, C. H. (1984). *An introduction to marital theory and therapy*. Pacific Grove, CA: Brooks/Cole.

Baruth, L. G., & Huber, C. H. (1985). *Counseling and psychotherapy: Theoretical analyses and skills applications*. Englewood Cliffs, NJ: Prentice Hall.

Baruth, L. G., & Manning, L. M. (1998). *Multicultural counseling and psychotherapy: A lifespan perspective* (2nd ed.). Upper Saddle River, NJ: Prentice Hall.

Basse, D. T., & Greenstreet, K. L. (1991). On counseling men. *The Journal of the Colorado Association for Counseling and Development, 19*, 3–6.

Basseches, M. (1984). *Dialectical thinking and adult development*. Norwood, NJ: Ablex.

Bateson, G., Jackson, D. D., Haley, J., & Weakland, J. H. (1956). Toward a theory of schizophrenia. *Behavioral Science, 1*, 251–274.

Baxter, N. J., Toch, M. U., & Perry, P. A. (1997). *Opportunities in counseling and development careers* (rev. ed.). Lincolnwood, IL: VGM Career Horizons.

Baxter, W. E. (1994). American psychiatry celebrates 150 years of caring. *The Psychiatric Clinics of North America, 17*(3), 683–693.

Beale, A. V. (1986). The history of guidance. *The School Counselor, 34*, 14–17.

Beck, A. T. (1972). *Depression: Causes and treatment*. Philadelphia: University of Pennsylvania Press.

Beck, A. T. (1976). *Cognitive therapy and the emotional disorders*. New York: International Universities Press.

Beck, A. T. (1987). Cognitive therapy. In J. K. Zeig (Ed.), *The evolution of psychotherapy* (pp. 149–178). New York: Brunner/Mazel.

Beck, A. T., & Weishaar, M. E. (2000). Cognitive therapy. In R. J. Corsini & D. Wedding (Eds.), *Current psychotherapies* (6th ed., pp. 229–261). Itasca, IL: Peacock.

Becker, R. E., & Harris, L. H. (1973). A school that grew. In W. L. Claiborn & R. Cohen (eds.), *School intervention*. New York: Behavioral Publications.

Becvar, D. S., & Becvar, R. J. (1999). *Systems theory and family therapy: A primer*. Washington, DC: University Press of America.

Becvar, D. S., & Becvar, R. J. (2000). *Family therapy: A systemic integration* (4th ed.). Boston, MA: Allyn & Bacon.

Bedell, K. B. (Ed.). (1996). *Yearbook of American and Canadian churches: 1996*. Nashville,TN: Abingdon Press.

Beer, M., & Spector, B. (1993). Organizational diagnosis: Its role in organizational learning.

Journal of Counseling and Development, 71, 642–651.

Beers, C. W. (1948). *A mind that found itself* (7th ed.). Garden City, NY: Doubleday.

Belenky, M. F., Clinchy, B. M., Goldberger, N. R., & Tarule, J. M. (1997). *Women's ways of knowing*. New York: Basic Books. (Original work published 1986)

Belgium, D. (1992). Guilt. In M. T. Burker & J. G. Miranti (Eds.). *Ethical and spiritual values in counseling*. Alexandria, VA: American Association for Counseling and Development.

Belkin, G. S. (1988). *Introduction to counseling* (3rd ed.). Dubuque, IA: William C. Brown Publishers.

Bell, P., & Evans, J. (1981). *Counseling the black client: Alcohol use and abuse in black America*. Center City, MN: Hazelden Educational Services.

Benack, S. (1984). Post-formal epistemologies and the growth of empathy. In M. Commons, F. A. Richards, & C. Armon (Eds.), *Beyond formal operations* (pp. 340–356). New York: Praeger.

Benack, S. (1988). Relativistic thought: A cognitive basis for empathy in counseling. *Counselor Education and Supervision, 27*(3), 216–232.

Benjamin, A. (1987). *The helping interview* (4th ed.). Boston: Houghton Mifflin.

Benkendorf, J., Callanan, N. P., Grobstein, R., & Schmerler, S. (1994). Code of ethics: Day-to-day applications. *Journal of Genetic Counseling, 3*(3), 245–261.

Bennett, G. K., Seashore, H. G., & Wesman, A. G. (1998). *The Differential Aptitude Test*. San Antonio: The Psychological Corporation.

Benshoff, J. M. (1994). *Peer consultation for professional counselors* (Report No. EDO-CG-92-10). Greensboro, NC: ERIC Clearinghouse on Counseling and Student Services. (ERIC Document Reproduction Service No. ED 347- 476).

Benson, H., & Klipper, M. S. (2000). *The relaxation response*. New York: Morrow Avon.

Bergin, A. E. (1985). Proposed values for guiding and evaluating counseling and psychotherapy. *Counseling and Values, 29*, 99–116.

Bernard, H. S. (2000). The future training and credentialing in group psychotherapy. *Group, 24*(2–3), 167–175.

Bernard, J. M. (1992). The challenge of psychotherapy-based supervision. Making the pieces fit. *Counselor Education and Supervision, 31*, 232–237.

Bernard, J. M. (1994). *Ethical and legal dimensions of supervision* (Report No. CG025751). Greensboro, NC: ERIC Clearinghouse on Counseling and Student Services. (ERIC Document Reproduction Service No. ED 342-349).

Bernard, J. M. (1997). The discrimination model. In C. E. Watkins. *Handbook of psychotherapy supervision* (pp. 310–327). New York: John Wiley & Sons.

Bernard, J. M., & Goodyear, R. K. (1992). *Fundamentals of clinical supervision*. Boston, MA: Allyn & Bacon.

Berne, E. (1964). *Games people play*. New York: Simon & Schuster.

Bertalanffy, L. von. (1934). *Modern theories of development: An introduction to theoretical biology*. London: Oxford University Press.

Bertalanffy, L. von. (1968). *General systems theory*. New York: Braziller.

Bertram, B. (1996). Careers in private practice. In B. B. Collison & N. J. Garfield (Eds.), *Careers in counseling and human services* (2nd ed., pp. 65–72). Washington, DC: Taylor & Francis.

Best, J. W., & Kahn, J. V. (1997). *Research in education* (8th ed.). Englewood Cliffs, NJ: Prentice Hall.

Betz, N. E., & Fitzgerald, L. F. (1995). Career assessment and intervention with racial and ethnic minorities. In F. T. Leong (Ed.), *Career development and vocational behavior of racial and ethnic minorities* (pp. 263–278). Mahway, NJ: Lawrence Erlbaum Associates.

Beutler, L. E. (1986). Systematic eclectic psychotherapy. In U. C. Norcross (Ed.), *Handbook of eclectic psychotherapy* (pp. 94–131). New York: Brunner/Mazel.

Biegeleisen, J. I. (1991). *Job resumes: How to write them, how to present them, preparing for interviews*. New York: Berkley Publishing Group.

Bingham, R. P., & Ward, C. M. (1996). Practical applications of career counseling with ethnic minority women. In M. L. Savickas & W. Bruce Walsh (Eds.), *Handbook of career counseling theory and practice* (pp. 291–313). Palo Alto, CA: Davies-Black Publishing.

Binswanger, L. (1962). *Existential analysis and psychotherapy*. New York: Dutton.

Binswanger, L. (1963). *Being-in-the-world. Selected papers*. New York: Basic Books.

Birchler, G. R., & Spinks, S. H. (1980). Behavioral-systems-marital-therapy: Integration and clinical application. *American Journal of Family Therapy, 8*, 6–29.

Black, C. (1979). Children of alcoholics. *Alcohol Health and Research World*, Fall, 23–27.

Blake, R. R., & Mouton, J. S. (1976). *Consultation*. Reading, MA: Addison-Wesley.

Blake, R. R., & Mouton, J. S. (1982). *Consultation* (2nd ed.). Reading, MA: Addison-Wesley.

Blasi, G. L. (1990). Social policy and social science research on homelessness. *Journal of Social Issues, 46*(4), 207–219.

Blocher, D. (1988). Developmental counseling revisited. In R. Hayes & R. Aubrey (Eds.), *New directions for counseling and human development* (pp. 13–21). Denver: Love Publishing Company.

Bloom, J. (1987). *HMOs: The revolution in health care*. Tuscon, AZ: The Body Press.

Bloom, J. (1997). *Credentialing Professional Counselors for the 21st Century*. (Report No. ISBN-1-56109-070-0). Greensboro, NC: ERIC Clearinghouse on Counseling and Counseling and Student Services. (ERIC Document Reproduction Service No. Ed 399- 498).

Bolles, R. N. (2001). *What color is your parachute? A practical manual for job-hunters & career changers* (rev. ed.). Berkeley, CA: Ten Speed Press.

Borders, L., & Drury, S. (1992). Comprehensive school counseling programs: A review for policymakers and practitioners. *Journal of Counseling and Development, 70*, 487–498.

Borders, L. D. (1994a). *Supervision: Exploring the effective components*. (Report No. EDO-CG-94-18). Greensboro, NC: ERIC Clearinghouse on Counseling and Student Services. (ERIC Document Reproduction Service No. ED 372-339).

Borders, L. D. (1994b). *The good supervisor* (Report No. EDO-CG-94-18). Greensboro, NC: ERIC Clearinghouse on Counseling and Student Services. (ERIC Document Reproduction Service No. ED 372-350).

Borders, L. D., & Cashwell, C. S. (1992). Supervision regulation in counselor licensure legislation. *Counselor Education and Supervision, 31*, 208–218.

Borders, L. D., & Fong, M. L. (1994). Cognitions of supervisors-in-training: An exploratory study. *Counselor Education and Supervision, 33*, 280–293.

Borders, L. D., & Larrabee, M. J. (1993). A *research perspective for the Journal of Counseling and Development, 72*, 5–6.

Borders, L. D., & Usher, C. H. (1992). Post-degree supervision: Existing and preferred practices. *Journal of Counseling and Development, 70*, 594–599.

Borstein, C. (2001, June). Verbal consultation with attorney Borstein following review of Lexus search re: parent's rights to children's records.

Boszormenyi-Nagy, I. (1973). *Invisible loyalties: Reciprocity in intergenerational family therapy*. New York: Harper & Row.

Boszormenyi-Nagy, I. (1987). *Foundations of contextual therapy*. New York: Brunner/Mazel.

Bowen, M. (1976). Theory in the practice of psychotherapy. In P. J. Guerin (Ed.), *Family therapy: Theory and practice* (pp. 42–90). New York: Gardner Press.

Bowen, M. (1978). *Family therapy in clinical practice*. New York: Jason Aronson.

Bowman, J. T., & Allen, B. R. (1988). Moral development and counselor trainee empathy. *Counseling and Values, 32*(2), 144–146.

Bowman, J. T., & Reeves, T. G. (1987). Moral development and empathy in counseling. *Counselor Education and Supervision, 26*(4), 293–299.

Boyers, R., & Orrill, R. (Eds.). (1971). *R. D. Laing & anti-psychiatry*. New York: Harper & Row.

Brace, K. (1992). Nonrelativist ethical standards for goal setting in psychotherapy. *Ethics & Behavior, 2*(1), 15– 38.

Brack, G., Jones, E. S., Smith, R. M., White, J., & Brack, C. J. (1993). A primer on consultation theory: Building a flexible worldview. *Journal of Counseling and Development, 71*, 619–628.

Bradey, J., & Post, P. (1991). Impaired students: Do we eliminate them from counselor education programs? *Counselor Education and Supervision, 31*, 100–108.

Bradley, F. O. (Ed.). (1991). *Credentialing in counseling*. Alexandria, VA: Association for Counselor Education and Supervision.

Bradley, L. J. (1995). Certification and licensure. *Journal of Counseling and Development, 74*, 185–186.

Bradley, L. J., & Gould, L. J. (1994). *Supervisee resistance* (Report No. EDO-CG-94-12). Greensboro, NC: ERIC Clearinghouse on Counseling and Student Services. (ERIC Document Reproduction Service No. ED 372-344).

Bradley, R. W. (1994). Tests and counseling: How did we ever become partners? *Measurement and Evaluation in Counseling, 26*(4), 224–226.

Brammer, L. M., & MacDonald, G. (1999). *The helping relationship* (7th ed.). Boston: Allyn & Bacon.

Brammer, L. M., Shostrom, E. L., & Abrego, P. L. (1989). *Therapeutic psychology: Fundamentals of counseling and psychotherapy* (5th ed.). Englewood Cliffs: NJ: Prentice Hall.

Brammer, L. M., Shostrom, E. L., & Abrego, P. L. (1993). *Therapeutic psychology: Fundamentals of counseling and psychotherapy* (6th ed.). Englewood Cliffs, NJ: Prentice Hall.

Breasted, J. H. (1930). *The Edwin Smith surgical papyrus*. Chicago: University of Chicago Press.

Breasted, J. H. (1934). *The dawn of conscience*. New York: Scribner's.

Brewer, J. M. (1932). *Education as guidance*. New York: Macmillan.

Brill, A. (1960). *Basic principles of psychoanalysis*. New York: Washington Square Press.

Britton, P. J. (2000). Staying on the roller coaster with clients: Implications of the new HIV/AIDS medical treatments for counseling. *Journal of Mental Health Counseling, 22*(1), 85–94.

Britton, P. J., Rak, C. F., Cimini, K. T., & Shepherd, J. B. (1999). HIV/AIDS education for counselors: Efficacy of training. *Counselor Education and Supervision, 39*, 53–65.

Brooks, D. K., & Gerstein, L. H. (1990). Counselor credentialing and interprofessional collaboration. *Journal of Counseling and Development, 68*, 477–484.

Brown, B. (1995). The process of inclusion and accommodation: A bill of rights for people with disabilities in group work. *The Journal for Specialists in Group Work, 71*(2), 71–75.

Brown, D. (1984). Trait and factor theory. In D. Brown & L. Brooks (Eds.), *Career choice and development, applying contemporary theories to practice* (Chap. 2). San Francisco: Jossey-Bass.

Brown, D. (1993). Training consultants: A call to action. *Journal of Counseling and Development, 72*, 139–143.

Brown, D., Pryzwansky, W. B., & Schulte, A. C. (1987). *Psychological consultation: Introduction to theory and practice*. Boston: Allyn & Bacon.

Brown, D., Spano, D. B., & Schulte, A. C. (1988). Consultation training in master's level counselor education programs. *Counselor Education and Supervision, 27*, 323–330.

Brown, D., & Srebalus, D. J. (1996). *Introduction to the counseling profession* (2nd ed.). Boston: Allyn & Bacon.

Brown, N. (1992). *Teaching group therapy: Process and practice*. New York: Praeger Press.

Brown, R. R. (1991). Fostering intellectual and personal growth: The student development role. In U. Delworth & G. Hanson (Eds.), *Student services* (2nd ed., pp. 284–303). San Francisco: Jossey-Bass.

Brown, S. P., & Espina, M. R. (2000). Report of the ACA Ethics Committee: 1989–1999. *Journal of Counseling and Development, 78*, 237–241.

Browning, C., Reynolds, A. L., & Dworkin, S. H. (1998). Affirmative psychotherapy for lesbian women. In D. R. Atkinson & G. Hackett (Eds.), *Counseling diverse populations* (2nd ed., 317–334). Boston: McGraw-Hill.

Bubenzer, D. L., Zimpfer, D. G., & Mahrle, C. L. (1990). Standardized individual appraisal in agency and private practice: A survey. *Journal of Mental Health Counseling, 12*(1), 51–66.

Budman, S. H. (Ed.), (1981). *Forms of brief therapy*. New York: Guilford Press.

Budman, S. H., & Gurman, A. S. (1988). *Theory and practice of brief therapy*. New York: The Guilford Press.

Burger, W. R., & Youkeles, M. (2000). *Human services in contemporary America* (5th ed.). Pacific Grove, CA: Brooks/Cole.

Burgess, R. G. (1995). *In the field: An introduction to field research*. New York: Routledge.

Burnett, J. W., Anderson, W. P., & Heppner, P. P. (1995). Gender roles and self-esteem: A consideration of environmental factors. *Journal of Counseling and Development, 73*, 319–322.

Buscaglia, L. (1972). *Love*. Thorofare, NJ: Slack.

Bussod, N., & Jacobson, N. S. (1986). Cognitive behavioral marital therapy. In R. F. Levant (Ed.), *Psychoeducational approaches to family therapy and counseling* (pp. 131–145). New York: Springer.

Byrne, R. H. (1995). *Becoming a master counselor: Introduction to the profession*. Pacific Grove, CA: Brooks/Cole.

CACREP (Council on Accreditation of Counseling and Related Educational Programs). (1994). *CACREP accreditation standards and procedures manual*. Alexandria, VA: Author.

CACREP (Council on Accreditation of Counseling and Related Educational Programs). (2000). *Director of accredited programs–2000*. Retrieved June 1, 2001, from the World Wide Web: http://www.counseling.org/cacrep/directory.htm.

CACREP (Council on Accreditation of Counseling and Related Educational Programs). (2001). *The 2001 standards [Online]*. Retrieved June 1, 2001, from the World Wide Web: http://www.counseling.org/cacrep/2001standards700.htm.

Cameron, S. C., & Wycoff, S. M. (1998). The destructive nature of the term *race*: Graowing beyond a false paradigm. *Journal of Counseling and Development, 76*(3), 277–285.

Campbell, D., Coldicott, T., & Kinsella, K. (1995). *Systemic work with organizations: A new model for managers and change agents*. London, UK: Karnac Books.

Campbell, D. P. (1968). The Strong vocational interest blank: 1927–1967. In P. McReynolds (Ed.), *Advances in psychological assessment* (Vol. 1, pp. 105–130). Palo Alto, CA: Science and Behavior Books.

Campbell, D. T., & Stanley, J. C. (1963). *Experimental and quasi-experimental designs for research*. Chicago: Rand McNally.

Caplan, G. (1970). *The theory and practice of mental health consultation*. New York: Basic Books.

Capshew, J. H. (1992). Psychologists on site: A reconnaissance of the historiography of the laboratory. *American Psychologists, 47*(2), 132–142.

Capuzzi, D., & Gross, D. R. (1998). Group counseling: An introduction. In D. Capuzzi & D. R. Gross (Eds.), *Introduction to group counseling* (2nd ed., pp. 3–30). Denver, CO: Love Publishing Company.

Career Guide to America's Top Industries (2nd ed.). (1999). Indianapolis, IN: JIST Works.

Carey, J. (1989). *Life-span developmental supervision*. Paper presented at the annual meeting of the American Association for Counseling and Development, Boston, MA.

Carkhuff, R. (1969). *Helping and human relations* (vol. 2). New York: Holt, Rinehart & Winston.

Carkhuff, R. (1983). *The art of helping* (5th ed.). Amherst, MA: Human Resource Development Press.

Carkhuff, R. (2000). *The art of helping* (8th ed.). Amherst, MA: Human Resource Development Press.

Carkhuff, R. R., & Berenson, B. G. (1977). *Beyond counseling and therapy* (2nd ed.). New York: Holt, Rinehart & Winston.

Carlson, J. (1993). Marriage and family counseling. In G. R. Walz & J. C. Bleuer (Eds.), *Counselor efficacy: Assessing and using counseling outcomes research* (pp. 69–83). (Report No. ISBN-1-56109-056-5). Ann Arbor, MI: ERIC Clearinghouse on Counseling and Personnel Services. (ERIC Document Reproduction Service No. Ed 362 821).

Carlson, J., & Sperry, L. (Eds.). (2000). *Brief therapy with individuals and couples*. Phoenix, AZ: Zeig, Tucker, and Theisen.

Carpenter, S. (1996). The philosophical heritage of student affairs. In A. Rentz (Ed.), *Student affairs practice in higher education* (2nd ed., pp. 3–27). Springfield, IL: Charles C Thomas.

Carson, A. D., & Altai, N. M. (1994). 1000 years before Parsons: Vocational psychology in classical Islam. *The Career Development Quarterly, 43*, 197–206.

Carter, R. T. (1990). The relationship between racism and racial identity among white Americans: An exploratory investigation. *Journal of Counseling and Development, 69*, 46–50.

Casas, J. M., Brady, S., & Ponterotto, J. G. (1983). Sexual preference biases in counseling: An information processing approach. *Journal of Counseling Psychology, 30*, 139–145.

Casey, J. A. (1999). Computer assisted simulation for counselor training of basic skills. *Journal of technology in counseling, 1*(1), 1–7.

Casey, J. A., Bloom, J. W., & Moan, E. R. (1994). *Use of technology of counselor supervision* (Report No. EDO-CG-94-25). Greensboro, NC: ERIC Clearinghouse on Counseling and Student Services. (ERIC Document Reproduction Service No. ED 372-357).

Cashwell, C. S. (1994). *Interpersonal process recall* (Report No. EDO-CG-94-10). Greensboro, NC: ERIC Clearinghouse on Counseling and Student Services. (ERIC Document Reproduction Service No. ED 372-342).

Cass, V. C. (1979). Homosexual identity formation: A theoretical model. *Journal of Homosexuality, 4*, 219–235.

Castex, G. M. (1998). Providing services to Hispanic/Latino populations: Profiles in diversity. In D. R. Atkinson, G. Morten, & D. W. Sue (Eds.), *Counseling American minorities* (5th ed., pp. 255–267). Boston: McGraw-Hill. (Original work published 1994)

Cayleff, S. E. (1986). Ethical issues in counseling, gender, race, and culturally distinct groups. *Journal of Counseling and Development, 64*, 345–347.

Centers for Disease Control. (2002). *Division of HIV/AIDS prevention*. Retrieved May 31, 2002, from the World Wide Web: http://www.cdc.gov/nchstp/od/news/At-a-Glance.pdf

Chandler, G. (1973). Providing training in behavior modification techniques for school personnel. In W. L. Claiborn & R. Cohen (Eds.), *School intervention*. New York: Behavioral Publications.

Chandras, K. V. (1991, April). *Changing role of father in the United States*. Paper presented at the Annual Convention of the American Association for Counseling and Development, Reno, NV.

Chaplin, J. P. (1975). *Dictionary of psychology* (2nd ed.). New York: Dell.

Charles, C. M., & Mertler, C. A. (2002). *Introduction to educational research* (4th ed.). Boston: Allyn and Bacon.

Chickering, A. W. (1969). *Education and identity*. San Francisco: Jossey-Bass.

Chickering, A. W., & Reisser, L. (1993). *Education and identity* (2nd ed.). San Francisco: Jossey-Bass.

Chopra, D. (1999). *Journey into healing*. New York: Harmony books.

Claiborn, C. D. (Ed.). (1991a). Multiculturalism as a fourth force in counseling [Special issue]. *Journal of Counseling and Development, 70*(1).

Claiborn, C. D. (1991b). The Buros tradition and the counseling profession. *Journal of Counseling and Development, 69*, 456–457.

Clark, A. (1992). Defense mechanisms in group counseling. *The Journal for Specialists in Group Work, 17*(3), 151–160.

COAMFTE (Commission on Accreditation for Marital and Family Therapy Education). (2001). *The AAMFT commission on accreditation for marriage and family therapy accreditation*. Retrieved June 1, 2001, from the World Wide Web: http://www.aamft.org/resources/coamfte.htm.

Cobia, D. C., Carney, J. S., & Shannon, D. M. (2000). In G. McAuliffe & K. Eriksen (Eds.), *Preparing counselors and therapists: Creating constructivist and developmental programs* (pp. 135–147). Virginia Beach, VA: The Donning Company.

Code of Virginia. (1950). *Communications between physicians and patients*. 8.01-399, p. 439.

Cohen, E. D. (1990). Confidentiality, counseling, and clients who have AIDS: Ethical foundations of a model rule. *Journal of Counseling and Development, 68*(3), 282–286.

Cohen, G. D. (1984). Counseling interventions for the late twentieth century elderly. *The Counseling Psychologist, 12*(2), 97–99.

Cole, J., & Pilisuk, M. (1976). Differences in the provision of mental health services by race. *American Journal of Orthopsychiatry, 46*, 520–525.

Cole, S. (1975). *The sociological method*. Chicago: Rand McNally.

Cole, W., Gorman, C., Barrett, L. I., & Thompson, D. (1993, April 26). The shrinking ten percent. *Time*, 27–29.

Coleman, H. L. K. (1995). Cultural factors and the counseling process: Implications for school counselors. *The School Counselor, 42*, 180–185.

Coll, K. M. (1995). Clinical supervision of community college counselors: Current and preferred practices. *Counselor Education and Supervision, 35*, 111–117.

Collins, B. G., Collins, T. M., Botyrius-Maier, G., & MacIntosh-Daeschler, S. (1994). Mental health professionals' perceptions of parent-professional collaboration. *Journal of Mental Health Counseling, 16*(2), 261–274.

Collison, B. B., & Garfield, N. J. (Eds.). (1996). *Careers in counseling and human development* (2nd ed.). Washington, DC: Taylor & Francis.

Comas-Diaz, L. (1993). Hispanic/Latino communities: Psychological implications. In D. R. Atkinson, G. Morten, & D. W. Sue, *Counseling American minorities: A cross-cultural perspective* (4th ed., pp. 245–263). Madison, WI: Brown & Benchmark. (Original work published 1988)

Committee on Government Operations (fourth report). (1991). *A citizen's guide on using the freedom of information act and the privacy act of 1974 to request government records*. (House Report 102-146). Washington, DC: U.S. Government Printing Office.

Comptons Encyclopedia. (December 14, 1996). Religion [Online]. Available: America Online.

Consulting Psychologists Press (1985). *The Myers-Briggs type indicator*. Stanford, CA: Author.

Consulting Psychologists Press (1994). *The Strong interest inventory*. Stanford, CA: Author.

Consulting Psychologists Press (1996). *The California psychological inventory* (3rd ed.). Palo Alto, CA: Author.

Conte, H., Plutchik, R., Wild, K., & Karasu, T. (1986). Combined psychotherapy and pharmacotherapy for depressions. *Archives of General Psychiatry, 38*, 471–479.

Cook, T. D., & Campbell, D. T. (1979). *Quasi-experimentation: Design and analysis issues for field settings*. Chicago: Rand McNally.

CORE (Council on Rehabilitation Education). (2001). Retrieved June 1, 2001, from the World Wide Web: http://core-rehab.org.

Corey, G. (2000a). *Theory and practice of counseling and psychotherapy* (6th ed.). Pacific Grove, CA: Brooks/Cole.

Corey, G. (2000b). *Theory and practice of group counseling* (5th ed.). Pacific Grove, CA: Brooks/Cole.

Corey, G., Corey, M., & Callanan, P. (1998). *Issues and ethics in the helping professions* (5th ed.). Pacific Grove, CA: Brooks/Cole.

Corey, M. S., & Corey, G. (2002). *Groups, process & practice* (6th ed.). Pacific Grove, CA: Brooks/Cole.

Cormier, W. H., & Cormier, L. S. (1998). *Interviewing strategies for fundamental skills and cognitive behavioral strategies* (4th ed.). Pacific Grove, CA: Brooks/Cole.

Corsini, R. J., & Wedding, D. (2000). *Current psychotherapies* (6th ed.). Itasca, IL: Peacock Publishers.

Costa, L. (1994). Reducing anxiety in live supervision. *Counselor Education and Supervision, 34*, 30–40.

Cottone, R. R. (2001). A social constructivism model of ethical decision making in counseling. *Journal of Counseling and Development, 79*(1), 39–45.

Cottone, R. R., & Claus, R. E. (2000). Ethical decision-making models: A review of the literature. *Journal of Counseling and Development, 78*, 275–283.

Couch, R. D. (1995). Four steps for conducting a pregroup screening interview. *The Journal for Specialists in Group Work, 20*(1), 10–25.

Council on Scientific Affairs. (1995). Female genital mutilation. *Journal of the American Medical Association, 274*, 1714–1716.

Coy, D. (1991). The role of the counselor in today's school. *NASSP Bulletin, 75*, 15–19.

CRCC (Commission on Rehabilitation Counselor Certification). (2000). *Code of professional ethics for certified rehabilitation counselors*. Retrieved June 1, 2001, from the World Wide Web: http://www.crccertification.org/html/code_of_professional_ethics.html.

CRCC (Certified rehabilitation counselor certification). (2001). Retrieved June 1, 2001, from the World Wide Web: http://www.crccertification.org/home.html.

Cross, K. P. (1976). *Accent on learning: Improving instruction and reshaping the curriculum*. San Francisco: Jossey-Bass.

Cummings, N. A. (1990). The credentialing of professional psychologists and its implication for the other mental health disciplines. *Journal of Counseling and Development, 68*, 490.

D'Andrea, M., & Daniels, J. (1991). Exploring the different levels of multicultural counseling training in counselor education. *Journal of Counseling and Development, 70*, 78–85.

D'Andrea, M., & Daniels, J. (1992). *The structure of racism: A developmental framework*. Paper presented at the Association for Counselor Education and Supervision National Conference, San Antonio, Texas.

D'Andrea, M., & Daniels, J. (1995). Helping students learn to get along: Assessing the effectiveness of a multicultural developmental guidance project. *Elementary School Guidance & Counseling, 30*, 143–153.

D'Andrea, M., & Daniels, J. (1999). Exploring the psychology of white racism through naturalistic inquiry, *Journal of Counseling and Development, 77*(1), 93–101.

Daniels, J., D'Andrea, M. D., & Kim, B. S. K. (1999). Assessing the barriers and changes of cross-cultural supervision: A case study. *Counselor Education and Supervision, 38*, 191–204.

Daniels, M. H. (1993). Renaming the association: Reorganizing Counseling and Value. *Counseling and Values, 38*(1), 2–3.

Danzinger, P. R., & Welfel, E. R. (2001). The impact of managed care on mental health counselors: A survey of perceptions, practices, and compliance with ethical standards. *Journal of Mental Health Counseling, 23*, 137–150.

Das, A. K. (1995). Rethinking multicultural counseling: Implications for counselor education. *Journal of Counseling and Development, 74*, 45–52.

Davidson, B. (1992). What can be the relevance of the psychiatric nurse to the life of a person who is mentally ill? *Journal of Clinical Nursing, 1*(4), 199–205.

Davis, F. J. (1978). *Minority-dominant relations: A sociological analysis*. Arlington Heights, IL: AHM Publishing.

Davis, H. V. (1969). *Frank Parsons: Prophet, innovator, counselor*. Carbondale: Southern Illinois University Press.

Davis, J. L., & Mickelson, D. J. (1994). School counselors: Are you aware of ethical and legal aspects of counseling? *School Counselor, 42*(1), 5–13.

Davis, T., & Ritchie, M. (1993). Confidentiality and the school counselor: A challenge for the 1990s. *The School Counselor, 41*, 23–30.

Davison, G., & Friedman, S. (1981). Sexual orientation stereotype in the distortion of clinical judgment. *Journal of Homosexuality*, 6, 37–44.

Davison, G. C., & Neale, J. M. (2001). *Abnormal psychology* (8th ed.). New York: John Wiley & Sons.

Dawis, R. V. (1992). The individual differences tradition in counseling psychology. *Journal of Counseling Psychology, 39*(1), 2–19.

Dean, L. A., & Meadows, M. E. (1995). College counseling: Union and intersection. *Journal of Counseling and Development, 74*, 139–141.

Dean, R. B., & Richardson, H. (1964). Analysis of MMPI profiles of 40 college-educated overt role homosexuals. *Journal of Consulting Psychology, 28*, 483–486.

Delworth, U., & Hanson, G. (Eds.). (1991a). *Student services* (2nd ed.). San Francisco: Jossey-Bass.

Delworth, U., & Hanson, G. (1991b). Future directions: A vision of student services in the 1990s. In U. Delworth & G. Hanson (Eds.), *Student services* (2nd ed., pp. 604–618). San Francisco: Jossey-Bass.

Derlega, V. J., Lovell, R., & Chaikin, A. L. (1976). Effects of therapist disclosure and its perceived appropriateness on client self-disclosure. *Journal of Consulting and Clinical Psychology, 44*, 866.

De Shazer, S. (1985). *Keys to solutions in brief therapy*. New York: Norton.

De Shazer, S. (1988). *Clues: Investigating solutions in brief therapy*. New York: Norton.

De Shazer, S. (1991). *Putting difference to work*. New York: Norton.

Deutsch, C. J. (1984). Self-reported sources of stress among psychotherapists. *Professional Psychology: Research & Practice, 15*(6), 833–845.

DeVoe, D. (1990). Feminist and nonsexist counseling: Implications for the male counselor. *Journal of Counseling and Development, 69*, 33–38.

Dewey, J. (1956). *School and society*. Chicago: University of Chicago Press. (Originally published 1900)

Dewey, J., & Bentley, A. F. (1960). *Knowing and the known*. Boston: Beacon Press.

DiLeo, J. H. (1996). *Child development: Analysis and synthesis*. New York: Bruner/Mazel.

Dinkmeyer, D. (1982a). *Developing understanding of self and others (DUSO-1)*. Circle Pine, MN: American Guidance Service.

Dinkmeyer, D. (1982b). *Developing understanding of self and others (DUSO-2)*. Circle Pine, MN: American Guidance Service.

Dinkmeyer, D., Dinkmeyer, D., Jr., & Sperry, L. (1987). *Adlerian counseling and psychotherapy* (2nd ed.). Columbus, OH: Merrill.

Donaho, M. W., & Meyer, J. L. (1990). *How to get the job you want: A guide to resumes, interviews, and job-hunting strategy*. Englewood Cliffs, NJ: Prentice Hall.

Donaldson v. O'Connor, 422 U.S. 563 (U.S. Supreme Ct., 1975).

Donley, R. J., Horan, J. J., & DeShong, R. L. (1990). The effect of several self-disclosure permutations on counseling process and outcome. *Journal of Counseling and Development, 67*, 408–412.

Donlon, P. T., Schaffer, C. B., Ericksen, S. E., Pepitone-Arreola-Rockwell, F., & Schaffer, L. C. (1983). *A manual of psychotropic drugs: A mental health resource*. Bowie, MD: Robert J. Brady.

Doster, J. A., & Nesbitt, J. G. (1979). Psychotherapy and self-disclosure. In J. Chelune and Associates (Eds.), *Self-disclosure: Origins, patterns, and implications of openness in interpersonal relationships* (pp. 177–242). San Francisco: Jossey-Bass.

Dougherty, A. M. (1990). *Consultation: practice and perspectives*. Pacific Grove, CA: Brooks/Cole.

Dougherty, A. M. (1992a). Ethical issues in consultation. *Elementary School Guidance & Counseling, 26*, 214–221.

Dougherty, A. M. (Ed.). (1992b). Special issues on consultation [Special issue]. *Elementary School Guidance & Counseling, 26*, 3.

Downing, N. E., & Roush, K. L. (1985). From passive acceptance to active commitment: A model of feminist identity development for women. *The Counseling Psychologist, 13*(4), 695–709.

Doyle, R. E. (1992). *Essential skills and strategies in the helping process*. Pacific Grove, CA: Brooks/Cole.

Dreikurs, R. R. (1953). *Fundamentals of Adlerian psychology*. Chicago: Alfred Adler Institute.

Drum, D. J. (1992). A review of Leo Goldman's article "Qualitative assessment: An approach for counselors." *Journal of Counseling and Development, 70*(5), 622–623.

Drummond, R. J. (2000). *Appraisal procedures for counselors and helping professionals* (4th ed.). Upper Saddle River, NJ: Merrill.

Dryden, W., & Feltham, C. (1992). *Brief counselling: A practical guide for beginning practitioners*. Philadelphia: Open University Press.

Dumont, F. (1993). Inferential heuristic in clinical problem formulation: Selective review of their strengths and weaknesses. *Professional Psychology: Research and Practice, 24*, 196–205.

Durkin, H. E. (1972). Analytic group therapy and general systems theory. In C. J. Sager & H. S. Kaplan (Eds.), *Progress in group and family therapy* (pp. 9–17). New York: Brunner/Mazel.

Dworkin, S. H., & Gutierrez, F. (1989). Counselors be aware: Clients come in every size, shape, color, and sexual orientation. *Journal of Counseling and Development, 68*, 6–8.

Dye, A. M. (1994). *The supervisory relationship* (Report No. EDO-CG-94-11). Greensboro, NC: ERIC Clearinghouse on Counseling and Student Services. (ERIC Document Reproduction Service No. 372-343).

Dye, H. A., & Borders, L. D. (1990). Counseling supervisors: Standards for preparation and practice. *Journal of Counseling and Development, 69*, 27–29.

Dykhuizen, G. (1973). *The life and mind of John Dewey*. Carbondale: Southern Illinois University Press.

Dyne, W. A. (Ed.). (1990). *Encyclopedia of Homosexuality: Volume 1*. New York: Garland Publishing.

Eberts, M., & Gisler, M. (1998). *Careers for good Samaritans & other humanitarian types* (2nd ed.). Lincolnwood, IL: VGM Career Horizons.

Educational Testing Services. (1993). *SIGI*. Princeton, NJ: Author.

Egan, G. (1975). *The skilled helper: A model for systematic helping and interpersonal relating*. Pacific Grove, CA: Brooks/Cole.

Egan, G. (1998). *The skilled helper: Model, skills, and methods for effective helping* (6th ed.). Pacific Grove, CA: Brooks/Cole.

Ehrenwald, J. (Ed.). (1976). *The history of psychotherapy: From healing magic to encounter*. New York: Aronson.

Ellis, A. (1962). *Reason and emotion in psychotherapy*. New York: Lyle Stuart.

Ellis, A. (1973). *Humanistic psychotherapy*. New York: Julian Press.

Ellis, A. (1988a). Are there "rationalist" and "constructivist" camps of the cognitive therapies? A response to Michael Mahoney. *Cognitive Behaviorist, 10*(2), 13–17.

Ellis, A. (1988b). *How to stubbornly refuse to make yourself miserable about anything, yes anything!* Secaucas, NJ: Lyle Stuart.

Ellis, A. (1990). Is rational-emotive therapy (RET) "rationalist" or "constructivist"? In W. Dryden (Ed.), *The essential Albert Ellis: Seminal writings on psychotherapy* (pp. 114–141). New York: Springer.

Ellis, A. (1993). Reflections on rational-emotive therapy. *Journal of Consulting and Clinical Psychology, 61*, 199–201.

Ellis, A., & Harper, R. A. (1961). *A guide to rational living*. Englewood Cliffs, NJ: Prentice Hall.

Ellis, A., & Harper, R. A. (1997). *A guide to rational living* (3rd ed.). North Hollywood, CA: Wilshire Book Company.

Ellwood, R. S. (1993). *Introducing religion from inside and outside*. Englewood Cliffs, NJ: Prentice Hall.

Elmore, P. B., Ekstrom, R. B., Diamond, E. E., & Whittaker, S. (1993). School counselors' test use patterns and practices. *The School Counselor, 41*(2), 73–80.

Encyclopedia of Black America. (1981). New York: McGraw-Hill.

Erikson, E. H. (1950). *Childhood and society*. New York: Norton.

Erikson, E. H. (1963). *Childhood and society* (2nd ed.). New York: Norton.

Erikson, E. H. (1968). *Identity: Youth and crisis*. New York: Norton.

Erikson, E. (1980). *Identity and the life cycle*. New York: Norton.

Erikson, E. H. (1982). *The life cycle completed*. New York: Norton.

Essandoh, P. K. (1996). Multicultural counseling as the "fourth force": A call to arms. *Counseling Psychologist, 24*, 126–138.

Evans, D. R., Hearn, M. T., Uhlemann, M. R., & Ivey, A. E. (1998). *Essential interviewing: A programmed approach to effective communication* (5th ed.). Pacific Grove, CA: Brooks/Cole.

Evans, G. W., & Howard, R. B. (1973). Personal space. *Psychological Bulletin, 80*, 334–344.

Evans, N.M., Forney, D. S., & Guido-Dibrito, F. (1998). *Student development in college: theory, research, and practice*. San Francisco: Jossey-Bass.

Evans, R. B. (1970). Sixteen personality factor questionnaire scores of homosexual men. *Journal of Consulting Psychology, 34*, 212–215.

Everett, C. A. (1990). The field of marital and family therapy. *Journal of Counseling and Development, 68*, 498–502.

Eysenck, H. J. (1952). The effects of psychotherapy: An evaluation. *Journal of Consulting Psychology, 16*, 319–324.

Eysenck, H. J., Wakefield, J. A., & Friedman, A. F. (1983). Diagnosis and clinical assessment: *The DSM-III*. *Annual Review of Psychology, 34*, 167–193.

Faith, M. S., Wong, F. Y., & Carpenter, K. M. (1995). Group sensitivity training: Update, meta-analysis, and recommendations. *Journal of Counseling Psychology, 42*, 390–399.

Faiver, C. M., O'Brien, E. M., & Ingersoll, R. E. (2000). Religion, guilt, and mental health, *Journal of Counseling and Development, 78*, 155–161.

Fall, M. (1995). Planning for consultation: An aid for the elementary school counselor. *The School Counselor, 43*, 151–157.

Fassinger, R. E. (1991). The hidden minority: Issues and challenges in working with lesbian women and gay men. *The Counseling Psychologist, 19*, 157–176.

Faust, V. (1968). *The counselor-consultant in the elementary school*. Boston: Houghton Mifflin.

Fava, G. A., & Sonino, N. (2000). Psychosomatic medicine: Emerging trends and perspectives. *Psychotherapy and Psychosomatics, 69*(4), 184–187.

Fawcett, J., & Busch, K. A. (1998). Stimulants in psychiatry. In A. F. Schatzberg & C. B. Nemeroff (Eds.), *Textbook of psychopharmacology* (2nd ed., pp. 503–522). Washington, DC: American Psychiatric Press.

FBI (Federal Bureau of Investigation). (1999). *Uniform crime reports: Hate crime statistics*. Retrieved June 1, 2001, from the World Wide Web: http://www.fbi.gov/ucr/99hate.pdf.

Federal Register (1977). Regulation implementing Education for All Handicapped Children Act of 1975 (PL94-142), *42*(163), 42474–42518.

Feitel, B. (1968). *Feeling understood as a function of a variety of therapist activities*. Unpublished doctoral dissertation. New York: Teacher's College, Columbia University.

Fenske, R. H., & Hughes, M. S. (1991). Current challenges: Maintaining quality amid increasing student diversity. In U. Delworth & G. Hanson (Eds.), *Student services* (2nd ed., pp. 584–603). San Francisco: Jossey-Bass.

Ferber, A., Mendelsohn, M., & Napier, A. (1972). *The book of family therapy*. New York: Jason Aronson.

Field, S. (2000). *100 best careers for the 21st century* (2nd ed.). New York: IDG Books Worldwide.

Finkel, N. J. (1994). History of clinical psychology. In *The encyclopedia of psychology* (2nd ed.). (vol. 2, pp. 127–129). New York: Wiley.

Finn, R. (1996). Biological determination of sexuality heating up as a research field. *The Scientist, 10*(1), 13, 16.

Fisher, P. (1991). *Alcohol, drug abuse and mental health problems among homeless persons: A Review of the Literature, 1980–1990*. National Institute on Alcohol Abuse and Alcoholism: March 1991.

Fitzgerald, L. F., & Nutt, R. (1998). The division 17 principles concerning the counseling/psychotherapy of women: Rationale and implementation. In D. R. Atkinson & G. Hackett (Eds.), *Counseling diverse populations* (2nd ed., pp. 229–261). Boston: McGraw-Hill.

Flavell, J. H. (1963). *The developmental psychology of Jean Piaget*. New York: Van Nostrand.

Flowers, J. V., Booraem, C. D., & Schwartz, B. (1993). Impact of computerized rapid assessment on counselors and client outcome. *Computers in Human Services, 10*(2), 9–18.

Fong, M., & Malone, C. M. (1994). Defeating ourselves: Common errors in counseling research. *Counselor Education and Supervision, 33*, 356–362.

Fong, M. L. (1994). *Multicultural issues in supervision* (Report No. EDO-CG-94-14). Greensboro, NC: ERIC Clearinghouse on Counseling and Student Services. (ERIC Document Reproduction Service No. ED372-346).

Fong, M. L. (1995). Assessment and DSM-IV diagnosis of personality disorders: A primer for counselors. *Journal of Counseling and Development, 73*, 635–639.

Foos, J. A., Ottens, A. J., & Hill, L. K. (1991). Managed mental health: A primer for counselors. *Journal of Counseling and Development, 69*, 332–336.

Ford, E. (1963). Being and becoming a psychotherapist: The search for identity. *American Journal of Psychotherapy, 17*, 472–482.

Forman, S. G. (1995). Organizational factors and consultation outcome. *Journal of Educational and Psychological Consultation, 6*, 191–195.

Forrest, D. V., & Stone, L. A. (1991). Counselor certification. In F. O. Bradley (Ed.), *Credentialing in counseling* (pp. 23–52). Alexandria, VA: Association for Counselor Education and Supervision.

Forrest, L. (1991). Guiding, supporting, and advising students: The counselor role. In U. Delworth & G. Hanson (Eds.), *Student services* (2nd ed., pp. 265–283). San Francisco: Jossey-Bass.

Foster, S., & Gurman, A. S. (1985). Family therapies. In S. J. Lynn & J. P. Garske (Eds.), *Contemporary psychotherapies: Models and methods* (pp. 377–418). Columbus, OH: Merrill.

Fouad, N. A., & Bingham, R. P. (1995). Career counseling with racial/ethnic minorities. In W. B. Walsh & S. H. Osipow (Eds.), *Handbook of vocational psychology* (2nd ed.). Hillsdale, NJ: Earlbaum.

Fowler, J. (1976). Stages in faith: The structural-developmental approach. In T. C. Hennessy (Ed.), *Values & Moral Development* (pp. 173–211). New York: Paulist Press.

Fowler, J. (1981). *Stages of faith: The psychology of human development and the quest for meaning*. New York: Harper & Row.

Fowler, J. (1991). The vocation of faith developmental theory. In J. W. Fowler, K. E. Nipkow, & F. Schweitzer (Eds.), *Stages of faith and religious development: Implications for church, education, and society* (pp.19–37). New York: Crossroad Publishing.

Fowler, J. (1995). *Stages of faith: The psychology of human development and the quest for meaning*. New York: Harper & Row. (Original work published 1981)

Fowler, J. W. (1984). *Becoming adult, becoming Christian: Adult development and Christian faith*. New York: Harper & Row.

Fox, T. (1987). *The essential Moreno: Writings on psychodrama, group method, and spontaneity*. New York: Springer.

Foxhall, K. (2000). Platform for a long-term push. *Monitor on Psychology, 39*(9). Retrieved June 1, 2001, from the World Wide Web: http://www.apa.org/monitor/oct00/push.html.

Frankl, V. (1963). *Man's search for meaning*. Boston: Beacon.

Fredrickson, R. H. (1982). *Career information*. Englewood Cliffs, NJ: Prentice Hall.

Freeman, S. C. (1992). C. H. Patterson on client-centered supervision: An interview. *Counselor Education and Supervision, 31*, 219–226.

French, M. (1993, April). *How to get the job you want: Using a portfolio*. Symposium conducted at the annual spring conference of the Southern Organization for Human Services Education. Port Richey, Florida.

Fretz, B., & Mills, D. (1980). *Licensing and certification of psychologists and counselors*. San Francisco: Jossey-Bass.

Freud, A. (1935). *Psycho-analysis for teachers and parents*. New York: Emerson Books.

Freud, S. (1969). *An outline of psycho-analysis* (rev. ed.) (J. Strachey, trans.). New York: Norton. (Original work published 1940)

Freud, S. (1975). *Group psychology and the analysis of the ego* (J. Strachey, trans.). New York: Norton. (Original work published 1922)

Freud, the hidden nature of man (1970). [Film]. Columbus, OH: Coronet/MTI Film & Video [distributor].

Friedman, M. (1989). Martin Buber and Ivan Boszormenyi-Nagy: The role of dialogue in contextual therapy. *Psychotherapy, 26*, 402–409.

Froehle, T. C., & Rominger, R. L. (1993). Directions in consultation research: Bridging the gap between science and practice. *Journal of Counseling and Development, 71*, 693–699.

Fry, P. S. (1992). Major social theories of aging and their implications for counseling concepts and practice: A critical review. *The Counseling Psychologist, 20*, 246–329.

Fukuyama, M. A. (1994). Multicultural training: If not now, when? If not you, who? *The Counseling Psychologist, 22*(2), 296–299.

Fuqua, D. R., & Kurpius, D. J. (1993). Conceptual models in organizational consultation. *Journal of Counseling and Development, 71*, 607–618.

Gabbard, G. O. (1995a). Are all psychotherapies equally effective? *The Menninger Letter, 3*(1), 1–2.

Gabbard, G. O. (1995b). What are boundaries in psychotherapy? *The Menninger Letter, 3*(4), 1–2.

Gallup. (1999/2000). *The Gallup Organization: Homosexual relations*. Retrieved June 1, 2001, from the World Wide Web: http://www.gallup.com/poll/indicators/indhomosexual.asp.

Gallup. (2001). *The Gallup Organization: Religion*. Retrieved June 1, 2001, from the World Wide Web: http://www.gallup.com/poll/indicators/indreligion.asp.

Garcia, A. (1990). An examination of the social work profession's efforts to achieve legal regulation. *Journal of Counseling and Development, 68*, 491–497.

Garcia, M. H., Wright, J. W., & Corey, G. (1991). A multicultural perspective in an undergraduate human services program. *Journal of Counseling and Development, 70*, 86–90.

Garfield, N. J., & Beaman, J. (1996). Careers in health care facilities. In B. B. Collison, & N. J. Garfield (Eds.), *Careers in counseling and human services* (2nd ed., pp. 95–110). Washington, DC: Taylor & Francis.

Garfield, S. L. (1977). Research of the training of professional psychotherapists. In A. S. Gurman & A. M. Razin (Eds.), *Effective psychotherapy: A handbook of research* (pp. 63–83). New York: Pergamon.

Garfield, S. L. (1982). Eclecticism and integration in psychotherapy. *Behavior Therapy, 13*, 610–623.

Garfield, S. L. (1998). *The practice of brief psychotherapy* (2nd ed.). New York: John Wiley & Sons.

Garfield, S. L., & Kurtz, R. (1976). Personal therapy for the psychotherapist: Some findings and issues. *Psychotherapy: Theory, research and practice, 13*(2), 188–192.

Garner, G. O. (2001). *Careers in social and rehabilitation services* (2nd ed.). Lincolnwood, IL: VGM Career Horizons.

Garretson, D. J. (1993). Psychological misdiagnosis of African Americans. *Journal of Multicultural Counseling and Development, 21*, 119–126.

Garvin, C. (1981). *Contemporary group work*. Englewood Cliffs, NJ: Prentice Hall.

Gay, L. R., & Airasian, P. (2000). *Educational research: Competencies for analysis and application* (6th ed.). Upper Saddle River, NJ: Merrill.

Gazda, G. M. (1989). *Group counseling: A developmental approach* (4th ed.). Boston: Allyn & Bacon.

Gazda, G. M., Asbury, F. R., Balzer, F. J., Childers, W. C., & Walters, R. P. (1977). *Human relations development: A manual for educators*. Boston: Allyn & Bacon.

Gelso, C. J. (1992). Realities and emerging myths about brief therapy. *The Counseling Psychologist, 20*(3), 464–471.

Gelso, C. J., & Carter, J. A. (1994). Components of the psychotherapy relationship: Their interaction and unfolding during treatment. *Journal of Counseling Psychology, 41*(3), 296–306.

George, R. L., & Cristiani, R. S. (1995). *Counseling theory and practice* (4th ed.). Boston: Allyn & Bacon.

Gerler, E. (1992). What we know about school counseling: A reaction to Borders and Drury. *Journal of Counseling and Development, 70*, 499–501.

Germain, C. B. (1981). The physical environment and social work practice. In A. N. Maluccio (Ed.), *Promoting competence in clients* (pp. 103–124). New York: Free Press.

Gerrig, R., & Zimbardo, P. G.,(2002). *Psychology and life* (14th ed.). Boston, MA: Allyn & Bacon.

Gert, B. (1988). *Morality*. New York: Oxford University Press.

Gesell, A., & Ilg, F. L. (1943). *Infant and child in the culture of today*. New York: Harper.

Getz, H. G., & Protinsky, H. O. (1994). Training marriage and family counselors: A family-of-origin approach. *Counselor Education and Supervision, 33*, 183–190.

Gibbs, A., & Szablewicz, J. J. (1994). Colleges' new liabilities. In A. L. Rentz (Ed.), *Student affairs: A profession's heritage* (pp. 643–652). Lanham, MD: American College Personnel Association and the University Press of America.

Gibson, R. L., & Mitchell, M. (1999). *Introduction to counseling and guidance* (5th ed.). Upper Saddle River, NJ: Merrill.

Gibson, W. T., & Pope, K. S. (1993). The ethics of counseling: A national survey of certified counselors. *Journal of Counseling and Development, 71*, 330–336.

Gilbert, S. P. (1989). The juggling act of the college counseling center: A point of view. *The Counseling Psychologist, 17*, 477–489.

Gilligan, C. (1982). *In a different voice*. Cambridge, MA: Harvard University Press.

Gilliland, B. E., James, R. K., & Bowman, J. T. (1994). Response to the Lazarus and Beutler article "On technical eclecticism." *Journal of Counseling and Development, 72*, 554–555.

Gingerich, W. J., & Eisengart, S. (2000). Solution focused brief therapy: A review of outcome research. *Family Process, 39*(4), 477–498.

Ginter, E. J. (1988). Stagnation in eclecticism: The need to recommit to a journey. *Journal of Mental Health Counseling, 10*, 3–8.

Ginter, E. J., Scalise, J. J., & Presse, N. (1990). The elementary school counselor's role: Perceptions of teachers. *The School Counselor, 38*(1), 19–23.

Ginzberg, E. (1972). Toward a theory of occupational choice: A restatement. *Vocational Guidance Quarterly, 20*, 169–176.

Ginzberg, E., Ginsburg, S. W., Axelrad, S., & Herma, J. (1951). *Occupational choice: An approach to a general theory*. New York: Columbia University Press.

Gladding, S. (1994). Teaching family counseling through the use of fiction. *Counselor Education and Supervision, 33*, 191–200.

Gladding, S. (1997). *Community and agency counseling*. Upper Saddle River, NJ: Prentice Hall.

Gladding, S. (2000). *Counseling: A comprehensive profession* (4th ed.). Upper Saddle River, NJ: Merrill.

Gladding, S., Remley, T. P., & Huber, C. H. (2001). *Ethical, legal, and professional issues in the practice of marriage and family therapy* (3rd ed.). Upper Saddle River, NJ: Merrill.

Gladding, S. T. (1999). *Group work: A counseling specialty* (3rd ed.). New York: Merrill.

Gladstein, G. (1983). Understanding empathy: Integrating counseling, developmental, and social psychology perspectives. *Journal of Counseling Psychology, 30*, 467–482.

Glaser, J. L. (1994). Clinical applications of Maharishi Ayur-Veda in chemical dependency disorders. Treating addictions using Transcendental Meditation and Maharishi Ayur-Veda: II. *Alcoholism Treatment Quarterly, 11*(3–4), 367–394.

Glasser, W. (1961). *Mental health or mental illness?* New York: Harper & Row.

Glasser, W. (1965). *Reality therapy: A new approach to psychiatry*. New York: Harper & Row.

Glasser, W. (1976). *Positive addiction*. New York: McGraw-Hill.

Glasser. W. (Ed.). (1989). *Control theory in the practice of reality therapy: Case studies*. New York: Harper & Row.

Glasser, W. (1994). *Control theory: A new explanation of how we control our lives*. New York: San Bernardino, CA: Millefleurs.

Glasser, W. (1999). *Choice theory: A new psychology of personal freedom*. New York: HarperCollins.

Glidewell, J. C., & Livert, D. E. (1992). Confidence in the practice of clinical psychology. *Professional Psychology: Research and Practice, 23*, 151–157.

Glosoff, H. L., Herlihy, B., & Spense, B. E. (2000). Privileged communication in the counselor–client relationship. *Journal of counseling and development, 78*(4), 454–462.

Goldenberg, I, & Goldenberg, H. (2000). *Family therapy: An overview* (5th ed.). Pacific Grove, CA: Brooks/Cole.

Goldenson, R. M. (Ed.). (1984). *Longman dictionary of psychology and psychiatry*. New York: Longman.

Goldman, L. (1971). *Using tests in counseling* (2nd ed.). Pacific Palisades, CA: Goodyear.

Goldman, L. (1992). Qualitative assessment: An approach for counselors. *Journal of Counseling and Development, 70*(5), 616–621.

Goldman, L. (1994). The marriage between tests and counseling redux: Summary of the 1972 article. *Measurement and Evaluation in Counseling and Development, 26*(4), 214–216.

Gompertz, K. (1960). The relation of empathy to effective communication. *Journalism Quarterly, 37*, 535–546.

Goncalves, O. F. (1995). A constructivist outline of human knowing processes. In M. J. Mahoney (Ed.), *Cognitive and constructive psychotherapies: Theory, research, and practice* (pp. 89–102). New York: Springer.

Goncalves, O. F., & Machado, P. P. (1995). Cognitive narrative psychotherapy: Research foundations. *Journal of Clinical Psychology, 55*(10), 1179–1191.

Gonzales, M., Castillo-Canez, I., Tarke, H., Soriano, F., Garcia, P., Velasquez, R. J. (1997). Promoting the culturally sensitive diagnosis of Mexican Americans: Some personal insights. *Journal of Multicultural Counseling & Development*, *25*(2), 156–161.

Good, B. J. (1997). Studying mental illness in context: Local, global, or universal. *Ethos*, *25*(2), 230–248.

Good, G. E., Gilbert, L. A., & Scher, M. (1990). Gender aware therapy: A synthesis of feminist therapy and knowledge about gender. *Journal of Counseling and Development*, *68*, 376–380.

Goodyear, R. K. (1981). Termination as a loss experience for the counselor. *Personnel and Guidance Journal*, *59*, 349–350.

Goodyear, R. K. (1984). On our journal's evolution: Historical developments, transitions, and future directions. *Journal of Counseling and Development*, *63*, 3–9.

Gooley, R. L. (1992). African American communities: A significant part of the whole. *Western Journal of Black Studies*, *16*(3), 113–122.

Gottfredson, G. D., Holland, J. L., & Ogawa, D. K. (1996). *Dictionary of Holland occupational codes*. Odessa, FL: Psychological Assessment Resources.

Gould, R. L. (1972). The phases of adult life: A study in developmental psychology. *American Journal of Psychiatry*, *129*, 521–539.

Gould, R. L. (1978). *Transformations: Growth and change in adult life*. New York: Simon & Schuster.

Graduate Record Examination (GRE) Guide. (1990). Princeton, NJ: Educational Testing Service.

Graham, D. L. R., Rawlings, E. I., Halpern, H. S., & Hermes, J. (1984). Therapists' needs for training in counseling lesbians and gay men. *Professional Psychology*, *15*, 482–496.

Granello, P. F. (2000). *Historical context: The relationship of computer technologies and counseling*. (Report No. EDO-CG-00-10). Greensboro, NC: ERIC Counseling and Student Services Clearinghouse. (ERIC Document Reproduction Service No. ED-99-CO-0014).

Granello, P. F., & Witmer, M. (1998). Standards of care: Potential implications for the counseling profession. *Journal of Counseling and Development*, *76*, 371–380.

Gray, J. (1998). *Men are from Mars, women are from Venus: A practical guide for improving communication and getting what you want in your relationships*. London, U.K.: Thorsons.

Green, S. L., & Hansen, J. C. (1986). Ethical dilemmas in family therapy. *Journal of Marital and Family Therapy*, *12*, 225–230.

Greenberg, L. S. (1994). What is "real" in the relationship? Comment on Gelso and Carter (1994). *Journal of Counseling Psychology*, *41*(3), 307–309.

Greenberg, R. P., & Staller, J. (1981). Personal therapy for therapists. *American Journal of Psychiatry*, *138*, 1461–1471.

Griggs v. Duke Power Company, 401 U. S. 424 (1971).

Gross, D. R., & Capuzzi, D. (1998). Group counseling: Theory and application. In D. Capuzzi & D. R. Gross (Eds.), *Introduction to group counseling* (2nd ed., pp. 75–98). Denver, CO: Love Publishing Company.

Grumpy, fearful neurotics appear to be short on a gene. (1996, November 29). *The New York Times*, pp. A1, B17.

Grunebaum, H. (1983). A study of therapists' choice of a therapist. *American Journal of Psychiatry*, *140*, 1336–1339.

Guerra, P. (1998, February). Revamping school counselor education: The Dewitt Wallace-Reader's Digest Fund. *Counseling Today*, pp. 19, 36.

Guest, C. L., & Dooley, K. (1999). Supervisor malpractice: Liability to the supervisee in clinical supervision. *Counselor Education and Supervision*, *38*, 269–279.

Guidano, V. F. (1995). Constructivist psychotherapy: A theoretical framework. In M. J. Mahoney (Ed.), *Cognitive and constructive psychotherapies: Theory, research, and practice* (pp. 89–102). New York: Springer.

Guterman, J. T., & Kirk, M. A. (1999). Mental health counselors and the Internet. *Journal of Mental Health Counseling*, *21*, 309–325.

Gutheil, I. A. (1991). The physical environment and quality of life in residential facilities for frail elders. *Adult Residential Care Journal*, *5*, 131–145.

Guy, J. D. (1987). *The personal life of the psychotherapist*. New York: Wiley.

Guy, J. D., & Liaboe, G. P. (1986). Personal therapy for the experienced psychotherapist: A discussion of its usefulness and utilization. *The Clinical Psychologist*, *39*(1), 20–23.

Gysbers, N., & Henderson, P. (2000). *Developing and managing your school guidance program* (3rd ed.). Alexandria, VA: American Counseling Association.

Hackney, H., & Cormier, L. S. (1996). *The professional counselor* (3rd ed.). Boston, MA: Allyn & Bacon.

Hackney, H., & Cormier, L. S. (2001). *The professional counselor* (4th ed.). Boston, MA: Allyn & Bacon.

Haley, A. (2001). *The autobiography of Malcolm X*. London, U.K.: Penguin.

Haley, J. (1973). *Uncommon therapy*. New York: Norton.

Haley, J. (1976). *Problem-solving therapy*. San Francisco: Jossey-Bass.

Haley, J. (1986). *The power tactics of Jesus Christ and other essays* (2nd ed.). Rockville, MD: The Triangle Press.

Hall, A. S., & Lin, M. (1994). An integrative consultation framework: A practical tool for elementary school counselors. *Elementary School Guidance and Counseling*, *29*, 17–27.

Hall, C. S. (1954). *A primer of Freudian psychology*. New York: Mentor.

Halley, A. A., Kopp, J., & Austin, M. J. (1998). *Delivering human services: A learning approach to practice* (4th ed.). New York: Longman.

Hammersmith, S. K., & Weinberg, M. S. (1973). Homosexual identity: Commitment, adjustment, and significant others. *Sociometry*, *36*, 56–79.

Hammond, L. A., & Fong, M. L. (1988, August). *Mediators of stress and role satisfaction in multiple role persons*. Paper presented at the annual Meeting of the American Psychological Association, Atlanta, GA.

Haney, H., & Leibsohn, J. (1999). *Basic counseling responses: A multimedia learning system for the helping professional*. Pacific Grove, CA: Brooks/Cole.

Hanna, F. J., Bemak, F., & Chung, R. C. (1999). Toward a new paradigm for multicultural counseling. *Journal of Counseling and Development*, *77*, 125–134.

Hanna, F. J., & Shank, G. (1995). The specter of metaphysics in counseling research and practice: The qualitative challenge. *Journal of Counseling and Development*, *74*, 53–59.

Hannon, J. W., Ritchie, M. R., & Rye, D. A. (1992, September). *Class: The missing dimension in multicultural counseling and counselor education*. Presentation made at the Association for Counselor Education and Supervision National Conference, San Antonio, TX.

Hansen, J. C. (1995). *Interest assessment* (Report No. EDO-CG-95-13). Greensboro, NC: ERIC Clearinghouse on Counseling and Student Services. (ERIC Document Reproduction Service No. ED 389-961.)

Hansen, J. C., Rossberg, R. H., Cramer, S. H. (1994). *Counseling: Theory and process* (5th ed.). Boston: Allyn & Bacon.

Hardiman, R. (1982). White identity development: A process oriented model for describing the racial consciousness of white Americans. *Dissertation Abstracts International*, *43*, 104A (University Microfilms No. 82-10330).

Harrington, T., & O'Shea, A. (2000). *Career decision-making system*. Circle Pines, MN: American Guidance Service.

Harrington, T. F. (1995). *Assessment of abilities* (Report No. EDO-CG-95-12). Greensboro, NC: ERIC Clearinghouse on Counseling and Student Services. (ERIC Document Reproduction Service No. ED 389-960.)

Harrison, R. (1972). Role negotiation: A touch mind approach to team development. In W. W. Burke & H. A. Hornstein (eds.), *The social technology of organization development*. Fairfax, VA: NTL Learning Resources.

Hartung, P. J. (1996). Transforming counseling courses: From monocultural to multicultural. *Counselor Education and Supervision, 36*, 6–13.

Hashimi, J. (1991). Counseling older adults. In P. K. H. Kim (Ed.), *Serving the elderly: Skills for practice* (pp. 33–51). New York: McGraw-Hill.

Havighurst, R. J. (1972). *Developmental tasks and education* (3rd ed.). New York: David McKay.

Hayes, B., & Paisley, P. O. (1996). Careers in business and industry. In B. B. Collison & N. J. Garfield (Eds.), *Careers in counseling and human services* (2nd ed., pp. 53–64). Washington, DC: Taylor & Francis.

Hayes, R. (1994). The legacy of Lawrence Kohlberg: Implications for counseling and human development. *Journal of Counseling and Development, 72*(3), 261–267.

Heinrich, R. K., Corbine, J. L., & Thomas, K. R. (1990). Counseling Native Americans. *Journal of Counseling and Development, 69*, 128–133.

Helms, J. E. (1984). Toward a theoretical model of the effects of race on counseling: A black and white model. *The Counseling Psychologist, 12*, 153–165.

Helms, J. E. (1990). Development of the white racial identity inventory. In J. E. Helms (Ed.), *Black and white racial identity: Theory, research, and practice* (pp. 67–80). Westport, CT: Greenwood Press.

Helms, J. E. (1994). How multiculturalism obscures racial factors in the therapy process: Comment on Ridely et al. (1994), Sodowsky et al. (1994), Ottavi et al. (1994), and Thompson et al. (1994). *Journal of Counseling Psychology, 41*(2), 162–165.

Helms, J. E. (1995). An update of white and people of color racial identity model. In J. G. Ponterotto, J. M. Casa, L. A. Suzuki, & C. M. Alexander (Eds.), *Handbook of multicultural counseling* (pp. 181–198). Thousand Oaks, CA: Sage.

Helwig, A. A. (1996). Careers in federal and state agencies. In B. B. Collison & N. J. Garfield (Eds.), *Careers in counseling and human services* (2nd ed., pp. 91–103). Washington, DC: Taylor & Francis.

Henderson, P. (1994). *Supervision of school counselors* (Report No. EDO-CG-94-21). Greensboro, NC: ERIC Clearinghouse on Counseling and Student Services. (ERIC Document Reproduction Service No. ED 372-353).

Heppner, P. P., Kivlighan, D. M., & Wampold, B. E. (1992). *Research design in counseling*. Pacific Grove, CA: Brooks/Cole.

Herlihy, B., & Remley, T. P. (1995). Unified ethical standards: A challenge for professionalism. *Journal of Counseling and Development, 74*, 130–134.

Herr, E. (1985a). *Why counseling?* (2nd ed.). Alexandria, VA: American Association for Counseling and Development.

Herr, E. (1985b). AACD: An association committed to unity through diversity. *Journal of Counseling and Development, 63*(7), 395–404.

Herr, E. L., & Cramer, S. H. (1996). *Career guidance and counseling through the life span: Systematic approaches* (5th ed.). Reading, MA: Addison-Wesley.

Hersen, M., & Van Hasselt, V. B. (2001). (Eds.). *Advanced abnormal psychology* (2nd ed). New York: Plenum Press.

Hershenson, D. B., & Berger, G. P. (2001). The state of community counseling: A survey of directors of CACPREP-accredited programs. *Journal of Counseling and Development, 79*, 188–193.

Hershenson, D. B., Power, P. W., & Waldo, M. (1996). *Community counseling: Contemporary theory and practice*. Boston: Allyn & Bacon.

Higgs, J. A. (1992). Dealing with resistance: Strategies for effective group. *The Journal for Specialists in Group Work, 17*(2), 67–73.

Highlen, P. S., & Hill, C. E. (1984). Factors affecting client change in individual counseling. In S. D. Brown & R. W. Lent (Eds.), *Handbook of counseling psychology* (pp. 334–396). New York: Wiley.

Hinkle, S. (1994a). *Psychodiagnosis for counselors: The DSM-IV* (Report No. MF01/PC01). Greensboro, NC: ERIC Clearinghouse on Counseling and Student Services. (ERIC Document Reproduction Service No. ED 366-890.)

Hinkle, S. (1994b). *The DSM-IV:* Prognosis and implications for mental health counselors. *Journal of Mental Health Counseling, 16*(2), 174–183.

Ho, M. K. (1987). *Family therapy and ethnic minorities*. Newbury Park, CA: Sage.

Hobson, S. M., & Kanitz, H. M. (1996). Multicultural counseling: An ethical issue for school counselors. *The School Counselor, 43*, 245–255.

Hohenshil, T. H. (1993a). Teaching the *DSM-III-R* in counselor education. *Counselor Education and Supervision, 32*, 267–275.

Hohenshil, T. H. (1993b). Assessment and diagnosis. *Journal of Counseling and Development, 72*, 7.

Hohenshil, T. H. (1994). *DSM-IV:* What's new. *Journal of Counseling and Development, 73*, 105–107.

Hohenshil, T. H. (2000). High tech counseling. *Journal of Counseling and Development*, 78, 365–368.

Holcomb-McCoy, C. C., & Myers, J. E. (1999). Multicultural competence and counselor training: A national survey. *Journal of Counseling and Development, 77*, 294–302.

Holland, J. L. (1973). *Making vocational choices: A theory of career*. Englewood Cliffs, NJ: Prentice Hall.

Holland, J. L. (1994). *The self-directed search* (rev. ed.). Odessa, FL: Psychological Assessment Resources.

Holland, J. L., & Gottfredson, G. D. (1976). Using a topology of persons and environments to explain careers: Some extensions and clarifications. *Counseling Psychologist, 6*, 20–29.

Hollis, J. W., & Dodson, T. A. (2000). *Counselor preparation 1999-2001: Programs, faculty, trends* (10th ed.). Philadelphia: Taylor & Francis.

Homan, M. S. (1994). *Promoting community change: Making it happen in the real world*. Pacific Grove, CA: Brooks/Cole.

Hooker, E. (1957). The adjustment of the male homosexual. *Journal of Projective Techniques, 21*, 18–31.

Horst, E. A. (1995). Reexamining gender issues in Erikson's stages of identity and intimacy. *Journal of Counseling and Development, 73*, 271–278.

Horwitz, A. V. (1982). *The social control of mental illness*. San Diego, CA: Academic Press.

Hosie, T. (1991). Historical antecedents and current status of counselor licensure. In F. O. Bradley (Ed.). *Credentialing in counseling* (pp. 23–52). Alexandria, VA: Association for Counselor Education and Supervision.

House, J. D., & Johnson, S. J. (1993a). Predictive validity of the Graduate Record Examination Advanced Psychology Test for graduate grades. *Psychological Reports, 73*(1), 184–186.

House, J. D., & Johnson, S. J. (1993b). Graduate Record Examination Scores and academic background variables as predictors of graduate degree completion. *Educational and Psychological Measurement, 53*(2), 551–556.

House, R., & Martin, P. (1999). Teaching school counselors to advocate for better futures for all students. In G. McAuliffe, K. Eriksen, & C. Lovell (Eds.), *Constructing counselor education: Transformative teaching practices*. New York: Teachers College Press.

Howard, G. S., Nance, D. W., & Myers, P. (1986). Adaptive counseling and therapy: An integrative, eclectic model. *Counseling Psychologist, 14*, 363–442.

Hoyt, K. (1993). Guidance is not a dirty word. *The school counselor*, 40(4), 267–274.

Hoyt, M. F. (1995). Introduction: Competency-based future-oriented therapy. In M. F. Hoyt (Ed.), *Constructive therapies* (pp. 1–11). New York: The Guilford Press.

Hoyt, M.F. (2000). *Some stories are better than others: Doing what works in brief therapy and managed care*. Philadelphia: Brunner/Mazel.

Huber, C. (1997). Time-limited counseling, invisible rationing, and informed consent. *Family Journal: Counseling & Therapy for Couples and Families*, 5(4), 325–327.

Hubert, M. (1995, December). Independence: An ethical consideration. *The ASCA Counselor*, 13.

Hubert, M. (1996, February). Confidentiality and the minor student. *The ASCA Counselor*, 20.

Huey, W. C. (1986). Ethical concerns in school counseling. *Journal of Counseling and Development*, 64, 321–322.

Huey, W. C. (1988). Ethical concerns in school counseling. In W. C. Huey & T. P. Remley (Eds.). *Ethical & legal issues in school counseling* (pp. 321–322). Alexandria,VA: American School Counseling Association.

Hughey, K. F. (Ed.). (2000). School violence and counselors [Special issue]. *Professional School Counseling*, 4(2).

Hughey, K. F. (Ed.). (2001). Comprehensive guidance and counseling programs [Special issue]. *Professional School Counseling*, 4(4).

Hutchens, T. A., Hamilton, S. E., Town, P. A., Gaddis, L. R., & Presley, R. J. (1991). *The stability of I.Q. in preschool years: A review.* Paper presented at the American Association for Counseling and Development, Reno, NV. (ERIC Document Reproduction Service No. ED 353-068.)

Hutchins, D. E., & Cole, C. G. (1997). *Helping relationships and strategies* (3rd ed.). Pacific Grove, CA: Brooks/Cole.

Hutchinson, R. L., & Bottorff, R. R. (1986). Selected high school counseling services: Student assessment. *The School Counselor*, 33(5), 350–354.

IAMFC (International Association of Marriage and Family Counselors). (2001). *Code of ethics.* Retrieved June 1, 2001, from the World Wide Web: http://www.iamfc.org/ethicalcodes.htm.

Ibrahim, F. A. (1996). A multicultural perspective on principle and virtue ethics. *The Counseling Psychologist*, 24(1), 78–85.

Ihle, G. M., Sodowsky, G. R., & Kwan, K. (1996). Worldviews of women: Comparisons between white American clients, white American counselors, and Chinese international students. *Journal of Counseling and Development*, 74, 300–306.

Ingersoll, R. E. (1994). Spirituality, religion, and counseling: Dimensions and relationships. *Counseling and Values*, 38, 98–111.

Ingersoll, R. E. (2000). Teaching a psychopharmacology course to counselors: Justification, structure, and methods. *Counselor Education and Supervision*, 40, 58–69.

Inhelder, B., & Piaget, J. (1958). *The growth of logical thinking: From childhood to adolescence.* New York: Basic Books.

Isaacs, M. L., & Stone, C. (1999). School counselors and confidentiality: Factors affecting professional choices. *Professional School Counseling*, 2, 258–266.

Isaacson, L. E. (1985). *Basics of career counseling.* Boston: Allyn & Bacon.

Isaacson, L. E., & Brown, D. (2000). *Career information, career counseling, and career development* (7th ed.). Boston MA: Allyn & Bacon.

Ivey, A. (1980). *Counseling and psychotherapy.* Englewood Cliffs, NJ: Prentice Hall.

Ivey, A. (1990). *Developmental counseling and therapy.* Monterey, CA: Brooks/Cole.

Ivey, A. (1993). *Developmental strategies for helpers.* Pacific Grove, CA: Brooks/Cole.

Ivey, A., & Gluckstein, N. (1974). *Basic attending skills: An introduction to microcounseling and helping.* North Amherst, MA: Microtraining Associates.

Ivey, A., & Goncalves, O. F. (1988). Developmental therapy: Integrating developmental processes into the clinical practice. *Journal of Counseling and Development*, 66, 406–413.

Ivey, A., & Ivey, M. (1998). Reframing *DSM-IV*: Positive strategies from developmental counseling and therapy. *Journal of Counseling and Development*, 76(3), 334–350.

Ivey, A., & Ivey, M. (1999). *Intentional interviewing and counseling: Facilitating client development in a multicultural society.* Pacific Grove, CA: Brooks/Cole.

Ivey, A., & Simek-Downing, L. (1987). *Counseling and psychotherapy: Integrating skills, theories, and practice.* Englewood Cliffs, NJ: Prentice Hall.

Ivey, A., Simek-Morgan, L., & Ivey, M. B. (1997). *Counseling and psychotherapy: A multicultural perspective* (4th ed.). Boston: Allyn & Bacon.

Jackson, D. N., & Hayes, D. H. (1993). Multicultural issues in consultation. *Journal of Counseling and Development*, 72, 144–147.

Jacobs, E. E., Masson, R. L., & Harvill, R. L. (2002). *Group counseling: Strategies and skills* (4th ed.). Pacific Grove, CA: Brooks/Cole.

Jacobson, E. (1938). *Progressive relaxation.* Chicago: University of Chicago Press.

Jaffee v. *Redmond*, 518 U.S. 1 (U.S. Supreme Ct., 1996).

Jagger, L., Neukrug, E., & McAuliffe, G. (1992). Congruence between personality traits and chosen occupation as a predictor of job satisfaction for people with disabilities. *Rehabilitation Counseling Bulletin*, 36(1), 53–60.

Janesick, B. J., & Goldsmith, K. L., 2000. *Managed dying.* Philadelphia: Xlibris Corporation.

Jayakar, P. (1986). *Krishnamurti: A biography.* New York: Harper & Row.

Jensen, J. P., Bergin, A. E., & Greaves, D. W. (1990). The meaning of eclecticism: New survey and analysis of components. Professional Psychology: *Research and Practice*, 21, 124–130.

Jereb, R. J. (1982). Assessing the adequacy of counseling theories for use with black clients. *Counseling and Values*, 27(1), 17–26.

Jetter, J. (2001, April 20). Global issues dog S. Africa on AIDS: Way is cleared for cheaper drugs, but market-medicine conflict remains. *Washington Post Foreign Service*, p. A01.

Jin, P. (1992). Efficacy of Tai Chi, brisk walking, meditation, and reading in reducing mental and emotional stress. *Journal of Psychosomatic Research*, 36(4), 361–370.

Johansson, C. B. (1996). *Career assessment inventory: Enhanced version.* Minnetonka, MN: National Computer Systems.

Johnson, L. (1995). Enhancing multicultural relations Intervention strategies for the school counselor. *The School Counselor*, 43, 103–113.

Jones, J., & Wilson, W. (1995). *An incomplete education* (rev. ed.). New York: Ballantine Books.

Jones, L. K. (1994). Frank Parsons' contribution to career counseling. *Journal of Career Development*, 20(4), 287–294.

Jongsma, A.E., Jr., & Peterson, L.M. (1999). *The complete adult psychotherapy treatment planner* (2nd ed.). New York: John Wiley & Sons.

Jordan, A. E., & Meara, N. M. (1990). Ethics and the professional practice of psychologists: The role of virtues and principles. *Professional Psychology: Research and Practice*, 21(2), 107–114.

Jordan, J. M., & Denson, E. L. (1990). Student service for athletes: A model for enhancing the student-athlete experience. *Journal of Counseling and Development*, 69, 95–97.

Jourard, S. M. (1971). *The transparent self: Self disclosure and well-being* (2nd ed.). Princeton, NJ: Van Nostrand Reinhold.

Juhnke, G. A., & Culbreth, J. R. (1994). *Clinical supervision in addictions counseling: Special challenges and solutions* (Report No. EDO-CG-94-23). Greensboro, NC: ERIC Clearinghouse on Counseling and Student Services. (ERIC Document Reproduction Service No. ED 372-355).

Jung, C. G. (1968). *Analytical psychology: Its theory and practice: The Tavistock lectures.* New York: Pantheon Books. (Original work published 1935)

Jung, C. G. (1975). Freud and Jung: Contrasts. In R. F. C. Hull (trans.). *Critiques of psychoanalysis.* (Extracted from *The Collected Works of C.G. Jung* [Vols. 4 and 18] by W. McGuire [Ed.], 1961. Princeton, NJ: Princeton University Press.) (Original work published 1929)

Kagan, N. (1980). Influencing human interaction Eighteen years with IPR. In A. I. Hess (Ed.), *Psychotherapy supervision:*

Theory, research, and practice (pp. 262–283). New York: Wiley.

Kahill, S. (1988a). Interventions for burnout in the helping professions: A review of the empirical evidence. *Canadian Journal of Counselling, 22*(3), 162–169.

Kahill, S. (1988b). Symptoms of professional burnout: A review of the empirical evidence. *Canadian Psychology, 29*(3), 284–297.

Kahn, M. (1997). *Between therapist and client: The new relationship* (rev. ed.). New York: W. H. Freeman.

Kain, C. D. (Ed.). (1989). *No longer immune: A counselor's guide to AIDS*. Alexandria, VA: American Association for Counseling and Development.

Kalat, J. W. (2001). *Biological psychology* (7th ed.). Pacific Grove, CA: Brooks Cole.

Kaplan, M., & Cuciti, P. L. (Eds.). (1986). *The Great Society and its legacy: Twenty years of U.S. social policy*. Durham, NC: Duke University Press.

Kaplan, R. M., & Saccuzzo, D. P. (1993). *Psychological testing: Principles, applications, and issues* (3rd ed.). Pacific Grove, CA: Brooks/Cole.

Katz, L. (1985). *A practical guide to psychodiagnostic testing*. Springfield, IL: Charles C Thomas.

Keck, P. E., & McElroy (1998). Antiepileptic drugs. In A. F. Schatzberg & C. B. Nemeroff (Eds.), *Textbook of psychopharmacology* (2nd ed., pp. 431–454). Washington, DC: American Psychiatric Press.

Kegan, R. (1982). *The evolving self*. Cambridge, MA: Harvard University Press.

Kegan, R. (1994). *In over our heads*. Cambridge, MA: Harvard University Press.

Keith-Spiegel, P. (1991). *The complete guide to graduate school admission: Psychology and related fields*. Hillsdale, NJ: Lawrence Erlbaum Associates.

Kelly, E. L. (1994). *History of clinical psychology*. In *The encyclopedia of psychology* (2nd ed.). (vol. 2, pp. 130–132). New York: Wiley.

Kelly, K. R. (1991). Theoretical integration is the future for mental health counseling. *Journal of Mental Health Counseling, 13*(1), 106–111.

Kelly, K. R., & Hall, A. S. (Eds.). (1992). Mental health counseling for men [Special issue]. *Journal of Mental Health Counseling, 19*(2).

Kemp, C. G. (1962). Influence of dogmatism on the training of counselors. *Journal of Counseling Psychology, 9*, 155–57.

King, P. M. (1978). William Perry's theory of intellectual and ethical development. In L. Knetelkamp, C. Widick, & C. L. Parker (Eds.), *Applying new developmental findings* (pp. 34–51). San Francisco: Jossey-Bass.

King, P. M. (1994). Theories of college student development: Sequences and consequences. *Journal of College Student Development, 35*(6), 413–421.

Kinsey, A. C., Pomeroy, W. B., & Martin, C. E. (1948). *Sexual behavior in the human male*. Philadelphia: Saunders.

Kinsey, A. C., Pomeroy, W. B., Martin, C. E., & Gebhard, P. H. (1953). *Sexual behavior in the human female*. Philadelphia: Saunders.

Kirschenbaum, H., & Henderson, V. L. (Eds.). (1989). *The Carl Rogers reader*. Boston: Houghton Mifflin.

Kitchener, K. S. (1984). Intuition, critical evaluation and ethical principles: The foundation for ethical decisions in counseling psychology. *The Counseling Psychologists, 12*(3), 43–45.

Kitchener, K. S. (1986). Teaching applied ethics in counselor education: An integration of psychological processes and philosophical analysis. *Journal of Counseling and Development, 64*(5), 306–311.

Kivlighan, D. M., Marsh-Angelone, M., & Angelone, E. O. (1994). Projection in group counseling: The relationship between members' interpersonal problems and their perception of the group leader. *Journal of Counseling Psychology, 41*(1), 99–104.

Klein, E. B., Gabelnick, F., & Herr, P. (Eds.). (2000). *Dynamic consultation in a changing workplace*. Madison, CT: International Universities Press.

Klein, M. (1975). *Psychoanalytic theory: An exploration of essentials*. New York: International Universities Press.

Kleinke, C. L. (1994). *Common principles of psychotherapy*. Pacific Grove, CA: Brooks/Cole.

Kluckhohn, C., & Murray, H. A. (1953). Personality formation: The determinants. In C. Kluckhohn, H. A. Murray, & D. M. Scheider (Eds.), *Personality in nature, society, and culture* (pp. 335–370). New York: Random House.

Knefelkamp, L. L., & Slepitza, R. (1976). A cognitive developmental model of career development: An adaptation of the Perry scheme. *The Counseling Psychologist, 6*(3), 53–58.

Knock, G. H., Rentz, A. L., & Penn, J. R. (1994). Our philosophical heritage: Significant influences on professional practice and preparation. In A. L. Rentz (Ed.), *Student affairs: A profession's heritage* (pp. 674–682). Lanham, MD: American College Personnel Association and the University Press of America.

Kohlberg, L. (1969). *Stages in the development of moral thought and action*. New York: Holt, Rinehart & Winston.

Kohlberg, L. (1984). *The psychology of moral development: The nature and validity of moral stages*. San Francisco: Harper & Row.

Kohut, H. (1984). *How does analysis cure?* Chicago: University of Chicago Press.

Kornetsky, C. (1976). *Pharmacology: Drugs affecting behavior*. New York: Wiley.

Koss, M. P., & Butcher, J. N. (1986). Research on brief psychotherapy. In S. L. Garfield & A. E. Bergin (Eds.), *Handbook of psychotherapy and behavior change* (3rd ed., pp. 627–670). New York: Wiley.

Kottler, J. A. (1994). *Advanced group leadership*. Pacific Grove, CA: Brooks/Cole.

Kottler, J. A, & Brown, R. W. (1999). *Introduction to therapeutic counseling* (4th ed.). Pacific Grove, CA: Brooks/Cole.

Krishnan, K. R. R. (1998). Monoamine oxidase inhibitors. In A. F. Schatzberg & C. B. Nemeroff (Eds.), *Textbook of psychopharmacology* (2nd ed., pp. 239–250). Washington, DC: American Psychiatric Press.

Krogman, W. M. (1945). The concept of race. In R. Linston (Ed.), *The science of man in world crisis* (pp. 38–62). New York: Columbia University Press.

Krumboltz, J. D. (1966a). Promoting adaptive behavior. In J. D. Krumboltz (Ed.), *Revolution in counseling* (pp. 3–26). Boston: Houghton Mifflin.

Krumboltz, J. D. (Ed.). (1966b). *Revolution in counseling*. Boston: Houghton Mifflin.

Krumboltz, J. D. (1994). Improving career development theory from a social learning perspective. In M. L. Savickas & R. W. Lent (Eds.), *Convergence in career development theories. Implications for science and practice* (pp. 9–31). Palo Alto, CA: CPP books.

Krumboltz, J. D., Mitchell, A. M., & Gelatt, H. B. (1975). Applications of social learning theory of careers selection. *Focus on Guidance, 8*(3), 1–16.

Krumboltz, J. D., Mitchell, A. M., & Jones, G. B. (1976). A social learning theory of career selection. *Counseling Psychologist, 6*, 71–81.

Kübler-Ross, E. (1969). *On death and dying*. New York: Macmillan.

Kuhn, T. S. (1962). *The structure of scientific revolutions*. Chicago: University of Chicago Press.

Kurpius, D. J. (1978). Consultation theory and process: An integrated model. *The Personnel and Guidance Journal, 56*, 335–338.

Kurpius, D. J. (1985). Consultation interventions: Successes, failures, and proposals. *The Counseling Psychologist, 13*, 368–369.

Kurpius, D. J., & Brubaker, J. C. (1976). *Psychoeducational consultation: Definitions-functions-preparation*. Bloomington: Indiana University.

Kurpius, D. J., & Fuqua, D. R. (1993a). Consultation: A paradigm for helping. Consultation I: Conceptual, structural, and operational dimensions [Special issue]. *Journal of Counseling and Development, 71*(6).

Kurpius, D. J., & Fuqua, D. R. (1993b). Consultation: A paradigm for helping.

Consultation II: Prevention, preparation, and key issues [Special issue]. *Journal of Counseling and Development, 72*(2).

Kurpius, D. J., & Fuqua, D. R. (1993c). Fundamental issues in defining consultation. *Journal of Counseling and Development, 71*, 598–600.

Kurpius, D. J., & Fuqua, D. R. (1993d). Introduction to the special issues (Special Issue: Consultation I). *Journal of Counseling and Development, 71*, 596–597.

Kurpius, D. J., Fuqua, D. R., & Rozecki, T. (1993). The consulting process: A multidimensional approach. *Journal of Counseling and Development, 71*, 601–606.

Kurpius, D. J., & Robinson, S. E. (1978). An overview of consultation. *Personnel and Guidance Journal, 56*, 321–323.

Ladany, N., & Friedlander, M. L. (1995). The relationship between the supervisor working alliance and trainee's experience of role conflict and role ambiguity. *Counselor Education and Supervision, 34*, 220–231.

LaFromboise, T. D. (1998). American Indian mental health policy. In D. R. Atkinson, G. Morten, & D. Sue (Eds.), *Counseling American minorities* (5th ed., pp. 137–158). Boston: McGraw-Hill.

LaFromboise, T. D., Trimble, J. E., & Mohatt, G. V. (1995). Counseling intervention and American Indian tradition: An integrative approach. In D. R. Atkinson, G. Morten, & D. Sue (Eds.), *Counseling American minorities* (5th ed., pp. 159–182). Boston: McGraw-Hill.

Laing, R. D. (1967). *The politics of experience*. New York: Ballantine.

Lamar, J. (1992). The problem with you people. *Esquire, 117*, 90–91, 94.

Lambert, M. J., & Bergin, A. E. (1983). Therapist characteristics and their contribution to psychotherapy outcome. In C. E. Walker (Ed.), *Handbook of psychotherapy and behavior change* (pp. 205–241). Homewood, IL: Dow Jones-Irwin.

Lambert, M. J., Ogles, B. M., & Masters, K. S. (1992). Choosing outcome assessment devices: An organizational and conceptual scheme. *Journal of Counseling and Development, 70*, 527–534.

Lambert, M. J., Shapiro, D. A., & Bergin, A. E. (1986). The effectiveness of psychotherapy. In S. L. Garfield & A. E. Bergin (Eds.), *Handbook of psychotherapy and behavior change* (pp. 157–211). New York: Wiley.

Lanci, J. R. (1997). *A new temple for Corinth: Rhetorical and archaeological approaches to Pauline imagery*. New York: Peter Lang Publishing.

Lanci, J. R. (1999). *Texts, rocks, and talk: Reclaiming biblical Christianity*. Collegeville, MN: Michael Glazier/Liturgical Press.

Lancy, D. F. (1993). *Qualitative research in education: An introduction to the major traditions*. New York: Longman.

Landis, L. L., & Young, M. E. (1994). The reflecting team in counselor education. *Counselor Education and Supervision, 33*, 210–219.

Langer, E. (2000). Mindful learning. *Current Directions in Psychological Science, 9*(6), 220–223.

Langer, J. (1969). *Theories of development*. New York: Holt, Rinehart, & Winston.

Lawrence, G., & Kurpius, S. E. R., (2000). Legal and ethical issues involved when counseling minors in nonschool settings. *Journal of Counseling and Development, 78*, 130–136.

Lazarus, A. A. (1971). *Behavior therapy and beyond*. New York: McGraw-Hill.

Lazarus, A. A. (1976). *The practice of multimodal therapy*. Baltimore: Johns Hopkins University Press.

Lazarus, A. A. (1986). Multimodal therapy. In U. C. Norcross (Ed.), *Handbook of eclectic psychotherapy* (pp. 65–93). New York: Brunner/Mazel.

Lazarus, A. A., & Beutler, L. E. (1993). On technical eclecticism. *Journal of Counseling and Development, 71*(4), 381–385.

Leahy, M. J., & Szymanski, E. M. (1995). Rehabilitation counseling: Evolution and current issues. *Journal of Counseling and Development, 74*(2), 163–166.

Leary, D. (1992). William James and the art of human understanding. *American Psychologist, 47*(2), 152–160.

Leary, M. R. (2001). *Introduction to behavioral research methods* (3rd ed.). Boston: Allyn & Bacon.

Leddick, G. R. (1994). *Models of clinical supervision* (Report No. EDO-CG-94-08). Greensboro, NC: ERIC Clearinghouse on Counseling and Student Services. (ERIC Document Reproduction Service No. ED 372-340).

Lee, C. C. (1994). Pioneers of multicultural counseling: A conversation with Clemmont E. Vontress. *Journal of Multicultural Counseling and Development, 22*, 66–78.

Lee, C. C. (2001). Culturally responsive school counselors and programs: Addressing the needs of all students. *Professional School Counseling, 4*, 257–262.

Lee, E. & Loeb, S. (1995). Where do head start attendees end up? One reason why preschool effects fade out. *Educational Evaluation & Policy Analysis, 17*(1), 62–82.

Lee, R. S. (1993). Effects of classroom guidance on student achievement. *Elementary School Guidance and Counseling, 27*, 163–171.

Lee, V. E., Brooks-Gunn, J., Schnur, E., & Liaw, F. (1990). Are Head Start effects sustained: A longitudinal follow-up comparison of disadvantaged children attending Head Start, no preschool, and other preschool programs. *Child Development, 61*, 495–507.

Lee, W. M. L., & Mixson, R. J. (1995). Asian and Caucasian client perceptions of the effectiveness of counseling. *Journal of Multicultural Counseling and Development, 23*, 48–56.

Leiby, J. (1978). *A history of social welfare and social work in the United States*. New York: Columbia University Press.

Lenox, R. H., & Manji, H. K. (1998). Lithium. In A. F. Schatzberg & C. B. Nemeroff (Eds.), *Textbook of psychopharmacology* (2nd ed., pp. 370–430). Washington, DC: American Psychiatric Press.

Leong, F. T. (1991). Career development of racial and ethnic minorities [Special issue]. *Career Development Quarterly*, 39.

Leong, F. T. (1995a). Introduction and overview. In F. T. Leong (Ed.), *Career development and vocational behavior of racial and ethnic minorities* (pp. 1–4). Mahway, NJ: Erlbaum.

Leong, F. T. (1995b). *Career development and vocational behavior of racial and ethnic minorities*. Mahway, NJ: Erlbaum.

Lesch, K., et al. (1996). Association of anxiety-related traits with a polymorphism in the serotonin transporter gene regulatory region. *Science, 274*, 1527–1531.

Levenson, H. & Davidovitz, D.(2000). Brief therapy prevalence and training: A national survey of psychologists. *Psychotherapy, 37*(4), 335–340.

Levinson, D. (1985). *The seasons of a man's life*. New York: Knopf.

Levinson, D. (1996). *The seasons of a woman's life*. New York: Knopf.

Lewandowski, D. G., & Saccuzzo, D. P. (1976). The decline of psychological testing: have traditional procedures been fairly evaluated? *Professional Psychology, 7*, 177–184.

Lewis, H. W. (1984). A structured group counseling program for reading-disabled elementary students. *School Counseling, 31*, 454–459.

Lightfoot-Klein, H. (1993). Disability in female immigrants with ritually inflicted genital mutilation. *Women & Therapy, 14*(3/4), 187–194.

Lipps, T. (1935). Empathy, inner-imitation of sense feelings. In *Radar: A modern book of esthetics*. New York: Holt.

Livingston, R. (1979). The history of rehabilitation counselor certification. *Journal of Applied Rehabilitation Counseling, 10*, 111–118.

Lloyd, A. P. (1992). The impact of the accreditation movement on one counselor education program: Idaho State University. *Journal of Counseling and Development, 70*, 673–676.

Locke, D. (1990). A not-so-provincial view of multicultural counseling. *Counselor Education and Supervision, 30*, 18–25.

Locke, D. (1992). Counseling beyond U.S. borders. *American Counselor, 1*, 13–17.

Locke, D. (1998). *Increasing multicultural understanding: A comprehensive model.* Thousand Oaks, CA: Sage Publications.

Loevinger, J. (1976). *Ego development*. San Francisco: Jossey-Bass.

Loewenberg, F., & Dolgoff, R. (2000). *Ethical decisions for social work practice* (6th ed.). Itasca, IL: F. E. Peacock.

Loganbill, C., Hardy, E., & Delworth, U. (1982). Supervision: A conceptual model. *The Counseling Psychologist, 10*, 3–42.

Lombana, J. H. (1989). Counseling persons with disabilities: Summary and projections. *Journal of Counseling and Development*, 68(2), 177–179.

Lonergan, E. C. (1994). Using theories of group therapy. In H. S. Bernard & K. R. MacKenzie, *Basics of Group Psychotherapy* (pp. 191–216). New York: Guilford Press.

Loulan, J. (1987). *Lesbian passion: Loving ourselves and each other.* San Francisco: Spinsters/Aunt Lute.

Lovell, C. (1999a). Empathic-cognitive development in students of counseling. *Journal of Adult Development*, 6(4), 195–203.

Lovell, C. (1999b). Supervisee cognitive complexity and the integrated developmental model. *Clinical Supervisor, 18*(1), 191–201.

Lovell, C. W. (1990, October). *Cognitive development (Perry scheme) in students of counseling: The national sample*. Paper presented at the annual meeting of the Southern Association for Counselor Education and Supervision, Norfolk, VA.

Luborsky, L., Crits-Christoph, P., Mintz, J., & Auerbach, A. (1988). *Who will benefit from psychotherapy? Predicting therapeutic outcomes*. New York: Basic Books.

Lum, D. (2000). *Social work practice & people of color: A process-stage approach* (4th ed.). Pacific Grove, CA: Brooks/Cole.

Lupton, M. L. (1994). Behaviour modification by genetic intervention: The law's response. *Medicine and Law, 13*(66), 417–431.

Lynch, R. T., & Lynch, R. K. (1996). Careers in residential treatment centers and community based support programs. In B. B. Collison & N. J. Garfield (Eds.), *Careers in counseling and human services* (2nd ed., pp. 111–121). Washington, DC: Taylor & Francis.

Lynn, S. J., & Garske, J. P. (Eds.). (1985). *Contemporary psychotherapies: Models and methods*. Columbus, OH: Merrill.

Mabe, A. R., & Rollin, S. A. (1986). The role of a code of ethical standards in counseling. *Journal of Counseling and Development*, 64(5), 294–297.

Macionis, J. J. (2001). *Sociology* (8th ed.). Upper Saddle River, NJ: Prentice Hall.

Madanes, C. (1981). *Strategic family therapy*. San Francisco: Jossey-Bass.

Magolda, M. B., & Porterfield, W. D. (1988). *Assessing intellectual development: The link between theory and practice*. Alexandria VA: American College Personnel Association.

Mahalik, J. R. (1990). Systematic eclectic models. *The Counseling Psychologist, 18*(4), 655–679.

Mahler, M. (1952). On child psychosis and schizophrenia. *The psychoanalytic study of the child*, Vol. 7 (pp. 286–305). New York: International Universities Press.

Mahler, M. (1971). *On child psychosis and schizophrenia. The psychoanalytic study of the child*. New York: International Universities Press.

Mahoney, M., Miller, H. M., & Arciero, G. (1995). Constructive metatheory and the nature of mental representation. In M. J. Mahoney (Ed.), *Cognitive and constructive psychotherapies: Theory, research, and practice* (pp. 195–208). New York: Springer.

Mahoney, M. J. (1974). *Cognition and behavior modification*. Cambridge, MA: Ballinger.

Mahoney, M. J. (1991). *Human change processes: The scientific foundation of psychotherapy*. New York: Basic Books.

Mahoney, M. J. (Ed.). (1995a). *Cognitive and constructive psychotherapies: Theory, research, and practice*. New York: Springer.

Mahoney, M. J. (1995b). Theoretical developments in the cognitive and constructive psychotherapies. In M. J. Mahoney (Ed.), *Cognitive and constructive psychotherapies: Theory, research, and practice* (pp. 3–19). New York: Springer.

Major religions of the world (2001). Retrieved June 1, 2001, from the World Wide Web: http://www.adherents.com/Religions_By_Adherents.html.

Majors, R., & Nikelly, A. (1983). Serving the black minority: A new direction for psychotherapy. *Journal of Non-White Concerns in Personnel and Guidance, 11*(4), 142–151.

Male, R. A. (1990). Careers in public and private agencies. In B. B. Collison & N. J. Garfield (Eds.), *Careers in counseling and human development* (2nd ed., pp. 81–89). Alexandria, VA: American Association for Counseling and Development.

Marder, S. R.(1998). Antipsychotic medications. In A. F. Schatzberg & C. B. Nemeroff (Eds.), *Textbook of psychopharmacology* (2nd ed., pp. 309-322). Washington, DC: American Psychiatric Press.

Martin, J., Slemon, A., Hiebert, B., Hallberg, E., & Cummings, A. (1989). Conceptualizations of novice and experienced counselors. *Journal of Counseling Psychology, 36*, 395–400.

Maslach, C. (1982). *Burnout: The cost of caring*. Englewood Cliffs, NJ: Prentice Hall.

Maslow, A. (1968). *Toward a psychology of being* (2nd ed.). Princeton, NJ: Van Nostrand.

Maslow, A. (1970). *Motivation and personality* (rev. ed.). New York: Harper & Row.

Masterson, J. F. (1981). *The narcissistic and borderline disorders: An integrated developmental approach*. New York: Brunner/Mazel.

Matarazzo, R. G., & Patterson, D. R. (1986). Methods of teaching therapeutic skill. In S. L. Garfield & A. E. Bergin, (Eds.), *Handbook of psychotherapy and behavior change* (3rd ed., pp. 821–845). New York: Wiley.

Matthews, C. O. (1992). An application of general system theory (GST) to group therapy. *The Journal for Specialists in Group Work, 17*(3), 161–169.

May, K. M., & Sowa, C. J. (1992). The relationship between a counselor's ethical orientation and stress experienced in ethical dilemmas. *Counseling and Values*, *36*(2), 150–159.

May, R. (1950). *The meaning of anxiety*. New York: Ronald Press.

May, R., Angel, E., & Ellenberger, H. F. (Eds.). (1958). *Existence: A new dimension in psychiatry and psychology*. New York: Basic Books.

McAuliffe, G. (1992a). A case presentation approach to group supervision for community college counselors. *Counselor Education and Supervision, 31*, 163–174.

McAuliffe, G. (1992b). Assessing and changing career decision making self-efficacy expectations. *Journal of Career Development, 19*, 25–36.

McAuliffe, G. (1993). Constructive development and career transition. Implications for counseling. *Journal of Counseling and Development, 72*, 29–36.

McAuliffe, G. (Ed.). (2001). *Working with troubled youth in schools: A guide for all school staff*. Westport, CT: Bergin and Garvey.

McAuliffe, G., & Eriksen, K. (1999). Toward a constructivist and developmental identity for the counseling profession: The context-phase-stage-style assessment model. *Journal of Counseling and Development, 77*(3), 267–280.

McAuliffe, G., & Eriksen, K. (Eds.). (2000). *Preparing counselors and therapists: Creating constructivist and developmental programs*. Virginia Beach, VA: The Donning Company.

McAuliffe, G., Neukrug, E., & Lovell, C. (1998). The cognitive development of counselor trainees. Unpublished manuscript.

McBride, B. C., & Martin, G. E. (1990). A framework for eclecticism: The importance of theory to mental health counseling. *Journal of Mental Health Counseling, 12*(4), 495–505.

McCormack, J. (1990). Careers in health care facilities. In B. B. Collison & N. J. Garfield (Eds.), *Careers in counseling and human development* (2nd ed., pp. 105–116). Alexandria, VA: American Association for Counseling and Development.

McDaniels, C., & Watts, G. A. (1994). Frank Parsons: Light, information, inspiration, cooperation [Special Issue]. *Journal of Career Development, 20*(4).

McFadden, J. (1996). A transcultural perspective: Reaction to C. H. Patterson's "Multicultural counseling: From diversity to universality." *Journal of Counseling and Development, 74*, 232–235.

McFadden, J. (Ed.). (1999). *Transcultural counseling* (2nd ed.). Alexandria, VA: American Counseling Association.

McGoldrick, M., Pearce, J. K., & Giordano, J. (Eds.). (1996). *Ethnicity and family therapy* (2nd ed). New York: Guilford Press.

McKean, K. (1985, October). Intelligence: Ways to measure the wisdom of man. *Discover*, 25–41.

McKenzie, K. (1999). Moving the misdiagnosis debate forward. *International Review of Psychiatry,11*(2–3), 153–161.

McMillan, J. H., & Schumacher, S. (1993). *Research in education: A conceptual introduction* (3rd. ed.). New York: HarperCollins.

McMillan, J. H., & Schumacher, S. (2001). *Research in education: A conceptual introduction* (5th ed.). New York: Addison Wesley Longman, Inc.

McNamara, K., & Rickard, K. M. (1989). Feminist identity development: Implications for feminist therapy with women. *Journal of Counseling and Development, 68*, 184–189.

McNeill, B. W., Stoltenberg, C. D., & Romans, J. S. C. (1992). The integrated developmental model of supervision: Scale development and validation procedures. *Professional Psychology: Research and Practice, 23*, 504–508.

Mead, M. (1961). *Coming of age in Samoa; a psychological study of primitive youth for western civilization*. New York: Morrow.

Medical Economics Staff (2001). *HMO/PPO directory, 2001*. Montvale, NJ: Author.

Mehr, J. (2001). *Human services: Concepts and intervention strategies* (8th ed.). Boston: Allyn & Bacon.

Mehrabian, A. (1972). *Nonverbal communication*. Chicago: Aldene-Atherton.

Mehrens, W. A. (1992). Leadership to researchers and practitioners. *Journal of Counseling and Development, 70*, 439–440.

Meichenbaum, D. (1977). *Cognitive behavior modification: An integrative approach*. New York: Basic Books.

Mendoza, D. W. (1993). A review of Gerald Caplan's theory and practice of mental health consultation. *Journal of Counseling and Development, 71*, 629–635.

Menninger, K. (1973). *Whatever became of sin?* New York: Hawthorne Books.

Mental Illness and Homelessness (1999). *National coalition for the homeless fact sheet number 5*. Retrieved June 1, 2001, from the World Wide Web: http://nch.ari.net/mental.html.

Merchant, N., & Dupuy, P. (1996). Multicultural counseling and qualitative research: Shared worldview and skills. *Journal of Counseling and Development, 74*, 537–541.

Merta, R. J., Johnson, P., & McNeil, K. (1995). Updated research on group work: Educators, course work, theory, and teaching methods. *The Journal for Specialists in Group Work, 20*(1), 132–142.

Mezzano, J. (1969). A note on dogmatism and counselor effectiveness. *Counselor Education and Supervision, 9*, 64–65.

Midgette, T. E., & Meggert, S. S. (1991). Multicultural counseling instruction: A challenge for faculties in the 21st century. *Journal of Counseling and Development, 70*, 136–141.

Miller, C. H. (1974). Career development theory in perspective. In E. L. Herr (Ed.), *Vocational guidance and human development*. Boston: Houghton Mifflin.

Miller, J. B. (1976). *Toward a new psychology of women*. Boston: Beacon Press.

Miller, G. (1999). The development of the spiritual focus in counseling and counselor education. *Journal of Counseling and Development, 77*, 598–601.

Minkoff, H. B., & Terres, C. K. (1985). ASCA perspectives: Past, present, and future. *Journal of Counseling and Development, 63*, 424–427.

Minuchin, S. (1974). *Families & family therapy*. Cambridge, MA: Harvard University Press.

Minuchin, S. (1981). *Family therapy techniques*. Cambridge, MA: Harvard University Press.

Mio, J. S., & Iwamasa, G. (1993). To do, or not to do: That is the question for white cross-cultural researchers. *The Counseling Psychologist, 21*(2), 197–212.

Moles, O. C. (1991). Guidance programs in American high schools: A descriptive portrait. *The School Counselor, 38*, 163–177.

Monson, R., & Brown, D. (1985). Secondary school counseling: A time for reassessment and revitalization. *NASSP Bulletin, 69*, 32–35.

Mood disorders in childhood and adolescence Part I (1993). *The Harvard Mental Health Letter, 10*(5), 1–4.

Moore, D., & Haverkamp, B. E. (1989). Measured increases in male emotional expressiveness following a structured group intervention. *Journal of Counseling and Development, 67*, 513–517.

Moore, D., & Leafgren, F. (Eds). (1990). *Problem solving strategies and interventions for men in conflict*. Alexandria, VA: ACA.

Morales, A., & Sheafor B. W. (1997). *Social work: A profession of many faces* (8th ed.). Boston: Allyn & Bacon.

Morrow, K. A., & Deidan, C. T. (1992). Bias in the Counseling Process: How to Recognize and Avoid It. *Journal of Counseling and Development, 70*(5), 571–77.

Morse, P. S., & Ivey, A. E. (1996). *Face to face: Communication and conflict resolution in the schools*. Thousand Oaks, CA: Corwin Press.

Moses, A. E., & Hawkins, R. (1986). *Counseling lesbian women and gay men*. Columbus, OH: Merrill.

Mowrer, O. H. (Ed.). (1967). *Morality and mental health*. Chicago: Rand McNally.

Muro, J. J., & Dinkmeyer, D. C. (1977). *Counseling in the elementary and middle schools: A pragmatic approach*. Dubuque, Iowa: William C. Brown.

Muro, J. J., & Kottman, T. (1995). *Guidance and counseling in the elementary schools: A practical approach*. Madison, WI: Brown & Benchmark.

Muth, J. L., & Cash, T. F. (1997). Body-image attitudes: What difference does gender make? *Journal of Applied Social Psychology, 27*(16),1438–1452.

Mwaba, K., & Pedersen, P. (1990). Relative importance of intercultural, interpersonal, and psychopathological attributions in judging critical incidents by multicultural counselors. *Journal of Multicultural Counseling and Development, 18*, 106–117.

Myers, D. G. (2001). *Psychology* (6th ed.). New York: Worth Publishers.

Myers, J. E. (1983). Gerontological counseling training: The state of the art. *Journal of Counseling and Development, 61*, 398–401.

Myers, J. E. (1995). Specialities in counseling: Rich heritage or force for fragmentation. *Journal of Counseling and Development, 74*, 115–116.

Myers, J. E., Loesch, L. D., & Sweeney., T. J., (1991). Trends in gerontological counselor preparation. *Counselor Education and Supervision, 30*, 194–204.

Myers, J. E., & Salmon, H. E. (1984). Counseling programs for older persons: Status, shortcomings, and potentialities. *The Counseling Psychologists, 12*(2), 39–53.

Myers, J. E., Sweeney, T. J., & Witmer, J. M. (2000). The wheel of wellness counseling for wellness: A holistic model for treatment planning. *Journal of Counseling and Development, 78*, 251–266.

Myrick, R. D. (1997). *Developmental guidance and counseling: A practical approach* (3rd ed.). Minneapolis: Educational Media Corporation.

Myrick, R. D., & Sabella, R. A. (1995). Cyberspace: New place for counselor supervision. *Elementary School Guidance and Counseling, 30*, 35–45.

NACFT (National Association of Certified Family Therapists). (2001). *National Association of Certified FamilyTherapists,Inc. (On-line)*. Available: http://www.nacft.com/.

Nance, D. W., & Myers, P. (1991). Continuing the eclectic journey. *Journal of Mental Health Counseling, 13*(1), 119–130.

Napier, A., & Whitaker, C. (1972). A conversation about co-therapy. In A. Ferber, M. Mendelsohn, & A. Napier (Eds.), *The book of family therapy* (pp. 480–506). New York: Jason Aronson.

Napier, A., & Whitaker, C. (1978). *The family crucible*. New York: Harper & Row.

NASW (National Association of Social Workers). (1999). *Code of ethics*. Retrieved June 1, 2001, from the World Wide Web: http://www.naswdc.org/code.htm.

National Institute of Mental Health (NIMH). (1990). *Mental health, United States, 1990*. (DHHS Publication No. ADM 90-1708.) Washington, DC: U.S. Government Printing Office.

National Institute of Mental Health (NIMH). (1995). *Decade of the brain* (3rd ed.). [Brochure]. Rockville, MD: Author.

National Law Center on Homelessness and Poverty (2001). *Homelessness and poverty in America*. Retrieved June 1, 2001, from the World Wide Web: http://www.nlchp.org/h&pusa.htm.

NBCC (National Board for Certified Counselors). (1997). *National board for certified counselors code of ethics*. Retrieved June 1, 2001, from the World Wide Web: http://www.nbcc.org/ethics/nbcc-code.htm.

NBCC (National Board for Certified Counselors). (2001). *NBCC Homepage [online]*. Available: www.nbcc.org/.

Neimeyer, G. J., Banikiotes, P. G., & Winum, P. C. (1979). Self-disclosure flexibility and counseling-related perceptions. *Journal of Counseling Psychology, 26*, 546–548.

Neimeyer, G. J., & Fong, M. L. (1983). Self-disclosure flexibility and counselor effectiveness. *Journal of Counseling Psychology, 30*, 258–261.

Neimeyer, R. A. (1995). An appraisal of constructivist psychotherapies. In M. J. Mahoney (Ed.), *Cognitive and constructive psychotherapies: Theory, research, and practice* (pp. 163–194). New York: Springer.

Neimeyer, R. A., & Mahoney, M. (Eds.). (1995). *Constructivism in psychotherapy*. Washington, DC: American Psychological Association.

Neukrug, E. (1980). *The effects of supervisory style and type of praise upon counselor trainees level of empathy and perception of supervisor*. Unpublished doctoral dissertation, University of Cincinnati, Ohio.

Neukrug, E. (1987). The brief training of paraprofessional counselors in empathic responding. *New Hampshire Journal for Counseling and Development, 15*(1), 15–19.

Neukrug, E. (1991). Computer-assisted live supervision in counselor skills training. *Counselor Education and Supervision, 31*, 132–138.

Neukrug, E. (1994). Understanding diversity in a pluralistic world. *The Journal of Intergroup Relations, XXI*(2), 3–12.

Neukrug, E. (1997). Support and challenge: Use of metaphor as a higher level empathic response. In. H. Rosenthal (Ed.), *Favorite counseling and therapy techniques*. Bristoll, PA: Accelerated Development.

Neukrug, E. (2000). *Theory, practice and trends in human services: An introduction to an emerging profession* (2nd ed.). Pacific Grove, CA: Brooks/Cole.

Neukrug, E. (2001). Medical breakthroughs: Genetic research and genetic counseling, psychotropic medications, and the mind-body connection. In T. McClam & M. Woodside (Eds.), *Human service challenges in the 21st century*. Birmingham, AL: Ebsco Media.

Neukrug, E. (2002). *Skills and techniques for human service professionals: Counseling environment, helping skills, treatment issues*. Pacific Grove, CA: Brooks/Cole.

Neukrug, E., Barr, C., Hoffman, L., & Kaplan, L. (1993). Developmental counseling and guidance: A model for use in your school. *The School Counselor, 40*, 356–362.

Neukrug, E., Herlihy, B., & Healy, M. (1992). Ethical practices of licensed professional counselors: An updated survey of state licensing boards. *Counselor Education and Supervision, 32*(2),130–141.

Neukrug, E., Lovell, C., & Parker, R. (1996). Employing ethical codes and decision-making models: A developmental process. *Counseling and Values, 40*, 98–106.

Neukrug, E., & McAuliffe, G. (1993). Cognitive development and human service education. *Human Service Education, 13*(1), 13–26.

Neukrug, E., Milliken, T., & Shoemaker, J. (2001). Counselor seeking behaviors of NOHSE practitioners, educators, and trainees. *Human Service Education, 21*, 45–58.

Neukrug, E., Milliken, T., & Walden, S. (2001). Ethical practices of credentialed counselors: An updated survey of state licensing boards. *Counselor Education and Supervision, 41*(1), 57–70.

Neukrug, E., & Williams, G. (1993). Counseling counselors: A survey of values. *Counseling and Values, 38*(1), 51–62.

Newman, J. A., & Lovell, M. (1993). A description of a supervisory group for group counselors. *Counselor Education and Supervision, 33*, 22–31.

Newman, J. L. (1993). Ethical issues in consultation. *Journal of Counseling and Development, 72*, 148–156.

Nichols, M., & Schwartz, R. C. (2001). *Family therapy: Concepts and methods* (5th ed.). Boston: Allyn & Bacon.

Niehoff, M. A. (1994). *Collective definition of practices causing dysfunction in children* (Report No. CG025992). Department of Human Resource Development. Portland: University of Southern Maine. (ERIC Document Reproduction Service No. ED 379554.)

Nigg, J. T., & Goldsmith, H. H. (1994). Genetics of personality disorders: Perspectives from personality and psychopathology research. *Psychological Bulletin, 115*, 346–380.

Niles, F. S. (1993). Issues in multicultural counselor education. *Journal of Multicultural Counseling and Development, 21*, 14–21.

Ninan, P. T., Cole, J. O., & Yonkers, K. A. (1998). Nonbenzodiazepine anxiolytics. In A. F. Schatzberg & C. B. Nemeroff (Eds.), *Textbook of psychopharmacology* (2nd ed., pp. 287–301). Washington, DC: American Psychiatric Press.

Nishino, S., Mignot, E., & Dement, W. C. (1998). Sedative-hypnotics. In A. F. Schatzberg & C. B. Nemeroff (Eds.), *Textbook of psychopharmacology* (2nd ed., pp. 487–502). Washington, DC: American Psychiatric Press.

Nixon, D. N., & Claiborn, C. D. (1987). A social influence approach to counselor supervision. In J. E. Maddux, C. D. Stoltenberg, & R. Rosenwein (Eds.), *Social processes in clinical and counseling psychology* (pp. 83–94). New York: Springer-Verlag.

NOHSE (National Organization of Human Service Education). (1995). *Ethical standards of human service professionals*. Fitchburg, MA: Author.

Norcross, J. C., Prochaska, J. O., & Gallagher, K. M. (1989). Clinical psychologists in the 1980s. Theory, research, and practice. *The Clinical Psychologist, 42*, 45–53.

Norcross, J. C., Strausser, D. J., & Faltus, F. J. (1988). The therapist's therapist. *American Journal of Psychotherapy, 42*(1), 53–66.

Norcross, J. C., Strausser-Kirtland, D., & Missar, C. D. (1988). The processes and outcomes of psychotherapists' personal treatment experiences. *Psychotherapy, 25*(1), 36–43.

Norden, M. J. (1996). *Beyond Prozac: Brain-toxic lifestyles, natural antidotes & new generation antidepressants* (2nd ed.). New York: ReganBooks.

Nova. (2000). *Cracking the code of life*. Burlington, Vt: Public Broadcasting, Nova.

NRCA. (National Rehabilitation Counseling Association). (1987). *Code of professional ethics for rehabilitation counselors*. Retrieved February 26, 2002, from the World Wide Web: http://www.nchrtm.okstate.edu/NRCA_files/code.html.

Nugent, F. A. (2000). *An introduction to the profession of counseling* (3rd ed.). Upper Saddle River, NJ: Merrill.

Nye, R. D. (1992). *The legacy of B. F. Skinner: Concepts and perspectives, controversies and misunderstandings*. Pacific Grove, CA: Brooks/Cole.

Nye, R. D. (2000). *Three psychologies* (6th ed.). Pacific Grove, CA: Brooks/Cole.

O'Bryant, B. (1991). Getting the most from your school counseling program. *NASSP Bulletin, 75*, 1–5.

Occupational Outlook Handbook. (2000-2001a). *Occupational outlook handbook, 2000-2001 edition*. Retrieved June 1, 2001, from the World Wide Web: http://www.bls.gov.oco.

Occupational Outlook Handbook. (2000-2001b). *Professional and technical occupations: Counselors*. Retrieved June 1, 2001, from the World Wide Web: http://www.bls.gov/oco/ocos067.htm.

O'Hanlon, W. H., & Weiner-Davis, M. (1989). *In search of solutions: A new direction in psychotherapy*: New York: Norton.

Ohlsen, M. M. (1983). Evaluation of the counselor's services. In M. M. Ohlsen (Ed.), *Introduction to counseling* (pp. 357–372). Itasca, IL: Peacock.

Ontario consultants for religious tolerance (October, 1997). *Variety of thought within Christendom*. http://www.religioustolerance.org/christ.htm.

Orlinsky, D. E., & Howard, K. I. (1986). Process and outcome in psychotherapy. In S. L. Garfield and A. E. Bergin (Eds.), *Handbook of psychotherapy and behavior change* (3rd ed., pp. 311–381). New York: Wiley.

Osherson, S. (1986). *Finding our fathers*. New York: Faucett Columbine.

Ossipow, S. (1996). *Theories of career development* (4th ed.). Boston: Allyn & Bacon.

Ossipow, S. H., & Littlejohn, E. M. (Eds.). (1995). Toward a multicultural theory of career development: Prospects and dilemmas. In F. T. Leong (Ed.), *Career development and vocational behavior of racial and ethnic minorities* (pp. 251–261). Mahway, NJ: Erlbaum.

Ottavi, T. M., Pope-Davis, D. B., & Dings, J. (1994). Relationship between white racial identity and self-reported multicultural competencies. *Journal of Counseling Psychology, 41*, 149–154.

Owens, M. J., & Risch, S. C. (1998). Atypical antipsychotics. In A. F. Schatzberg & C. B. Nemeroff (Eds.), *Textbook of psychopharmacology* (2nd ed., pp. 323–348). Washington, DC: American Psychiatric Press.

Paisley, P., & Borders, L. (1995). School counseling: an evolving specialty. *Journal of Counseling and Development, 74*, 150–153.

Palazzoli, S. M., Boscolo, L., Cecchin, G., & Prata, G. (1978). *Paradox and counter-paradox*. New York: Jason Aronson.

Palmer, C. J., & Shuford, B. (1996). Multicultural affairs. In A. Rentz (Ed.), *Student affairs practice in higher education* (2nd ed., pp. 214–238). Springfield, IL: Charles C Thomas.

Parham, T. A. (1993). White researchers conducting multicultural counseling research: Can their efforts be "Mo Betta"? *The Counseling Psychologist, 21*(2), 250–256.

Parsons, F. (1909). *Choosing a vocation*. Boston: Houghton Mifflin.

Parsons, F. (1989). *Choosing a vocation*. Garrett Park, MD: Garrett Park. (Reprint of 1909 original version)

Partin, R. L. (1993). School counselors' time: Where does it go? *The School Counselor, 40*, 274–281.

Pascarella, E. T., & Terenzini, P. T. (1991). *How college affects students: Findings and insights from twenty years of research*. San Francisco: Jossey-Bass.

Passons, W. R. (1975). *Gestalt approaches in counseling*. New York: Holt, Rinehart & Winston.

Pate, R. H. (1995). Certification of specialities: Not if, but how. *Journal of Counseling and Development, 74*, 181–184.

Patterson, C. H. (1973). *Theories of counseling and psychotherapy* (2nd ed.). New York: Harper & Row.

Patterson, C. H. (1984). Empathy, warmth, and genuineness in psychotherapy: A review of reviews. *Psychotherapy, 21*, 431–438.

Patterson, C. H. (1985). New light for counseling theory. *Journal of Counseling and Development, 63*, 349–350.

Patterson, C. H. (1986). *Theories of counseling and psychotherapy* (4th ed.). New York: HarperCollins.

Patterson, C. H. (1996). Multicultural counseling: From diversity to universality. *Journal of Counseling and Development, 74*, 227–231.

Pearson, Q. M. (2001). A case in clinical supervision: A framework for putting theory into practice. *Journal of Mental Health Counseling, 23*, 174–183.

Peavy, R. V. (1994). A constructivist perspective for counseling. *Education and Vocational Guidance Bulletin, 55*, 31.

Pedersen, P. B. (1991a). Introduction to the special issue on multiculturalism as a fourth force in counseling. *Journal of Counseling and Development, 70*, 4.

Pedersen, P. B. (1991b). *Developing multicultural awareness*. North Amherst, MA: Microtraining Associates.

Pedersen, P. B. (1996a). *The search for a "third choice": The cultural context of ethical assumptions in the ACA code of ethics*. Paper presented at the American Counseling Association's conference, Pittsburgh, PA.

Pedersen, P. B. (1996b). The importance of both similarities and differences in multicultural counseling: Reaction to C. H. Patterson. *Journal of Counseling and Development, 74*, 236–237.

Pedersen, P. B. (2000). *A handbook for developing multicultural awareness* (3rd ed.). Alexandria, VA: American Counseling Association.

Pedersen, P. B. (2001). Triad counseling. In R. Corsini (Ed.), *Handbook of innovative psychotherapies* (2nd ed., pp. 704–714). New York: John Wiley & Sons.

Pedersen, P. B, & Carey, J. C. (1994). *Multicultural counseling in schools: A practical handbook*. Boston: Allyn & Bacon.

Pedersen, P. B., Draguns, J. G., Lonner, W. J., & Trimble, J. E. (1996). *Counseling across cultures* (4th ed.). Thousand Oaks, CA: Sage.

Pelligrini, A. D., Perlmutter, J. C., Galda, L., & Brody, G. H. (1990). Joint reading between black Head Start children and their mothers. *Child Development, 61*, 443–453.

Pelsma, D. M., & Borgers, S. B. (1986). Experience-based ethics: A developmental model of learning ethical reasoning. *Journal of Counseling and Development, 64*(5), 311–314.

Pencarinha, D. F., Bell, N. K., Edwards, J. G., & Best, R. G. (1992). Ethical issues in genetic counseling: A comparison of M.S. counselor and medical geneticist perspectives. *Journal of Genetic Counseling, 1*(1), 19–30.

Pence, G. E. (1990). *Classic cases in medical ethics: Accounts of the cases that have shaped medical ethics, with philosophical, legal, and historical backgrounds*. New York: McGraw-Hill.

Pennebaker, J. W., Colder, M., & Sharp, L. K. (1990). Accelerating the coping process. *Journal of Personality and Social Psychology, 58*, 528–537.

Pennebaker, J. W., & Susman, J. R. (1988). *Disclosure of traumas and psychosomatic processes. Social Science and Medicine, 26*, 327–332.

Perls, F. (1969). *Gestalt therapy verbatim*. Moab, UT: Real People Press.

Perry, M. A., & Furukawa, M. J. (1986). Modeling methods. In F. H. Kanfer & A. P. Goldstein (Eds.), *Helping people change: A textbook of methods* (3rd ed., pp. 66–110). New York: Pergamon Press.

Perry, W. G. (1970). *Forms of intellectual and ethical development in the college years: A scheme*. New York: Holt, Rinehart, & Winston.

Peters, T. (1999). *Thriving on chaos*. New York: Park Avenue Press.

Peterson, G. W., Sampson, J. P., & Reardon, R. C. (1991). *Career development and services: A cognitive approach*. Pacific Grove, CA: Brooks/Cole.

Phelps, R. E., Taylor, J. D., & Gerard, P. A. (2001). Cultural mistrust, ethnic identity, racial identity, and self-esteem among ethnically diverse black university students. *Journal of Counseling and Development, 79*, 209–216.

Piaget, J. (1954). The construction of reality in the child. New York: Basic Books.

Piercy, F. P., Sprenkle, D. H., & Wetchler, J. L. (1996). *Family therapy sourcebook* (2nd ed.). New York: Guilford Press.

Pinkerton, R. S., & Rockwell, W. J. K. (1994). Very brief psychological interventions with university students. *Journal of American College Health, 42*, 156–161.

Pinney, E. L. (1970). *A first group psychotherapy book*. Springfield, IL: Charles C Thomas.

Pirodsky, D. M., & Cohn, J. S. (1992). *Clinical primer of psychopharmacology*. (2nd ed.). New York: McGraw-Hill.

Plake, B. S., & Conoley, J. C. (1995). *Using Buros Institute of Mental Measurements materials in counseling and therapy*. Greensboro, NC: ERIC Clearinghouse on Counseling and Student Services. (ERIC Document Reproduction Service No. ED 391–987.)

Plake, B. S., Conoley, J. C., Kramer, J. J., & Murphy, L. (1991). The Buros Institute of mental measurements: Comment to the tradition of excellence. *Journal of Counseling and Development, 69*, 449–455.

Pollak, J., Levy, S., & Breitholtz, T. (1999). Screening for medical and neurodevelopmental disorders for the professional counselor. *Journal of Counseling and Development, 77*, 350–356.

Ponterotto, J. G. (1988). Racial consciousness development among white counselor trainees: A stage model. *Journal of Multicultural Counseling and Development, 16*(4), 145–156.

Ponterotto, J. G., Alexander, C. M., & Grieger, I. (1995). A multicultural competency checklist for counseling programs. *Journal of Multicultural Counseling & Development, 23*, 11–20.

Pope, K. S. (1987). Preventing therapist patient sexual intimacy: Therapy for a therapist at risk. *Professional Psychology: Research and Practice, 18*(6), 624–628.

Pope, K. S., & Tabachnik, B. G. (1994). Therapists as patients: A national survey of psychologist's experiences, problems, and beliefs. *Professional Psychology Research and Practice, 25*(3), 247–258.

Pope, M. (1995). The "salad bowl" is big enough for us all: An argument for the inclusion of lesbians and gay men in any definition of multiculturalism. *Journal of Counseling and Development, 73*, 301–303.

Posthuma, B. W. (1988). *Small groups in therapy settings: Process and leadership*. Boston: Allyn & Bacon.

Poston, W. S. C., Craine, M., & Atkinson, D. R. (1991). Counselor dissimilarity, confrontation, client cultural mistrust, and willingness to self-disclose. *Journal of Multicultural Counseling and Development, 19*, 65–73.

Potter, W. Z., Manji, H. K., & Rudorfer, M. (1998). Tricyclics and tetracyclics. In A. F. Schatzberg & C. B. Nemeroff (Eds.), *Textbook of psychopharmacology* (2nd ed., pp. 199–218). Washington, DC: American Psychiatric Press.

Pottick, K. J. (1988). Jane Addams revisited: Practice theory and social economics. *Social Work with Groups, 11*, 11–26.

Prediger, D. J. (1994). Multicultural assessment standards: A compilation for counselors. *Measurement and Evaluation in Counseling and Development, 27*, 68–73.

Pressly, P. K., & Heesacker, M. (2001). The physical environment and counseling: A review of theory and research. *Journal of Counseling and Development, 79*(2), 148–160.

Preston, J., & Johnson, J. (2001). *Clinical psychopharmacology made ridiculously simple* (4th ed.). Miami: MedMaster.

Prieto, L. R. (1996). Group supervision: Still widely practiced but poorly understood. *Counselor Education and Supervision, 35*, 295–307.

Pritts, T. A., Wang, Q., Sun, X., Moon, M. R., Fischer, D. R., Fischer, J. E., Wong, H. R., & Hasselgren, P. O. (2000). Induction of the stress response in vivo decreases nuclear factor-kappa B activity in jejunal mucosa of endotoxemic mice. *Archives of Surgery, 135*(7), 860–866.

Prochaska, J., & DiClemente, C. (1986). The transtheoretical approach. In U. C. Norcross (Ed.), *Handbook of eclectic psychotherapy* (pp. 163–200). New York: Brunner/Mazel.

Prochaska, J. O., & Norcross, J. C. (1983). Contemporary psychotherapists: A national survey of characteristics, practices, orientations, and attitudes. *Psychotherapy: Theory, Research and Practice, 20*(2), 161–173.

Proshansky, H. M., Ittleson, W. H., & Rivlin, L. G. (1970). The influence of the physical environment on behavior: Some basic assumptions. In H. M. Proshansky, W. H. Ittleson, & L. G. Rivlin (Eds.), *Environmental psychology: Man and his physical setting* (pp. 27–37). New York: Holt, Rinehart & Winston.

Pryzwansky, W. B. (1993). The regulation of school psychology: A historical perspective on certification, licensure, and accreditation. *Journal of School Psychology, 31*, 219–235.

Purkey, W. W., & Schmidt, J. J. (1996). *Invitational counseling: A self-concept approach to professional practice*. Pacific Grove, CA: Brooks/Cole.

Purton, C. (1993). Philosophy and counseling. In B. Thorne and W. W. Dryden (Eds.). *Counseling: Interdisciplinary perspectives* (pp. 152–161). Philadelphia, PA: Open University Press.

Quintana, S. M., & Bernal, M. E. (1995). Ethnic minority training in counseling psychology: Comparison with clinical psychology and proposed standards. *The Counseling Psychologist, 23*(1), 102–121.

Rabinowitz, F. E. (1991). The male-to-male embrace: Breaking the touch taboo in a men's therapy group. *Journal of Counseling and Development, 69*, 574–576.

Raskind, M. A., & Peskind, E. R. (1998). Treatment of noncognitive symptons in Alzheimer's disease and other dementias. In A. F. Schatzberg & C. B. Nemeroff (Eds.), *Textbook of psychopharmacology* (2nd ed., pp. 791–802). Washington, DC: American Psychiatric Press.

Ray, D., & Altekruse, M. (2000). Effectiveness of group supervision versus combined group and individual supervision. *Counselor Education and Supervision, 40*, 19–30.

Raymond, A. G. (1994). *The HMO health care companion: A consumer's guide to managed-care networks*. New York: HarperCollins.

Reeves, T. G., Bowman, J. T., & Cooley, S. L. (1989). Relationship between the client's moral development level and empathy of the counseling student. *Counselor Education and Supervision, 28*(4), 299–305.

Regulations Governing the Practice of Professional Counseling, VA, Stat. §54.1-2400.6. (2000). (Online). Available: http://www.dhp.state.va.us/counseling/leg/Licensed%20 Professional%20Counselor%204-12-00.doc.

Remen, N., May, R., Young, D., & Berland, W. (1985). The wounded healer. *Saybrook Review, 5*, 84–93.

Remley, R. P., Herlihy, B., & Herlihy, S. B. (1997). The U.S. Supreme Court decision in *Jaffe* v. *Redmond:* Implications for counselors. *Journal of Counseling and Development, 75*, 213–218.

Remley, T. P. (1988). The law and ethical practices in elementary and middle schools. In W. C. Huey & T. P. Remley, *Ethical and legal issues in school counseling* (pp. 95–105). Alexandria, VA: American School Counseling Association.

Remley, T. P. (1991). An argument for credentialing. In F. O. Bradley (Ed.), *Credentialing in counseling* (pp. 81–85). Alexandria, VA: Association for Counselor Education and Supervision.

Rentz, A. L. (1994). (Ed.). *Student affairs: a profession's heritage*. Lanham, MD: American College Personnel Association and the University Press of America.

Rentz, A. L. (1996). A history of student affairs. In A. Rentz (Ed.), *Student affairs practice in higher education* (2nd ed., pp. 28–55). Springfield, IL: Charles C Thomas.

Rest, J. R. (1984). Research on moral development: Implications for training counseling psychologists. *The Counseling Psychologist, 12*, 19–29.

Reynolds, J. F., Mair, D. C., & Fischer, P. C. (1995). *Writing and reading mental health records: Issues and analysis in professional writing and scientific rhetoric*. Mahwah, NJ: Lawrence Erlbaum Associates.

Rice, F. P. (1983). *Human development: A life-span approach* (3rd ed.). Upper Saddle River, NJ: Prentice Hall.

Rice, F. P. (2001). *Human development: A life-span approach* (4th ed.). Upper Saddle River, NJ: Prentice Hall.

Riordan, R. J., & Walsh, L. (1994). Guidelines for professional referral to Alcoholics Anonymous and other twelve step groups. *Journal of Counseling and Development, 72*, 351–355.

Riverside Publishing Company (1992). *Guidance information system*. Chicago: Author.

Robertiello, R. C., & Schoenewolf, G. (1987). *Common therapeutic blunders: Countertransference and counterresistance in psychotherapy*. Northvale, NJ: Jason Aronson.

Robiner, W. N., Arbisi, P., & Edwall, G. E. (1994). The basis of the doctoral degree for psychology licensure. *Clinical Psychology Review, 14*, 227–254.

Robinson, B. B. (1990). Careers working with special populations. In B. B. Collison & N. J. Garfield (Eds.), *Careers in counseling and human development* (2nd ed., pp. 129–137). Alexandria, VA: American Association for Counseling and Development.

Rockwell, P. J., & Rothney, W. M. (1961). Some social ideas of pioneers in the guidance movement. *Personnel and Guidance Journal, 40*, 349–354.

Rockwood, G. F. (1993). Edgar Schein's process versus content consultation models. *Journal of Counseling and Development, 71*(6), 636–638.

Rodgers, R. F. (1980). Theories underlying student development. In D. Creamer (Ed.), *Student development in higher education* (pp. 10–96). Cincinnati, OH: ACPA.

Roe, A. (1956). *The psychology of occupations*. New York: Wiley.

Roe, A., & Siegelman, M. (1964). *The origin of interests. APGA Inquiry Studies No. 1*. Washington, DC: American Personnel and Guidance Association.

Rogers, C. (1957). The necessary and sufficient conditions of therapeutic personality change. *Journal of Counseling Psychology, 21*(2), 95–103.

Rogers, C. (1959). A theory of therapy, personality and interpersonal relationships as developed in the client-centered framework. In S. Koch (Ed.), *Psychology: A study of science (vol. 3). Formulations of the person and the social context* (pp. 184–256). New York: McGraw-Hill.

Rogers, C. (1961). Ellen West and Loneliness. In H. Kirschenbaum & V. L. Henderson (Eds.), *The Carl Rogers reader* (pp. 157–167). Boston: Houghton Mifflin.

Rogers, C. (1970). *Carl Rogers on encounter groups*. New York: Harper & Row.

Rogers, C. (1980a). Client-centered psychotherapy. In A. M. Freedman, H. I. Kaplan, & B. J. Sadoc (Eds.), *Comprehensive textbook of psychiatry* (3rd ed.). Baltimore: Williams & Wilkins.

Rogers, C. (1980b). *A way of being*. Boston: Houghton Mifflin.

Rogers, C. (1986). Reflection of feelings. *Person-Centered Review, 1*(4), 375–377.

Rogers, C. (1989a). A client-centered/person-centered approach to therapy. In H. Kirschenbaum (Ed.), *The Carl Rogers reader* (pp. 135–152). Boston: Houghton Mifflin. (Original work published 1986)

Rogers, C. (1989b). Reinhold Niebuhr's *The self and the dramas of history*: Review by Carl Rogers. In H. Kirschenbaum (Ed.), *Carl Rogers: Dialogues* (pp. 208–211). Boston: Houghton Mifflin. (Original work published 1956)

Rogers, C. R. (1939). *The clinical treatment of the problem child*. Boston: Houghton Mifflin.

Rogers, C. R. (1942). *Counseling and psychotherapy: New concepts in practice*. Boston: Houghton Mifflin.

Rogers, C. R. (1951). *Client-centered therapy: Its current practice, implications and theory*. Boston: Houghton Mifflin.

Rogers, C. R. (1989c). A therapist's view of the good life: The fully functioning person. In H. Kirschenbaum & V. Henderson (Eds.), *The Carl Rogers reader* (pp. 127–134). Boston: Houghton Mifflin. (Original work published 1961)

Rokeach, M. (1960). *The open and closed mind*. New York: Basic Books.

Romano, G. (1992). Description of D. Locke's "Counseling beyond U.S. borders." *American Counselor, 1*(2), 13–17.

Root, M. P. P. (1998). Facilitating therapy with Asian American clients. In D. R. Atkinson, G. Morten, & D. W. Sue, *Counseling American minorities: A cross-cultural perspective* (5th ed., pp. 214–234). Boston: McGraw-Hill.

Rose, P. I. (1964). *They and we: Racial and ethnic relations in the United States*. New York: Random House.

Rosenhan, T. (1973). On being sane in insane places. *Science, 179*(19), 250–258.

Rosenthal, H. (Ed.). (1997). *Favorite counseling and therapy techniques*. Bristoll, PA: Accelerated Development.

Rosenthal, H. (Ed.). (2001). *Favorite counseling and therapy homework assignments: Leading therapists share their most creative strategies*. Philadelphia: Brunner-Routledge.

Ross, G. L. (1993). Peter Block's flawless consulting and the homunculus theory: Within each person is a perfect consultant. *Journal of Counseling and Development, 71*, 639–742.

Rossi, P. H. (1990). The old homeless and the new homelessness in historical perspective. *American Psychologist, 45*(8), 954–959.

Rowe, W., Murphy, H. B., & De Csipkes, R. A. (1975). The relationship of counseling characteristics and counseling effectiveness. *Review of Educational Research, 45*, 231–46.

Rubenstein, G. (1973). Towards authenticity in the consulting process. In W. L. Claiborn & R. Cohen (Eds.), *School intervention* (pp. 32–50). New York: Behavioral Publications.

Russo, J. R., Kelz, J. W., & Hudon, G. R. (1964). Are good counselors open-minded? *Counselor Education and Supervision, 3*, 74–77.

Rychalk, J. F. (1985). Eclecticism in psychological theorizing: Good and bad. *Journal of Counseling and Development, 63*, 351–353.

Ryff, C. D., & Singer, B. (1996). Psychological well-being: Meaning, measurement, and implications for psychotherapy research. *Psychotherapy & Psychosomatics, 65*(1), 14–23.

Sabnani, H. B., Ponterotto, J. G., & Borodovsky, L. G. (1991). White racial identity development and cross-cultural counselor training: A stage model. *The Counseling Psychologist, 19*(1), 76–102.

Sabshin, M. (1990). Turning points in twentieth-century American psychiatry. *The American Journal of Psychiatry, 147*(10), 1267–1274.

Safran, J. D., & Muran, J. C. (2000). *Negotiating the therapeutic alliance: A relational treatment guide*. New York: Guilford Press.

Safran, J. D., & Segal, Z. V. (1990). *Interpersonal processes in cognitive therapy*. New York: Basic Books.

Samovar, L. A., & Porter, R. E. (2001). *Intercultural communication: A reader* (9th ed.). Belmont, CA: Wadsworth.

Sampson, J. P., Jr. (1990). Computer-assisted testing and the goals of counseling psychology. *The Counseling Psychologist, 18*, 227–239.

Sampson, J. P., Jr. (1995). *Computer-assisted testing in counseling and therapy*. Greensboro, NC: ERIC Clearinghouse on Counseling and Student Services. (ERIC Document Reproduction Service No. ED 391–983.)

Sampson, J. P., Kolodinsky, R. W., & Greeno, B. P. (1997). Counseling on the information highway: Future possibilities and potential problems. *Journal of Counseling and Development, 75*, 203–212.

Sandberg, D. N., Crabbs, S. K., & Crabbs, M. A. (1988). Legal issues in child abuse: Questions and answers for counselors. In W. C. Huey & T. P. Remley, *Ethical and legal issues in school counseling* (pp. 173–181). Alexandria, VA: American School Counseling Association.

Sanders, J. R. (1994). *The program evaluation standards: How to assess evaluations of educational programs* (2nd ed.). Thousand Oaks, CA: Sage Publications.

Sandhu, D. S. (1995). Pioneers of multicultural counseling: A conversation with Paul B. Pedersen. *Journal of Multicultural Counseling and Development, 23*, 198–211.

Sang, B. E. (1989). New directions in lesbian research, theory, and education. *Journal of Counseling and Development, 68*, 92–96.

Sartre, J. P. (1962). *Existential psychoanalysis*. Chicago: Henry Regnery Company.

Sarwer-Foner, G. J. (1993). The relationship between psychotherapy and pharmacotherapy: An introduction. *American Journal of Psychotherapy, 47*, 387–392.

Satir, V. (1967). *Conjoint family therapy*. Palo Alto, CA: Science and Behavior Books.

Satir, V. (1972a). *Peoplemaking*. Palo Alto, CA: Science and Behavior Books.

Satir, V. (1972b). Family systems and approaches to family therapy. In G. D. Erickson & T. P. Hogan (Eds.), *Family therapy: An introduction to theory and technique* (2nd ed., pp. 211–225). Pacific Grove, CA: Brooks/Cole. (Original work published 1967)

Savage, D. (1992, November 10). Court lets firms cut health care. *Los Angeles Times*, Section A, pp. 1, 18–19.

Schaef, A. W. (1981). *Women's reality: An emerging female system in the white male society*. Minneapolis: Winston Press.

Schafer, W. D. (1995). *Assessment skills for school counselors* (Report No. EDO-CG-95-2). Washington, DC: ERIC Clearinghouse on Assessment and Evaluation. (ERIC Document Reproduction Service No. ED 387-709.)

Schatzberg, A. F., & Nemeroff, C. B. (1998). *Textbook of psychopharmacology* (2nd ed.). Washington, DC: American Psychiatric Press.

Schein, R. (1969). *Process consultation: Its role in organization development*. Reading, MA: Addison-Wesley.

Scher, M. (1979). On counseling men. *Personnel and Guidance Journal, 57*, 252–254.

Scher, M. (1981). Men in hiding. *Personnel and Guidance Journal, 60*, 199–202.

Schlossberg, N. K., Waters, E. B., & Goodman, J. (1995). *Counseling adults in transition* (2nd ed.). New York: Springer.

Schmidt, J. J. (1991). *A survival guide for the elementary/middle school counselor.* West Nyack, NY: The Center for Applied Research in Education.

Schmidt, J. J. (1999). Two decades of CACREP and what do we know? *Counselor Education and Supervision, 39*(1), 34–45.

Schofield, J. W., & Anderson, K. M. (1984). *Integrating quantitative components into qualitative studies: Problems and possibilities for research on intergroup relations in educational settings* (Report No. TM 840-489). Washington, DC: National Institute of Education. (ERIC Document Reproduction Service No. ED 248-250.)

Schuh, J. H. (1999). Duty to warn and foreseen danger created by nonstudents: Challenges for colleges and universities. *Journal of College Student Development, 40*, 178–184.

Schumacher, B. (1983). Rehabilitation counseling. In M. M. Ohlsen (Ed.), *Introduction to counseling* (pp. 313–324). Itasca, IL: Peacock.

Schwitzer, A. M. (1996). Using the inverted pyramid heuristic in counselor education and supervision. *Counselor Education and Supervision, 35*, 258–267.

Schwitzer, A. M. (1997). The inverted pyramid framework applying self psychology constructs to conceptualizing college student psychotherapy. *Journal of College Student Psychotherapy 11*, 29–48.

Schwitzer, A. M., Griffin, O. T., Ancis, J. R., & Thomas, C. R. (1999). School adjustment experiences of African American college students. *Journal of Counseling and Development, 77*, 189–197.

Scissons, E. D. (1993). *Counseling for results*. Pacific Grove, CA: Brooks/Cole.

Sears, S. (1982). A definition of career guidance terms: A national vocational guidance association perspective. *Vocational Guidance Quarterly, 31*(2), 137–143.

Sears, S. J. (1993). The changing scope of practice of the secondary school counselor. *The School Counselor, 40*, 384–388.

Seem, S. R., & Johnson, E. (1998). Gender bias among counseling trainees: A study of case conceptualization. *Counselor Education and Supervision, 37*, 257–268.

Segal, D. L., & Coolidge, F. L. (2001). Diagnosis and classification. In M. Hersen & V. B. Van Hasselt, (Eds.), *Advanced abnormal psychology* (2nd ed., pp. 5–22). New York: Kluwer Academic/Plenum Publishers.

Segal-Andrews, A. M. (1994). Understanding student behavior in one fifth-grade classroom as contextually defined. *The Elementary School Journal, 95*(2), 183–197.

Seiler, G. (1999). AMHCA after 20 years: Transformations for beyond the year 2000. *Journal of Mental Health Counseling, 21*, 295–301.

Seligman, L. (1996). *Diagnosis and treatment planning in counseling* (2nd ed). New York: Plenum Press.

Seligman, L. (1999). Twenty years of diagnosis and the DSM. *Journal of Mental Health Counseling, 21*, 229–239.

Selye, H. (1956). *The stress of life*. New York: McGraw-Hill.

Selye, H. (1974). *Stress without distress*. New York: Lippincott.

Senge, P. (1990). *The fifth discipline: The art and practice of the learning organization*. New York: Doubleday.

Sexton, T. (1993). A review of the counseling outcome research. In G. R. Walz and J. C. Bleuer (Eds.). *Counselor efficacy: Assessing and using counseling outcomes research*. (Report No. ISBN-1-56109-056-5). Ann Arbor, MI: ERIC Clearinghouse on Counseling and Personnel Services. (ERIC Document Reproduction Service No. Ed 362 821).

Sexton, T., & Whiston, S. C. (1991). A review of the empirical basis for counseling: Implications for practice and training. *Counselor Education and Supervision, 30*, 330–354.

Sexton, T., & Whiston, S. C. (1994). The status of the counseling relationship: An empirical review, theoretical implications, and research directions. *The Counseling Psychologist, 22*, 6–78.

Shaffer, J. B. P., & Galinsky, M. D. (1974). *Models of group therapy and sensitivity training*. Englewood Cliffs, NJ: Prentice Hall.

Shannon, J. W., & Woods, W. J. (1998). Affirmative psychotherapy for gay men. In D. R. Atkinson & G. Hackett (Eds.), *Counseling diverse populations* (2nd ed., pp. 317–334). Boston: McGraw-Hill.

Shapiro, A. E. (1994). A core problem in psychology: Response to Robiner, Arbisi, and Edwall's "The basis of the doctoral degree for psychology licensure." *Clinical Psychology Review, 14*(4), 255–259.

Sharf, R. S. (1993). *Occupational information overview*. Pacific Grove, CA: Brooks/Cole.

Sharkin, B. S. (1993). Anger and gender: Theory, research, and implications. *Journal of Counseling and Development, 71*, 386–389.

Sheehy, G. (1976). *Passages: Predictable crises of adult life*. New York: Bantam Books.

Sheehy, G. (1995). *New passages: Mapping your life across time*. New York: Random House.

Sheridan, E. P., Matarazzo, J. D., & Nelson, P. D. (1995). Accreditation of psychology's graduate professional education and training programs: An historical perspective. *Professional Psychology, Research and Practice, 26*, 386–392.

Shostrum, E. (1974). *Manual for the Personal Orientation Inventory: An inventory for the measurement of self-actualization*. San Diego: Educational and Instructional Testing Service.

Sieber, J. E. (1992). *Planning ethically responsible research*. Applied Social Research Methods Series. Newbury Park, CA: Sage.

Siegel, B. (1988). *Love, medicine, & miracles*. New York: Harper & Row.

Simmons, J. (2001). ARCA, NRCA join to form one group. *Counseling Today, 43*(11), 1, 18.

Simon, G. M. (1991). Theoretical eclecticism: A goal we are obliged to pursue. *Journal of Mental Health Counseling, 13*(1), 112–118.

Simon, L., Gaul, R., Friedlander, M. L., & Heatherington, L. (1992). Client gender and sex role: Predictors of counselors' impressions and expectations. *Journal of Counseling and Development, 71*, 48–52.

Singer, B. L., & Deschamps, D. C. (1994). *Gay and lesbian stats: A pocket guide to facts and figures*. New York: New Press.

Skillings, J. H., & Dobbins, J. E. (1991). Racism as a disease: Etiology and treatment implications. *Journal of Counseling and Development, 70*, 206–215.

Skinner, B. F. (1938). *The behavior of organisms: An experimental analysis*. New York: Appleton.

Skinner, B. F. (1960). Pigeons in a pelican. *American Psychologist, 15*, 28–37.

Skinner, B. F. (1971). *Beyond freedom and dignity*. New York: Knopf.

Skinner, B. F. (1972). *Cumulative record: A selection of papers* (3rd ed.). New York: Appleton-Century-Crofts.

Skynner, A. C. R. (1976). *Systems of marital and family psychotherapy*. New York: Brunner/Mazel.

Skynner, A. C. R. (1981). An open-systems, group-analytic approach to family therapy. In A. S. Gurman & D. P. Kniskern (Eds.), *Handbook of family therapy* (pp. 39–84). New York: Brunner/Mazel.

Smaby, M. H., & D'Andrea, L. M. (1995). CACREP Standards: Will we make the grade? *Journal of Counseling and Development, 74*, 105–109.

Smith, H. B. (1999). Managed care: A survey of counselor educators and counselor practitioners. *Journal of Mental Counseling, 21*, 270–284.

Smith, H. B., & Robinson, R. P. (1995). Mental health counseling: Past, present, and future. *Journal of Counseling and Development, 74*, 158–162.

Smith, R. L. (1994). Directions in marriage and family graduate level training. *Counselor Education and Supervision, 33*, 180–183.

Smith, R. L., Carlson, J., Stevens-Smith, P., & Dennison, M. (1995). Marriage and family counseling. *Journal of Counseling and Development, 74*, 154–157.

Snarey, J. (1985). Cross-cultural universality of social-moral development. *Psychological Bulletin*, 97(2), 202–232.

Sodowsky, G. R., & Taffe, R. C. (1991). Counselor trainees' analysis of multicultural counseling videotapes. *Journal of Multicultural Counseling and Development, 19*, 115–129.

Sokal, M. M. (1992). Origins and early years of the American Psychological Association, 1890-1906. *American Psychologist, 47*(2), 111–122.

Solomon, A. (1992). Clinical diagnosis among diverse populations: A multicultural perspective. Families in Society: *The Journal of Contemporary Human Services, 73* (6), 371–377.

Sommer, B., & Sommer, R. (1997). *A practical guide to behavior research: Tools and techniques*. New York: Oxford University Press.

Sommer, R. (1959). Studies in personal space. *Sociometry, 22*, 247–260.

Southern Regional Educational Board (SREB). (1969). *Roles and functions for different levels of mental health workers*. Atlanta, GA: Author.

Special Committee on Aging, U.S. Senate. (1983). *Developments in aging. 1983*. Washington, DC: U.S. Government Printing Office.

Speight, S. L., Myers, J., Cox, C. I., & Highlen, P. S. (1991). A redefinition of multicultural counseling. *Journal of Counseling and Development, 70*, 29–36.

Spiegler, M. D. (1998). *Contemporary behavior therapy*. Pacific Grove, CA: Brooks/Cole.

Spinks, S. H., & Birchler, G. R. (1982). Behavioral systems marital therapy: Dealing with resistance. *Family Process, 21*, 169–186.

Spokane, A. R. (1985). A review of research on person-environment congruence in Holland's theory of careers. *Journal of Vocational Behavior, 26*, 306–343.

Sprinthall, R. C., Sprinthall, N. A., & Oja, S. N. (1998). *Educational psychology: A developmental approach* (7th ed.). New York: McGraw-Hill.

Spruill, D. A. (1994). Use of videotaped initial family interviews in training beginning family therapists. *Counselor Education and Supervision, 33*, 201–210.

Spruill, D. A., & Benshoff, J. M. (1996). The future is now: Promoting professionals among counselors-in-training. *Journal of Counseling and Development, 74*(5), 486–471.

Spruill, D. A., & Benshoff, J. M. (2000). Helping beginning counselors develop a personal theory of counseling. *Counselor Education and Supervision, 40*, 58–69.

Stage, F. K., & Downey, J. P. (1999). Hate crimes and violence on college and university campuses. *Journal of Student Development, 40*, 3–9.

Stanard, R. P., Sandhu, D. S., & Painter, L. C. (2000). Assessment of spirituality in counseling. *Journal of Counseling and Development, 78*, 204–210.

Steenbarger, B. N. (1993). A multicontextual model of counseling: Bridging brevity and diversity. *Journal of Counseling and Development, 72*, 8–15.

Steenbarger, B. N., & Smith, H. B. (1996). Assessing the quality of counseling services: Developing accountable helping systems. *Journal of Counseling and Development, 75*, 145–150.

Steinem, G. (1992). *Revolution from within: A book on self-esteem*. Boston: Little, Brown.

Stevens-Smith, P., Hinkle, J. S., & Stahmann, R. F. (1993). A comparison of professional accreditation standards in marriage and family counseling therapy. *Counselor Education and Supervision, 33*, 116–126.

Sting (1991). *Mad about you*. Hollywood, CA: Regatta Music.

Stoltenberg, C. D., & Delworth, U. (1987). *Supervising counselors and therapists*. San Francisco: Jossey-Bass.

Stone, G. L., & Archer, J. (1990). College and university counseling centers in the 1990s: Challenges and limits. *The Counseling Psychologist, 18*, 539–607.

Stricker, L. J., & Burton, N. W. (1996). Using the SAT and high school record in academic guidance. *Educational and Psychological Measurement, 56*(4), 626–641.

Strong, S. R. (1991). Theory-driven science and naive empiricism in counseling psychology. *Journal of Counseling Psychology, 38*(2), 204–210.

Strupp, H. H. (1955). The effect of the psychotherapist's personal analysis upon his techniques. *Journal of Consulting Psychology, 19*(3), 197–204.

Student wins $900,000 from school in gay-bashing case. (1997, January). *Our Own, (21)*4, A8.

Subich, L. M. (1996). Addressing diversity in the process of career assessment. In M. L. Savickas & W. Bruce Walsh (Eds.), *Handbook of career counseling theory and practice* (pp. 277–289). Palo Alto, CA: Davies-Black Publishing.

Sue, D. (1978). Counseling across cultures. *Personnel and Guidance Journal, 56*, 451.

Sue, D. W. (1992). The challenge of multiculturalism: The road less traveled. *American Counselor, 1*(1), 6–15.

Sue, D. W., Arredondo, P., & McDavis, R. J. (1992). Multicultural counseling competencies and standards: A call to the profession. *Journal of Counseling and Development, 70*(4), 477–486.

Sue, D. W., Bernier, J. E., Durran, A., Feinberg, L., Pedersen, P., Smith, E. J., & Vasquez-Nuttall, E. (1982). Professional forum: Position paper: Cross-cultural counseling competencies. *The Counseling Psychologist, 10*(2), 45–52.

Sue, D. W., & Sue, D. (1998). The Interplay of Sociocultural Factors on the Psychological Development of Asians in America. In D. R. Atkinson, G. Morten, & D. W. Sue, *Counseling American minorities: A cross-cultural perspective* (5th ed., pp. 205-213). Dubuque, IA: McGraw-Hill.

Sue, D. W., & Sue, D. (1999). *Counseling the culturally different: Theory and practice* (3rd ed.). New York: John Wiley & Sons.

Sugarman, A. (1986). Self-experience and reality testing: Synthesis of an object relations and ego psychological model on the Rorschach. In M. Kissen (Ed.), *Assessing object relations*. Madison, CT: International Universities Press.

Sumerel, M. B. (1994). *Parallel process in supervision* (Report No. EDO-CG-94-15). Greensboro, NC: ERIC Clearinghouse on Counseling and Student Services. (ERIC Document Reproduction Service No. ED 372-347).

Super, D. E. (1953). A theory of vocational development. *American Psychologist, 8*(2), 185–190.

Super, D. E. (1957). *The psychology of careers*. New York: Harper & Row.

Super, D. E. (1976). *Career education and the meaning of work. Monographs on Career Education*. Washington, DC: The Office of Career Education, U.S. Dept. of Education.

Super, D. E. (1984). Career and life development. In D. Brown, L. Brooks, & Associates (Eds.), *Career choice and development*. San Francisco: Jossey-Bass.

Super, D. E. (1990). A life-span, life-space approach to career development. In D. Brown, L. Brooks, & Associates (Eds.), *Career choice and development: Applying contemporary theories to practice* (2nd ed.). San Francisco: Jossey-Bass.

Super, D. E., & Hall, D. T. (1978). Career development: Person, position, and process. *Counseling Psychologist, 1*, 2–9.

Swanson, J. L. (1994). The theory is the practice: Trait-and-factor/person-environment fit counseling. In M. L. Savickas & W. Bruce Walsh (Eds.), *Handbook of career counseling theory and practice* (pp. 93–108). Palo Alto, CA: Davies-Black Publishing.

Sweeney, T. J. (1991). Counselor credentialing: Purpose and origin. In F. O. Bradley (Ed.), *Credentialing in counseling* (pp. 81–85). Alexandria, VA: Association for Counselor Education and Supervision.

Sweeney, T. J. (1992). CACREP: Precursors, promises, and prospects. *Journal of Counseling and Development, 70*(6), 667–672.

Sweeney, T. J. (1995). Accreditation, credentialing, professionalization: The role of specialities. *Journal of Counseling and Development, 74*, 117–125.

Swenson, L. C. (1997). *Psychology and law for the helping professions* (2nd ed.). Pacific Grove, CA: Brooks/Cole.

Szasz, T. (1961). *The myth of mental illness*. New York: Paul B. Hoeber.

Szasz, T. (Speaker). (1990). *A conversation with an officially documented schizophrenic patient*. (Cassette Recording No. PC289-W9AD.) Phoenix, AZ: The Milton H. Erickson Foundation.

Szasz, T. S. (1970). *Ideology and insanity: Essays on the psychiatric dehumanization of man*. New York: Anchor Books.

Taeuber, D. M. (1996). *Statistical handbook on women in America* (2nd ed.). Phoenix, AZ: The Oryx Press.

Tafoya, T. (1996). New heights in human services: Multiculturalism. Keynote address at National Organization of Human Services Annual Conference. St. Louis, MO.

Tallent, N. (1993). *Psychological report writing* (4th ed.). Englewood Cliffs, NJ: Prentice Hall.

Taylor, C. B. (1998). Treatment of anxiety disorders. In A. F. Schatzberg & C. B. Nemeroff (Eds.), *Textbook of psychopharmacology* (2nd ed., pp. 775–790). Washington, DC: American Psychiatric Press.

Teglasi, H. (1995). *Assessment of temperament* (Report No. EDO-CG-95-15). Washington, DC: Office of Educational Research and Improvement. (ERIC Document Reproduction Service No. ED 389-963.)

Tennyson, W. W., & Strom, S. M. (1986). Beyond professional standards: Developing responsibleness. *Journal of Counseling and Development, 64*(5), 298–302.

Thomas, C. M., & Martin, V. (1998). Group counseling with the elderly and their caregivers. In D. Capuzzi & D. R. Gross (Eds.), *Introduction to group counseling* (2nd ed., pp. 389–414). Denver, CO: Love Publishing Company.

Thomas, K. R. (1991). Oedipal issues in counseling psychology. *Journal of Counseling and Development, 69*, 203– 205.

Thomas, R. M. (1990). *Counseling and life-span development*. New York: Sage.

Thomason, T. C. (1993). Counseling Native Americans: An introduction for non-native American counselors. In D. R. Atkinson, & G. Hackett (Eds.), *Counseling diverse populations* (pp. 171–181). Madison, WI: Brown & Benchmark. (Original work published 1988)

Thompson, B. (1993). The use of statistical significance in research: Bootstrap and other alternatives. *Journal of Experimental Education, 61*(4), 361–367.

Thompson, B. (1995a). *Inappropriate statistical practices in counseling research: Three pointers for readers of research literature* (Report No. EDO-CG-95-33). Greensboro, NC: ERIC Clearinghouse on Counseling and Student Services. (ERIC Document Reproduction Service No. ED 392-990.)

Thompson, B. (1995b). Publishing your research results: Some suggestions and counsel. *Journal of Counseling and Development, 73*, 342–345.

Thompson, J. J. (1973). *Beyond words: Nonverbal communication in the classroom*. New York: Citation Press.

Thorndike, R. M. (1997). *Measurement and evaluation in psychology and education* (6th ed.). Upper Saddle River, NJ: Simon & Schuster.

Tiedeman, D. V. (1983). Flexible filing, computers, and growing. *The Counseling Psychologist, 11*, 33–47.

Tiedeman, D. V., & Miller-Tiedeman, A. (1984). Career decision making: An individualistic perspective. In D. Brown & L. Brooks (Eds.), *Career choice and development: Applying contemporary theories to practice* (Chap. 10). San Francisco: Jossey-Bass.

Tiedeman, D. V., & O'Hara, R. P. (1963). *Career development: Choice and adjustment*. New York: College Entrance Examination Board.

Tillitski, C. J. (1990). A meta-analysis of estimated effect sizes for group versus individual versus control treatments. *International Journal of Group Psychotherapy, 40*(2), 215–224.

Todd, J., & Bohart, A. C. (1999). *Foundations of clinical and counseling psychology* (3rd ed.). New York: Longman.

Tolbert, E. L. (1982). *An introduction to guidance: The professional counselor* (2nd ed.). Boston: Little, Brown.

Tollefson, G. D., & Rosenbaum, J. R. (1998). Selective serotonin reuptake inhibitors. In A. F. Schatzberg & C. B. Nemeroff (Eds.), *Textbook of psychopharmacology* (2nd ed., pp. 219–238). Washington, DC: American Psychiatric Press.

Tompkins, L., & Mehring, T. (1993). Client privacy and the school counselor: Privilege, ethics, and employer practices. *The School Counselor, 40*, 335–342.

Toseland, R. W., & Siporin, M. (1986). When to recommend group treatment: A review of the clinical and research literature. *International Journal of Group Psychotherapy, 36*, 171–201.

Tosi, D. J. (1970). Dogmatism within the counselor-client dyad. *Journal of Counseling Psychology, 17*, 284–288.

Trotzer, J. P. (1999). *The counselor and the group:Integrating theory, training, and practice* (3rd ed.). Philadelphia: Accelerated Development.

Truax, C. B., & Mitchell, K. M. (1961). Research on certain therapist interpersonal skills in relation to process and outcome. In A. E. Bergin & S. L. Garfield (Eds.), *Handbook of psychotherapy and behavior change: An empirical analysis* (3rd ed.). New York: Wiley.

Tryon, G. S. (1996). Supervisee development during the practicum year. *Counselor Education and Supervision, 35*, 287–294.

Tuckman, B. W., & Jensen, M. A. C. (1977). Stages of small-group development revisited. *Group and Organizational Studies, 2*, 419–427.

Turkington, C. (1985). Analysts sued for barring non-MDs. *APA Monitor, 16*(5), 2.

Tyler, L. E. (1969). *The work of the counselor* (3rd ed.). Englewood Cliffs, NJ: Prentice Hall.

United Nations. (2000). *United Nations statistics division: The world's women 2000: Trends and statistics*. Retrieved June 1, 2001 from the World Wide Web: http://www.un.org/Depts/unsd/gender/.

U. S. Census Bureau. (2000a). *Historical poverty tables. Table 2. Poverty status of people by family relationship, race, and Hispanic origin: 1959 to 1999*. Retrieved June 1, 2001, from the World Wide Web: http://www.census.gov/hhes/poverty/histpov/hstpov2.html.

U. S. Census Bureau. (2000b). *Historical poverty tables: Table 18. Workers as a proportion of all poor people: 1978 to 1999*. Retrieved June 1, 2001, from the World Wide Web: http://www.census.gov/hhes/poverty/histpov/hstpov18.html.

U. S. Census Bureau. (2000c). *Historical poverty tables. Table 3. Poverty status of people, by age, race, and Hispanic origin:1959 to 1999*. Retrieved June 1, 2001, from the World Wide Web: http://www.census.gov/hhes/poverty/histpov/hstpov3.html.

U. S. Census Bureau. (2000d). *Historical poverty tables. Table 14. Distribution of the poor by race and Hispanic origin:1966 to 1999*. Retrieved June 1, 2001, from the World Wide Web: http://www.census.gov/hhes/poverty/histpov/hstpov14.html.

U. S. Census Bureau. (2000e). *Resident population estimates of the United States by age and sex: April 1, 1990 to July 1, 1999, with short-term projection to November 1, 2000*. Retrieved June 1, 2001, from the World Wide Web: http://www.census.gov/population/estimates/nation/intfile2-1.txt.

U. S. Census Bureau. (2000f). *Projections of the total resident population by 5-year age groups, and sex with special age categories: middle series, 2025 to 2045*. Retrieved June 1, 2001, from the World Wide Web: http://www.census.gov/population/projections/nation/summary/np-t3-f.txt.

U. S. Census Bureau. (2000g). Quick tables. Retrieved February 21, 2002, from the World Wide Web: http://factfinder.census.gov/servlet/QTTable?ds_name=DEC_2000_SF1_U&geo_id=01000US&qr_name=DEC_2000_SF1_U_DP1

U. S. Census Bureau. (2001a). *Resident population estimates of the United States by sex, race, and Hispanic origin: April 1, 1990 to July 1, 1999, with short-term projection to November 1, 2000*. Retrieved June 1, 2001, from the World Wide Web: http://www.census.gov/population/estimates/nation/intfile3-1.txt.

U. S. Census Bureau (2001b). *Projections of the resident population by race, Hispanic origin, and nativity: Middle series, 2050 to 2070*. Retrieved June 1, 2001, from the World Wide Web: http://www.census.gov/population/projections/nation/summary/np-t5-g.txt.

U. S. Census Bureau. (2001c). *Immigrants, fiscal year 1998*. Retrieved June 1, 2001, from the World Wide Web: http://www.ins.usdoj.gov/graphics/aboutins/statistics/imm98.pdf.

U. S. Census Bureau. (2001d). *The American Indian, Eskimo, and Aleut population*. Retrieved June 1, 2001, from the World Wide Web: http://www.census.gov/population/www/pop-profile/amerind.html.

U. S. Census Bureau. (2001e). *Table 1. Prevalence of disability by age, sex, race, and Hispanic origin: 1997*. Retrieved June 1, 2001, from the World Wide Web: http://www.census.gov/hhes/www/disable/sipp/disab97/ds97tl.html.

U. S. Census Bureau. (2002). *Quick tables*. Retrieved February 21, 2002, from the World Wide Web: http://factfinder.census.gov/servlet/QTTable?ds_name=DEC_2000_SF1_U&geo_id=01000US&qr_name=DEC_2000_SF1_U_DP1

U.S. Department of Commerce (1991). *Statistical abstracts of the United States* (111th ed.). Washington, DC: Bureau of Census. Government Printing Office.

U.S. Department of Commerce (1992). *Current population reports: Poverty in the United States* (Series P-60, No. 181). Washington, DC: Bureau of Census. Government Printing Office.

U.S. Department of Commerce (2000). *National Telecomunications and Information Administration. Percent of U.S. households with a computer and internet access*. Retrieved, June 1, 2001, from the World Wide Web: http://www.ntia.doc.gov/ntiahome/fttn00/chartscontents.html.

U.S. Department of Health and Human Services (1992). *Medications: Mental health/mental illness: Decade of the brain* (revised). [Brochure]. Washington, DC: Author.

U.S. Department of Health and Human Services (2000). *Health and human services fact sheet: Substance abuse*. Retrieved June 1, 2001, from the World Wide Web: http://www.hhs.gov/news/press/2000pres/00fsmtf.html.

U.S. Department of Justice (1992). *American with Disabilities Act requirements fact sheet*. Washington, DC: Civil Rights Division, Coordination and Review Section.

U.S. Department of Justice (2001). *Correction statistics*. Retrieved June 1, 2001, from the World Wide Web: http://www.ojp.usdoj.gov/bjs/pub/pdf/cj-3.pdf.

U.S. Department of Labor (1993). *Office of Disability Employment Policy: Americans with disability act: Focus on key provisions*. Retrieved June 1, 2001, from the World Wide Web: http://www50.pcepd.gov/pcepd/pubs/adabro/keypro.htm.

U.S. Department of Labor (1999). *Dictionary of occupational titles* (4th ed.). Indianapolis, IN: JIST Publishing.

Usher, C. H. (1989). Recognizing cultural bias in counseling theory and practice: The case of Rogers. *Journal of Counseling and Development, 17*(2), 62–71.

Usher, C. H., & Borders, L. D. (1993). Practicing counselors' preferences for supervisory style and supervisory emphasis. *Counselor Education and Supervision, 33*, 66–80.

Vacc, N. A. (1982). A conceptual framework for continuous assessment of clients. *Measurement and Evaluation in Guidance, 15*(1), 40–47.

Vaillant, G. E. (1977). *Adaptation to life*. Boston: Little, Brown.

Vander Kolk, C. J. (1990). *Introduction to group counseling and psychotherapy*. Prospect Heights, IL: Waveland Press.

Van Hoose, W. H. (1980). Ethics and counseling. *Counseling and Human Development, 13*, 1–12.

Van Hoose, W. H., & Paradise, L. V. (1979). Ethics in counseling and psychotherapy. Cranston, RI: Carroll Press.

VanZandt, C. D. (1990). Professionalism: A matter of personal initiatives. *Journal of Counseling and Development, 68*, 243–245.

Verny, T. R. (1974). *Inside groups: A practical guide to encounter groups and group therapy*. New York: McGraw-Hill.

Viney, L. L., Allwood, K., Stillson, L., & Walmsley, R. (1992). Caring for the carers: A note on counseling for the wider impact of AIDS. *Journal of Counseling and Development, 70*(3), 442–444.

Virginia Board of Counseling (2001). *Regulations governing the practice of marriage and family therapy*. Retrieved June 1, 2001, from the World Wide Web: http://www.dhp.state.va.us/counseling/leg/Marriage%20and%20Family%20Therapist%204-12-00.doc.

Vontress, C. E. (1988). An existential approach to cross-cultural counseling. *Journal of Multicultural Counseling and Development, 16*, 73–84.

Wahler, R. G. (1976). Deviant child behavior within the family: Developmental speculations and behavior change strategies. In H. Leitenberg (Ed.), *Handbook of behavior modification and therapy*. Englewood Cliffs, NJ: Prentice Hall.

Wakefield, J. C. (1992). The concept of mental disorder: On the boundary between biological facts and social values. *American Psychologist, 47*, 373–388.

Walker, A. (1993). *Warrior marks: Female genital mutilation and the sexual blinding of women* (pp. 516–543). New York: Harcourt Brace.

Wallen, J. (1993). *Addiction in human development: Developmental perspectives on addiction and recovery*. New York: Haworth Press.

Wallerstein, J. S., & Blakeslee, S. (1989). *Second chances: Men, women, and children a decade after divorce*. New York: Ticknor & Fields.

Walsh, W. B., & Betz, N. E. (2001). *Tests and assessment* (4th ed.). Upper Saddle River, NJ: Prentice Hall.

Walsh, W. B., & Osipow, S. H. (Eds.). (1988). *Career decision making*. Hillsdale, NJ: Earlbaum.

Wampler, L. D., & Strupp, H. H. (1976). Personal therapy for students in clinical psychology: A matter of faith? *Professional Psychology, 7*(2), 195–202.

Ward, D. E. (1982). A model for the more effective use of theory in group work. *Journal for Specialists in Group Work, 7*, 224–230.

Ward, D. E. (1984). Termination of individual counseling: Concepts and strategies. *Journal of Counseling and Development, 63*, 21–25.

Warnath, C. F. (1975). Vocational theories: Direction to nowhere. *Personnel and Guidance Journal, 53*, 422–428.

Watkins, C. E. (1983). Counselor acting out in the counseling situation: An exploratory analysis. *Personnel and Guidance Journal, 61*(7), 417–423.

Watkins, C. E. (1990). The testing the test section of the *Journal of Counseling and Development:* Historical, contemporary, and future perspectives. *Journal of Counseling and Development, 66*,70–74.

Watkins, C. E., Jr., & Campbell, V. L. (1990). Testing and assessment in counseling psychology: Contemporary developments and issues. *The Counseling Psychologist, 18*(2), 189–197.

Watson, J. B. (1925). *Behaviorism*. New York: Norton.

Watson, J. B., & Raynor, R. (1920). Conditioned emotional reactions. *Journal of Experimental Psychology, 3*, 1–14.

Watts, G. A. (1994). Frank Parsons: Promoter of a progressive era. *Journal of Career Development, 20*(4), 265–286.

Watts, R. E., & Pietrzak, D. (2000). Adlerian "encouragment" and the therapeutic process of solution-focused brief therapy. *Journal of Counseling and Development 78*(4), 442–447.

Watzlawick, P., Beavin, J. H., & Jackson, D. D. (1967). *Pragmatics of human communication: A study of interactional patterns, pathologies, and paradoxes*. New York: Norton.

Watzlawick, P., Weakland, J. H., & Fisch, R. (1974). *Change: Principles of problem formation and problem resolution study of interactional patterns, pathologies, and paradoxes*. New York: Norton.

Waxman, L. D., & Reyes, L. M. (1988). *A status report on hunger and homelessness in America's cities: A 27 city survey*. Washington, DC: United States Conferences of Mayors. (ERIC Document Reproduction Service No. ED 315465.)

Webb, W. (1999). *Solutioning: Solution-focused interventions for counselors*. Philadelphia: Accelerated Development.

Weinberg, G. (1970). The male homosexual: Age-related variations in social and psychological characteristics. *Social Problems, 17*, 527–537.

Weininger, O. (1992). *Melanie Klein, from theory to reality*. New York: Karnac Books, 1992.

Weinrach, S. G. (1991). CACREP: The need for a mid-course correction. *Journal of Counseling and Development, 69*, 491–494.

Weinrach, S. G., & Thomas, K. R. (1993). The national board for certified counselors: The good, the bad, and the ugly. *Journal of Counseling and Development, 72*, 105–109.

Weinrach, S. G., & Thomas, K. R. (1996). The counseling profession's commitment to diversity-sensitive counseling: A critical reassessment. *Journal of Counseling and Development, 74*, 472–477.

Welfel, E. R. (1998). *Ethics in counseling and psychotherapy: Standards, research, and emerging issues*. Pacific Grove: Brooks/Cole.

Welfel, E. R., & Lipsitz, N. E. (1983). Ethical orientation of counselors: Its relationship to moral reasoning and level of training. *Counselor Education and Supervision, 23*(1), 33–45.

Werner, M., & Tyler, M. (1993). Community-based interventions: A return to community mental health centers' origins. *Journal of Counseling and Development, 71*, 689–692.

Werstlein, P. (1994). *Fostering counselors' development in group supervision* (Report No. EDO-CG-94-19). Greensboro, NC: ERIC Clearinghouse on Counseling and Student Services. (ERIC Document Reproduction Service No. ED 372-351).

Wertheimer, M. (1978). *A brief history of psychology*. New York: Holt, Rinehart & Winston.

West, J. D., Bubenzer, D. L., Pinsoneault, T., & Holeman, V. (1993). Three supervision modalities for training marital and family counselors. *Counselor Education and Supervision, 33*, 127–138.

West, J. D., Hosie, T. W., & Mackey, J. A. (1987). Employment and roles of counselors in mental health agencies. *Journal of Counseling and Development, 66*, 135–138.

West, J. D., Hosie, T. W., & Mackey, J. A. (1988). The counselor's role in mental health: An evaluation. *Counselor Education and Supervision, 27*, 233–239.

West, J. D., & Idol, L. (1993). The counselor as consultant in the collaborative school. *Journal of Counseling and Development, 71*, 678–683.

Westbrook, F. D., Kandell, J. J., Kirkland, S. E., Phillips, P. E., Regan, A. M., Medvene, A., & Oslin, Y. D. (1993). University campus consultation: Opportunities and limitations. *Journal of Counseling and Development, 71*, 684–688.

Westwood, M. J. & Ishiyama, F. I. (1990). The communication process as a critical intervention for client change in cross-cultural counseling. *Journal of Multicultural Counseling and Development, 18*, 163–171.

Wheeler, S. (1991). Personal therapy: An essential aspect of counsellor training, or a distraction from focusing on the client? *Journal for the Advancement of Counselling, 14*, 193–202.

Whiston, S. C. (1996). Accountability through action research: Research methods for practitioners. *Journal of Counseling and Development, 74*, 616–623.

Whiston, S. C., & Coker, J. K. (2000). Reconstructing clinical training: Implications from research. *Counselor Education and Supervision, 39*, 228–253.

Whit, E. J., Carnaghi, J. E., Matkin, J., Scalese-Love, P., & Nestor, D. (1994). Believing is seeing: Alternative perspectives on a statement of professional philosophy for student affairs. In A. L. Rentz (Ed.), *Student affairs: A profession's heritage* (pp. 683–692). Lanham, MD: American College Personnel Association and the University Press of America.

Whitaker, C. (1976). The hindrance of theory in clinical work. In P. J. Guerin (Ed.), *Family therapy* (pp. 154–164). New York: Gardner Press.

White, P. E., & Franzoni, J. B. (1990). A multidimensional analysis of the mental health graduate counselors in training. *Counselor Educational and Supervision, 29*(4), 258–267.

Whiteley, J. M. (1984). A historical perspective on the development of counseling psychology as a profession. In S. D. Brown & R. W. Lent (Eds.), *Handbook of counseling psychology*. New York: Wiley.

Whitfield, D. (1994). Toward an integrated approach to improving multicultural counselor education. *Journal of Multicultural Counseling and Development, 22*, 227–238.

Whitfield, W., McGrath, P., & Coleman, V. (1992, October). *Increasing multicultural sensitivity and awareness*. Symposium presented at the Annual Conference of the National Organization for Human Service Education, Alexandria, VA.

Whitledge, J. (1994). Cross-cultural counseling: Implications for school counselors in enhancing student learning. *The School Counselor, 41*, 314–318.9

Wicks, R. J. (1977). *Counseling strategies and interventions techniques for the human services*. New York: Lippincott.

Widick, C. (1975). The counselor as a developmental instrument. *Counselor Education and Supervision 14*(4), 286–296.

Widick, C. (l977). The Perry scheme: A foundation for developmental practice. *The Counseling Psychologist, 6*(4), 35–38.

Wilgus, E., & Shelley, V. (1988). The role of the elementary-school counselor: Teacher perceptions, expectations, and actual functions. *The School Counselor, 35*(4), 259–266.

Williams, M. E., & Buboltz, W. C. (1999). Content analysis of the *Journal of Counseling and Development:* Volumes 67 to 74. *Journal of Counseling and Development, 77,* 344–349.

Williams, R. C., & Myer, R. A. (1992). The men's movement: An adjunct to traditional counseling approaches. *Journal of Mental Health Counseling, 14,* 393–404.

Williamson, E. G. (1950). *Counseling adolescents.* New York: McGraw-Hill.

Williamson, E. G. (1958). Value orientation in counseling. *Personnel and Guidance Journal, 37,* 520–528.

Williamson, E. G. (1964). An historical perspective of the vocational guidance movement. *Personnel and Guidance Journal, 42,* 854–859.

Wilson, F. R. (1995). Internet information sources for counselors. *Counselor Education and Supervision, 34*(4), 369–387.

Wilson, F. R., Conyne, R. K., & Ward, D. (1994). The general status of group work training in accredited counseling programs. *The Journal for Specialists in Group Work, 19*(3), 140–154.

Wilson, L. L., & Stith, L. L. (1991). Culturally sensitive therapy with black clients. *Journal of Multicultural Counseling and Development, 19,* 32–43.

Winston, R. B. (1991). Counseling and advising. In U. Delworth & G. Hanson (Eds.), *Student services* (2nd ed., pp. 371–400). San Francisco: Jossey-Bass.

Wise, R., Charner, I., & Randour, M. A. (1978). A conceptual framework for career awareness in career decision-making. In J. Whiteley & A. Resnikoff (Eds.), *Career counseling* (pp. 216–231). Monterey, CA: Brooks/Cole.

Wittenberg, R. (1997). *Opportunities in social work.* Lincolnwood, IL: VGM Career Horizons.

Woititz, J. G. (1983). *Adult children of alcoholics.* Hollywood, FL: Health Communications.

Wolf, A., & Schwartz, E. K. (1972). Psychoanalysis in groups. In H. I. Kaplan & B. J. Sadock, *The origins of group psychoanalysis* (pp. 41–100). New York: Jason Aronson.

Wolf, A., Schwartz, E. K., McCarty, G. J., & Goldberg, I. A. (1972). Psychoanalysis in groups: Comparison with other group therapies. In C. J. Sager & H. S. Kaplan (Eds.), *Progress in group and family therapy* (pp. 47–53). New York: Brunner/Mazel.

Wolfgang, A. (1985). The function and importance of nonverbal behavior in intercultural counseling. In P. B. Pedersen (Ed.), *Handbook of cross-cultural counseling and therapy.* Westport, CT: Greenwood Press.

Wolpe, J. (1958). *Psychotherapy by reciprocal inhibition.* Stanford, CA: Stanford University Press.

Wolpe, J. (1969). *The practice of behavior therapy.* New York: Pergamon Press.

Wolpe, J., & Lazarus, A. (1966). *Behavior therapy techniques.* New York: Pergamon.

Woodside, M., & McClam, T. (1990). *An introduction to human services.* Pacific Grove, CA: Brooks/Cole.

Worell, J. (1980). New directions in counseling women. *Personnel and Guidance Journal, 58,* 477–484.

World Almanac (1997). New York: Scripps Howard Company.

World Health Organization (2001). *AIDS epidemic update: December 2000.* Retrieved June 1, 2001, from the World Wide Web: http://www.unaids.org/wac/2000/wad00/files/WAD_epidemic_report.htm.

Worthen, B. R., & Sanders, J. R. (1987). *Educational evaluation: Alternative approaches and practical guidelines.* New York: Longman.

Wright, W. (1975). Counselor dogmatism, willingness to disclose, and clients empathy ratings. *Journal of Counseling Psychology, 22,* 390–394.

Wylie, M. S. (1995, September/October). The new visionaries. *The Family Therapy Networker,* pp. 20–29, 32–35.

Yalom, I. D. (1995). *The theory and practice of group psychotherapy* (4th ed.). New York: Basic Books.

Yeaton, W. H. (1994). The development and assessment of valid measures of service delivery to enhance inference in outcome-based research: Measuring attendance at self-help group meetings. *Journal of Consulting and Clinical Psychology, 62,* 686–694.

Young, F. A. (1992). APA and (AP)2. *Professional Psychology: Research and Practice, 23,* 436–438.

Young, M. E. (1992). *Counseling methods & techniques: An eclectic approach.* New York: Macmillan.

Yutrzenka, B. A. (1995). Making a case for training in ethnic and cultural diversity in increasing treatment efficacy. *Journal of Consulting and Clinical Psychology, 63*(2), 197–296.

Zimbardo, P. G., & Gerrig, R. (1996). *Psychology and life* (12th ed.). Reading, MA: Addison-Wesley.

Zinker, J. (1978). *Creative process in Gestalt therapy.* New York: Random House (Vintage).

Zinker, J. (1994). *In search of good form: Gestalt therapy with couples and families.* San Francisco: Jossey-Bass.

Zinnbauer, B. J., & Pargament, K. I. (2000). Working with the sacred: Four approaches to religion and spiritual issues in counseling. *Journal of Counseling and Development, 78,* 162–171.

Zins, J. E. (1993). Enhancing consultee problem-solving skills in consultative interactions. *Journal of Counseling and Development, 72,* 185–190.

Zunker, V. G. (2001). *Career counseling: Applied concepts of life planning* (6th ed.). Pacific Grove, CA: Brooks/Cole.

Zwelling, S. S. (1990). *Quest for a cure: The public hospital in Williamsburg, Virginia, 1773–1885.* Williamsburg, VA: The Colonial Williamsburg Foundation.

Zytowski, D. G. (1972). Four hundred years before Parsons. *Personnel and Guidance Journal, 50,* 443–450.

Zytowski, D. G. (1982). Assessment in the counseling process for the 1980s. *Measurement and Evaluation in Guidance, 15,* 15–21.

Zytowski, D. G. (1994). Tests and counseling: We are still married and living in discriminant analysis. *Measurement and Evaluation in Guidance, 15,* 15–21.

APPENDIX A

American Counseling Association Code of Ethics

Preamble

The American Counseling Association is an educational, scientific and professional organization whose members are dedicated to the enhancement of human development throughout the life span. Association members recognize diversity in our society and embrace a cross-cultural approach in support of the worth, dignity, potential, and uniqueness of each individual.

The specification of a code of ethics enables the association to clarify to current and future members, and to those served by members, the nature of the ethical responsibilities held in common by its members. As the code of ethics of the association, this document establishes principles that define the ethical behavior of association members. All members of the American Counseling Association are required to adhere to the Code of Ethics and the Standards of Practice. The Code of Ethics will serve as the basis for processing ethical complaints initiated against members of the association.

ETHICAL STANDARDS

Section A: The Counseling Relationship

A.1. CLIENT WELFARE

a. *Primary Responsibility*. The primary responsibility of counselors is to respect the dignity and to promote the welfare of clients.

b. *Positive Growth and Development*. Counselors encourage client growth and development in ways that foster the clients' interest and welfare; counselors avoid fostering dependent counseling relationships.

c. *Counseling Plans*. Counselors and their clients work jointly in devising integrated, individual counseling plans that offer reasonable promise of success and are consistent with abilities and circumstances of clients. Counselors and clients regularly review counseling plans to ensure their continued viability and effectiveness, respecting clients' freedom of choice. (See A.3.b.)

d. *Family Involvement*. Counselors recognize that families are usually important in clients' lives and strive to enlist family understanding and involvement as a positive resource, when appropriate.

e. *Career and Employment Needs*. Counselors work with their clients in considering employment in jobs and circumstances that are consistent with the clients' overall abilities, vocational limitations, physical restrictions, general temperament, interest and aptitude patterns, social skills, education, general qualifications, and other relevant characteristics and needs. Counselors neither place nor participate in placing clients in positions that will result in damaging the interest and the welfare of clients, employers, or the public.

A.2. RESPECTING DIVERSITY

a. *Nondiscrimination*. Counselors do not condone or engage in discrimination based on age, color, culture, disability, ethnic group, gender, race, religion, sexual orientation, marital status, or socioeconomic status. (See C.5.a., C.5.b., and D.1.i.)

b. *Respecting Differences*. Counselors will actively attempt to understand the diverse cultural backgrounds of the clients with whom they work. This includes, but is not limited to, learning how the counselor's own cultural/ethnic/racial identity impacts her/his values and beliefs about the counseling process. (See E.8. and F.2.i.)

A.3. CLIENT RIGHTS

a. *Disclosure to Clients*. When counseling is initiated, and throughout the counseling process as necessary, counselors inform clients of the purposes, goals, techniques, procedures, limitations, potential risks and benefits of services to be performed, and other pertinent information. Counselors take steps to ensure that clients understand the implications of diagnosis, the intended use of tests and reports, fees, and billing arrangements. Clients have the right to expect confidentiality and to be provided with an explanation of its limitations, including supervision and/or treatment team professionals; to obtain clear information about their case records; to participate in the ongoing counseling plans; and to refuse any recommended services and be advised of the consequences of such refusal. (See E.5.a. and G.2.)

b. *Freedom of Choice*. Counselors offer clients the freedom to choose whether to enter into a counseling relationship and to determine which professional(s) will provide counseling. Restrictions that limit choices of clients are fully explained. (See A.1.c.)

c. *Inability to Give Consent*. When counseling minors or persons unable to give voluntary informed consent, counselors act in these clients' best interests. (See B.3.)

A.4. CLIENTS SERVED BY OTHERS

If a client is receiving services from another mental health professional, counselors, with client consent, inform the professional persons already involved and develop clear agreements to avoid confusion and conflict for the client. (See C.6.c.)

A.5. PERSONAL NEEDS AND VALUES

a. *Personal Needs*. In the counseling relationship, counselors are aware of the intimacy and responsibilities inherent in the counseling relationship, maintain respect for clients, and avoid actions that seek to meet their personal needs at the expense of clients.

b. *Personal Values*. Counselors are aware of their own values, attitudes, beliefs, and behaviors and how these apply in a diverse society, and avoid imposing their values on clients. (See C.5.a.)

A.6. DUAL RELATIONSHIPS

a. *Avoid When Possible*. Counselors are aware of their influential positions with respect to clients, and they avoid exploiting the trust and dependency of clients. Counselors make every effort to avoid dual relationships with clients that could impair professional judgment or increase the risk of harm to clients. (Examples of such relationships include, but are not limited to, familial, social, financial, business, or close personal relationships with clients.) When a dual relationship cannot be avoided, counselors take appropriate professional precautions such as informed consent, consultation, supervision, and documentation to ensure that judgment is not impaired and no exploitation occurs. (See F.1.b.)

b. *Superior/Subordinate Relationships*. Counselors do not accept as clients superiors or subordinates with whom they have administrative, supervisory, or evaluative relationships.

A.7. SEXUAL INTIMACIES WITH CLIENTS

a. *Current Clients*. Counselors do not have any type of sexual intimacies with clients and do not counsel persons with whom they have had a sexual relationship.

b. *Former Clients*. Counselors do not engage in sexual intimacies with former clients within a minimum of two years after terminating the counseling relationship. Counselors who engage in such relationship after two years following termination have the responsibility to thoroughly examine and document that such relations did not have an exploitative nature, based on factors such as duration of counseling, amount of time since counseling, termination circumstances, client's personal history and mental status, adverse impact on the client, and actions by the counselor suggesting a plan to initiate a sexual relationship with the client after termination.

A.8. MULTIPLE CLIENTS

When counselors agree to provide counseling services to two or more persons who have a relationship (such as husband and wife, or parents and children), counselors clarify at the outset which person or persons are clients and the nature of the relationships they will have with each involved person. If it becomes apparent that counselors may be called upon to perform potentially conflicting roles, they clarify, adjust, or withdraw from roles appropriately. (See B.2. and B.4.d.)

A.9. GROUP WORK

a. *Screening*. Counselors screen prospective group counseling/therapy participants. To the extent possible, counselors select members whose needs and goals are compatible with goals of the group, who will not impede the group process, and whose well-being will not be jeopardized by the group experience.

b. *Protecting Clients*. In a group setting, counselors take reasonable precautions to protect clients from physical or psychological trauma.

A.10. FEES AND BARTERING
(See D.3 a. and D.3.b.)

a. *Advance Understanding*. Counselors clearly explain to clients, prior to entering the counseling relationship, all financial arrangements related to professional services including the use of collection agencies or legal measures for nonpayment. (A.11.c.)

b. *Establishing Fees*. In establishing fees for professional counseling services, counselors consider the financial status of clients and locality. In the event that the established fee structure is inappropriate for a client, assistance is provided in attempting to find comparable services of acceptable cost. (See A.10.d., D.3.a., and D.3.b.)

c. *Bartering Discouraged*. Counselors ordinarily refrain from accepting goods or services from clients in return for counseling services because such arrangements create inherent potential for conflicts, exploitation, and distortion of the professional relationship. Counselors may participate in bartering only if the relationship is not exploitive, if the client requests it, if a clear written contract is established, and if such arrangements are an accepted practice among professionals in the community. (See A.6.a.)

d. *Pro Bono Service*. Counselors contribute to society by devoting a portion of their professional activity to services for which there is little or no financial return (pro bono).

A.11. TERMINATION AND REFERRAL

a. *Abandonment Prohibited*. Counselors do not abandon or neglect clients in counseling. Counselors assist in making appropriate arrangements for the continuation of treatment, when necessary, during interruptions such as vacations, and following termination.

b. *Inability to Assist Clients*. If counselors determine an inability to be of professional assistance to clients, they avoid entering or immediately terminate a counseling relationship. Counselors are knowledgeable about referral resources and suggest appropriate alternatives. If clients decline the suggested referral, counselors should discontinue the relationship.

c. *Appropriate Termination*. Counselors terminate a counseling relationship, securing client agreement when possible, when it is reasonably clear that the client is no longer benefiting, when services are no longer required, when counseling no longer serves the client's needs or interests, when clients do not pay fees charged, or when agency or institution limits do not allow provision of further counseling services. (See A.10.b. and C.2.g.)

A.12. COMPUTER TECHNOLOGY

a. *Use of Computers*. When computer applications are used in counseling services, counselors ensure that: (1) the client is intellectually, emotionally, and physically capable of using the computer application; (2) the computer application is appropriate for the needs of the client; (3) the client understands the purpose and operation of the computer applications; and (4) a follow-up of client use of a computer application is provided to correct possible misconceptions, discover inappropriate use, and assess subsequent needs.

b. *Explanation of Limitations*. Counselors ensure that clients are provided information as a part of the counseling relationship that adequately explains the limitations of computer technology.

c. *Access to Computer Applications*. Counselors provide for equal access to computer applications in counseling services. (See A.2.a.)

Section B: Confidentiality

B.1. RIGHT TO PRIVACY

a. *Respect for Privacy.* Counselors respect their clients' right to privacy and avoid illegal and unwarranted disclosures of confidential information. (See A.3.a. and B.6.a.)

b. *Client Waiver.* The right to privacy may be waived by the client or their legally recognized representative.

c. *Exceptions.* The general requirement that counselors keep information confidential does not apply when disclosure is required to prevent clear and imminent danger to the client or others or when legal requirements demand that confidential information be revealed. Counselors consult with other professionals when in doubt as to the validity of an exception.

d. *Contagious, Fatal Diseases.* A counselor who receives information confirming that a client has a disease commonly known to be both communicable and fatal is justified in disclosing information to an identifiable third party, who by his or her relationship with the client is at a high risk of contracting the disease. Prior to making a disclosure the counselor should ascertain that the client has not already informed the third party about his or her disease and that the client is not intending to inform the third party in the immediate future. (See B.1.c. and B.1.f.)

e. *Court Ordered Disclosure.* When court ordered to release confidential information without a client's permission, counselors request to the court that the disclosure not be required due to potential harm to the client or counseling relationship. (See B.1.c.)

f. *Minimal Disclosure.* When circumstances require the disclosure of confidential information, only essential information is revealed. To the extent possible, clients are informed before confidential information is disclosed.

g. *Explanation of Limitations.* When counseling is initiated and throughout the counseling process as necessary, counselors inform clients of the limitations of confidentiality and identify foreseeable situations in which confidentiality must be breached. (See G.2.a.)

h. *Subordinates.* Counselors make every effort to ensure that privacy and confidentiality of clients are maintained by subordinates including employees, supervisees, clerical assistants, and volunteers. (See B.1.a.)

i. *Treatment Teams.* If client treatment will involve a continued review by a treatment team, the client will be informed of the team's existence and composition.

B.2. GROUPS AND FAMILIES

a. *Group Work.* In group work, counselors clearly define confidentiality and the parameters for the specific group being entered, explain its importance, and discuss the difficulties related to confidentiality involved in group work. The fact that confidentiality cannot be guaranteed is clearly communicated to group members.

b. *Family Counseling.* In family counseling, information about one family member cannot be disclosed to another member without permission. Counselors protect the privacy rights of each family member. (See A.8., B.3., and B.4.d.)

B.3. MINOR OR INCOMPETENT CLIENTS

When counseling clients who are minors or individuals who are unable to give voluntary, informed consent, parents or guardians may be included in the counseling process as appropriate. Counselors act in the best interests of clients and take measures to safeguard confidentiality. (See A.3.c.)

B.4. RECORDS

a. *Requirement of Records.* Counselors maintain records necessary for rendering professional services to their clients and as required by laws, regulations, or agency or institution procedures.

b. *Confidentiality of Records.* Counselors are responsible for securing the safety and confidentiality of any counseling records they create, maintain, transfer, or destroy whether the records are written, taped, computerized, or stored in any other medium. (See B.1.a.)

c. *Permission to Record or Observe.* Counselors obtain permission from clients prior to electronically recording or observing sessions. (See A.3.a.)

d. *Client Access.* Counselors recognize that counseling records are kept for the benefit of clients, and therefore provide access to records and copies of records when requested by competent clients, unless the records contain information that may be misleading and detrimental to the client. In situations involving multiple clients. access to records is limited to those parts of records that do not include confidential information related to another client. (See A.8., B.1.a., and B.2.b.)

e. *Disclosure or Transfer.* Counselors obtain written permission from clients to disclose or transfer records to legitimate third parties unless exceptions to confidentiality exist as listed in Section B.1. Steps are taken to ensure that receivers of counseling records are sensitive to their confidential nature.

B.5. RESEARCH AND TRAINING

a. *Data Disguise Required.* Use of data derived from counseling relationships for purposes of training, research, or publication is confined to content that is disguised to ensure the anonymity of the individuals involved. (See B.1.g. and G.3.d.)

b. *Agreement for Identification.* Identification of a client in a presentation or publication is permissible only when the client has reviewed the material and has agreed to its presentation or publication. (See G.3.d.)

B.6. CONSULTATION

a. *Respect for Privacy.* Information obtained in a consulting relationship is discussed for professional purposes only with persons clearly concerned with the case. Written and oral reports present data germane to the purposes of the consultation, and every effort is made to protect client identity and avoid undue invasion of privacy.

b. *Cooperating Agencies.* Before sharing information, counselors make efforts to ensure that there are defined policies in other agencies serving the counselor's clients that effectively protect the confidentiality of information.

Section C: Professional Responsibility

C.1. STANDARDS KNOWLEDGE

Counselors have a responsibility to read, understand, and follow the Code of Ethics and the Standards of Practice.

C.2. PROFESSIONAL COMPETENCE

a. *Boundaries of Competence.* Counselors practice only within the boundaries of their competence, based on their education, training, supervised experience, state and national professional credentials, and appropriate professional experience. Counselors will demonstrate a commitment to gain knowledge, personal awareness, sensitivity, and skills pertinent to working with a diverse client population.

b. *New Specialty Areas of Practice*. Counselors practice in specialty areas new to them only after appropriate education, training, and supervised experience. While developing skills in new specialty areas, counselors take steps to ensure the competence of their work and to protect others from possible harm.

c. *Qualified for Employment*. Counselors accept employment only for positions for which they are qualified by education, training, supervised experience, state and national professional credentials, and appropriate professional experience. Counselors hire for professional counseling positions only individuals who are qualified and competent.

d. *Monitor Effectiveness*. Counselors continually monitor their effectiveness as professionals and take steps to improve when necessary. Counselors in private practice take reasonable steps to seek out peer supervision to evaluate their efficacy as counselors.

e. *Ethical Issues Consultation*. Counselors take reasonable steps to consult with other counselors or related professionals when they have questions regarding their ethical obligations or professional practice. (See H.1.)

f. *Continuing Education*. Counselors recognize the need for continuing education to maintain a reasonable level of awareness of current scientific and professional information in their fields of activity. They take steps to maintain competence in the skills they use, are open to new procedures, and keep current with the diverse and/or special populations with whom they work.

g. *Impairment*. Counselors refrain from offering or accepting professional services when their physical, mental or emotional problems are likely to harm a client or others. They are alert to the signs of impairment, seek assistance for problems, and, if necessary, limit, suspend, or terminate their professional responsibilities. (See A.11.c.)

C.3. ADVERTISING AND SOLICITING CLIENTS

a. *Accurate Advertising*. There are no restrictions on advertising by counselors except those that can be specifically justified to protect the public from deceptive practices. Counselors advertise or represent their services to the public by identifying their credentials in an accurate manner that is not false, misleading, deceptive, or fraudulent. Counselors may only advertise the highest degree earned which is in counseling or a closely related field from a college or university that was accredited when the degree was awarded by one of the regional accrediting bodies recognized by the Council on Postsecondary Accreditation.

b. *Testimonials*. Counselors who use testimonials do not solicit them from clients or other persons who, because of their particular circumstances, may be vulnerable to undue influence.

c. *Statements by Others*. Counselors make reasonable efforts to ensure that statements made by others about them or the profession of counseling are accurate.

d. *Recruiting through Employment*. Counselors do not use their places of employment or institutional affiliation to recruit or gain clients, supervisees, or consultees for their private practices. (See C.5.e.)

e. *Products and Training Advertisements*. Counselors who develop products related to their profession or conduct workshops or training events ensure that the advertisements concerning these products or events are accurate and disclose adequate information for consumers to make informed choices.

f. *Promoting to Those Served*. Counselors do not use counseling, teaching, training, or supervisory relationships to promote their products or training events in a manner that is deceptive or would exert undue influence on individuals who may be vulnerable. Counselors may adopt textbooks they have authored for instruction purposes.

g. *Professional Association Involvement*. Counselors actively participate in local, state, and national associations that foster the development and improvement of counseling.

C.4. CREDENTIALS

a. *Credentials Claimed*. Counselors claim or imply only professional credentials possessed and are responsible for correcting any known misrepresentations of their credentials by others. Professional credentials include graduate degrees in counseling or closely related mental health fields, accreditation of graduate programs, national voluntary certifications, government-issued certifications or licenses, ACA professional membership, or any other credential that might indicate to the public specialized knowledge or expertise in counseling.

b. ACA *Professional Membership*. ACA professional members may announce to the public their membership status. Regular members may not announce their ACA membership in a manner that might imply they are credentialed counselors.

c. *Credential Guidelines*. Counselors follow the guidelines for use of credentials that have been established by the entities that issue the credentials.

d. *Misrepresentation of Credentials*. Counselors do not attribute more to their credentials than the credentials represent, and do not imply that other counselors are not qualified because they do not possess certain credentials.

e. *Doctoral Degrees from Other Fields*. Counselors who hold a master's degree in counseling or a closely related mental health field, but hold a doctoral degree from other than counseling or a closely related field do not use the title "Dr." in their practices and do not announce to the public in relation to their practice or status as a counselor that they hold a doctorate.

C.5. PUBLIC RESPONSIBILITY

a. *Nondiscrimination*. Counselors do not discriminate against clients, students, or supervisees in a manner that has a negative impact based on their age, color, culture, disability, ethnic group, gender, race, religion, sexual orientation, or socioeconomic status, or for any other reason. (See A.2.a.)

b. *Sexual Harassment*. Counselors do not engage in sexual harassment. Sexual harassment is defined as sexual solicitation, physical advances, or verbal or nonverbal conduct that is sexual in nature, that occurs in connection with professional activities or roles, and that either: (1) is unwelcome, is offensive, or creates a hostile workplace environment, and counselors know or are told this; or (2) is sufficiently severe or intense to be perceived as harassment to a reasonable person in the context. Sexual harassment can consist of a single intense or severe act or multiple persistent or pervasive acts.

c. *Reports to Third Parties*. Counselors are accurate, honest, and unbiased in reporting their professional activities and judgments to appropriate third parties including courts, health insurance companies, those who are the recipients of evaluation reports, and others. (See B.1.g.)

d. *Media Presentations*. When counselors provide advice or comment by means of public lectures, demonstrations, radio or television programs, prerecorded tapes, printed articles, mailed material, or other media, they take reasonable precautions to ensure that (1) the statements are based on appropriate professional counseling literature and practice; (2) the statements are otherwise consistent with the Code of Ethics and the Standards of Practice; and (3) the recipients of the information are not encouraged to infer that a professional counseling relationship has been established. (See C.6.b.)

e. *Unjustified Gains*. Counselors do not use their professional positions to seek or receive unjustified personal gains, sexual favors, unfair advantage, or unearned goods or services. (See C.3.d.)

C.6. RESPONSIBILITY TO OTHER PROFESSIONALS

a. *Different Approaches*. Counselors are respectful of approaches to professional counseling that differ from their own. Counselors know and take into account the traditions and practices of other professional groups with which they work.

b. *Personal Public Statements*. When making personal statements in a public context, counselors clarify that they are speaking from their personal perspectives and that they are not speaking on behalf of all counselors or the profession. (See C.5.d.)

c. *Clients Served by Others*. When counselors learn that their clients are in a professional relationship with another mental health professional, they request release from clients to inform the other professionals and strive to establish positive and collaborative professional relationships. (See A.4.)

Section D: Relationships with Other Professionals

D.1. RELATIONSHIPS WITH EMPLOYERS AND EMPLOYEES

a. *Role Definition*. Counselors define and describe for their employers and employees the parameters and levels of their professional roles.

b. *Agreements*. Counselors establish working agreements with supervisors, colleagues, and subordinates regarding counseling or clinical relationships, confidentiality, adherence to professional standards, distinction between public and private material, maintenance and dissemination of recorded information, workload, and accountability. Working agreements in each instance are specified and made known to those concerned.

c. *Negative Conditions*. Counselors alert their employers to conditions that may be potentially disruptive or damaging to the counselor's professional responsibilities or that may limit their effectiveness.

d. *Evaluation*. Counselors submit regularly to professional review and evaluation by their supervisor or the appropriate representative of the employer.

e. *In-Service*. Counselors are responsible for in-service development of self and staff.

f. *Goals*. Counselors inform their staff of goals and programs.

g. *Practices*. Counselors provide personnel and agency practices that respect and enhance the rights and welfare of each employee and recipient of agency services. Counselors strive to maintain the highest levels of professional services.

h. *Personnel Selection and Assignment*. Counselors select competent staff and assign responsibilities compatible with their skills and experiences.

i. *Discrimination*. Counselors, as either employers or employees, do not engage in or condone practices that are inhumane, illegal, or unjustifiable (such as considerations based on age, color, culture, disability, ethnic group, gender, race, religion, sexual orientation, or socioeconomic status) in hiring, promotion, or training. (See A.2.a. and C.5.b.)

j. *Professional Conduct*. Counselors have a responsibility both to clients and to the agency or institution within which services are performed to maintain high standards of professional conduct.

k. *Exploitive Relationships*. Counselors do not engage in exploitive relationships with individuals over whom they have supervisory, evaluative, or instructional control or authority.

l. *Employer Policies*. The acceptance of employment in an agency or institution implies that counselors are in agreement with its general policies and principles. Counselors strive to reach agreement with employers as to acceptable standards of conduct that allow for changes in institutional policy conducive to the growth and development of clients.

D.2. CONSULTATION

(See B.6.)

a. *Consultation as an Option*. Counselors may choose to consult with any other professionally competent persons about their clients. In choosing consultants, counselors avoid placing the consultant in a conflict of interest situation that would preclude the consultant being a proper party to the counselor's efforts to help the client. Should counselors be engaged in a work setting that compromises this consultation standard, they consult with other professionals whenever possible to consider justifiable alternatives.

b. *Consultant Competency*. Counselors are reasonably certain that they have or the organization represented has the necessary competencies and resources for giving the kind of consulting services needed and that appropriate referral resources are available.

c. *Understanding with Clients*. When providing consultation, counselors attempt to develop with their clients a clear understanding of problem definition, goals for change, and predicted consequences of interventions selected.

d. *Consultant Goals*. The consulting relationship is one in which client adaptability and growth toward self-direction are consistently encouraged and cultivated. (See A.1.b.)

D.3. FEES FOR REFERRAL

a. *Accepting Fees from Agency Clients*. Counselors refuse a private fee or other remuneration for rendering services to persons who are entitled to such services through the counselor's employing agency or institution. The policies of a particular agency may make explicit provisions for agency clients to receive counseling services from members of its staff in private practice. In such instances, the clients must be informed of other options open to them should they seek private counseling services. (See A.10.a., A.11.b., and C.3.d.)

b. *Referral Fees*. Counselors do not accept a referral fee from other professionals.

D.4. SUBCONTRACTOR ARRANGEMENTS

When counselors work as subcontractors for counseling services for a third party, they have a duty to inform clients of the limitations of confidentiality that the organization may place on counselors in providing counseling services to clients. The limits of such confidentiality ordinarily are discussed as part of the intake session. (See B.1.e. and B.1.f.)

Section E: Evaluation, Assessment, and Interpretation

E.1. GENERAL

a. *Appraisal Techniques*. The primary purpose of educational and psychological assessment is to provide measures that are objective and interpretable in either comparative or absolute terms. Counselors recognize the need to interpret the statements in this section as applying to the whole range of appraisal techniques, including test and nontest data.

b. *Client Welfare*. Counselors promote the welfare and best interests of the client in the development, publication, and utilization of educational and psychological assessment techniques. They do not misuse assessment results and interpretations and take reasonable steps to prevent others from misusing the information these techniques provide. They respect the client's right to know the results, the interpretations made, and the bases for their conclusions and recommendations.

E.2. COMPETENCE TO USE AND INTERPRET TESTS

a. *Limits of Competence*. Counselors recognize the limits of their competence and perform only those testing and assessment services for which they have been trained. They are familiar with reliability, validity, related standardization, error of measurement, and proper application of any technique utilized. Counselors using computer-based test interpretations are trained in the construct being measured and the specific instrument being used prior to using this type of computer application. Counselors take reasonable measures to ensure the proper use of psychological assessment techniques by persons under their supervision.

b. *Appropriate Use*. Counselors are responsible for the appropriate application, scoring, interpretation, and use of assessment instruments, whether they score and interpret such tests themselves or use computerized or other services.

c. *Decisions Based on Results*. Counselors responsible for decisions involving individuals or policies that are based on assessment results have a thorough understanding of educational and psychological measurement, including validation criteria, test research, and guidelines for test development and use.

d. *Accurate Information*. Counselors provide accurate information and avoid false claims or misconceptions when making statements about assessment instruments or techniques. Special efforts are made to avoid unwarranted connotations of such terms as IQ and grade equivalent scores. (See C.5.c.)

E.3. INFORMED CONSENT

a. *Explanation to Clients*. Prior to assessment, counselors explain the nature and purposes of assessment and the specific use of results in language the client (or other legally authorized person on behalf of the client) can understand, unless an explicit exception to this right has been agreed upon in advance. Regardless of whether scoring and interpretation are completed by counselors, by assistants, or by computer or other outside services, counselors take reasonable steps to ensure that appropriate explanations are given to the client.

b. *Recipients of Results*. The examinee's welfare, explicit understanding, and prior agreement determine the recipients of test results. Counselors include accurate and appropriate interpretations with any release of individual or group test results. (See B.1.a. and C.5.c.)

E.4. RELEASE OF INFORMATION TO COMPETENT PROFESSIONALS

a. *Misuse of Results*. Counselors do not misuse assessment results, including test results, and interpretations, and take reasonable steps to prevent the misuse of such by others. (See C.5.c.)

b. *Release of Raw Data*. Counselors ordinarily release data (e.g., protocols, counseling or interview notes, or questionnaires) in which the client is identified only with the consent of the client or the client's legal representative. Such data are usually released only to persons recognized by counselors as competent to interpret the data. (See B.1.a.)

E.5. PROPER DIAGNOSIS OF MENTAL DISORDERS

a. *Proper Diagnosis*. Counselors take special care to provide proper diagnosis of mental disorders. Assessment techniques (including personal interview) used to determine client care (e.g., locus of treatment, type of treatment, or recommended follow-up) are carefully selected and appropriately used. (See A.3.a. and C.5.c.)

b. *Cultural Sensitivity*. Counselors recognize that culture affects the manner in which clients' problems are defined. Clients' socioeconomic and cultural experience is considered when diagnosing mental disorders.

E.6. TEST SELECTION

a. *Appropriateness of Instruments*. Counselors carefully consider the validity, reliability, psychometric limitations, and appropriateness of instruments when selecting tests for use in a given situation or with a particular client.

b. *Culturally Diverse Populations*. Counselors are cautious when selecting tests for culturally diverse populations to avoid inappropriateness of testing that may be outside of socialized behavioral or cognitive patterns.

E.7. CONDITIONS OF TEST ADMINISTRATION

a. *Administration Conditions*. Counselors administer tests under the same conditions that were established in their standardization. When tests are not administered under standard conditions or when unusual behavior or irregularities occur during the testing session, those conditions are noted in interpretation, and the results may be designated as invalid or of questionable validity.

b. *Computer Administration*. Counselors are responsible for ensuring that administration programs function properly to provide clients with accurate results when a computer or other electronic methods are used for test administration. (See A.12.b.)

c. *Unsupervised Test-Taking*. Counselors do not permit unsupervised or inadequately supervised use of tests or assessments unless the tests or assessments are designed, intended, and validated for self-administration and/or scoring.

d. *Disclosure of Favorable Conditions*. Prior to test administration, conditions that produce most favorable test results are made known to the examinee.

E.8. DIVERSITY IN TESTING

Counselors are cautious in using assessment techniques, making evaluations, and interpreting the performance of populations not represented in the norm group on which an instrument was standardized. They recognize the effects of age, color, culture, disability, ethnic group, gender, race, religion, sexual orientation, and socioeconomic status on test administration and interpretation and place test results in proper perspective with other relevant factors. (See A.2.a.)

E.9. TEST SCORING AND INTERPRETATION

a. *Reporting Reservations*. In reporting assessment results, counselors indicate any reservations that exist regarding validity or reliability because of the circumstances of the assessment or the inappropriateness of the norms for the person tested.

b. *Research Instruments*. Counselors exercise caution when interpreting the results of research instruments possessing insufficient technical data to support respondent results. The specific purposes for the use of such instruments are stated explicitly to the examinee.

c. *Testing Services*. Counselors who provide test scoring and test interpretaion services to support the assessment process confirm the validity of such interpretations. They accurately describe the purpose, norms, validity, reliability, and applications of the procedures and any special qualifications applicable to their use. The public offering of an automated test interpretations service is considered a professional-to-professional consultation. The formal responsibility of the consultant is to the consultee, but the ultimate and overriding responsibility is to the client.

E.10. TEST SECURITY

Counselors maintain the integrity and security of tests and other assessment techniques consistent with legal and contractual obligations. Counselors do not appropriate, reproduce, or modify published tests or parts thereof without acknowledgment and permission from the publisher.

E.11. OBSOLETE TESTS AND OUTDATED TEST RESULTS

Counselors do not use data or test results that are obsolete or outdated for the current purpose. Counselors make every effort to prevent the misuse of obsolete measures and test data by others.

E.12. TEST CONSTRUCTION

Counselors use established scientific procedures, relevant standards, and current professional knowledge for test design in the development, publication, and utilization of educational and psychological assessment techniques.

Section F: Teaching, Training, and Supervision

F.1. COUNSELOR EDUCATORS AND TRAINERS

a. *Educators as Teachers and Practitioners*. Counselors who are responsible for developing, implementing, and supervising educational programs are skilled as teachers and practitioners. They are knowledgeable regarding the ethical, legal, and regulatory aspects of the profession, are skilled in applying that knowledge, and make students and supervisees aware of their responsibilities. Counselors conduct counselor education and training programs in an ethical manner and serve as role models for professional behavior. Counselor educators should make an effort to infuse material related to human diversity into all courses and/or workshops that are designed to promote the development of professional counselors.

b. *Relationship Boundaries with Students and Supervisees*. Counselors clearly define and maintain ethical, professional, and social relationship boundaries with their students and supervisees. They are aware of the differential in power that exists and the student's or supervisee's possible incomprehension of that power differential. Counselors explain to students and supervisees the potential for the relationship to become exploitive.

c. *Sexual Relationships*. Counselors do not engage in sexual relationships with students or supervisees and do not subject them to sexual harassment. (See A.6. and C.5.b.)

d. *Contributions to Research*. Counselors give credit to students or supervisees for their contributions to research and scholarly projects. Credit is given through coauthorship, acknowledgment, footnote statement, or other appropriate means, in accordance with such contributions. (See G.4.b. and G.4.c.)

e. *Close Relatives*. Counselors do not accept close relatives as students or supervisees.

f. *Supervision Preparation*. Counselors who offer clinical supervision services are adequately prepared in supervision methods and techniques. Counselors who are doctoral students serving as practicum or internship supervisors to master's level students are adequately prepared and supervised by the training program.

g. *Responsibility for Services to Clients*. Counselors who supervise the counseling services of others take reasonable measures to ensure that counseling services provided to clients are professional.

h. *Endorsement*. Counselors do not endorse students or supervisees for certification, licensure, employment, or completion of an academic or training program if they believe students or supervisees are not qualified for the endorsement. Counselors take reasonable steps to assist students or supervisees who are not qualified for endorsement to become qualified.

F.2. COUNSELOR EDUCATION AND TRAINING PROGRAMS

a. *Orientation*. Prior to admission, counselors orient prospective students to the counselor education or training program's expectations, including but not limited to the following: (1) the type and level of skill acquisition required for successful completion of the training, (2) subject matter to be covered, (3) basis for evaluation, (4) training components that encourage self-growth or self-disclosure as part of the training process, (5) the type of supervision settings and requirements of the sites for required clinical field experiences, (6) student and supervisee evaluation and dismissal policies and procedures, and (7) up-to-date employment prospects for graduates.

b. *Integration of Study and Practice*. Counselors establish counselor education and training programs that integrate academic study and supervised practice.

c. *Evaluation*. Counselors clearly state to students and supervisees, in advance of training, the levels of competency expected, appraisal methods, and timing of evaluations for both didactic and experiential components. Counselors provide students and supervisees with periodic performance appraisal and evaluation feedback throughout the training program.

d. *Teaching Ethics*. Counselors make students and supervisees aware of the ethical responsibilities and standards of the profession and the students' and supervisees' ethical responsibilities to the profession. (See C.1. and F.3.e.)

e. *Peer Relationships*. When students or supervisees are assigned to lead counseling groups or provide clinical supervision for their peers, counselors take steps to ensure that students and supervisees placed in these roles do not have personal or adverse relationships with peers and that they understand they have the same ethical obligations as counselor educators, trainers, and supervisors. Counselors make every effort to ensure that the rights of peers are not compromised when students or supervisees are assigned to lead counseling groups or provide clinical supervision.

f. *Varied Theoretical Positions*. Counselors present varied theoretical positions so that students and supervisees may make comparisons and have opportunities to develop their own positions. Counselors provide information concerning the scientific bases of professional practice. (See C.6.a.)

g. *Field Placements*. Counselors develop clear policies within their training program regarding field placement and other clinical experiences. Counselors provide clearly stated roles and responsibilities for the student or supervisee, the site supervisor, and the program supervisor. They confirm that site supervisors are qualified to provide supervision and are informed of their professional and ethical responsibilities in this role.

h. *Dual Relationships as Supervisors*. Counselors avoid dual relationships such as performing the role of site supervisor and training program supervisor in the student's or supervisee's training program. Counselors do not accept any form of professional services, fees, commissions, reimbursement, or remuneration from a site for student or supervisee placement.

i. *Diversity in Programs*. Counselors are responsive to their institution's and program's recruitment and retention needs for training program administrators, faculty, and students with diverse backgrounds and special needs. (See A.2.a.)

F.3. STUDENTS AND SUPERVISEES

a. *Limitations*. Counselors, through ongoing evaluation and appraisal, are aware of the academic and personal limitations of students and supervisees that might impede performance. Counselors assist students and supervisees in securing remedial assistance when needed, and dismiss from the training program supervisees who are unable to provide competent service due to academic or personal limitations. Counselors seek professional consultation and document their decision to dismiss or refer students or supervisees for assistance. Counselors assure that students and supervisees have recourse to address decisions made, to require them to seek assistance, or to dismiss them.

b. *Self-Growth Experiences*. Counselors use professional judgment when designing training experiences conducted by the counselors themselves that require student and supervisee self-growth or self-disclosure. Safeguards are provided so that students and supervisees are aware of the ramifications their self-disclosure may have, on counselors whose primary role as teacher, trainer, or supervisor requires acting on ethical obligations to the profession. Evaluative components of experiential training experiences explicitly delineate predetermined academic standards that are separate and not dependent on the student's level of self-disclosure. (See A.6.)

c. *Counseling for Students and Supervisees*. If students or supervisees request counseling, supervisors or counselor educators provide them with acceptable referrals. Supervisors or counselor educators do not serve as counselor to students or supervisees over whom they hold administrative, teaching, or evaluative roles unless this is a brief role associated with a training experience. (See A.6.b.)

d. *Clients of Students and Supervisees*. Counselors make every effort to ensure that the clients at field placements are aware of the services rendered and the qualifications of the students and supervisees rendering those services. Clients receive professional disclosure information and are informed of the limits of confidentiality. Client permission is obtained in order for the students and supervisees to use any information concerning the counseling relationship in the training process. (See B.1.e.)

e. *Standards for Students and Supervisees*. Students and supervisees preparing to become counselors adhere to the Code of Ethics and the Standards of Practice. Students and supervisees have the same obligations to clients as those required of counselors. (See H.1.)

Section G: Research and Publication

G.1. RESEARCH RESPONSIBILITIES

a. *Use of Human Subjects*. Counselors plan, design, conduct, and report research in a manner consistent with pertinent ethical principles, federal and state laws, host institutional regulations, and scientific standards governing research with human subjects. Counselors design and conduct research that reflects cultural sensitivity appropriateness.

b. *Deviation from Standard Practices*. Counselors seek consultation and observe stringent safeguards to protect the rights of research participants when a research problem suggests a deviation from standard acceptable practices. (See B.6.)

c. *Precautions to Avoid Injury*. Counselors who conduct research with human subjects are responsible for the subjects' welfare throughout the experiment and take reasonable precautions to avoid causing injurious psychological, physical, or social effects to their subjects.

d. *Principal Researcher Responsibility*. The ultimate responsibility for ethical research practice lies with the principal researcher. All others involved in the research activities share ethical obligations and full responsibility for their own actions.

e. *Minimal Interference*. Counselors take reasonable precautions to avoid causing disruptions in subjects' lives due to participation in research.

f. *Diversity*. Counselors are sensitive to diversity and research issues with special populations. They seek consultation when appropriate. (See A.2.a. and B.6.)

G.2. INFORMED CONSENT

a. *Topics Disclosed*. In obtaining informed consent for research, counselors use language that is understandable to research participants and that: (1) accurately explains the purpose and procedures to be followed; (2) identifies any procedures that are experimental or relatively untried; (3) describes the attendant discomforts and risks; (4) describes the benefits or changes in individuals or organizations that might be reasonably expected; (5) discloses appropriate alternative procedures that would be advantageous for subjects; (6) offers to answer any inquiries concerning the procedures; (7) describes any limitations on confidentiality; and (8) instructs that subjects are free to withdraw their consent and to discontinue participation in the project at any time. (See B.1.f.)

b. *Deception*. Counselors do not conduct research involving deception unless alternative procedures are not feasible and the prospective value of the research justifies the deception. When the methodological requirements of a study necessitate concealment or deception, the investigator is required to explain clearly the reasons for this action as soon as possible.

c. *Voluntary Participation.* Participation in research is typically voluntary and without any penalty for refusal to participate. Involuntary participation is appropriate only when it can be demonstrated that participation will have no harmful effects on subjects and is essential to the investigation.

d. *Confidentiality of Information.* Information obtained about research participants during the course of an investigation is confidential. When the possibility exists that others may obtain access to such information, ethical research practice requires that the possibility, together with the plans for protecting confidentiality, be explained to participants as a part of the procedure for obtaining informed consent. (See B.1.e.)

e. *Persons Incapable of Giving Informed Consent.* When a person is incapable of giving informed consent, counselors provide an appropriate explanation, obtain agreement for participation, and obtain appropriate consent from a legally authorized person.

f. *Commitments to Participants.* Counselors take reasonable measures to honor all commitments to research participants.

g. *Explanations after Data Collection.* After data are collected, counselors provide participants with full clarification of the nature of the study to remove any misconceptions. Where scientific or human values justify delaying or withholding information, counselors take reasonable measures to avoid causing harm.

h. *Agreements to Cooperate.* Counselors who agree to cooperate with another individual in research or publication incur an obligation to cooperate as promised in terms of punctuality of performance and with regard to the completeness and accuracy of the information required.

i. *Informed Consent for Sponsors.* In the pursuit of research, counselors give sponsors, institutions, and publication channels the same respect and opportunity for giving informed consent that they accord to individual research participants. Counselors are aware of their obligation to future research workers and ensure that host institutions are given feedback information and proper acknowledgment.

G.3. REPORTING RESULTS

a. *Information Affecting Outcome.* When reporting research results, counselors explicitly mention all variables and conditions known to the investigator that may have affected the outcome of a study or the interpretation of data.

b. *Accurate Results.* Counselors plan, conduct, and report research accurately and in a manner that minimizes the possibility that results will be misleading. They provide thorough discussions of the limitations of their data and alternative hypotheses. Counselors do not engage in fraudulent research, distort data, misrepresent data, or deliberately bias their results.

c. *Obligation to Report Unfavorable Results.* Counselors communicate to other counselors the results of any research judged to be of professional value. Results that reflect unfavorably on institutions, programs, services, prevailing opinions, or vested interests are not withheld.

d. *Identity of Subjects.* Counselors who supply data, aid in the research of another person, report research results, or make original data available take due care to disguise the identity of respective subjects in the absence of specific authorization from the subjects to do otherwise. (See B.1.g. and B.5.a.)

e. *Replication Studies.* Counselors are obligated to make available sufficient original research data to qualified professionals who may wish to replicate the study.

G.4. PUBLICATION

a. *Recognition of Others.* When conducting and reporting research, counselors are familiar with and give recognition to previous work on the topic, observe copyright laws, and give full credit to those to whom credit is due. (See F.1.d. and G.4.c.)

b. *Contributors.* Counselors give credit through joint authorship, acknowledgment, footnote statements, or other appropriate means to those who have contributed significantly to research or concept development in accordance with such contributions. The principal contributor is listed first and minor technical or professional contributions are acknowledged in notes or introductory statements.

c. *Student Research.* For an article that is substantially based on a student's dissertation or thesis, the student is listed as the principal author. (See F.1.d. and G.4.a.)

d. *Duplicate Submission.* Counselors submit manuscripts for consideration to only one journal at a time. Manuscripts that are published in whole or in substantial part in another journal or published work are not submitted for publication without acknowledgment and permission from the previous publication.

e. *Professional Review.* Counselors who review material submitted for publication, research, or other scholarly purposes respect the confidentiality and proprietary rights of those who submitted it.

Section H: Resolving Ethical Issues

H.1. KNOWLEDGE OF STANDARDS

Counselors are familiar with the Code of Ethics and the Standards of Practice and other applicable ethics codes from other professional organizations of which they are members, or from certification and licensure bodies. Lack of knowledge or misunderstanding of an ethical responsibility is not a defense against a charge of unethical conduct. (See F.3.e.)

H.2. SUSPECTED VIOLATIONS

a. *Ethical Behavior Expected.* Counselors expect professional associates to adhere to the Code of Ethics. When counselors possess reasonable cause that raises doubts as to whether a counselor is acting in an ethical manner, they take appropriate action. (See H.2.d. and H.2.e.)

b. *Consultation.* When uncertain as to whether a particular situation or course of action may be in violation of the Code of Ethics, counselors consult with other counselors who are knowledgeable about ethics, with colleagues, or with appropriate authorities.

c. *Organization Conflicts.* If the demands of an organization with which counselors are affiliated pose a conflict with the Code of Ethics, counselors specify the nature of such conflicts and express to their supervisors or other responsible officials their commitment to the Code of Ethics. When possible, counselors work toward change within the organization to allow full adherence to the Code of Ethics.

d. *Informal Resolution.* When counselors have reasonable cause to believe that another counselor is violating an ethical standard, they attempt to first resolve the issue informally with the other counselor if feasible, providing that such action does not violate confidentiality rights that may be involved.

e. *Reporting Suspected Violations*. When an informal resolution is not appropriate or feasible, counselors, upon reasonable cause, take action such as reporting the suspected ethical violation to state or national ethics committees, unless this action conflicts with confidentiality rights that cannot be resolved.

f. *Unwarranted Complaints*. Counselors do not initiate, participate in, or encourage the filing of ethics complaints that are unwarranted or intend to harm a counselor rather than to protect clients or the public.

H.3. COOPERATION WITH ETHICS COMMITTEES
Counselors assist in the process of enforcing the Code of Ethics. Counselors cooperate with investigations, proceedings, and requirements of the ACA Ethics Committee or ethics committees of other duly constituted associations or boards having jurisdiction over those charged with a violation. Counselors are familiar with the ACA Policies and Procedures and use it as a reference in assisting the enforcement of the Code of Ethics.

STANDARDS OF PRACTICE

All members of the American Counseling Association (ACA) are required to adhere to the Standards of Practice and the Code of Ethics. The Standards of Practice represent minimal behavioral statements of the Code of Ethics. Members should refer to the applicable section of the Code of Ethics for further interpretation and amplification of the applicable Standard of Practice.

Section A: The Counseling Relationship

STANDARD OF PRACTICE ONE (SP-1)
NONDISCRIMINATION
Counselors respect diversity and must not discriminate against clients because of age, color, culture, disability, ethnic group, gender, race, religion, sexual orientation, marital status, or socioeconomic status. (See A.2.a.)

STANDARD OF PRACTICE TWO (SP-2)
DISCLOSURE TO CLIENTS
Counselors must adequately inform clients, preferably in writing, regarding the counseling process and counseling relationship at or before the time it begins and throughout the relationship. (See A.3.a.)

STANDARD OF PRACTICE THREE (SP-3)
DUAL RELATIONSHIPS
Counselors must make every effort to avoid dual relationships with clients that could impair their professional judgment or increase the risk of harm to clients. When a dual relationship cannot be avoided, counselors must take appropriate steps to ensure that judgment is not impaired and that no exploitation occurs. (See A.6.a. and A.6.b.)

STANDARD OF PRACTICE FOUR (SP-4)
SEXUAL INTIMACIES WITH CLIENTS
Counselors must not engage in any type of sexual intimacies with current clients and must not engage in sexual intimacies with former clients within a minimum of two years after terminating the counseling relationship. Counselors who engage in such relationship after two years following termination have the responsibility to thoroughly examine and document that such relations did not have an exploitative nature.

STANDARD OF PRACTICE FIVE (SP-5)
PROTECTING CLIENTS DURING GROUP WORK
Counselors must take steps to protect clients from physical or psychological trauma resulting from interactions during group work. (See A.9.b.)

STANDARD OF PRACTICE SIX (SP-6)
ADVANCE UNDERSTANDING OF FEES
Counselors must explain to clients, prior to their entering the counseling relationship, financial arrangements related to professional services. (See A.10.a-d. and A.11.c.)

STANDARD OF PRACTICE SEVEN (SP-7)
TERMINATION
Counselors must assist in making appropriate arrangements for the continuation of treatment of clients, when necessary, following termination of counseling relationships. (See A.11.a.)

STANDARD OF PRACTICE EIGHT (SP-8)
INABILITY TO ASSIST CLIENTS
Counselors must avoid entering or immediately terminate a counseling relationship if it is determined that they are unable to be of professional assistance to a client. The counselor may assist in making an appropriate referral for the client. (See A.11.b.)

Section B: Confidentiality

STANDARD OF PRACTICE NINE (SP-9)
CONFIDENTIALITY REQUIREMENT
Counselors must keep information related to counseling services confidential unless disclosure is in the best interest of clients, is required for the welfare of others, or is required by law. When disclosure is required, only information that is essential is revealed and the client is informed of such disclosure. (See B.1.a.-f.)

STANDARD OF PRACTICE TEN (SP-10)
CONFIDENTIALITY REQUIREMENTS FOR SUBORDINATES
Counselors must take measures to ensure that privacy and confidentiality of clients are maintained by subordinates. (See B.1.h.)

STANDARD OF PRACTICE ELEVEN (SP-11)
CONFIDENTIALITY IN GROUP WORK
Counselors must clearly communicate to group members that confidentiality cannot be guaranteed in group work. (See B.2.a.)

STANDARD OF PRACTICE TWELVE (SP-12)
CONFIDENTIALITY IN FAMILY COUNSELING
Counselors must not disclose information about one family member in counseling to another family member without prior consent. (See B.2.b.)

STANDARD OF PRACTICE THIRTEEN (SP-13)
CONFIDENTIALITY OF RECORDS
Counselors must maintain appropriate confidentiality in creating, storing, accessing, transferring, and disposing of counseling records. (See B.4.b.)

STANDARD OF PRACTICE FOURTEEN (SP-14)
PERMISSION TO RECORD OR OBSERVE
Counselors must obtain prior consent from clients in order to electronically record or observe sessions. (See B.4.c.)

STANDARD OF PRACTICE FIFTEEN (SP-15)
DISCLOSURE OR TRANSFER OF RECORDS
Counselors must obtain client consent to disclose or transfer records to third parties, unless exceptions listed in SP-9 exist. (See B.4.e.)

STANDARD OF PRACTICE SIXTEEN (SP-16)
DATA DISGUISE REQUIRED
Counselors must disguise the identity of the client when using data for training, research, or publication. (See B.5.a.)

Section C: Professional Responsibility

STANDARD OF PRACTICE SEVENTEEN (SP-17)
BOUNDARIES OF COMPETENCE
Counselors must practice only within the boundaries of their competence. (See C.2.a.)

STANDARD OF PRACTICE EIGHTEEN (SP-18)
CONTINUING EDUCATION
Counselors must engage in continuing education to maintain their professional competence. (See C.2.f.)

STANDARD OF PRACTICE NINETEEN (SP-19)
IMPAIRMENT OF PROFESSIONALS
Counselors must refrain from offering professional services when their personal problems or conflicts may cause harm to a client or others. (See C.2.g.)

STANDARD OF PRACTICE TWENTY (SP-20)
ACCURATE ADVERTISING
Counselors must accurately represent their credentials and services when advertising. (See C.3.a.)

STANDARD OF PRACTICE TWENTY-ONE (SP-21)
RECRUITING THROUGH EMPLOYMENT
Counselors must not use their place of employment or institutional affiliation to recruit clients for their private practices. (See C.3.d.)

STANDARD OF PRACTICE TWENTY-TWO (SP-22)
CREDENTIALS CLAIMED
Counselors must claim or imply only professional credentials possessed and must correct any known misrepresentations of their credentials by others. (See C.4.a.)

STANDARD OF PRACTICE TWENTY-THREE (SP-23)
SEXUAL HARASSMENT
Counselors must not engage in sexual harassment. (See C.5.b.)

STANDARD OF PRACTICE TWENTY-FOUR (SP-24)
UNJUSTIFIED GAINS
Counselors must not use their professional positions to seek or receive unjustified personal gains, sexual favors, unfair advantage, or unearned goods or services. (See C.5.e.)

STANDARD OF PRACTICE TWENTY-FIVE (SP-25)
CLIENTS SERVED BY OTHERS
With the consent of the client, counselors must inform other mental health professionals serving the same client that a counseling relationship between the counselor and client exists. (See C.6.c.)

STANDARD OF PRACTICE TWENTY-SIX (SP-26)
NEGATIVE EMPLOYMENT CONDITIONS
Counselors must alert their employers to institutional policy or conditions that may be potentially disruptive or damaging to the counselor's professional responsibilities, or that may limit their effectiveness or deny clients' rights. (See D.1.c.)

STANDARD OF PRACTICE TWENTY-SEVEN (SP-27)
PERSONNEL SELECTION AND ASSIGNMENT
Counselors must select competent staff and must assign responsibilities compatible with staff skills and experiences. (See D.1.h.)

STANDARD OF PRACTICE TWENTY-EIGHT (SP-28)
EXPLOITIVE RELATIONSHIPS WITH SUBORDINATES
Counselors must not engage in exploitive relationships with individuals over whom they have supervisory, evaluative, or instructional control or authority. (See D.1.k.)

Section D: Relationship with Other Professionals

STANDARD OF PRACTICE TWENTY-NINE
(SP-29) ACCEPTING FEES FROM AGENCY CLIENTS
Counselors must not accept fees or other remuneration for consultation with persons entitled to such services through the counselor's employing agency or institution. (See D.3.a.)

STANDARD OF PRACTICE THIRTY (SP-30)
REFERRAL FEES
Counselors must not accept referral fees. (See D.3.b.)
Section E: Evaluation, Assessment, and Interpretation

STANDARD OF PRACTICE THIRTY-ONE (SP-31)
LIMITS OF COMPETENCE
Counselors must perform only testing and assessment services for which they are compotent. Counselors must not allow the use of psychological assessment techniques by unqualified persons under their supervision. (See E.2.a.)

STANDARD OF PRACTICE THIRTY-TWO (SP-32)
APPROPRIATE USE OF ASSESSMENT INSTRUMENTS
Counselors must use assessment instruments in the manner for which they were intended. (See E.2.b.)

STANDARD OF PRACTICE THIRTY-THREE
(SP-33) ASSESSMENT EXPLANATIONS TO CLIENTS
Counselors must provide explanations to clients prior to assessment about the nature and purposes of assessment and the specific uses of results. (See E.3.a.)

STANDARD OF PRACTICE THIRTY-FOUR (SP-34)
RECIPIENTS OF TEST RESULTS
Counselors must ensure that accurate and appropriate interpretations accompany any release of testing and assessment information. (See E.3.b.)

STANDARD OF PRACTICE THIRTY-FIVE (SP-35)
OBSOLETE TEST AND OUTDATED TEST RESULTS
Counselors must not base their assessment or intervention decisions or recommendations on data or test results that are obsolete or outdated for the current purpose. (See E.11.)

Section F: Teaching, Training, and Supervision

STANDARD OF PRACTICE THIRTY-SIX (SP-36)
SEXUAL RELATIONSHIPS WITH STUDENTS OR SUPERVISEES

Counselors must not engage in sexual relationships with their students and supervisees. (See F.1.c.)

STANDARD OF PRACTICE THIRTY-SEVEN (SP-37)
CREDIT FOR CONTRIBUTIONS TORESEARCH

Counselors must give credit to students or supervisees for their contributions to research and scholarly projects. (See F.1.d.)

STANDARD OF PRACTICE THIRTY-EIGHT (SP-38)
SUPERVISION PREPARATION

Counselors who offer clinical supervision services must be trained and prepared in supervision methods and techniques. (See F.1.f.)

STANDARD OF PRACTICE THIRTY-NINE (SP-39)
EVALUATION INFORMATION

Counselors must clearly state to students and supervisees in advance of training, the levels of competency expected, appraisal methods, and timing of evaluations. Counselors must provide students and supervisees with periodic performance appraisal and evaluation feedback throughout the training program. (See F.2.c.)

STANDARD OF PRACTICE FORTY (SP-40)
PEER RELATIONSHIPS IN TRAINING

Counselors must make every effort to ensure that the rights of peers are not violated when students and supervisees are assigned to lead counseling groups or provide clinical supervision. (See F.2.e.)

STANDARD OF PRACTICE FORTY-ONE(SP-41)
LIMITATIONS OF STUDENTS AND SUPERVISEES

Counselors must assist students and supervisees in securing remedial assistance, when needed, and must dismiss from the training program students and supervisees who are unable to provide competent service due to academic or personal limitations. (See F.3.a.)

STANDARD OF PRACTICE FORTY-TWO (SP-42)
SELF-GROWTH EXPERIENCES

Counselors who conduct experiences for students or supervisees that include self-growth or self disclosure must inform participants of counselors' ethical obligations to the profession and must not grade participants based on their nonacademic performance. (See F.3.b.)

STANDARD OF PRACTICE FORTY-THREE (SP-43)
STANDARDS FOR STUDENTS AND SUPERVISEES

Students and supervisees preparing to become counselors must adhere to the Code of Ethics and the Standards of Practice of counselors. (See F.3.e.)

Section G: Research and Publication

STANDARD OF PRACTICE FORTY-FOUR (SP-44)
PRECAUTIONS TO AVOID INJURY IN RESEARCH

Counselors must avoid causing physical, social, or psychological harm or injury to subjects in research. (See G.1.c.)

STANDARD OF PRACTICE FORTY-FIVE (SP-45)
CONFIDENTIALITY OF RESEARCH INFORMATION

Counselors must keep confidential information obtained about research participants. (See G.2.d.)

STANDARD OF PRACTICE FORTY-SIX (SP-46)
INFORMATION AFFECTING RESEARCH OUTCOME

Counselors must report all variables and conditions known to the investigator that may have affected research data or outcomes. (See G.3.a.)

STANDARD OF PRACTICE FORTY-SEVEN (SP-47)
ACCURATE RESEARCH RESULTS

Counselors must not distort or misrepresent research data, nor fabricate or intentionally bias research results. (See G.3.b.)

STANDARD OF PRACTICE FORTY-EIGHT (SP-48)
PUBLICATION CONTRIBUTORS

Counselors must give appropriate credit to those who have contributed to research. (See G.4.a. and G.4.b.)

Section H: Resolving Ethical Issues

STANDARD OF PRACTICE FORTY-NINE (SP-49)
ETHICAL BEHAVIOR EXPECTED

Counselors must take appropriate action when they possess reasonable cause that raises doubts as to whether counselors or other mental health professionals are acting in an ethical manner. (See H.2.a.)

STANDARD OF PRACTICE FIFTY (SP-50)
UNWARRANTED COMPLAINTS

Counselors must not initiate, participate in, or encourage the filing of ethics complaints that are unwarranted or intended to harm a mental health professional rather than to protect clients or the public. (See H.2.f.)

STANDARD OF PRACTICE FIFTY-ONE (SP-51)
COOPERATION WITH ETHICS COMMITTEES

Counselors must cooperate with investigations, proceedings, and requirements of the ACA Ethics Committee or ethics committees of other duly constituted associations or boards having jurisdiction over those charged with a violation. (See H.3.)

References

The following documents are available to counselors as resources to guide them in their practices. These resources are not a part of the Code of Ethics and the Standards of Practice.

AMERICAN ASSOCIATION FOR COUNSELING AND DEVELOPMENT

Association for Measurement and Evaluation in Counseling and Development. (1989). *The responsibilities of users of standardized tests* (revised). Washington, DC: Author.

American Counseling Association. (1988). *American Counseling Association Ethical Standards*. Alexandria, VA: Author.

American Psychological Association. (1985). *Standards for educational and psychological testing* (revised). Washington, DC: Author.

American Rehabilitation Counseling Association, Commission on Rehabilitation Counselor Certification, and National Rehabilitation Counseling Association. (1995). *Code of professional ethics for rehabilitation counselors*. Chicago, IL: Author.

American School Counselor Association. (1992). *Ethical standards for school counselors*. Alexandria, VA: Author.

Joint Committee on Testing Practices. (1988). *Code of fair testing practices in education*. Washington, DC: Author.

National Board for Certified Counselors. (1989). *National Board for Certified Counselors Code of Ethics*. Alexandria, VA: Author.

Prediger, D.J. (Ed.). (1993, March). *Multicultural assessment standards*. Alexandria, VA: Association for Assessment in Counseling.

STATE CREDENTIALING REQUIREMENTS

Education, Experience & Examination Requirements of Credentialed Counselors as Dictated by State Statutes

The information presented is from the statutes of the District of Columbia and 42 states that, as of March 11, 1997, have passed some form of counselor credentialing legislation. When CACREP (Council for the Accreditation of Counseling and Related Educational Programs) is referred to under the column "Minimum Education Requirements," most states accept equivalent coursework. Please contact regulatory boards for further information on specific coursework required. The title(s) listed is the primary one(s) granted to professional counselors in each state. Many states grant associated licenses to persons who meet the education and exam requirements but have not yet had the supervised experience required. For additional information, clarification of terminology, or statutory interpretation, please contact the state regulatory board.

ACRONYMS:

CMHCE	Clinical Mental Health Counselors Examination (used by the National Board for Certified Counselors [NBCC] for certification of Certified Clinical Mental Health Counselors [CCMHCs])
CCMHC	Certified Clinical Mental Health Counselor
CRCE	Certified Rehabilitation Counselor Examination (used by Commission on Rehabilitation Counselor Certification [CRCC])
NCE	National Counselor Examination (used by NBCC)
NCCE	National Career Counselor Examination (used by NBCC for certification as a National Certified Career Counselor)

As noted on page 1, many states grant associate licenses to persons who are working on completing certain requirements. In addition to the titles noted, which relate to the regulation of professional counselors, some states grant licenses to persons in specialty areas such as marriage and family therapy, pastoral counseling, and rehabilitation. Please contact the state regulatory board for the availability, requirements, scopes of practice, and further information regarding licensure in these specialty areas as well as information on requirements for an associate license.

APPENDIX B

Selected Web Sites for Organizations

AAMFT (American Association of Marriage and Family Therapy): www.aamft.org

AAPC (American Association of Pastoral Counselors): www.aapc.org

ACA (American Counseling Association): www.counseling.org

Access all of the following from ACA homepage, www.counseling.org

- American College Counseling Association (ACCA)
- American Mental Health Counselors Association (AMHCA)
- American Rehabilitation Counselor Association (ARCA)
- American School Counselor Association (ASCA)
- Association for Adult Development and Aging (AADA)
- Association for Counselor Education and Supervision (ACES)
- Association for Assessment in Counseling (AAC)
- Association for Counselors and Educators in Government (ACEG)
- Association for Gay, Lesbian and Bisexual Issues in Counseling (AGLBIC)
- Association for Multicultural Counseling and Development (AMCD)
- Association for Spiritual, Ethical, and Religious Values in Counseling (ASERVIC)
- Association for Specialists in Group Work (ASGW)
- Counseling Association for Humanistic Education and Development (C-AHEAD)
- Counselors for Social Justice (CSJ)
- International Association of Addictions and Offender Counselors (IAAOC)
- International Association of Marriage and Family Counselors (IAMFC)
- National Career Development Association (NCDA)
- National Employment Counseling Association (NECA)

ACA Listservs: www.counseling.org/resources/listservs.htm

ACPA (American College Personnel Association): www.acpa.nche.edu

ACLU (American Civil Liberties Union): www.aclu.org

ACSW (Academy of Certified Social Workers): www.naswdc.org/credentials/acsw.asp

AATA (American Art Therapy Association): www.arttherapy.org

APA (American Psychiatric Association): www.psych.org

APA (American Psychological Association): www.apa.org

APNA (American Psychiatric Nurses Association): www.apna.org

APSA (American Psychoanalytical Association): www.apsa.org

ASWB (Association of Social Work Boards): www.aswb.org

ACPE (Association for Clinical Pastoral Education): www.acpe.edu

CACREP (Council on Accreditation of Counseling and Related Educational Programs): www.counseling.org/cacrep

COAMFTE (Commission on Accreditation for Marital and Family Therapy Education): www.aamft.org/about/COAMFTE/AboutCOAMFTE.htm

CORE (Council on Rehabilitation Education): www.core-rehab.org

CSWE (Council on Social Work Education): www.cswe.org

CRCC (Commission on Rehabilitation Counselor Certification): www.crccertification.com

NACFT (National Academy of Certified Family Therapists): www.iamfc.org/nacft.htm

NASP (National Association of School Psychologists): www.nasponline.org

NASW (National Association of Social Workers): www.naswdc.org

NBCC (National Board for Certified Counselors): www.nbcc.org

NCRE (National Council on Rehabilitation Education): www.nchrtm.okstate.edu/ncre

NOHSE (National Organization of Human Service Education: www.nohse.com

NRCA (National Rehabilitation Counseling Association): www.nationalrehab.org/website/divs/nrca.html

Credits

This page constitutes an extension of the copyright page. We have made every effort to trace the ownership of all copyrighted material and to secure permission from copyright holders. In the event of any question arising as to the use of any material, we will be pleased to make the necessary corrections in future printings. Thanks are due to the following authors, publishers, and agents for permission to use the material indicated.

TEXT AND FIGURE CREDITS

Figure 1.2, p. 17: Adapted from "Counseling Across Cultures," by D. W. Sue, 1978, *Personnel and Guidance Journal, 56*, p. 460. Copyright © 1978 ACA. Reprinted with permission. No further reproduction authorized without written permission of the American Counseling Association.

Box 2.2, p. 37: Army Alpha Test from "Intelligence: New Ways to Measure the Wisdom of Man," by Kevin McKean. In *Discover*, October 1985. Reprinted with permission of the author.

Table 3.1, p. 53: From "Ethics of Counseling: A National Survey of Certified Counselors," by W. T. Gibson and K. S. Pope, 1993, *Journal of Counseling and Development, 71*, pp. 330–336. Copyright © 1993 ACA. Reprinted with permission. No further reproduction authorized without written permission.

Table 4.3, p. 108: From *Theory and Practice of Brief Therapy*, by S. H. Budman and A. S. Gurman, p. 11. Copyright 1988 The Guilford Press. Reprinted with permission.

Figure 5.3, p. 132: Adapted from "Using the Inverted Pyramid Heuristic," by A. M. Schwitzer, 1996, *Counselor Education and Supervision, 35*, p. 260. Copyright © 1996 ACA. Reprinted with permission. No further reproduction authorized without written permission.

Figure 9.2, p. 241: From *The Seasons of a Man's Life*, by Daniel Levinson, copyright © 1978 by Daniel J. Levinson. Used by permission of Alfred A. Knopf, a division of Random House, Inc.

Table 9.2, p. 242: From *Human Development: A Life-span Approach*, 3rd ed., by F. Philip Rice, © 1983. Adapted by permission of Prentice-Hall, Inc., Upper Saddle River, NJ.

Table 10.2, p. 270: Reprinted with permission from the *Diagnostic and Statistical Manual of Mental Disorders*, Fourth Edition, Text Revision. Copyright 2000 American Psychiatric Association.

Table 11.1, p. 282: From *Career Guidance and Counseling Through the Lifespan*, 5th ed., by E. L. Herr and S. H. Cramer, p. 70. Copyright © 1996 by Allyn & Bacon. Reprinted by permission.

Box 11.1, p. 286: Reproduced by special permission of the Publisher, Psychological Assessment Resources, Inc., from *Making Professional Choices*, copyright 1973, 1985, 1992, 1997 by Psychological Assessment Resources, Inc. All rights reserved.

Figure 11.1, p. 287: Reproduced by special permission of the Publisher, Psychological Assessment Resources, Inc., from *Making Professional Choices*, copyright 1973, 1985, 1992, 1997 by Psychological Assessment Resources, Inc. All rights reserved.

Figure 11.3, p. 288: From "The Origins of Interests," by A. Roe and M. Siegelman in *APGA Inquiry Studies No. 1*. Copyright © 1964 ACA. Reprinted with permission. No further reproduction authorized without written permission.

Figure 11.4, p. 290: From Donald E. Super, *New Dimension in Adult Vocational and Career Counseling*, Columbus, Ohio: The Center on Education and Training for Employment (formerly NCRVE), The Ohio State University. Copyright 1985. Used with permission.

Table 13.1, page 335: From *Research in Education: A Conceptual Introduction*, 5th ed., by J. H. McMillan and S. Schumacher. Published by Allyn and Bacon, Boston, MA. Copyright © 2001 Pearson Education. Reprinted by permission of the publisher.

Table 13.3, p. 357: From *Educational Evaluation: Alternative Approaches and Practical Guidelines*, by B. R. Worthen and J. R. Sanders, p. 36. Copyright © 1987. Reprinted by permission of Allyn & Bacon.

Figure 14.1, p. 375: From "A Redefinition of Multicultural Counseling," by S. L. Speight, J. Myers, C. F. Fox, and P. S. Highlen, 1991, *Journal of Counseling and Development, 70*, 29–36. Copyright 1991 ACA. Reprinted by permission. No further reproduction authorized without written permission.

Table 14.2, p. 377: From *Counseling American Minorities: A Cross-Cultural Perspective*, 5th ed., by D. R. Atkinson, G. Morten, and D. W. Sue (Eds.), p. 35. Copyright © 1998 The McGraw-Hill Companies. Reprinted by permission of The McGraw-Hill Companies.

Table 14.3, p. 379: From H. B. Sabnani, J. G. Ponterotto, and L. G. Borodovsky, *The Counseling Psychologist 19*(1), pp. 76–102, copyright

© 1991 by Sage Publications, Inc. Reprinted by permission of Sage Publications, Inc.

Box 15.2, p. 401: From *Counseling Diverse Populations*, 2nd ed., by D. R. Atkinson and G. Hackett, pp. 229–261. Copyright © 1998 The McGraw-Hill Companies. Reprinted by permission of The McGraw-Hill Companies.

Figure 16.1, p. 428: From "Developmental Counseling and Guidance: A Model for Use in Your School," by E. S. Neukrug, C. G. Barr, L. R. Hoffman, and L. S. Kaplan in *The School Counselor, 40*, pp. 356–362. Copyright © 1993 ACA. Reprinted with permission. No further reproduction authorized without written permission.

Table 16.1, p. 429: From "School Counselors' Time: Where Does It Go?" by R. L. Partin in *The School Counselor, 40*, p. 278. Copyright © 1993 ACA. Reprinted with permission. No further reproduction authorized without written permission.

Box 16.9, p. 441: From "Tips for Counselors." Copyright © 1998 American School Counselors Association. Reprinted with permission.

Box 19.2, p. 494: Adapted with permission from the *Diagnostic and Statistical Manual of Mental Disorders*, Fourth Edition, Text Revision. Copyright © 2000 American Psychiatric Association.

Box 19.3, p. 497: From "Counseling on the Information Highway: Future Possibilities and Potential Problems," by J. P. Sampson, R. W. Kolodinsky, and B. P. Greeno in *Journal of Counseling and Development, 75*, p. 211. Copyright © 1997 ACA. Reprinted with permission. No further reproduction authorized without written permission.

Figure 19.1, p. 503: From *The Wheel of Wellness*, by J. M. Witmer, T. J. Sweeney, and J. E. Meyers, p. 10. Greensboro, NC: Authors. Copyright © 1998 by Witmer et al. Reprinted with permission.

Appendix A, p. 531: Copyright © 1995 ACA. Reprinted with permission. No further reproduction authorized without written permission.

PHOTO CREDITS

Chapter 1, p. 15: Natalie Rogers

Chapter 2, p. 24: © Bettmann/CORBIS; **p. 29:** Photo Researchers

Chapter 4, p. 77: © Bettmann/CORBIS; **p. 80:** Photo Researchers; **p. 84:** © Bettmann/CORBIS; **p. 87:** Natalie Rogers; **p. 90:** Paul Herbert, Esalen Institute; **p. 93:** Courtesy of the Harvard University Archives; **p. 97:** Arnold Lazarus; **p. 98:** The William Glasser Institute Website; **p. 100:** Albert Ellis

Chapter 6, p. 160: Used with permission of AVANTA, The Virginia Satir Network, 2104 SW 152nd Street, #2, Burien, WA 98166, www.avanta.net. All rights reserved.

Chapter 7, p. 179: © CORBIS

Chapter 9, p. 228: Edward Neukrug; **p. 233:** Courtesy of the Harvard University Archives; **p. 234:** Republished with permission of Globe Newspaper Company, Inc., from the July 27, 1997, issue of *The Boston Globe*, © 1997

Chapter 14, p. 382: Derald Sue

Chapter 16, p. 430: Anne Christie; **p. 432:** Joyce Beamon; **p. 436:** Randy Sowala

Chapter 17, p. 453: Kathy Walsh Moore; **p. 454:** Michael Nahl; **p. 459:** Bill Austin

Chapter 18, p. 475: Bruce Lynch; **p. 477:** Kevin Kelz; **p. 478:** Carretta Cooke

Author Index

Subject Index